COMMON PAIN CONDITIONS

A CLINICAL GUIDE TO NATURAL TREATMENT

COMMON PAIN CONDITIONS

A CLINICAL GUIDE TO NATURAL TREATMENT

MARC S. MICOZZI, MD, PhD
Adjunct Professor
Department of Physiology & Biophysics,
Department of Pharmacology
Georgetown University School of Medicine
Washington, DC

Former Director
Center for Integrative Medicine
Thomas Jefferson University Hospital,
Philadelphia, Pennsylvania

SEBHIA MARIE DIBRA
Editorial Board Member
European Journal of Physics Education
Kayseri, Turkey

Member, Biophysical Society
Rockville, Maryland

Research Collaborator and Chief Editor
Resonance Science Foundation
San Clemente, California

Managing Editor
Hawaii Institute of Unified Physics
Kauai, Hawaii

Biofeedback Retreat Facilitator
Academy of Wellness
Toronto, Canada

With foreword by
JAMES L. OSCHMAN, PhD
Nature's Own Research Association,
Dover, New Hampshire

ELSEVIER

ELSEVIER

3251 Riverport Lane
St. Louis, Missouri 63043

COMMON PAIN CONDITIONS, A CLINICAL
GUIDE TO NATURAL TREATMENT

ISBN: 978-0-323-41370-1

Notices

Knowledge and best practice in this field are constantly changing. As new research and experience broaden our understanding, changes in research methods, professional practices, or medical treatment may become necessary.

Practitioners and researchers must always rely on their own experience and knowledge in evaluating and using any information, methods, compounds, or experiments described herein. In using such information or methods they should be mindful of their own safety and the safety of others, including parties for whom they have a professional responsibility.

With respect to any drug or pharmaceutical products identified, readers are advised to check the most current information provided (i) on procedures featured or (ii) by the manufacturer of each product to be administered, to verify the recommended dose or formula, the method and duration of administration, and contraindications. It is the responsibility of practitioners, relying on their own experience and knowledge of their patients, to make diagnoses, to determine dosages and the best treatment for each individual patient, and to take all appropriate safety precautions.

To the fullest extent of the law, neither the Publisher nor the authors, contributors, or editors, assume any liability for any injury and/or damage to persons or property as a matter of products liability, negligence or otherwise, or from any use or operation of any methods, products, instructions, or ideas contained in the material herein.

Library of Congress Cataloging-in-Publication Data

Names: Micozzi, Marc S., 1953- author. | Dibra, Sebhia M., 1988- author.
Title: Common pain conditions : a clinical guide to natural treatment / Marc
S. Micozzi, Sebhia Marie Dibra.
Description: St. Louis, Missouri : Elsevier, [2017] | Includes
bibliographical references.
Identifiers: LCCN 2016046014 | ISBN 9780323413701 (pbk.)
Subjects: | MESH: Pain Management–methods | Complementary Therapies–methods
Classification: LCC RB127 | NLM WL 704.6 | DDC 616/.0472–dc23 LC record available at
https://lccn.loc.gov/2016046014

Senior Content Strategist: Linda Woodard
Content Development Manager: Ellen Wurm-Cutter
Senior Content Development Specialist: Maria Broeker
Publishing Services Manager: Jeff Patterson
Senior Project Manager: Mary Pohlman
Designer: Renee Duenow

Printed in the United States of America.
Last digit is the print number: 9 8 7 6 5 4 3 2 1

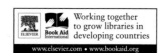

Working together
to grow libraries in
developing countries

www.elsevier.com • www.bookaid.org

Foreword

Pain is probably the most prodigious problem facing modern medicine. Consequently, this compendium is one of the most important medical books available today. The treatment of pain is a daunting challenge in the practice of medicine, which has led to outcries for safer alternatives that work for pain. Fortunately, complementary and alternative medicine (CAM) approaches to pain have been maturing steadily and now provide an important opportunity to fill the vacuum created by the withdrawal of the (formerly) best pain drugs. The CAM approaches not only work very well, they are extremely attractive to patients. There are important reasons for the effectiveness and attractiveness: these approaches gently, effectively, and inexpensively treat the causes of pain, which is the opposite of approaches that mask pain.

The level of detail and scholarship in this volume is truly remarkable. Such a richly rewarding and easy-to-read resource could only come from a research physician with a background in medical anthropology and forensic medicine. The book is also very readable and fascinating. It is a book unlike any I have seen! Do a test for me: pick any chapter at random and read a bit of it. I predict that you will be enthralled and that you may not be able to put it down.

An attitude that has slowed the clinical application of CAM approaches is the widespread belief among physicians that there is no scientific basis for them. This attitude may have had some justification years ago, but the situation has changed dramatically. Remember the words of a great American sage:

All generalizations are false, including this one.

—Mark Twain

This book is a remarkable compilation of the research basis for a wide range of CAM approaches, which include literally thousands of individual treatment modalities not taught in medical schools. Here you will find a snapshot of the burgeoning scientific literature on CAM. Many of the CAM methods actually have better scientific support than a large percentage of the methods routinely used in hospitals as standard care. The *British Medical Journal* analyzed common medical treatments to determine which are supported by sufficient, reliable evidence. They evaluated approximately 2500 treatments, and the results were as follows:

- 13% were found to be beneficial.
- 23% were likely to be beneficial.
- 8% were as likely to be harmful as beneficial.

- 6% were unlikely to be beneficial.
- 4% were likely to be harmful or ineffective.

This analysis left the largest category, 46%, as unknown in their effectiveness. In other words, when you take your sick child to the hospital or clinic, there is only a 36% chance that he or she will receive a treatment that has been reliably, scientifically demonstrated to be either beneficial or likely to be beneficial (Dossey, Chopra, & Roy, 2010).

A huge turning point in pain management came on October 1, 2004, when one of the world's most widely used pain medications, Vioxx, was withdrawn from the market by its manufacturer, Merck, because of concerns about increased risk of heart attack and stroke associated with long-term, high-dosage use. This action was the largest prescription drug recall in history. Worldwide, more than 80 million people had been prescribed Vioxx at one time or another. Merck voluntarily withdrew the drug after disclosures that it had improperly withheld information about the risks from doctors and patients for over 5 years, resulting in between 88,000 and 140,000 cases of serious heart disease. The value of shares in Merck plummeted, and several manufacturing facilities had to be closed. Soon several other extremely popular nonsteroidal anti-inflammatory drugs (NSAIDs) were also withdrawn from the market. The ensuing congressional investigations led to the public admission by the US Food and Drug Administration (FDA) that they do not, in fact, have the means to evaluate the toxic side effects and other dangers of new drugs, as the public had widely believed.

The FDA is criticized from many different perspectives (Hawthorne, 2005). Public statements are nearly always harshly critical to the point of blame and outrage from organizations that have long argued that the FDA impedes the advancement of medical science and practice. For example, there is a widely held belief that the pharmaceutical industry "rules" the FDA. Whether or not this picture is accurate, such appearances of conflict of interest are very destructive to the image of the FDA and to the vital spirit of medical innovation.

Criticism may not be agreeable, but it is necessary. It fulfills the same function as pain in the human body. It calls attention to an unhealthy state of things.

—Winston Churchill

The FDA is one of the most powerful government agencies when it comes to health and medical practice, and it has a key role in protecting the public health by ensuring the safety, efficacy, and security of human and veterinary drugs, biological products, medical devices, the food supply, cosmetics, and products that emit radiation. This scope represents a vast bureaucratic enterprise, with all its inherent limitations, yet remains crucial to the future advancement of medicine and affects public health worldwide. The FDA employs thousands of scientists and other staff, many of whom are competent and dedicated. With a budget of about $4 billion, the FDA is responsible for oversight of more than $2 trillion in foods, medications, medical devices, cosmetics, dietary supplements, and other consumer goods. Given the criticisms of the FDA bureaucracy and its key roles in protecting the public health, the organization urgently needs to be radically redesigned to be more transparent, efficient, and effective. A modern civilization that has been able to put men on the moon and to develop the atomic bomb certainly has the capability of creating a much more efficient effective regulatory process and agency. Congress could mandate and fund such a restructuring, calling on the expertise of the National Academy of Sciences, the National Science Foundation, philanthropic organizations, and the US military, to name a few.

The Vioxx affair and the sad sequence of developments that followed left many pain patients completely in the lurch, asking their physicians what they could do. Marc Micozzi and Sebhia Dibra provide a remarkably in-depth exploration of CAM approaches to pain. Here you will find extraordinarily thoughtful and detailed explanations of the best natural, nondrug alternatives and their fascinating history, scientific basis, and practical applications.

A characteristic of many CAM approaches to pain and healing is expressed in the statements "small is powerful," and "less is more" (the latter is a mantra of homeopathy, as well as other natural approaches).

To an observer who has never experienced remarkable pain relief from some of the biofield or consciousness-based therapies such as Reiki, acupuncture, healing touch, therapeutic touch, polarity therapy, cranial sacral therapy, or BodyTalk, to name a few, it may not look as if the practitioner is doing anything at all. In some cases, the therapist is not even touching the patient. In terms of classical Newtonian physics, they may be doing very little, except for introducing field effects described by classical electrodynamics. There is one reason why "less is more" becomes profoundly important. We generally have the idea in modern medicine that, when an intervention is not working, we need to try harder, push harder or longer, increase the dose, and so on. However, many CAM interventions act informationally. "They utilize stimuli that are extremely low in intensity. They are small nudges that act in accordance with the organism's natural system dynamics to restore balance and harmony. Examples of such medical modalities include acupuncture, homeopathy, bioelectromagnetic interventions, and, in fact, a large number of CAM modalities" (Rubik, 2002).

The nature of these "nudges" has become clearer from bioelectromagnetic research that has repeatedly demonstrated something surprising: extremely low-intensity, nonionizing electromagnetic fields, having even less energy content than the physical thermal noise limit, can produce biologic effects (Adey & Bawin, 1977; Rubik, Becker, Flower, Hazlewood, Liboff, & Walleczek, 1994). At these extremely low levels, the energy content of the signal is less than the random energy of molecular motions at body temperature. Such extremely low-level fields are probably delivering information rather than energy.

The mystery of these subtle effects has been resolved by Martin L. Pall in one of the most important papers in recent years (Pall, 2013). Professor Pall studied 116 papers in the literature concerning effects of exposure to minute electromagnetic fields. In what has to be a classic statement about the state of current science, Pall said:

How do EMFs composed of low-energy photons produce non-thermal biological changes, both pathophysiological and, in some cases, potentially therapeutic, in humans and higher animals? It may be surprising that the answer to this question has been hiding in plain sight in the scientific literature. However, in this era of highly focused and highly specialized science, few of us have the time to read the relevant literature, let alone organize the information found within it in useful and critical ways.

Pall concluded that voltage-gated calcium channels in cell membranes are responsible for the effects of extremely minute signals. This makes good sense, as calcium channels regulate a vast array of cellular processes. In many cases the effects of electromagnetic fields on calcium channels are virtually instantaneous. The concept fits well with the emerging biophotonic model of physiological regulations. Cyril Smith has pointed out that "if a physical parameter can produce a chemical effect, quantum physics must be involved since chemistry cannot be described through classical physics" (Smith, 2013).

There is another biophysical basis for these phenomena. It is termed a frequency–power window or a frequency–power–density "window" or "response surface" for an effect of an intervention.

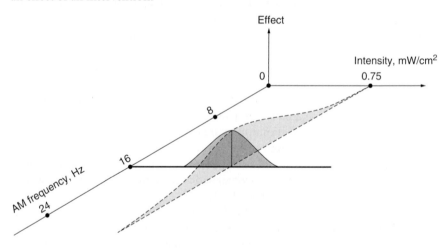

In the classic example illustrated here, the measured response was calcium ion efflux from chick forebrain tissue. A high-frequency signal was amplitude modulated at various frequencies and intensities. Brain tissue has maximum frequency sensitivity in the extremely low frequency (ELF) range between 6 and 20 cycles per second (Hz) and intensity of 10^{-7} V/cm. This is the remarkably low intensity level associated with navigation and prey detection in marine vertebrates and with control of human biological rhythms, as observed by generations of naturalists. The intensity window is about 10^{-1} V/cm, corresponding to the level of the electroencephalogram (EEG) fields in brain tissue (Adey & Bawin, 1977; Blackman, Elder, Weil, Benane, Eichinger, & House, 1979). For a long time, the EEG fields were thought to be useless by-products of brain functioning, but we now know that they have major roles in regulating neural activity throughout the body.

It is obviously important to gather the best evidence that can be used to support the selection of the best medical approaches that are available. This path is not always straightforward, and conflicts of interest abound. Ultimately, a key component is effective and accurate communication that enables a patient to make an educated decision about the methods being employed for her or his treatment. Such communications must meet the highest ethical standards. At present there is a growing awareness among patients that they cannot always rely on healthcare businesses, doctors, and the FDA to protect them from potentially harmful chemicals or treatments. Both toxicology and homeopathy teach that even a very tiny dose of a substance can have a big effect on a patient, and this also means that a tiny trace of a poison in a cosmetic or shampoo, for example, can likewise have a big effect on physiology (Blanc, 2007; Schapiro, 2007).

One reason for the slow pace of incorporating CAM approaches in clinical practice is the lack of understanding of basic physics and quantum physics and their application to biology and medicine. It is widely thought that careful research can reveal the mechanisms and safety of particular medical approaches. The mature scientist recognizes that there is no such thing as absolute proof of a concept or discovery. The scientific methodology used to research any medical approach is forever open to examination, reexamination, and reinterpretation. Many rely on the idea that once a technique has been published in a peer-reviewed journal and approved by the FDA, the patient and physician can be assured that the method is safe and effective.

However, research into any question is never finished. Careful and ethical research requires attention to every step of the investigation—selecting the topic, methods, and ways of reporting the results; making certain that the results are not distorted when they are reported to the public; and ensuring that the information is made available to both clinicians and patients. The US Congress has demanded that pharmaceutical companies publish all studies that found no benefits from new drugs they wish to bring to market, but this has not happened. Correcting the causes of this kind of practice is essential for the future of our medicine.

It is widely held that reliable results are achieved by following the scientific method. In fact, there are a number of scientific methods. The context of a research project should be stated, including the personal background of the investigator that has led him or her to select the topic to be investigated and the methods and interpretations to be applied. It is also widely held that the randomized controlled clinical trial (RCT) is the best approach; it is "the gold standard." However, the RCT was developed to test the effectiveness of drugs, and it only gives an idea of the percentage of the population (often small) that will respond to a particular treatment as compared to a placebo. The RCT has limited application to many CAM approaches because CAM therapists often develop patient-specific treatments rather than relying on "standard dosage forms" and statistical averages (O'Meara, 2009). Likewise, the concept of "evidence-based medicine" sounds appropriate, but things are not so simple (Gupta, 2003; Sackett, Rosenberg, Gray, Haynes, & Richardson, 1996; Timmermans & Mauck, 2005).

Awareness of both the dominant paradigms and the anomalies is valuable in understanding any branch of biomedicine. Anomalies are often taken as an indication that the investigator is incompetent or has made an experimental error. Although they are often rejected at first, anomalies often prove to be the real stepping stones toward truly new discoveries.

Some hold that being open to new ideas can be dangerous, and that once a scientific consensus has been reached about a particular topic, one can count on its accuracy. However, agreement among experts, although helpful, is no criterion for accuracy. Openness to new ideas and skepticism are both essential ingredients in any biomedical inquiry. Beware of the ways concepts are labeled. Ideas that are completely unacceptable for one generation often become dominant in the next. When you hear that science has said the last word on a particular subject, be cautious.

Models that represent (literally re-present) a phenomenon are widely used in science, and many believe they can be relied upon. However, beware of when just a model of a phenomenon, or a set of equations representing the phenomenon, is investigated instead of observing the phenomenon itself. CAM approaches often enable a clinician to identify the root cause of a medical issue and specify how and where the most appropriate treatments can be applied. This medical model is different from naming a condition on the basis of symptoms and then generically treating those symptoms.

To conclude, this is a very special and exciting time for CAM in general and particularly for CAM and natural approaches to pain. We have never had a book like the one you are holding in your hands. Thank you, Marc Micozzi and Sebhia Dibra, for your scholarship and your dedication to being "always on the side of science."

JAMES L. OSCHMAN, PhD
Author of Energy Medicine: The Scientific Basis

REFERENCES

Adey, W. R., & Bawin, S. M. (1977). Brain interactions with weak electric and magnetic fields. *Neuroscience Research Program Bulletin, 15,* 1–129.

Blackman, C. F., Elder, J. A., Weil, C. M., Benane, S. G., Eichinger, D. C., & House, D. E. (1979). Induction of calcium-ion efflux from brain tissue by radio-frequency radiation: Effects of modulation frequency and field strength. *Radio Science, 14*(6S), 93–98.

Blanc, P. D. (2007). *How everyday products make people sick. Toxins at home and in the workplace.* Berkeley, CA: University of California Press.

Dossey, L., Chopra, D., & Roy, R. (7 January 2010). The mythology of science-based medicine. *The Huffington Post.*

Gupta, M. (2003). A critical appraisal of evidence based medicine: Some ethical considerations. *Journal Evaluation in Clinical Practice, 9,* 111–121.

Hawthorne, F. (2005). *Inside the FDA. The business and politics behind the drugs we take and the food we eat.* Hoboken, NJ: John Wiley & Sons.

O'Meara, A. (2009). *Chasing medical miracles. The promise and perils of clinical trials.* New York: Walker.

Pall, M. L. (2013). Electromagnetic fields act via activation of voltage-gated calcium channels to produce beneficial or adverse effects. *Journal Cell Molecular Medicine, 17*(8), 958–965. http://onlinelibrary.wiley.com/doi/10.1111/jcmm.12088/full.

Rubik, B. (2002). The biofield hypothesis: Its biophysical basis and role in medicine. *Journal of Alternative and Complementary Medicine, 8*(6), 703–717.

Rubik, B., Becker, R. O., Flower, R. G., Hazlewood, C. F., Liboff, A. R., & Walleczek, J. (1994). Bioelectromagnetics applications in medicine. In *Alternative medicine: expanding medical horizons.* (NIH Publication No. 94-066, pp. 45–65) Washington DC: US Government Printing Office.

Sackett, D. L., Rosenberg, W. M. C., Gray, J. A. M., Haynes, R. B., & Richardson, W. S. (1996). Evidence-based medicine: What it is and what it isn't (Editorial). *BMJ, 312*(7023), 71–72.

Schapiro, M. (2007). *Exposed. The toxic chemistry of everyday products and what's at stake for American power.* White River Junction, VT: Chelsea Green.

Smith, S. (2013). Comments on "Electromagnetic fields act via activation of voltage-gated calcium channels to produce beneficial or adverse effects" by Martin L. Pall. Personal communication to Jim Oschman, 7 August 2013.

Timmermans, S., & Mauck, A. (2005). The promises and pitfalls of evidence-based medicine. *Health Affairs (Millwood), 24*(1), 18–28.

About the Authors

Marc S. Micozzi is a physician-anthropologist who has created broadly science-based tools for the health professions to be better informed and productively engaged in the fields of complementary and alternative medicine (CAM) and natural medicine. He was the founding editor-in-chief of the first US journal in CAM, *Journal of Alternative and Complementary Medicine: Research on Paradigm, Practice, and Policy* (1994), and the first review journal in CAM, *Seminars in Integrative Medicine* (2002). He also edited the classic survey textbook in the field, *Fundamentals of Complementary and Alternative Medicine*, in continuous print for 20 years through five editions. He has served as series editor for Churchill-Livingstone/Elsevier's *Medical Guides to Complementary and Alternative Medicine*, with 18 titles on a broad range of CAM therapies and natural approaches. He organized and chaired six international continuing education conferences on the theory, science, and practice of CAM and has spoken at many others.

Dr. Micozzi published original research on diet, nutrition, and chronic disease as a senior investigator at the National Institutes of Health from 1984 to 1986, when he was appointed associate director of the Armed Forces Institute of Pathology and founding director of the National Museum of Health and Medicine. In 1992, he was jointly appointed as a Distinguished Scientist in the American Registry of Pathology. He has published more than 300 articles in the medical, scientific, and technical literature.

From 1995 to 2002, he served as executive director of the College of Physicians of Philadelphia. There, he opened the C. Everett Koop Community Health Information Center (Koop CHIC), which provides information to consumers on health and wellness, including CAM. The White House Commission on CAM recognized his work on behalf of consumer health in 2001.

Dr. Micozzi actively collaborated with former US Surgeon General C. Everett Koop (1915–2013) for more than 25 years. As a medical and scientific advisor to Dr. Koop LifeCare Corporation, he worked on new developments with the US Food and Drug Administration (FDA) regarding review of dietary supplements. Over many years Dr. Micozzi developed his own formulations for dietary, herbal, and nutritional supplements for a variety of applications and has reviewed thousands of publications on hundreds of nutritional supplements and herbal remedies, including bringing to light little-known herbal remedies from the African continent.

In 2002, he was the founding director for the Policy Institute for Integrative Medicine in Washington, DC, educating the US Congress, policymakers, the health professions, and the general public about needs and opportunities for CAM and integrative medicine. From 2003 to 2005, he accepted an additional interim appointment as executive director of the Center for Integrative Medicine at Thomas Jefferson University Hospital in Philadelphia. He has served as adjunct professor in the Department of Medicine at the University of Pennsylvania and in the Departments of Pharmacology and Physiology & Biophysics at Georgetown University. In 2012 he became editor-in-chief at www.drmicozzi.com, where he writes a daily column on natural health and medicine, a monthly newsletter, and periodic monographs and special reports on current healthcare issues. Contact e-mail: marcsmicozzi@gmail.com.

Sebhia Marie Dibra is an established author with a unique 21st-century perspective on energetics and spiritual dimensions in health and healing, as well as contemporary and timely health and wellness issues, including life cycle and healthy aging. Her contributions help bring the book into the 21st century for a new generation of readers. She is an author of several books, including *Overcoming Acute and Chronic Pain: Keys to Treatment Based on Your Emotional Type* and *Complementary and Alternative Treatments in the Community – An Introduction for Public Health, Nursing, and Social Work.*

Ms. Dibra is a contributor for a number of online and print publications, for the Resonance Science Foundation, NYC CAAF, and Pennsylvania State University. She has innovative ideas that help conceptualize foundations in biophysics, neuroscience, applied earth sciences, psychology, nutrition, meditation, and mindfulness. She has a degree in psychology with a minor in public health from Pennsylvania State University.

Bridging the world of biology and physics (biophysics), Sebhia is a leader in health and fundamental concepts of energy medicine. She is an advocate of teaching innovative, mindful-base strategies to heal emotional pain.

Sebhia also works with her uncle, Bash Dibra, a celebrity animal behaviorist who has been featured on *The Tonight Show, Animal Planet, Jay Leno*; in major film productions; and on media outlets such as CNN, NBC, CBS, and ABC. He has also worked closely with celebrities such as Jennifer Aniston, Ralph Lauren, Mariah Carey, Mathew Broderick, Joan Rivers, Jennifer Lopez, Ron Howard, Bryce Dallas Howard, Georgina Chapman, and Sarah Jessica Parker.

Reviewers

David. A. Bray, R.AC, R.TCMP, Dipl. C.H. (NCCAOM)
Acupuncture and Traditional Chinese Medicine Practitioner
Doctor of Acupuncture and Traditional Chinese Medicine
Toronto, Ontario

Yoon Hang Kim, MD, MPH
Diplomate, American Board of Medical Acupuncture
Diplomate, American Board of Holistic and Integrative Medicine
Director, Georgia Integrative Medicine
Tyrone, Georgia

John O'Leary, JD
Principle, Zaccheus Press
Bethesda Public Library
Bethesda, Maryland

Jongbae Jay Park, KMD, PhD, NCCAOM
Associate Professor
Department of Anesthesiology
Duke University School of Medicine
Durham, North Carolina

Preface

Original insights gained from editing and co-authoring six consecutive editions of *Fundamentals of Complementary and Alternative Medicine* with today's Elsevier Health Sciences, over the past 20 years, together with 40 years' experience investigating and researching natural and complementary/alternative treatments for **pain, inflammation, and pain-related conditions**, led to preparation of this clinical guide as a background and interactive tool (Appendix I) for health professionals and their patients seeking safe, effective, and individualized pain relief.

Fundamentals of Complementary and Alternative Medicine was the most frequently requested textbook of Elsevier Health Sciences at the annual meeting of the American Academy of Pain Medicine in 2011, which helped prompt a 5-year project to compile this new textbook, *Common Pain Conditions: A Clinical Guide to Natural Treatment*. This terrain includes the **inflammation** that typically accompanies **pain** and for which there are many effective natural treatments. More broadly, research is recognizing that many of the modern chronic diseases that challenge contemporary healthcare and medical practice are related to states of **chronic inflammation**— and again, natural approaches have much to offer. The most promising natural approaches to **diseases of chronic inflammation** are also covered in this text.

In addition to the promise of natural approaches to pain relief, there are serious problems with current approaches to managing pain with drugs.

The epidemic of unsafe narcotic pain-relieving prescription drugs in the United States has led to government calls for reducing our dependence on them, as well as reducing the many health and social hazards of abuse and dependency. After a century of improving health and declining death rates among US women, the US Urban Institute in spring 2015 released a study showing dramatically increasing death rates among these women. The increases are due primarily to the increase in use of these dangerous narcotic pain-relieving drugs.

Perhaps even more shocking is data from the US National Academy of Sciences, and analysis by the 2015 Nobel laureate in Economics, showing that death rates among white, middle-aged, middle-class people have increased by 22% in just the past 15 years. No group of people anywhere in the world has shown increases in death rates in our modern era, and historically no population in history has shown a 22% increase in death rates over just 15 years short of a disease or ecological calamity of global proportions. The leading cause of death in white, middle-aged, middle-class people is intentional or accidental overdose of narcotic drugs, as well as alcohol.

In addition, popular over-the-counter pain relievers such as acetaminophen have long been known to be the leading cause of fatal liver toxicity in the United States; even more alarming is recent research showing they are not even effective for back pain and other common pain conditions.

Fortunately, there are safe, affordable alternatives, readily available today, that have been hiding in plain sight. To know which choices will work best for your patients, it is important to understand a psychometric indicator developed over several decades at Tufts University Medical Center in Boston by the late Ernst Hartmann, MD, called "personality boundary type." This concept is presented in the current fifth edition of *Fundamentals of Complementary and Alternative Medicine* in Chapters 1 co-authored with Michael Jawer of the American Academy of Naturopathic Physicians. We have coined the term "your emotional type" for this psychometric scale to predict susceptibility to various alternative treatments. The concept is based on the hypnotic susceptibility or suggestibility scales of Spiegel, which have proven so useful in predicting which 10% of patients are highly benefitted by hypnosis (covered in this text), which 10% are impervious, and which 80% fall on a scale in between.

The interactive tools needed to determine each individual's "boundary" or "emotional" psychometric type, together with an assessment for matching individual type to the most effective treatments for that type, are provided in Appendix I. The sequential sections and chapters in this book will help you learn about the available natural approaches and alternatives that will work for pain.

Appendix I, *Psychometrics of Pain* is an interactive, individualized patient evaluation that may be completed by your clients online. Appendix II, *Patient Monitoring Pain and Related Symptoms*, is a guide for the individual patient to describe their pain experiences over time, that can be completed at home or in the waiting room. Appendices I and II are provided on the companion website micozzipainconditions.com. The website also contains Suggested Readings for chapters that provide additional resources for further information.

Contents

Appendix I, Psychometrics of Pain is an interactive, individualized patient
evaluation that may be completed by your clients online. Appendix II,
Patient Monitoring Pain and Related Symptoms, is a guide for the
individual patient to describe their pain experiences over time, that
can be completed at home or in the waiting room. Appendices I and II
are provided on the companion website micozzipainconditions.com.
The website also contains Suggested Readings for chapters that provide
additional resources for further information.

Section I

FUNDAMENTALS AND BASIC SCIENCES

Chapter 1

The Problem of Pain and Pain Management

Why Natural Alternatives Are Needed

As Earth's population grows, so do numbers of acute and chronic pain sufferers. The US Census Bureau's annual projections for the United States in 2015 will well exceed 320 million people and the rest of the planet will total over 7.2 billion (Census Bureau, 2014). In 2011 the Institute of Medicine reported over 100 million Americans suffering from chronic pain and pain costs the United States approximately $700 billion per year (Institute of Medicine Report from the Committee on Advancing Pain Research, Care, and Education, 2011; Gaskin & Richard, 2012). These numbers have continued to drastically rise annually because the treatment of pain in America is clearly a major public health challenge that accounts for large and increasing burdens for the health care system in more than 70% of the United States.

It has been 20 years since the first US medical textbook on complementary and alternative medicine (CAM) and natural approaches to health, *Fundamentals of Complementary & Alternative Medicine* (*FCAM*, currently going into its 6th edition), was published with Elsevier Health Sciences (originally Churchill Livingstone). Since then there has been growing awareness that one of the major motivations for learning, seeking, and applying what has been termed "complementary" or "alternative" medicine is to address the prodigious problem of pain. Indeed, *FCAM, 5th edition* has been the publisher's most requested book at the annual meetings of the American Association for Pain Management, although that basic text is a foundational survey of CAM approaches that was not particularly focused on pain itself. This new text is the first to address CAM and natural approaches specifically for pain.

THE PROBLEM OF PAIN AND THE PROBLEMS OF PAIN TREATMENTS

The dimensions and parameters of the pain problem have only expanded during the past 20 years with an aging and changing population. There are many daunting new challenges in the practice of medicine generally and specifically with respect to pain, as well as the looming problems of misuse and abuse of both legal pain medications and illegal narcotic drugs. These overwhelming issues for public health, law enforcement, and public policy have become evident across most states in the United States, the entire country, and worldwide—leading to a renewed outcry for safer alternatives that work for pain.

In my former consulting practice in forensic medicine (Micozzi), we see many cases of deaths from drug overdose (usually pain drugs). These overdoses are intentional (suicide), accidental, or even, rarely, homicidal in manner of death. From an insurance standpoint, the main concern is not in determining the manner of death but whether or not the levels of drugs detected could have been consistent with following the physician's prescription!

NEW MODELS AND MISSES

Meanwhile there have been large shifts in the accepted paradigm for health, healing, and medical practice over the last generation when it comes to elucidation, understanding, and acceptance of a *bioenergetic* model of biology and pathophysiology, as well as the *consciousness* dimension of human medicine. An expanded paradigm is being incorporated or "integrated" in some places into medical practice (typically not well, effectively, or cost-effectively), all under the rubric of so-called "integrative medicine." In terms of this integration, medical practice and patient care is confronted with an often bewildering array of different "CAM" therapies, originating from more than 20 different major healing traditions, ranging from single, simple techniques, to entire "alternative" systems of medical practice and health care, which represent essentially parallel universes when it comes to functional systems of human health care. There has been virtually no effort to systematize and select such different approaches in actual health care structure, organization, training, or practice—outside of the pages of a few textbooks.

BRINGING PSYCHOMETRIC ASSESSMENTS TO NATURAL MEDICINE AND PAIN TREATMENT

A useful development during the prior 5 years has been our application of a time-tested psychometric evaluation associated with the susceptibility of different individuals to chronic medical conditions, notably including pain, that have been shown to be treatable by CAM therapies. Such assessments have been routine for decades in consulting practices, education, vocational training, management, human resources, and other major areas of human endeavor. They have been sorely needed for true "individualized" medical care and for the often bewildering array of "alternative and complementary" natural treatments available. With the notable exception of Spiegel Hypnotic Susceptibility Scales, there has been no science-based, evidence-based clinical tool for helping physicians and patients find the right natural treatments that will work for each individual.

Finally, there are new psychometrics assessments available that are able to predict which CAM therapies will work best for different individual patients. Working with Michael Jawer (presently with the American Association of Naturopathic Physicians), one of the authors (Micozzi) of this new text adapted the "personality boundary scale" psychometric assessment developed over several decades by Ernst Hartmann at Tufts University Medical Center, Boston, to determine susceptibility of different individuals to different CAM therapies. This new tool was discussed in a medical text in the current edition of *FCAM, 5th ed* (2015) and will be presented in detail, together with interactive assessment tools, in Appendix I (pp. 572–579).

CHOICES IN HEALING PAIN

From among the many different CAM options there are many safe and effective natural alternatives to the drug treatment of pain. Nature's original pain medication from the opium poppy (morphine, named from the Greek god of sleep, *Morpheus*) has been largely supplanted by synthetic or semisynthetic prescription and illegal drugs (e.g., diacetyl morphine, or heroin), some of which are many times more powerful (and dangerous) than can be found anywhere in nature (e.g., fentanyl). The development of drug approaches to pain relief and to addiction and dependence on pain drugs has led to its own industry and social institutions, such as networks of methadone clinics, which in turn have spawned additional problems for medicine, public health, and public safety.

Both the domain of "mind-body" approaches and that of herbal remedies, diet and nutrition, and plant oils (aromatherapy) have been studied and applied for pain treatment and management and are discussed in this text. Natural approaches generally and herbal pain remedies specifically are typically less potent (and also safer) than pain drugs. However, there are many examples in which the appropriate micronutrient doses of herbal remedies are *more* effective in direct clinical trial comparisons to the standard drug treatments for certain pain conditions. In addition, different herbal remedies effective for pain, when used in combination, show marked positive synergies that allow the doses of the individual components to be reduced while maintaining the same effectiveness. More such research on synergistic herb interactions needs to be performed—in contrast to the emphasis on cataloguing drug-drug and drug-herb interactions, which typically show added toxicities as opposed to synergistic benefits. Some long-standing prescription drugs (e.g., Darvon) and over-the-counter (OTC) drugs (e.g., acetaminophen) are also being shown to be completely ineffective for common pain conditions—to which must be added their significant toxicities.

CONSCIOUSNESS OF PAIN AND SUFFERING

The drug-oriented approach to pain management is being challenged by the emerging perspective on bioenergy and the consciousness model, which offers a new frontier for noninvasive pain and medical management. These innovative nondrug approaches are often able to account more completely for clinical observations, as well as taking into account newer findings in the basic sciences and in neuroscience and neurophysiology. This new approach to pain processing may perhaps borrow and expand on an important concept from the original medical subspecialty of one of the authors (Micozzi), forensic medicine. The term "conscious pain and suffering" for medical-legal analysis, proceedings, and jurisprudence may be seen more broadly as "conscious*ness of* pain *and* suffering" as more commensurate with an expanded view. A consciousness approach to pain and pain treatments is emphasized throughout this book.

BETTER IDEAS

Students and scholars of the origins and development of new technologies among human societies and civilizations down through the ages have often observed that the *discovery* of innovative ideas and approaches long precedes their *acceptance* and application, eventually supplanting older, less effective practices. Usually the old approaches and practices are not replaced with "a better idea" until they are overwhelmed by problems and limitations that overcome them and threaten the society. Such is the time we are now in when it comes to drug approaches to pain. The time may be right to finally improve on the old approaches to pain and all its attendant medical and social problems.

Fortunately, CAM and natural therapies offer a new world of opportunities for nondrug pain treatments that are time tested and increasingly demonstrated by modern clinical trials and substantiated by new discoveries in the basic sciences. This text provides the background and science that support the use of natural therapies and CAM approaches, organized in five major sections: (1) basic fundamentals and sciences; (2) mind-body approaches; (3) energetic, bodywork, and biophysical approaches; (4) Asian medical systems; and (5) natural nutritional and plant-based remedies. Finally, the psychometric evaluation appendix puts some interactive tools in the hands of practitioners, students, and patients to get on the right specific path and begin the healing journey here and now.

REFERENCES

Census Bureau. (2014). Census Bureau's annual projections for the United States in 2015 will well exceed 320 million people and the rest of the planet will total over 7.2 billion. http://www.census.gov/newsroom/press-releases/2014/cb14-tps90.html.

Gaskin, D. J. & Richard, P. (2012). The economic costs of pain in the United States. *Journal of Pain, 13*(8), 715.

Institute of Medicine Report from the Committee on Advancing Pain Research, Care, and Education. (2011). *Relieving pain in America: A blueprint for transforming prevention, care, education and research.* Washington DC: The National Academies Press. http://books.nap.edu/openbook.php?record_id=13172&page=1.

Suggested Readings can be found on the companion website, http://www.micozzipainconditions.com.

Chapter 2

Bioenergetic Foundations of Pain and Inflammation

If you don't get what you want, you suffer; if you get what you don't want, you suffer; even when you get exactly what you want, you still suffer because you can't hold on to it forever. Your mind is your predicament. It wants to be free of change. Free of pain, free of the obligations of life and death. But change is law and no amount of pretending will alter that reality.

(Socrates, 470–399 BC, 5th century BC)

As a concept, pain has been a continued topic of exploration since its emergence in ancient writings, as long as 5000 years ago, and can be traced back as long as pain has been consciously expressed in humans. The quote about pain and suffering from Socrates, a founder of Western philosophy, may remind one of the sayings of his 5th-century BC contemporary, Siddhartha Gautama, or Buddha (d. 400 BC), a founder of Eastern philosophy.

Pain is the most common reason that people sought medical attention in earlier times and continue to seek it today. Biologically, pain is the common cue that something is wrong in the body and thus has great adaptive value when it motivates actions to alleviate pain (as long as the treatment addresses the cause[s] and does not simply masques the symptoms). All humans on Earth have lived through painful experiences. Spiritual teachings and philosophical traditions dating back thousands of years speak of pain, as in Buddhism (Siddhartha Gautama, commonly known as the Buddha, and after what he called himself, "the awakened one") as well as his contemporary Greek philosophers such as Socrates. The burgeoning field of mindfulness-based interventions (MBI) in medicine focuses on the ever-changing present moment, and how to be present in that moment and "in the now." MBI techniques have contributed to a more simple understanding of how to experience and manage life experiences to achieve lessened or absent pain and suffering (McCown, Reibel, & Micozzi, 2017).

In Chapter 4, we will discuss how pain is communicated in the brain through multiple mechanisms of the central nervous system. Later, we will discuss the perception of pain. In this chapter, pain is addressed in bioenergetic terms. We will discuss ways that patients may observe the positive changes in their physical and emotional pain by unblocking pain-energy obstructions throughout the body's natural energy pathways. The treatments that are presented in this chapter, as in this textbook, are noninvasive.

BRIEF OVERVIEW OF ENERGY MEDICINE

Early practices of energy medicine (EM; electromagnetic therapy) were recorded in 2750 BC, when a human illness was treated by exposure to the shocks from electric eels (Oschman, 2015). Around 400 BC, the Greek philosopher Thales of Miletus rubbed amber and obtained static electricity that he believed to cure afflictions. (Note: there is more history in Chapter 10 on electromagnetic therapies.)

In 1929, Yale anatomy professor Harold Saxton Burr (1889–1973) undertook study of electricity and its role in disease. Burr measured human energy fields with standard detectors. Today, researchers have confirmed Burr's concrete findings that healthy and unhealthy people produce electrical charges and changes in their magnetic fields (MFs). From the late 1920s until the 1970s, scientists such as Einthoven developed different energy techniques and made discoveries including the galvanometer to record heart and skin electricity and electrocardiogram (EKG), used as a standard instrument for medical diagnosis. As seen in today's medical practices, EKGs and electroencephalograms (EEGs) have long been used to record the electrical energy or electromagnetic frequencies (EMFs) of the heart and brain for diagnostic purposes.

Medical doctors also use the other forms of energy, such as radiation, for therapeutic purposes. This application of energy has long been considered a standard oncologic treatment of many cancers, sometimes treating tumors without making an incision. Radiation therapy can be used for men with prostate cancer in contrast to surgery (National Institutes of Health, 2013). Ionizing radiation, focused energy that is beamed through the skin and tissue, is used for breast cancer and cervical cancer in women and other cancers in both sexes. However, these radiation energies have been shown in multiple studies to cause secondary, untreatable cancers and involve a number of other health risks. There are other well-established uses of measurable energy fields in the diagnosis and treatment of illness and disease. Some of these include magnetic resonance imaging (MRI), laser eye correction surgery, cardiac pacemakers, ultraviolet (UV) light therapies, and light therapy for psoriasis and seasonal affective disorder (Mayo Clinic, 2013).

HEALING ENERGY

While aspects of these energies are utilized in hospitals and by medical professionals, there are likely other areas of energy that need to be explored. It may be that many commonly observed "healing energies" may be set at a particular frequency or set of frequencies that cannot be measured because we do not use the right instruments at this point in time. By stating a "particular frequency," it would mean defining a measurement of a frequency that a "healer" would need to emit in order to effectively heal another person. For example, a healthy human being is vibrating at a certain level of frequency. As a whole, what is this frequency measurement at the healthiest state? In contrast, an unhealthy person is vibrating at another certain frequency. What is this measurement and how does it differ from the healthy person's overall frequency? Thus, what is the specific measurement of frequency that a "healer" would need to emit that would affect a patient's own frequency and heal them? Mainstream science presents limits to measuring these "healing" energies. There are few applicable studies on healing energy and intention of healing (Connor & Schwartz, 2007; Syldona & Rein, 1999; see Chapter 9)

Conflicts of interest with pharma and government-subsidized research may exist, as they say there is no reason to create a device that can measure or even influence human healing energy frequencies or the putative energies we *currently* cannot measure conventionally. During the 1990s, one of the authors (Micozzi) had encouraged the late Sen. Arlen Specter of Pennsylvania, Chair of the Senate Appropriations Committee on Health and Human Services, to provide funding to the National Institutes of Health (NIH) to study human healing energy, or bioenergy. NIH responded to him that they do not believe in bioenergy.

Veritable energy is defined based on frequencies used as energy-based therapies. They employ specific, measurable wavelengths and frequencies to treat patients. The wavelength is the inverse of the frequency, and early 20th-century fundamental physicist Max Planck calculated the constant ("Planck's Constant") for converting the wavelength/frequency to its energy content.

Veritable energies are considered to be bioelectromagnetic-based therapies. These energies consist of vibrations and their forces, or waves, such as sound, light, and magnetism—all of which have measurable wavelengths and frequencies. In the case of sound, it has a mechanical component based on successive compressions and rarefactions of the medium through which it travels as sound in air, water, or solid medium.

Putative energy uses electromagnetic fields generated by material objects and subtle energetic processes from humans such as "energy work." It is also known as "biofield therapy." The field of EM involving putative energy fields is based on a fundamental premise that all physical *objects* (bodies) as well psychological *processes* (thoughts, emotions, beliefs, mind-sets, and attitudes; consciousness) are expressions of energy. Putative, from the Late Latin word *putat*, translates to "thought," and from Greek translates to "thought to be," or "assumed to exist." These approaches are based on the idea that humans contain subtle forms of energies within them. Harnessing these energies may involve healing abilities within oneself, or applied to others, as observed in practitioners who use energy that radiates off of their hands (no touch) to apply as healing energy; see Chapters 4, 13, and 17.

The "healing touch," in which the therapist is purported to identify imbalances and correct a patient's energy by passing his or her hands over the patient, can be seen in some accounts of the Bible and today in reiki and Johrei, which are ascribed to ancient Japanese origins. A related, well-documented, and well-known ancient

Chinese practice is called "qigong." A different kind of healing "touch" is invoked in intercessory prayer, through which people pray on behalf of themselves or others for "healing at a distance" (see Chapter 4). It should be noted that "prayer" does not require touch and is different from meditation and mindfulness practices. Prayer is connection to a putative higher divine power, whereas meditation and mindfulness are connecting to one's own "higher self." *Higher self* is a term for where the field of knowledge can enter easily when the mind is in a balanced and relaxed state. In addition, it is where deliberate and intentional actions are executed with heightened awareness.

"THE FORCE" THAT MAY BE WITH YOU

Healing energy, life-force, or vital energy has been known throughout history by different names. In Chinese Medicine, life-force is referred to as "qi" or "chi"; it is known as "ki" to the Japanese and "prana" in Indian Ayurvedic medicine. Among other terms are "mana," "etheric energy," "fohat," "orgone," "odic force," and "homeopathic resonance" (Esmail, 2007). In the Judeo-Christian tradition, it is called "spirit." "Vital force" came into popularity during the 17th–18th century (and again recently) and is of European origin. Vital energy is believed by many to flow throughout the entire human body; it is believed that people are able to work with this subtle energy field to help influence health. Furthermore, all bodies are assumed to be permeated with a "subtle" energy or life-force.

BRIEF TIMELINE OF ENERGY

HOW WAS ENERGY FORMED?

Energy in the Universe

Among scientific theorists, all would have to agree that there exists the basic concept of energy. In light of energy-matter equivalence, energy is ultimately what makes up the earth, the sun's massive forces, the planets in our solar system, the galaxies and stars, and all the matter (and antimatter) of the universe.

For the purpose of energy exploration from the "beginning," we address only in some detail the Big Bang Theory. This theory is a primary scientific concept that has garnered some evidence rendering its vast principles and explains the universe at its precise infinitesimal moment of creation. The universe started with a small "singularity," then "inflated," or dispersed over the next 13.8 billion years into the infinite energy-filled cosmos that we know today. Seconds after the big bang, an immense collision of energy expanded, or "inflated," and there were billions and billions of particles floating around space, often referred to as an "energetic soup." It is important to note here that some cosmologists also suggest the expansion happened (or was guided) by way of "cosmic strings" (Bennett & Bouchet, 1990). One may be tempted to ask, if there were cosmic strings, what or who was the cosmic puppeteer?

This "energetic soup" formed just seconds after the big bang and consisted of protons and neutrons that were moving so fast they could not stick together. The cosmos eventually contained a vast array of fundamental particles such as neutrons, electrons, and protons. As the universe became gradually cooler with expansion, these particles, through a process known as "nucleosynthesis," decayed or combined. Some of the protons and neutrons collided and stuck together, forming elements heavier than hydrogen (atomic number 1), such as helium (atomic number 2; NASA, 2014). These particles (atoms), relatively heavy by comparison to subatomic particles, are known as "baryons." Almost all the things in life (i.e., the "stuff" and objects we see every day on Earth) are mostly made up of baryons, which are essentially combinations of protons, neutrons, and electrons of various atomic masses.

Atoms are the basic units of matter and the defining structure of elements. Atoms are made up of three particles: protons, neutrons, and electrons. You, this textbook, and the air we breathe—as well as the planets and stars in the universe—are all made up of protons, neutrons, and electrons. Energy exists within and without the formation of the objects seen and *unseen* on Earth and the in rest of the universe.

Energy in Everyday Experience

Forces like electricity, heat, light, and sound are all forms of energy. Energy produces changes in matter. Electrical energy can run a motor, a lightbulb, or send your voice over thousands of miles of space, as when we make phone calls.

Chemical energy heats your home and runs your car (also seen with heat energy), and the mechanism of atomic energy has become very well known and often feared (as in nuclear reactors and atomic and hydrogen bombs).

A turbine sustains the energy of movement from wind or water. This kind of energy converts kinetic energy (energy of an object due to its motion—the motion/force in a medium like water or wind) into mechanical energy. An electromagnetic generator (such as a turbine) converts kinetic energy to electrical energy generally by moving a coil of wires in a magnetic field. The most compact and efficient method is rotating an electrical coil in place through a magnetic field. Vehicles, when in motion, have kinetic energy from the conversion of heat energy (chemical internal combustion energy) into mechanical energy. In an electric motor or vehicle, the concept of the electromagnetic generator is reversed by using an electric current from a battery or current source to turn electromagnets, converting the energy into mechanical motion.

Bioenergy

EM therapy is a major category of what has been labeled *complementary and alternative medicine* (CAM). Such therapies typically involve low-level energy field interactions. They include human energy therapies, homeopathy (according to one prominent theory), acupressure, acupuncture, magnet therapy, bioelectromagnetic therapy, sound therapy, microcurrent therapy, and emotional freedom technique (tapping), among others. EM therapy is a subdiscipline of CAM that deals with energies of two types: *veritable,* which can be measured, and *putative,* which science has yet to identify. In the absence of definitive evidence that putative energy exists, supporters imply that *all* energy, whether or not its existence can be verified, is nearly identical. For example, putative energy in physics is known as "putative energy fields." Veritable energies include mechanical vibrations and sound vibrations (as seen in cymatics, the study of visible sound in combination with its vibration) and electromagnetic forces (including visible light, magnetism, monochromatic radiation [laser beams], and rays from other parts of the electromagnetic spectrum).

The electromagnetic spectrum comprises types of waves that have low frequencies (long wavelengths) in a continuum to high frequencies (short wavelengths). Radio waves and microwaves are low frequencies, and x-rays and gamma rays are high frequencies. Energy content is directly related to frequency (i.e., the higher the frequency, and shorter the wavelength, the higher the energy). All of the different electromagnetic waves run on the same kind of vibrations but at different frequencies. Electromagnetic waves are vibrations of magnetic and electric fields, so they do not need air or another conduction medium, unlike a sound wave, in order to travel. Sound waves travel through air or another physical medium because it is the *air particles* that are vibrating. Electromagnetic waves do not need a medium in order to sustain themselves, thus traveling the "vacuum" of the universe at the speed of light.

Wavelength means "the length of one wave," and frequency in terms of waves is defined as "how many waves per second." Frequency can be measured in hertz (1 Hz = 1 wave per second) and also in kilohertz (1 kHz = 1000 waves per second), megahertz (1 MHz = 1 million waves per second), and gigahertz (1 GHz = billion waves per second). These numbers in the range of frequency of "radio waves" appear as the numbers on your radio dial, for example.

EARTH, HEART, AND BRAIN: ELECTROMAGNETIC FIELDS

In geophysical sciences, the Earth's magnetic field has been measured, and the Earth's extremely low frequencies are deemed the *Schumann resonances*. This ongoing, veritable energy state is powered by the "heart" or center of the planet, first discovered in the early 1950s by Winfried Otto Schumann. Rhythms in the Earth's magnetic field have been observed to be associated with changes in brain and nervous system activity; the performance of tasks (sports, memory, energetic sensitivity); the synthesis of micronutrients in plants and algae; traffic violations and accidents; mortality from heart attacks; and vascular disease, depression and suicide, and strokes (McCraty, n.d.). This rhythm not only affects us unidirectionally; we also affect the Earth's rhythm and frequency (McCraty, 2009) Geosynchronous operational environmental satellites showed a disruption and clear correlation with the Earth's geomagnetic field at the time of the terrorist attack on September 11, 2001. Magnetic patterns of the Earth's field that immediately followed the attack were irregular and observed as more erratic than the previous magnetic waves (HeartMath Institute, 2015a; Humpel, 2013; NOAA, 2016; Princeton University, 2009).

Scientists have been able to record electrical currents in human hearts and brains and measure their electromagnetic fields. Willem Einthoven (1860–1927), born in the Dutch East Indies (today's Indonesia), discovered that heart electricity could be recorded with a galvanometer. Einthoven won the Nobel Prize in Physiology of

Medicine in 1924 for his discovery of heart electricity. Hans Berger showed that smaller electrical fields could be recorded from the brain using electrodes attached to the scalp, now known as the "electroencephalograph" (EEG). Today, the EEG is used to in medical practices to help categorize states of consciousness, health status, and diseases of the brain. This low voltage is measured due to fluctuations in the ionic current flows among neurons or brain cells. In the 1940s, Hodgkin and Huxley's study showed that neuronal membranes have voltage-dependent permeability, which means that there is an electrical potential (voltage) between the interior and the exterior of a biological cell, also known as "cellular membrane potential."

The heart has by far the largest and most powerful electromagnetic field of the entire body, far surpassing that of the brain. The heart's EMF is 5000 times more powerful than the electromagnetic field created by the brain. The heart manifests subtle, nonlocal effects that travel within these forms of energy. The heart generates over 50,000 femtoteslas (a measure of EMF, in tesla units, or "T"), compared to less than 10 femtoteslas recorded from the brain. Studies in developmental biology have indicated where EMFs are located in the action potentials of nerves, within heart tissue, and in skeletal muscle vibrations, with frequencies elicited by rhythmic activities of the entire heart organism. Endogenous EMFs are normally in the range of extremely low (5–60 Hz; Funk, Monsees, & Ozkucur, 2009). The electrical field of the heart as measured in an ECG is about 60 times greater than the brain waves recorded in an EEG. HeartMath Institute studies show the heart's powerful electromagnetic field can be detected and measured several feet away from a person's body and between two individuals in close proximity (HeartMath Institute, 2015b). These effects can be measured by electronic sensors and also sensed routinely by other human beings, and probably by pets and other animals.

Another property of the heart appears to be an ability to think, feel, and remember, as well as a capability of deep intuitive-knowing. These properties, far from being counterintuitive vis-à-vis the brain, have been sensed and ascribed to the heart by every tradition in every known culture and society through antiquity. The heart, in this context coming to be considered as the heart-brain (or "mind-body"), is composed of about 40,000 neurons that can sense, feel, learn, and remember. The heart sends messages directly to the brain about how the body feels, along with other components. For the majority of the 20th century, scientists believed that the brain sent messages and commands to the heart and the heart was the least responsible organism for any type of knowledge. Today, scientists now understand that it works *both* ways—and therefore the heart can "think" independently from (although preferably in concert with) the brain (McCraty, Atkinson, Tomasino, & Trevor Bradley, 2009). This phenomenon, for example, is described in essence in the Ayurvedic concept of the energy chakras of the mind-body (see Chapter 18).

The heart has the ability to send important subtle energy messages to the brain. Scientists now know that the heart is made up of an intricate and systematic nervous system with the same type of vast network of neurons as found in the brain, with neurotransmitters, neuropeptides, and supporting cells. One significant way that the heart communicates with the brain is through its natural beating rhythm. When the heart is beating at a stable interval, the body and the brain attain higher-order cognitive abilities, such as greater mental clarity and decision-making processes ("executive decision making" in cognitive terms) and may be better able to cope with stress (rather than submitting to primeval "fight-flight" or "alarm-defense" brainstem/spinal reflex reactions). There is also a significant increase in intuitive abilities (HeartMath Institute, 2015a).

In terms of the heart's coherence, another way of looking at these energetic intervals is through the order distribution of the heart. This coherence is also recognized in physics as a pattern of action generated by a single system known as a stable energy in a perfect wave form. An example is a *sine* wave, which is a completely perfect wave. (The EKG recognizes the "normal *sinus rhythm*" of the heart under stable conditions.) The more stable the frequency, amplitude, and shape of the waveform, the higher the degree of *coherence*. The degree of order and stability in physiological processes are reflected in the rhythmic activity generated by a single oscillatory cycle such as the heart's rhythmic activity, which also can be measured in beats per minute (BPM). As we will see in the next paragraph, when stability and overall coherence is increased in a single system that is coupled to other systems, such as other major organs in the body, it can pull or gather the other systems into coherence, or *entrainment*. Such entrainment corresponds with increased cross-coherence in the activity of the other systems, even across different time scales of activity. Entrainment can also manifest among different members of a species of the same organism, and even potentially among different organisms and species (HeartMath Institute, 2015b; Mayor & Micozzi, 2012).

The heart and brain are in constant communication, yet we can *intentionally* instruct the heart to communicate to the brain and increase the benefits of overall brain and body (being). When humans experience sincere, authentic, and honest emotions, such as compassion or appreciation, the heart processes these emotions independently and the heart's rhythm becomes ever more harmonious, coherent, and stable. When these "feelings" are intentionally positively driven, they increase harmony in the heart's rhythms and improve balance in the nervous system. Negative emotions, such as hostility, anger, and feelings of lack of self-worth, lead to havoc and increased stress on the heart and other bodily organs and are therefore more stressful on the body's systems (HeartMath Institute, 2015a). These emotional and behavioral influences can also be referred to as *psychophysiological coherence*.

The heart, as the most powerful generator of rhythmic information patterns of the entire body, acts more as a symphonic generator to promote balance and to influence conditions and states of the brain and body. For example, the heart affects physical health and significantly influences perceptual processing (such as pain), emotional experience, and intentional, voluntary behaviors (McCraty et al., 2009). The heart is a highly complex and self-organized information processing center that affects the cranial brain by ways of the nervous system, hormonal system, and other pathways. The heart thereby influences brain function and most of the body's major organs, which in essence affects and determines one's quality of life and one's own perception of it (like the pain and suffering described by Socrates and Buddha).

The information we process in the heart, such as continual reading and monitoring of emotional experiences and feelings that influence cognitive function, are sent to the brain and the *entire body*—neurologically, biochemically, biophysically, and energetically (McCraty et al., 2009). Humans conventionally conceive that we are using our brains to make decisions and think logically. The role of the heart provides further insight into understanding why we like certain people right away or we receive a "download" of information about people without really "consciously knowing" from whence it came. Psychologists have long recognized and referred to this ability as "stereotyping" or "profiling," a functional, adaptive, "labor-saving" device that we use to protect ourselves and not to have to relearn the same life lessons over and over again, which can be quite costly to ourselves, our communities, and our society.

For example, feelings or the "vibes" we get from people may in fact just be the combination of electromagnetic fields from both parties' heart energy. Therefore, we can think of both the heart *and* the brain as having magnetic and electrical currents and (unhinged) unique healing capabilities that run through our bodies at different intervals and speeds to continually create and sustain a surrounding energetic field—which acts as a "force field" and even a "shield."

Clinical studies show that being in this coherent state has many health benefits (McCraty, n.d.):

1. High blood pressure and hypertension—20% reduction in diastolic and systolic blood pressure
2. Diabetes—30% increase in quality of life metrics; 1.1% reduction in HbA1c in type 2 diabetes (LifeScan, division of Johnson & Johnson)
3. Congestive heart failure—14% improvement in functional capacity (Stanford Hospital)
4. Heart arrhythmias—75% of patients had significantly fewer episodes of atrial fibrillation and 20% were able to stop medication altogether (Kaiser Permanente)
5. Asthma—Over 50% of patients experienced a decrease in airway impedance, symptom severity, and medication consumption (Robert Wood Johnson Medical School)

McCraty, Heart-Brain Dynamics Study

A study conducted in 2010 by a team of researchers discovered that the higher EMFs distributed by hand-held mobile devices actually changed the overall behavior of the cardiovascular system significantly and the "degree of chaos" created on heart rate variability (HRV) increased the higher the EMF (Yılmaz & Yıldız, 2010). If overall EMF affects HRV, it is probably best to hold or keep any mobile devices away from the center of the chest where they may affect the heart.

Meditation From the "Heart"

In addition to the heart-brain connection, the heart's intelligence during meditation is able to emit photoelectrical activity, or photons, that are radiated during meditations *specific to the heart*. For example, this "internal light" has been observed when meditating *through* the heart and with the heart, just as one "loves with the heart." A study in Witzenhousen, Germany, showed it is possible to produce visible light from the chest area with meditation that is focused on the heart center and is not transcendent. Sustained light emissions of 100,000 photons per second were measured and steadily recorded, whereas a normal count of 20 photons per second was observed without meditation (Bair, 1997). This type of meditation is most likely to promote positive emotions, and these positive emotions, when the intention is to be processed by the heart, may increase the probability of a more harmonious and coherent heart rate (HeartMath Institute, 2015a).

VERITABLE ENERGY THERAPIES

ELECTROMAGNETIC THERAPY

Electromagnetic therapies can be dispersed as either low-frequency or high-frequency stimulations. However, clinically used EMFs are usually in the range of extremely low (5–60 Hz; Funk et al., 2009). As studies have observed, the effects of mobile devices on the heart, higher EMFs (900–1800 MHz) EMF are not the same frequencies generated with electromagnetic therapy.

EMF treatment has a coherent, "intelligent," energetic ability to communicate with cells in a way that has higher-order processing attributes. For example, EMF stimulates neuronal cells to differentiate overtly into neurons and send out neurites. The term *neurite* refers to any extension from the cell body of a neuron. This projection can be either an axon or a dendrite (Robinson, 1985). There are also increasing findings of intracellular communication, instructions, and repositioning of cells in the body when this treatment has been applied (Robinson, 1985). Remember, each cell in the human body has permeability to electricity. EMF treatment depends on how cells can generate EMF both endogenously (substances within an organism or cell) and exogenously (outside an organism or cell; Robinson, 1985).

Well-known mechanisms of cell-to-cell interaction from EMF also play an important role, as with chemical and electrical signaling of cells. Interestingly, *entrainment* of this resonance influences the effects of EMF on cells and tissues and has been shown to affect various cell functions. These normal cell functions include cell proliferation, differentiation, apoptosis, DNA synthesis, RNA transcription, gene transcription, and protein expression, among many others (Foletti, Lisi, Ledda, de Carlo, & Grimaldi, 2009; Goodman et al., 1988; Phillips, 2004; Seeliger et al., 2014; Tian et al., 2002). Another specific example of these interactions is thereby signaling the release or modulation of calcium, which is an important second messenger for many cellular processes, including synthesis and assembly of DNA, RNA, and proteins (Gartzke & Lange, 2002).

Clinical use of electromagnetic therapy treatments, especially in recent years, is reported to repair many different types of cells and tissues through membrane and cytoskeletal organizations. In addition, this type of treatment is noninvasive, low-cost, immediately available, and has ease of localized application, rare if any side effects, and an indefinite shelf life. Immunity studies show that even low-intensity

EMF can affect and influence interactions in cells and tissues (Ross & Harrison, 2015). This approach benefits any individual with inflammation conditions and wound healing in particular. Within the immune system, phagocyte cells aid the immune system against bacterial growth by ingesting harmful bacteria and foreign particles, and with extremely low-frequency (ELF) EMF, the properties and conditions of these cells are enhanced greatly. The role of EMF plays a huge part in the immune system because of its effect on these cells and the growth rate of bacteria. Clinical practices are subject to prescribing medicine when patients are adhering to mainstream antibiotics that are resistant to bacteria. These EM factors may greatly enhance the fields of disease pathology, biomedicine, and tissue engineering and regenerative medicines.

Electromagnetic Field Therapy and Inflammation

Inflammation is usually the initial protective activation response to infection, burn, irritation, or injury. Inflammation involves immune cells, heat, blood, and other mediators. Forty years of research has contributed to the knowledge we have today about EMF and its benefits for inflammation in individuals, providing safe and easy methods to treat sources of pain, injury, and inflammation (Markov et al., 2001). Without an acute inflammatory response, the body would not be able to repair and regenerate tissue. Enduring and long-lasting chronic inflammation from poor diet, exercise, injury, minor illnesses, and other factors contributes to the long-term consequences of chronic inflammation, which can cause serious chronic illness and disease in the body in its own right (Després, 2012).

Inflammation plays a role in the development of diseases such as heart disease, diabetes, arthritis, Alzheimer's disease, obesity, irritable bowel syndrome (IBS), Parkinson's disease, cancer, HIV/AIDS, lack of vitamins in individuals such as vitamin D, and all autoimmune diseases (Camilleri et al., 2012; High et al., 2012; Johnson et al., 2012; Knevel et al., 2013; Laird et al., 2012; Matarese et al., 2012; Moretti et al., 2012; Nielsen & Bendtzen, 2012; Rosen et al., 2012; Tufekci et al., 2012; Zilka et al., 2012).

Heart disease is affected by inflammation for a major reason, involving the immune system and its attack on low-density lipoprotein (LDL) cholesterol, which is in the tissue of the arterial walls. Chronic inflammation of these areas will damage major arteries, potentially causing them to burst (Hovland, Lappegård, & Mollnes, 2012).

Inflammation disorders involve pathogenic processes in such disorders as pulmonary disease, Crohn's disease, rheumatoid arthritis, osteoarthritis, atherosclerosis, asthma, gout, psoriasis, ulcerative colitis, and multiple sclerosis, among others such as sarcoidosis (chronic lung disease; Nathan, 2002). Inflammation can also contribute largely to a number of microbial toxicities in diseases such as influenza, cystic fibrosis, pneumonitis, hepatitis C, influenza, viral pneumonia, leprosy, sepsis, and tuberculosis (Nathan, 2002). Accordingly with diabetes, inflammation is heavily linked and attacks beta cells that produce insulin (Nielson et al., 2012). Evidently, it has been recorded in early research that chronic inflammation can promote cancer growth (Sakurai, 2012).

Magnetic Therapy

The use of magnetic energy for healing dates back thousands of years. The word magnet comes from the ancient Greeks. It is thought to derive from *Magnes lithos,* meaning "Magnesia stone," in an area of Greece near the Aegean Sea that was known for its volcanic rocks with magnetic properties. The Greek philosopher Aristotle spoke about using magnets as a healing therapy.

Essentially, magnets are placed on different parts of the body to relieve pain. One of the earliest written medical texts published in China, *The Yellow Emperor's Book of Internal Medicine,* mentions the application of magnetic stones to correct health imbalances, including the relief of pain, dating back to around 2000 BC (Chernyak & Sessler, 2005; Rosch, 2015). The ancient Egyptians were apparently acquainted with the power of magnets. Egyptian legends claim to have seen Cleopatra sleep with a magnetic stone on her forehead to preserve her youthful appearance.

During the 16th century, William Gilbert, physician to Elizabeth I of England, published the early Western scientific treatise on magnetism, *De Magnete.* This book summarized the current knowledge about magnetism, showing, for example, the first signs of a compass by the fact that steel holds a magnetic charge better than iron and that there is a distinction between magnetism and electricity. Gilbert helped start the era of modern geophysics since he was the first to describe the Earth as a huge magnet with magnetic poles close to the geographic North and South Poles. The discovery of the electron at the end of the 19th century moved electromagnetism to the atomic level, demonstrating that all matter (where electrons are gravitating within atoms) is electrical or energetic in nature.

The magnetic measurement of strength is described in terms of "gauss" and "tesla." Carl Friedrich Gauß (Gauss in German; 1777–1855) was a mathematician, worked on magnetism, and later developed the gauss measurement. Nikola Tesla (1856–1943) was a multidisciplinary genius who discovered the AC power system still used today. A tesla is equal to 10,000 gauss. Therapeutic magnets are most often in the range of 200–10,000 gauss. Typical household magnets, such as refrigerator magnets, are typically around 200 gauss.

Human blood is made up of 4% iron, carried in the hemoglobin and red corpuscles; therefore, some have speculated magnets have the ability to influence these and other charged molecules in the blood and other parts of the body. Many scientific studies on pain have been completed with people who have neuropathic pain conditions, and people with this condition may find this method helpful. It is important to note that scientific evidence on this therapy is inconclusive and conflicting. A study of carpel tunnel syndrome found no statistical difference between magnets and a placebo, although the authors of the study noted, "Although this study did not show magnets to be more effective than the placebo, the reduction in pain with this simple intervention was remarkable" (Carter et al., 2002).

People wear magnets to treat other painful conditions such as lower back pain, chronic fatigue syndrome, migraine headaches, multiple sclerosis (MS), menstrual periods, carpel tunnel syndrome, and sports injuries. The most effective forms of magnetic therapy demonstrated are for nerve pain caused by diabetes (diabetic neuropathic) and osteoarthritis (Mert, Gunay, Gocmen, Kaya, & Polat, 2006; Weintraub & Cole, 2004; Weintraub et al., 2003; see Chapter 10).

SOUND ENERGY THERAPY

Sound energy therapy, also referred to as vibrational therapy, is a therapeutic modality that eases physical pain, promotes emotional healing, and induces the relaxation response in individuals. It may involve tones or using tuning forks to create certain healing sound frequencies that resonate with the body to promote healing. Music therapy is another type of sound energy therapy. Listening to music has been shown to lower blood pressure and to reduce chronic pain and anxiety (Nauert, 2011). When used in combination with biofeedback techniques, music can reduce tension and facilitate the relaxation response (Thoma et al., 2013).

The first findings on the physiological effects of music date back to 1923. The cardiovascular, pulse rate, and blood pressure responses to music were studied by Hyde in 1924. He concluded that people are generally psychologically and physiologically affected by music, which is harmonic and rich in tone, and benefits the cardiovascular system, influences muscle tone, enhances endurance, and aids digestion (Hyde, 1924).

Sound therapy has been shown to decrease pain in patients who suffer from tinnitus in more than one study (Hoare, Searchfield, El Refaie, & Henry, 2014). In addition, Joudry and Joudry (1999) conducted a 3-year survey of 388 respondents where 45% to 100% of subjects showed less symptoms of tinnitus. Participants also improved in hearing loss, stress, fatigue, sleep problems, learning difficulties, speech problems, depression, headaches, and overall well-being. Nearly the entire group of subjects observed some positive results in at least one area.

Plants and Sound

A study, conducted in 2004, suggesting that sound vibrations (music and noise) as well as biofields (bioelectromagnetic and healing intention) both directly affect living biologic systems. The "intention" was that a certain group of seeds would sprout faster than the other group of seeds. The researchers found that sound vibrations and the energetic intentions ultimately affected seed germination and that germination bioassay has the sensitivity to detect various applied energetic conditions, such as sound, music, and noise. Therefore, sound and intention had a highly statistically significant effect on the number of seeds sprouted compared to the untreated seed group (Creath & Schwartz, 2004). This observation suggests that our minds and our intentions have powerful effects on the world around us. If our intention to speed the germination process has these types of effects, perhaps we could speed our own healing process. And, as we have discussed previously, plants' abilities are also affected by the Earth's electromagnetic field (HeartMath Institute, 2015a).

The Energy of Thought

Every thought we have is energy that can be measured. Whether it is a negative thought or a positive thought, it is based on our internal feelings while having this thought. Some people are not even aware of their internal feelings and general constitution while they are thinking. By being completely aware of our thoughts, as in every single thought that enters our mind, we slow down what we are thinking about and overrule automatic processes. And by slowing down our minds, we are able to transition our awareness to leverage our thoughts. We can slow down our thoughts and focus on "good" or "bad" thoughts. If we start "catching" thoughts and knowing "This is a bad thought" versus "This is a good thought," we can start implementing positive-driven thoughts as well as appropriate actions. How can we do this? By recreating the neural structure of our brains. When thinking negative thoughts, our brains are wired to do so. We never learned that by repeatedly thinking negative thoughts, we have been creating a series of neural networks that are familiar to us, and therefore familiar and easy for our brains. Think of traveling to work every single day. Chances are you know how to get to work very easily because you have walked or driven countless times. However, if you took a different route to work one day, you would likely be more engaged, and your brain would put a bit more effort into understanding the new images involved, the new smells, and the overall sensory awareness that your new reality is creating. By going the "new way," your brain starts rewiring itself through new neuronal pathways that are made to remember and more easily apply this new way of thinking.

Catch Your Thoughts

One way to understand pain is to understand human thought. What are we humans constantly thinking about? Are we thinking mostly negative, positive, or neutral thoughts? Are we even *aware* of what thoughts we are thinking? Unregulated and uncontrolled thoughts can be one reason that teachers have gradually reintroduced mindfulness and meditation into Western civilizations. The existence of unnatural thought processes explains the popularity of meditation, which has also brought about a very important awareness of the power of "no thought." It has also given us a deeper understanding of the awareness behind human thoughts, emotions, and actions in everyday life. One way to achieve this awareness is by practicing mindfulness. Simply put, meditation is no thought, and mindfulness is the awareness of the thought and an acceptance of it (see Chapter 5).

Thoughts may induce pain and emotional suffering in us. What purpose do these negative-feeling thoughts serve? It is possible that we actually choose to experience pain and suffering in order to overcome them? If that is so, then how do we overcome our pain, and what will life be like if our thoughts did not include emotions tied to our painful past?

As we have seen, pain centers have complex neurological functions and are involved with many mechanisms along the central nervous system. These topics will be discussed in the remaining chapters and sections.

REFERENCES

Bair, P. (1997). *Case study: Visible light radiated from the heart with heart rhythm meditation*. http://journals.sfu.ca/seemj/index.php/seemj/article/viewFile/56/44.

Bennett, D.P & Bouchet, F.R. (1990). High-resolution simulations of cosmic-string evolution. i Network evolution. http://journals.aps.org/prd/abstract/10.1103/PhysRevD.41.2408.

Camilleri, M., Lasch, K., & Zhou, W. (2012). Irritable bowel syndrome: Methods, mechanisms, and pathophysiology. The confluence of increased permeability, inflammation, and pain in irritable bowel syndrome. *American Journal of Physiology. Gastrointestinal and Liver Physiology, 303*(7), G775–G795.

Carter, R., Hall, T., & Aspy, C. B. (2002). The effectiveness of magnet therapy for treatment of wrist pain attributed to carpal tunnel syndrome. *Journal of Family Practice, 51*(1), 38–40.

Chernyak, G. V. & Sessler, D. I. (2005). Perioperative acupuncture and related techniques. *Anesthesiology, 102*(5), 1031–1078. http://www.acupunctuurjolandanijenhuis.nl/wp-content/uploads/2014/09/Perioperative-setting-kopie.pdf.

Connor, M. & Schwartz, G. (2007). Measuring ELF magnetic fields. In G. Schwartz (Ed.), *Research findings at the University of Arizona Center for frontier medicine in biofield science: A summary report*. http://lach.web.arizona.edu/CFMBS_Report.pdf.

Creath, K. & Schwartz, G. E. (2004). Measuring effects of music, noise, and healing energy using a seed germination bioassay. *Journal of Alternative and Complementary Medicine, 10*(1), 113–122. http://www.ncbi.nlm.nih.gov/pubmed/15025885.

Després, J. P. (2012). Abdominal obesity and cardiovascular disease: is inflammation the missing link? http://www.ncbi.nlm.nih.gov/pubmed/22889821.

Esmail, M. (2007). *Complementary and alternative medicine in Canada: Trends in use and public attitudes, 1997–2006*. http://www.fraserinstitute.org/uploadedFiles/fraser-ca/Content/research-news/research/publications/complementary-alternative-medicine-in-canada-2007.pdf.

Foletti, A., Lisi, A., Ledda, M., de Carlo, F., & Grimaldi, S. (2009). Cellular ELF signals as a possible tool in informative medicine. *Electromagnetic Biology and Medicine, 28*(1), 71–79. http://www.ncbi.nlm.nih.gov/pubmed/19337897.

Funk, R. H., Monsees, T., & Ozkucur, N. (2009). *Electromagnetic effects - From cell biology to medicine*. http://www.ncbi.nlm.nih.gov/pubmed/19167986.

Gartzke, J. & Lange, K. (2002). *Cellular target of weak magnetic fields: Ionic conduction along actin filaments of microvilli*. http://www.ncbi.nlm.nih.gov/pubmed/12372794.

Goodman, R. & Henderson, A. (1988). Exposure of salivary gland cells to low-frequency electromagnetic fields alters polypeptide synthesis. *Proceedings of the National Academy of Sciences of the United States of America, 85*, 3928.

HeartMath Institute. (2015a). *Global coherence research*. https://www.heartmath.org/research/global-coherence/.

HeartMath Institute. (2015b). *Science of the heart: Exploring the role of the heart in human performance*. https://www.heartmath.org/resources/downloads/science-of-the-heart/?submenuheader=3.

High, K. P., Brennan-Ing, M., Clifford, D. B., et al. (2012). *HIV and aging: State of knowledge and areas of critical need for research*. A report to the NIH Office of AIDS Research by the HIV and Aging Working Group. http://www.ncbi.nlm.nih.gov/pubmed/22688010.

Hoare, D. J., Searchfield, G. D., El Refaie, A., & Henry, J. A. (2014). Sound therapy for tinnitus management: Practicable options. *Journal of the American Academy of Audiology, 25*(1), 62–75. http://www.ncbi.nlm.nih.gov/pubmed/24622861.

Hovland, A., Lappegård, K. T., & Mollnes, T. E. (2012). LDL apheresis and inflammation—Implications for atherosclerosis. *Scandinavian Journal of Immunology, 76*(3), 229–236. http://www.ncbi.nlm.nih.gov/pubmed/22670805.

Humpel, N. (2013). *Journey to the truth: An introduction to the reality of ourselves and the world* (pp. 34–36). Calwell: ACT Inspiring Publishers.

Hyde, I. H. (1924). Effects of music upon electrocardiograms and blood pressure. *Journal of Experimental Psychology, 7*(3), 213–224. http://dx.doi.org/10.1037/h0073580.

Johnson, A. R., Milner, J. J., & Makowski, L. (2012). *The inflammation highway: Metabolism accelerates inflammatory traffic in obesity*. http://www.ncbi.nlm.nih.gov/pmc/articles/PMC3422768/.

Joudry, P. & Joudry, R. (1999). *Sound therapy music to recharge your brain*. Sydney, Australia: Sound Therapy Australia.

Knevel, R., van Nies, J. A., le Cessie, S., Huizinga, T. W., Brouwer, E., & van der Helm-van Mil, A. H. (Aug 17 2013). Evaluation of the contribution of cumulative levels of inflammation to the variance in joint destruction in rheumatoid arthritis. *Annals of the Rheumatic Diseases*, 2012.

Laird, E., et al. (2012). *Vitamin D deficiency is associated with inflammation in older Irish adults*. http://press.endocrine.org/doi/abs/10.1210/jc.2013-3507.

Markov, M. & Colbert, A. P. (2001). Magnetic and electromagnetic field therapy. *Journal of Back and Musculokeletal Rehabilitation*, 15, 17.

Matarese, G., et al. (2012). *At the crossroad of T cells, adipose tissue, and diabetes*. http://www.ncbi.nlm.nih.gov/pubmed/22889219.

Mayo Clinic. (2013). *Tests and procedures: Light therapy*. http://www.mayoclinic.org/tests-procedures/light-therapy/basics/definition/prc-20009617.

Mayor, D. M. & Micozzi, M. S. (2012). *Energy medicine east and west*. London and St Louis: Elsevier.

McCown, D., Reibel, D. K., & Micozzi, M. S. (2017). *Teaching mindfulness* (2nd ed.). New York, NY: Springer.

McCraty, R. (n.d.) *The relationship between heart-brain dynamics, positive emotions, coherence, optimal health and cognitive function*. http://www.coherenceinhealth.nl/usr-data/general/verslagen/Verlsag_Rollin_McCraty.pdf.

McCraty, R., Atkinson, M., Tomasino, D., & Bradley, R. T. (2009). The coherent heart heart-brain interactions, psychophysiological coherence, and the emergence of system-wide order. *Integral Review*, 5(2). http://www.heartmathbenelux.com/doc/McCratyeal_article_in_integral_review_2009.pdf.

Mert, T., Gunay, I., Gocmen, C., Kaya, M., & Polat, S. (2006). Regenerative effects of pulsed magnetic field on injured peripheral nerves. *Alternative Therapies in Health and Medicine*, 12(5), 42–49. http://www.ncbi.nlm.nih.gov/pubmed/17017754.

Moretti, M., Bennett, J., Tornatore, L., Thotakura, A. K., & Franzoso, G. (2012). *Cancer: NF-kB regulates energy metabolism*. http://www.ncbi.nlm.nih.gov/pubmed/22903018.

Nathan, C. (2002). *Points of control in inflammation*. http://www.direct-ms.org/pdf/ImmunologyGeneral/PointsOfControl.pdf.

National Aeronautics and Space Administration (NASA). (2014). *What is the universe made of?*. http://map.gsfc.nasa.gov/universe/uni_matter.html.

National Oceanic and Atmospheric Administration (NOAA). (2016). *NOAA goes satellite mission*. Retrieved from: http://spidr.ngdc.noaa.gov/spidr/help.do?group=GOES.

National Institutes of Health. (2013). *Prostate cancer*. https://report.nih.gov/nihfactsheets/ViewFactSheet.aspx?csid=60.

Nauert, R. (2011). *Music soothes anxiety, reduces pain*. http://psychcentral.com/news/2011/12/23/music-soothes-anxiety-reduces-pain/32952.html.

Nielsen, C. H. & Bendtzen, K. (2012). *Immunoregulation by naturally occurring and disease-associated autoantibodies: Binding to cytokines and their role in regulation of T-cell responses*. http://www.pubfacts.com/detail/22903670/Immunoregulation-by-naturally-occurring-and-disease-associated-autoantibodies-:-binding-to-cytokines.

Oschman, J. (2015). *Energy medicine: The scientific basis*. https://goo.gl/olzGjI.

Phillips, J. L. (2004). *Effects of electromagnetic field exposure on gene transcription*. http://onlinelibrary.wiley.com/wol1/doi/10.1002/jcb.2400510401/abstract.

Princeton University. (2009). *Extended analysis: September 11 2001 in context*. http://noosphere.princeton.edu/extended.analysis.html.

Robinson, K. R. (1985). The responses of cells to electrical fields: A review. *Journal of Cell Biology*, 101, 2023–2027. http://jcb.rupress.org/content/101/6/2023.full.pdf.

Rosch, P. J. (2015). *Bioelectromagnetic and subtle energy medicine* (2nd ed., pp. 17–18). Boca Raton, FL: CRC Press.

Rosen, C. J., Adams, J. S., Bikle, D. D., et al. (2012). The nonskeletal effects of vitamin D: An Endocrine Society scientific statement. *Endocrine Reviews*, 33, 456–492. Article.

Ross, C. L. & Harrison, B. S. (2015). *An introduction to electromagnetic field therapy and immune function: A brief history and current status.* http://inter-use.com/Journals/JSAB/2015/Volume_03_Issue_02/2015/0302/86.html.

Sakurai, H. (2012). Targeting of TAK1 in inflammatory disorders and cancer. *Trends in Pharmacological Sciences, 33*(10), 522–530. http://www.ncbi.nlm.nih.gov/pubmed/22795313.

Seeliger, C., Falldorf, K., Sachtleben, J., & van Griensven, M. (2014). *Low-frequency pulsed electromagnetic fields significantly improve time of closure and proliferation of human tendon fibroblasts.* http://www.ncbi.nlm.nih.gov/pmc/articles/PMC4096547/.

Syldona, M. & Rein, G. (1999). The use of DC electrodermal potential measurements and healer's felt sense to assess the energetic nature of qi. *Journal of Alternative and Complementary Medicine, 5*(4), 329–347. http://www.ncbi.nlm.nih.gov/pubmed/10471013.

Thoma, M. V., et al. (2013). *The effect of music on the human stress response.* http://www.ncbi.nlm.nih.gov/pmc/articles/PMC3734071/.

Tian, F., Nakahara, T., Yoshida, M., Honda, N., Hirose, H., Miyakoshi, J. (2002). Exposure to power frequency magnetic fields suppresses X-ray-induced apoptosis transiently in Ku80-deficient xrs5 cells. *292*(2), 355–361. http://www.ncbi.nlm.nih.gov/pubmed/11906169.

Tufekci, K. U., Meuwissen, R., Genc, S., & Genc, K. (2012). *Inflammation in Parkinson's disease.* http://www.ncbi.nlm.nih.gov/pubmed/22814707.

Weintraub, M. I. & Cole, S. P. (2004). Pulsed magnetic field therapy in refractory neuropathic pain secondary to peripheral neuropathy: Electrodiagnostic parameters—Pilot study. *Neurorehabilitation and Neural Repair, 18*(1), 42–46. http://www.ncbi.nlm.nih.gov/pubmed/15035963.

Weintraub, M. I., Wolfe, G. I., Barohn, R. A., Cole, S. P., Parry, G. J., Hayat, G., et al. (2003). Static magnetic field therapy for symptomatic diabetic neuropathy: A randomized, double-blind, placebo-controlled trial. *Archives of Physical Medicine and Rehabilitation, 84*(5), 736–746. http://www.ncbi.nlm.nih.gov/pubmed/12736891.

Yılmaz, D. & Yıldız, M. (2010). Analysis of the mobile phone effect on the heart rate variability by using the largest Lyapunov exponent. *Journal of Medical Systems, 34*(6), 1097–1103. http://www.ncbi.nlm.nih.gov/pubmed/20703598.

Zilka, N., Kazmerova, Z., Jadhav, S., Neradil, P., et al. (2012). *Who fans the flames of Alzheimer's disease brains? Misfolded tau on the crossroad of neurodegenerative and inflammatory pathways.* http://www.jneuroinflammation.com/content/9/1/47.

Suggested Readings can be found on the companion website, http://www.micozzipainconditions.com.

Chapter *3*

Geophysical and Biophysical Energy in Pain and Inflammation

Energy in our solar system comes from the sun and is transmitted and conserved through the Earth to plants and eventually to all living organisms. The sun and Earth serve as good fundamental starting points for a basic 21st-century "grounding" in the forms of geophysical and biophysical energy that may influence pain, inflammation, and chronic pain conditions.

THE SUN, SOLAR RADIATION, AND VISIBLE LIGHT

In light of the electromagnetic spectrum, visible light has many health and other benefits. New research shows that red, white, and blue light—all part of the visible spectrum of sunlight—may help to treat a variety of medical problems. Light, air, and water are fundamental to human life and health. The air we breathe contains oxygen, which fuels every cell in the body. Water is the fluid for blood and tissues. Plant life takes the carbon dioxide from the air humans exhale and, together with light, manufactures food and oxygen. This process called "photosynthesis" puts oxygen back into the air. It may sound like simple elementary earth science, but it is truly a miraculous cycle of life. Sometimes modern medicine loses sight of these basic elements of life for good health. Natural light provides a full spectrum of the sun's radiation, which reaches the Earth and penetrates through the atmosphere, but not all solar radiation is hospitable to life.

Approximately 300 million years ago the Earth's atmosphere had accumulated enough oxygen (contributed by marine plants) and ozone to filter out harmful cosmic radiation. Before that time, life on Earth flourished only in the oceans because the water blocked and filtered deadly cosmic and solar radiation, but there was no such protection on the land. Then, over millions and millions of years, marine plants produced enough oxygen through photosynthesis to increase oxygen levels in the atmosphere high enough (~20%) to then form the protective ozone layer. Deadly radiation was blocked by the critical ozone layer—and life emerged from the sea onto the land—first plant life then arthropods from the sea (insects). During this geologic era (Carboniferous Era) exuberant plant and insect life covered the land for millions and millions of years. Then they successively died, fossilized, and laid down the huge deposits of coal and oil ("fossil fuels") still found in the Earth today.

It makes sense that exposure to full-spectrum solar light would also have numerous health benefits because life on Earth eventually flourished because of exposure to it. First and foremost, exposure to natural sunlight activates vitamin D production in your skin. In addition to the well-known benefits of vitamin D (see Chapters 20 and 21), exposure to full-spectrum light seems to improve mood and reduce anxiety. Studies show it improves attitude and performance in the classroom and workplace. It also improves attendance and achievement.

Studies show specific "light therapy" can help a variety of health problems, including seasonal affective disorder (SAD), depression, Parkinson's disease, and dementia. In addition, new research shows that light therapy reduces back pain and premenstrual syndrome (PMS), epilepsy, and even halitosis (bad breath). Of course, the best "light therapy" involves spending more time outside in Nature, but one can also benefit from sitting in front of a light box. In addition, make sure the light *inside* your home comes from "full-spectrum" bulbs. The old-fashioned incandescent bulb, originally invented by Thomas Edison in the 19th century, provides a full spectrum of light similar to what the sun provides. For a long time this incandescent light bulb had been the most effective product for the most affordable price.

THE DIM BULBS OF THE ENVIRONMENTAL PROTECTION AGENCY

The government Environmental Protection Agency has recently required us to install (which in a private residence can total almost $1000 worth of) new compact fluorescent (CFL) bulbs. CFLs are very *inefficient,* at least in terms of practical daily living. It takes many minutes for these bulbs to actually provide light after you switch them on. They start out very dim and then slowly begin to provide the promised illumination. So in many cases, people stumble around in the dark trying to maneuver or locate something and by the time these lights really come on, you do not need them anymore. Does that sound very efficient? The problems associated with these CFL bulbs get much worse. These bulbs emit unhealthy levels of ultraviolet radiation and can also reportedly catch fire and even burn the skin. CFL bulbs also release chemical toxins, including naphthalene ("moth balls") and styrene, both of which other government agencies classify as likely human carcinogens. Some people have even observed a kind of electrical "smog" that develops around these lamps. They also contain mercury, which is prohibited from being dumped in landfills. The government has created another problem that we literally cannot get rid of.

LIGHT THERAPY FOR THE MOST COMMON CAUSE OF PAIN

When treating back pain, like all medical problems, the most sensible approach is to try the least dangerous, least expensive treatments first and reserve the dangerous, expensive treatments as the last resort. Research shows spinal manual therapy (SMT) should be the first choice for the vast majority of people. It is presently the most available, effective, and cost-effective treatment for back pain (see Chapter 12). Acupuncture (see Chapter 15) and massage (see Chapter 13) also show great promise.

European researchers have also used blue light to treat back pain. (This blue-light research began in Europe. In these countries the governments pay for all health care and needs to avoid expensive, ineffective and dangerous back surgeries.)

European doctors recently developed an innovative patch that emits a blue light. Blue light, seen at the end of the visible *spectrum* (e.g., the colors of light produced when a light beam is passed through a prism), has higher energy according to the Planck equation:

$$E = h\text{v}; \text{ where } E \text{ equals energy, and } h \text{ is Planck's constant}$$

The Greek letter nu *(v)* is frequency, which is inversely proportional to wavelength. Blue light has smaller wavelengths, thus greater frequency and greater energy, in the visible spectrum. The speed of a wave is the product of wavelength (λ) and frequency *(v)*.

Doctors place the light patch over the area of back pain. The light painlessly penetrates the skin and activates metabolic pathways in cells that produce nitric oxide. This potent chemical dilates blood vessels by relaxing the smooth muscle cells that line the blood vessels (a bit like the effects of a "micromassage" without the hands). As a result it increases the amount of blood flow and oxygen in cells and helps to carry away metabolic by-products and toxins that cause cell damage. By locally increasing blood flow to painful areas, it also increases the amount of the body's own pain-relieving compounds that are present. It even appears to reduce muscle spasms by relaxing muscle fibers. Blue-light devices are available for purchase in the United States. You can find them on the Internet for approximately $100. Blue-light waves are also present in the visible spectrum of solar radiation, which has also been shown to release nitric oxide, thus dilating blood vessels and reducing high blood pressure (see Chapter 11).

SHEDDING LIGHT ON PAINFUL PEPTIC ULCERS

Peptic ulcers are also a common and painful gastrointestinal (GI) condition. Blue light also appears to help to treat painful stomach ulcers thought to be caused by harmful *Helicobacter pylori* bacteria. A study found that shining a blue light *inside* the stomach (with an endoscopic device) for less than 1 hour killed 91% of the bacteria. In one test reported by the National Institutes of Health, some patients reduced their *H. pylori* bacteria by 99%. Light therapy presents a safe treatment option for stomach ulcers, and it does not expose patients to the dangers and GI disruptions of standard antibiotics or contribute to the public health hazard of antibiotic resistance.

SINKING YOUR TEETH INTO LIGHT THERAPY

Dental problems are another very common cause of severe pain too often not addressed by routine medical care or covered by health insurance. Interestingly, dentists use blue light to whiten teeth cosmetically. It also kills the bacteria that cause bad breath and even appears to treat periodontitis. (Periodontitis is a bacterial infection of the gums that can lead to the loss of teeth and bone in the jaw, as well as dangerous brain abscesses that can be fatal.)

Researchers at the Hebrew University and Hadassah School of Dental Medicine in Israel exposed their patients to particular wavelengths of blue light. They discovered that the blue light killed a large percentage of bacteria within seconds.

Full Spectrum of Benefits: Migraine Headache and Premenstrual Syndrome

As mentioned earlier, blue is not the only wavelength of light showing health benefits. Researchers are also finding uses for other parts of the visible and invisible spectrum of sunlight. In one study, researchers at San Diego State University flashed red light into the eyes of people who were in the middle of a serious migraine headache attack. Migraines immediately eased in 93% of the participants, and 72% of the patients said their migraines completely vanished within 1 hour. London's Royal Postgraduate Medical School conducted another migraine headache study using light therapy. They found that photic stimulation (pulsed light shone into closed eyes) shortened migraine attacks in all study participants, and up to 55% reported an increase in the interval before suffering another migraine attack.

At the same institution, researchers found that photic stimulation effectively treated women with PMS. Women reduced their symptoms by 76%, on average. They also felt positive "side effects," such as improved sleep, fewer food cravings, and weight loss.

INFRARED LIGHT FOR STROKE AND EPILEPSY

Other studies explored the benefits of using infrared light. This kind of light is invisible to the naked eye. It also has longer wavelengths than those of visible light. It is still an important part of the spectrum of light emitted from the sun and carries a lot of heat.

Infrared light appears to help stroke victims with their recovery when exposed within 18 hours after suffering a stroke. Researchers believe the red light may reinvigorate brain cells or accelerate the release of protective antioxidants. One study found that infrared light helped 70% of stroke patients.

Finally, a growing body of evidence suggests that light therapy may help people with epilepsy. In the past, many experts believed that flashing red lights would bring on a seizure in someone with epilepsy, but white light appears to help. However, in London, which has a lot of cloudy days, a study found that people suffer fewer seizures on sunny compared to overcast days. Researchers at the University College London are currently planning to use light therapy on epilepsy patients. They plan to shine bright white light emitted by a light box at epilepsy patients for 30 minutes a day for 3 months. This potential epilepsy treatment could one day reduce or eliminate the need for dangerous and debilitating drugs now used for this condition. The foregoing information provides an introductory sampling of the clinical significance and opportunities afforded by energy in light. The detailed science, research, and clinical applications are provided in Chapters 10 and 11.

MICROCURRENT STIMULATION

Microcurrent therapy (MCT) is performed with a US Food and Drug Administration (FDA)-approved neuromuscular stimulator that uses extremely low electrical microcurrent stimulation throughout the body. This type of stimulation has been used in complementary medicine for the treatment of nerve and muscle pain, fracture and delayed healing, inflammation, and other health difficulties. It has been deemed a "novel" treatment in pain reduction specifically (e.g., back pain) (Koopman, Vrinten, & van Wijck, 2009). Each tissue and nerve cell in the body, as discussed in Chapters 1 and 2, has its own electrical frequency. This electrical frequency can change, resulting in, alternatively, negative impacts on the body or increasing overall coherence and balance. MCT restores normal frequencies (intensity in microamps, millionths of an amp) within cells, resulting in remarkable improvements in pain, level of pain perception, inflammation, and overall functionality. This type of therapy has also been found to help with soft-tissue disorders.

McMakin appears to have published more studies on this matter in intervals that seem to explain how this therapy has worked for chronic pain patients. She has completed studies showing improvement in head, neck, and facial pain (e.g., temporomandibular joint disorder [TMJ]), chronic low back pain, and fibromyalgia associated with cervical spine trauma. Most recent studies indicate there was a reduction in inflammatory cytokines, an increase in beta-endorphins, as well as subjective reports of pain relief in fibromyalgia (Mayor & Micozzi, 2012).

In one study, specific-frequency microcurrent treatment of fibromyalgia caused by spine trauma significantly decreased pain. Frequency of microcurrent between 40 Hz and 10 Hz reduced substance P, which belongs to a group called neurokinins and are found throughout the nervous system in relationship to inflammation. MCT reduced pain from an average of 7.3 out of 10 to 1.3 out of 10 in 90 minutes.

ELECTRICAL CELLS

At the cellular level, MCT stimulates a dramatic increase in adenosine triphosphate (ATP), the energy that fuels all biochemical functions in the body. ATP is a nucleotide and the chemical substance that serves as the currency of energy in a cell. ATP is responsible for the major energy currency of the cell, supporting all of the cells activities, which in turn influence the entire body's functions by becoming more balanced. Microcurrent stimulation increases ATP generation by almost 500% and enhances amino acid transport and protein synthesis (Chang et al., 1982). The increase in protein synthesis is necessary for tissue repair. It decreases inflammation, increases blood flow, and improves range of motion.

Microcurrents are exceptionally weak, so people do not feel variable shock sensations when this treatment is applied. This course of treatment usually involves several sessions, and benefits are usually felt after a few sessions. Typically women who are pregnant or people with pacemakers are not recommended to adhere to any such treatment.

THE EARTH AND EARTHING

The Earth creates its own energy as a constant electric potential, and human energies become harmonious, coherent, and balanced when this energy is able to penetrate through the skin and enter the body. The body functions optimally when there is an adequate supply of electrons, which may be easily and naturally obtained by barefoot contact with the Earth. People often report warming or tingling sensations in the legs when "earthing," especially after they have not had barefoot contact with the earth for an extended period of time. These earthing feelings are associated with dilation of blood vessels in the legs and the thinning of the blood, which is a result of standing barefoot, as blood plasma, blood cells, and vascular walls experience an increase in negative electrical charge.

The Earth has a *negative potential,* and any skin contact with the ground (sitting, laying, or being barefoot) enables electron conduction from the Earth into the body. This application is one of the newest "energy" medicines of the 21st century being demonstrated in mainstream science. One of the daily human interactions with the environment is a *capacitive* one, in which the body is able to store an electrical charge. The word *capacitance* in electrical terms extracts its origin from the word *capacity,* meaning here the capacity of that object to hold electrons and, in this light, to store electric charges.

In recent decades, stress-related chronic illness, immune disorders, and inflammatory diseases (as well chronic inflammation that leads to a host of other diseases) have increased dramatically. Biophysical medicine proposes that our increasing disconnection from the Earth is a likely contributing cause. Earthing is an important new natural modality for complementary and alternative medicine, especially because it has inescapably reached scientific review in mainstream academia in 2011.

ANCIENT HISTORY

Insights From Ancient Egypt and Greece

Earthing, by whatever name, and its importance to health have been entertained in various accounts throughout history. In Greek mythology there was a unique tale told between Antaeus and Hercules in Libya. Antaeus was son of Poseidon, God of the sea. Poseidon was considered a massive giant with the capability of superior and unexcelled strength when his bare feet were placed on the ground or the seabed. He always challenged anyone to enter a battle if they came through ancient Libya. Prior to fighting Hercules, who lifted him off the ground to be able to ultimately defeat and conquer him, he had never lost a battle.

The first recorded historical texts for how "beds" specifically raised "off the floor" were in the accounts of the Pharoahs in Egypt. These beds were a sign of wealth and power if designed with gold sheaths. During the Bronze Age (3000–1000 BC), craftsman had constructed beds mainly out of wood with animal shaped "legs" (along with the base for a person to sleep on), which would usually be covered in wool or other soft materials. This design is in line with Tutankhamun's bed that was discovered by archeologists (Partridge, 2011).

19TH–20TH CENTURY

In the late 19th century, in the German "nature cure" and "water cure" hygienic movement, it was stated that there are many health benefits from being barefoot outdoors, especially in cold weather. This hygienic concept also led to the idea that people, by earthing (in contemporary terms) and walking barefoot, would be literally "taking a step towards nature" and that this step would help to conquer chronic disease (Just, 1903). In 1929, George White, a medical doctor, had written many books on natural (the term alternative did not exist then) medicine, such as the importance of light as a cure and the effects of electricity and magnetism on human health. He also investigated the practice of sleeping on the "ground" after being informed by some individuals that they could not sleep properly. These individuals, when either sleeping on the ground or when they slept with copper wires attached to Earth, reported better sleep (Oschman & Rosch, 2015).

In the 1960s, Nobel Prize physicist Richard Feynman described the Earth's subtle energies in his famous *Lectures on Physics*. These subtle energies are blocked when wearing shoes or standing on an insulating surface—and the measurement of energy on such surfaces is reduced significantly. Approximately 350 volts (electrical potential) of electric charge is found between the Earth and just below or to the top of a human head when under insulating conditions. However, when people are barefoot, the 350-volt potential is raised *above* the head significantly, creating an "umbrella effect." The Earth's energy is then able to pass through the body and increasingly surround the body. Skin contact with the Earth creates an unbroken stream of electric charge that creates a protective barrier from the charged energy, which is then pushed out into the surrounding area *around* the head (Applewhite, 2004). Earth's qi, or energy, is absorbed when people do not wear shoes. This might be the reason why more exercises, especially in modern times, have stressed the importance of strengthening the body and relaxing the mind (t'ai chi, yoga, massage, qigong) without any type of footwear.

Footwear dating back 10,000 years has been found by anthropologists. One of the earliest shoes worn by humans—and most likely the most intelligent footwear—is made from leather. Because leather is conductive, leather-soled shoes allow you to be grounded while walking, whereas modern neoprene- or rubber-soled shoes insulate and disconnect you from the earth and inhibit electron transfer. Global health problems have started to make people aware that our disconnection from Earth is one reason to blame.

FREE ELECTRONS: WHAT ARE FREE ELECTRONS, AND HOW ARE THEY ABSORBED?

The natural energy of the Earth and its energy frequencies are abundant with "free electrons." The surface of the planet is electrically conductive, whether wet or dry. There is an abundance of static electricity when there is low humidity, and fewer water molecules to conduct current, so it builds up on surfaces until discharged (Williams & Heckman, 1993).

Electrons have a negative charge. Research has suggested that being disconnected from the Earth by shod feet being blocked (usually by *insulators,* which are materials through which free electrons cannot pass) are causes of physiological dysfunction and unwellness. Insulators include many "human-made" materials, some of these being fabricated of plastic, rubber, glass, and wood. When people walk barefoot on the ground, it has been shown to improve sleep and reduce pain, something that cannot be as readily achieved in an insulating environment (Chevalier, Sinatra, Oschman, Sokal, & Sokal, 2012).

CONDUCTORS, SEMICONDUCTORS, AND INSULATORS

Earthing or grounding benefits can be attained from walking barefoot and laying down outside or by sitting, working, or sleeping indoors connected to *conductive systems* that transfer the Earth's electrons from the ground into the body. Moist grounds, such as wet grass or sand, are excellent conductors and overall greatly enhance the process. *Conductors* were discussed in this light in the book of *Earthing,* released in 2010, and investigated in studies on earthing barefoot, and in-home conductors. In general, conductors help to achieve or create equilibrium in the body with the electric potentiality that stabilizes every level—from the micro to macro level—of the human body. Surfaces that allow for proper grounding and that are conducive include sand, grass, bare dirt, brick, ceramic tile, and usually concrete, such as a basement floor. *Semiconductors* are in-between insulators and conductors, sometimes conducting and other times not conducting (insulators do not conduct, and conductors can easily pick up electricity). Semiconductors prosper in modern electrical equipment because their abilities can be controlled by mainstream applications and thus can turn on and off effortlessly. Natural forms of semiconductors, such as silicone or germanium, are substances in which atoms or molecules are arranged in such a way that they form a pattern. For example, all semiconductors have a crystalline structure. When observed under a microscope, geranium's atoms make a structure and pattern that is strictly uniform and repetitive.

An interesting and unique finding from researchers at HeartMath Institute is that heart electrical coherence (see Chapter 2) actually changed the structure and order of saliva and influenced the information encoded in it. The study found that the overall structure of the *crystalline pattern* in the saliva of participants who had high heart coherence and saliva changed in 18 of the 20 participants. This finding could ultimately mean that positive emotions that affect the heart, such as compassion and love, can ultimately affect and *change* the encoded information in cells and body fluids. These harmonious feelings can be found after earthing and when stress is reduced.

MICROCOSM AND MACROCOSM

Because the Earth's energy has the ability to affect the entire human structure, including the Earth's own structure, we are essentially looking at "microcosm," to "macrocosm" as these ancient words and concepts describe the overall representations seen in nature from the "large scale" to the "small scale." An example of this correspondence is how the Earth is made up of an estimated average of 70% to 75% water, and the human body composition is the same. The Earth would serve as the macrocosm, and the human body would in correspondence be the microcosm. In addition, like the Earth, body and tissue fluids are made up of minerals, such as many different types of electrolytes (salts), and water.

Free electrons pushed into the human body are originally fed by natural events that occur every day, such as solar radiation, "magnetic" energy generated from inside Earth's "magma" core, and electricity. Electricity, in the form of lightning, hits the Earth from the clouds above at various points on the planet at a rate of approximately 100 times per second. This discharge can then change the electrical field of the planet, combined with solar radiation during the day (when diurnal—versus nocturnal—organisms are more productive, therefore cycling more energy), and it all helps to energize the electrical fields within the body.

WHEN LIGHTNING STRIKES

Lightning is probably the most powerful display of electrostatic charge in nature. This "naturalistic" event can also be projected down into the microcosm and seen in electrical interactions and communications between cells, as well as in *microcurrent therapy* (see earlier). The gas molecules that make up the clouds (and also that compose the surrounding air) are turned into a soup of positive ions and free electrons. The insulating air is transformed into conductive **plasma (electrically conductive and affected by magnetic fields)**. The ability of a storm cloud's electric fields to transform air into a conductor makes charge transfer (in the form of a lightning bolt) from the cloud to the ground (or even to other clouds). When lightning strikes the Earth, lightning in the immediate vicinity is "cleaning" the air by creating additional oxidants (like bleaching), and it is very hot. The heat it generates in the surrounding air is instantaneously five times hotter than the sun. Because of the high heat intensity, it causes the air exposed to this heat to rapidly expand and *vibrate* with kinetic energy, which then forms *sound waves*—the reason there is thunder after lightning strikes.

CELLULAR REACTIONS

Earthing has also been shown to have a blood-thinning effect, contributing to easier flow in capillaries and overall improved circulation within the body. In general, cells regulate and communicate through electrical currents by releasing and receiving energy. Cells perform specific biochemical reactions that are constantly adjusting and shifting to maintain an overall state of flow or balance in the human system. Any living being or creature we can see and touch consists of many cells and groups of cells. Each of these cells or groups of cells are aligned with the organism's overall "energetic microbiome" to perform particular functions. The heart, brain, nervous system, muscles, immune system, and bones are communicating and functioning in part because of electrical systems operating bioelectrically in the body, all made up of cells and components of cells.

The cells that make up the human body include mobile cells in the blood circulation that are not anchored but literally *circulate*, such as red and white blood cells. In addition, there are human parenchymal tissue, muscle, cartilage, and mucosal cells. Groups of cells similar in size, shape, and function make up tissues; thus, nerve cells working together form nerve tissue.

Cells in the blood have also a wide variety of benefits, and proper circulation of blood *plasma* transports nutrients, proteins, and hormones throughout the body. Blood plasma has been discovered to contain both properties of a solid and a liquid, as found by researchers at Saarland University in Saarbrücken, Germany, and additional experiments at the University of Pennsylvania. When isolated, blood plasma makes up 55% of the blood in the body and is yellow in its appearance. Plasma also contains salts (electrolytes) and enzymes (proteins), creating electrical communications within cells and also creating a synchronous chain of communication among other cells. Note: *Salts (electrolytes) can help cells to use electricity. Cells contain sodium and potassium ions. Sodium and potassium ions in cells help to create voltage differences and affect how the cells perform and communicate. The voltage inside cells has a slightly negative charge and effects electrical potential.*

For decades researchers had assumed that blood plasma flows like water because blood is made up of 92% water. Researchers at Saarland University, Germany, and at the University of Pennsylvania have discovered unique abilities of blood plasma and have deemed it a "non-Newtonian fluid" because its behavior is unlike water mechanistically or hydrologically. Blood has been shown to flow differently than water, and these fluids have flow properties that change depending on environmental conditions, with some becoming more viscous and others becoming less viscous. For example, blood is a "thinning fluid" that becomes less viscous with increasing pressure and more viscous with less pressure. This amazing property allows blood to flow into and through the narrowest of capillaries in the human body. According to these findings, the complex flow behavior of blood plasma plays a crucial role with respect to vascular wall deposits, aneurysms, and blood clots. The results of this research may well help to improve computer simulations of this kind of pathological process. It also appears that through earthing, these effects help to speed the process of overall blood thinning, as well as preventing cardiovascular disease.

TRANSDIFFERENTIATION IN CELLS

Science also now understands that under certain circumstances in nature, one cell can potentially redifferentiate to become a completely different cell, such as a nerve cell becoming a muscle cell. This process is called "transdifferentiation", when mature cells that have already been ontogenetically assigned a function become *different* cells. This discovery in recent years is associated with the *Turritopsis dohrnii*, which is biologically rendered to be an "immortal" jellyfish. It has the capability, when injured or under some kind of stress, to return to an earlier and younger state because of its ability to communicate with its own cells and instruct itself to regenerate, transdifferentiate, and heal.

PAIN AND INFLAMMATION

Research indicates that electrons from the Earth have antioxidant effects that can protect your body from pain and inflammation, which has many documented health consequences.

Scientific studies have concluded that inflammation (including reduced pain, decreased stress, better sleep, a shift from sympathetic to parasympathetic tone in the autonomic nervous system [ANS], and a blood-thinning effect) is reduced significantly when earthing (Ghaly & Teplitz, 2004). In addition, being grounded reduces inflammation and pain by thinning the blood—reducing blood viscosity—with ultimately a large effect on reversing symptoms that could turn into cardiovascular disease (Chevalier, Sinatra, Oschman, & Delany, 2013).

In the late 1990s, one of the authors (Micozzi) proposed that cortisol might also be considered an aging hormone (Seaton & Micozzi, 1998). Cortisol also reduces inflammation. In small amounts, it is normal; however, prolonged cortisol excretion is correlated with issues of sleep, pain, stress, anxiety, and aging (Chevalier et al., 2012; Seaton & Micozzi, 1998). In one study, participants who complained of sleep dysfunction, pain, and stress were grounded to Earth during sleep in their own beds using a conductive mattress pad for 8 weeks (Ghaly & Teplitz, 2004).

The number of inflammation studies performed from 1967 to 2012 has grown significantly. The number of inflammation studies in 1967 were recorded at 5000, and in 2012, studies had grown to almost 30,000 (Oschman, Chevalier, & Brown, 2015). There are scientific studies showing that inflammation is a contributory cause of more than 80 chronic diseases, including cancer (Khansari, Shakiba, & Mahmoudi, 2009; Ober, Sinatra, & Zucker, 2010a). Inflammation can also be caused by chronic psychological, emotional, or physical—such as *negative thoughts* (see the "Thought Field Therapy" section). Lack of sleep, poor nutrition, and consumption of junk foods also may impact inflammation. Many studies have shown that spending time out in nature can actually combat some of these harmful effects that promote inflammation (Gladwell, Brown, Wood, Sandercock, & Barton, 2013). Inflammation has also been costly; the US economy has spent over $1 trillion annually on managing the most severe inflammatory conditions.

Indeed, it has been believed over the past 40 years until recently that cholesterol was responsible for cardiovascular health and the cause of heart disease. This distorted the public perception of "good" cholesterol intake and healthy foods, such as butter, eggs, meat, and shellfish. Other foods, such as coconut oil, a saturated fat, and organic butter, such as ghee, have the ability to regulate "good" cholesterol potentially through effects on inflammation.

Inflammation thrives when blood is thicker and when there are resulting increases in free radical stress. One of the functions of the immune system is to release chemicals to combat foreign cells, some of which destroy invading cells by free radical oxidation. In chronic inflammation, an imbalanced, overactive immune system can release a constant cascade of toxic chemicals and free radicals that are harmful to normal cells.

Recent observers have categorized earthing as an excellent "antioxidant" for combating free radicals. Free radicals can exist independently from cells. There are harmful free radicals that are present in one's body usually as a result of pollution, pesticides, and radiation, as well as being by-products of immune cells and cellular metabolism. Free radicals can eventually lead to mutation and DNA damage, thereby being theorized as a strong factor in cancer and age-related diseases in humans (Khansari et al., 2009). The cellular damage that results from free radicals, due to *oxidative stress,* can cause decreases in energy level and slow performance. Effects on the central nervous system are thought to ultimately lead to cognitive and emotional problems. Natural products are abundant in antioxidants because all plants are exposed to the atmosphere and protect themselves against oxidizing effects of cosmic and solar radiation. For example, according to one study on blueberry supplementation, antioxidants in foods can increase your memory and improve overall cognitive function (Krikorian et al., 2011; see Section V).

WOUND HEALING, REPAIR, AND RECOVERY

A study of American cycling teams at the Tour de France showed that participants in these races usually experienced slow wound healing from accidents during the race. A study was conducted in which they would ground to earth after the cycling competitions. They reported less illness, better sleep, increased speed of wound healing, and dramatic recovery from the day's race (Ober, Sinatra & Zucker, 2010b).

BONE AND MUSCLE PAIN, ARTHRITIS, AND AUTOIMMUNE CONDITIONS

A study conducted in 2015 found that delayed onset of muscle soreness could be used to monitor the immune response of patients who were grounding versus not grounding. Patients who grounded had significantly reduced pain. This study also found that grounding participants altered the number of circulating neutrophils and lymphocytes and affected other chemicals within the body related to inflammation (Oschman et al., 2015).

Ober, et al. (2010a) and Sokal & Sokal (2011) indicated that regular earthing may improve blood pressure and cardiovascular arrhythmias, as well as autoimmune conditions, such as lupus, multiple sclerosis, and rheumatoid arthritis. Earthing also influenced many related physiological processes, such as affecting the serum concentrations of iron and increasing thyroid-stimulating hormone.

In a blind pilot study, Ober recruited 60 subjects (22 males and 28 females) who for at least 6 months had suffered from self-described sleep disturbances and chronic muscle and joint pains (Ober et al., 2010). Participants were randomly divided for the month-long study in which both groups slept on conductive mattress pads. Half the pads were connected to a specific part of the Earth (ground outside each subject's bedroom window), whereas the other half were not connected to the Earth. Most grounded subjects described symptomatic improvement, whereas most in the control group did not. Some subjects reported significant relief from asthmatic and respiratory conditions, rheumatoid arthritis, PMS, sleep apnea, and hypertension while sleeping *grounded*.

BRAIN AND NERVOUS SYSTEM

A study conducted by Chevalier and Mori (2007) at the California Institute of Human Science found that earthing has an extraordinary impact on the brain and nervous system. Fifty-eight healthy adults underwent brain and muscle measurements during grounding and nongrounding individual sessions. The experiment was a double-blind, controlled, randomized research study, so the researchers and the participants did not know which group was assigned to real versus "sham" grounding (the sham group that was not grounding were still attached to a "placebo" conducive wire that was detached from the ground outside), and randomly set up by different groups. The researchers did not learn who was in the grounding versus the nongrounding group until the study was completed.

Each person was placed under electroencephalography (EEG), used to measure electrical activity of the brain, and electromyography (EMG), used to measure electrical voltage of muscle cells and skeletal muscles. Chevalier and Mori (2007) found that grounding significantly impacted the electrical activity of the brain and of the muscles within *2 seconds* of earthing. Earthing appeared to have a major relaxing effect in the brain because there was a dramatic decrease in overall activity, seen especially on the left side of the brain. In addition, participants who had muscle tension were found to have significantly decreased tension. Lastly, the grounded participants were the only group to have very slow brain wave oscillations, which prior to this study had not been seen before. Slow oscillations (slow waves) have been found to affect brain cell activity during sleep and increase memory consolidation (Mölle, Marshall, Gais, & Born, 2002; Mölle & Born, 2011).

The results of studies on earthing indicate that the clinical potential of barefoot and skin contact with the earth's ground is systematic. Ongoing research suggests the Earth's remarkable benefits may contribute beyond general pain reduction, anti-inflammatory properties, and physiological balance.

EARTH AND BODY MERIDIANS OR CHANNELS
MERIDIAN POINT THERAPIES
Acupressure
Acupressure has sometimes been referred to as "acupuncture without needles." Numerous studies have demonstrated the effectiveness of acupuncture for pain, a sophisticated healing system that has been in use for 2000 years (see Chapter 15). Now there is mounting evidence supporting the efficacy of energy psychology using the meridian points, or channels, of acupuncture and acupressure to help to increase the overall coherence and flow of energy in the body.

Acupressure involves manipulating energy "points" in channels on the body by physical stimulation and is one of many Asian bodywork therapies (ABTs) that have roots in the traditional medicine of China. This practice is very much related to acupuncture and most likely was practiced even prior to the ancient discovery of placing needles on different meridian points on the body. Studies have shown that the needle placement can vary and benefits still accrue. The following energy techniques combine ancient Chinese acupressure and modern psychology.

Acupoints or meridian points are used to distinguish the location of needles in acupuncture and acupressure. In acupressure, the physical pressure can be placed by hands, elbows, knuckles, fingers, and other body parts to apply pressure to a specific area(s). This pressure, in essence, relieves the body of energy blockages and increases the natural, harmonic flow of energy within the body.

ACUPOINTS AND THE BRAIN

Research at Harvard University in 2013 has shown that stimulation of selected meridian acupoints decreases activity in the limbic system of the brain, such as the amygdala and hippocampus, and various parts of the brain associated with the emotion of fear (Claunch et al., 2013). Researchers also observed differences in the spatial distribution and degree of deactivation in the medial prefrontal cortex, medial parietal cortex, and medial temporal lobe in direct response to three specific acupoints. This observation suggests that acupoint stimulation can elicit specific brain responses that directly affect neural activity in relation to proposed neurological functions, such as emotional response and decision making, declarative memory (long-term memory, such as remembering events and facts), and attention (Baumann & Mattingley, 2010; Behrmann, Geng, & Shomstein, 2004; Squire, Stark, & Clark, 2004). Detailed discussions on ethnomedical and scientific background and clinical research and applications are provided in Section IV.

ENERGY PSYCHOLOGY

ENERGY BLOCKAGES AND PAIN

Energy flows through meridians or channels in the body much the same way blood flows through the blood vessels. When a person receives a physical injury or emotional shock, a blockage occurs in the meridian system and disruption in energy flow results. Negative emotions are not created by the event itself; they are created by the disruption in the energy system that occurs as a result of the event. The negative emotion can then be re-experienced whenever that event comes back to mind. If the blockage is not removed or rebalanced, it can result in causing anything from depression, stress, and other emotional problems, to physical problems, such as muscle tension, pain, or even in some cases contribute to cancer or heart disease.

By releasing emotional blockages, negative emotions and undesired responses can be rebalanced for the overall coherence of the body and how it communicates energetically and physically. Cognitively these issues may still reside in memory but do not have the intense emotional responses, for example, which can be seen in patients with posttraumatic stress disorder (PTSD) because they are essentially re-experiencing the event emotionally and mentally as if it were happening again at that moment of remembrance.

EMOTIONAL FREEDOM TECHNIQUES

Emotional Freedom Techniques (EFTs), known as a branch of energy psychology, is a psychological counseling intervention that draws on various theories of medicine, including acupuncture, neurolinguistic programming, and energy medicine. EFT also branches into other areas of similar approaches, including *Meridian Tapping Techniques (MTTs), Thought Field Therapy (TFT),* and *Energy Tapping,* which use related techniques as a means of simplified integration for self-help therapies. These names can be considered "umbrella terms."

For the purposes of this discussion, EFT appears to be the origin of most modernized "tapping" techniques. EFT has distinguished itself to reduce emotional trauma and pain using combined approaches (such as exposure, cognitive restructuring, waking hypnosis, and physical relaxation) while tapping gently on a sequence of pressure points, intentionally working on a specific area of emotional discomfort or pain, and repeating specific phrases out loud. The mechanism of action used in these sequences is unknown. However, researchers have suggested that physical stimulation of certain pressure points during exposure, or re-exposure, to an emotional trauma may send deactivating signals directly to the amygdala, or the "fear center" of the brain, resulting in rapid reduction of maladaptive fear. Maladaptive fear may include expected or unrealistic fears that affect and determine outcomes that may not be satisfactory or in alignment with one's true intentions or motives. This situation results when the person is making decisions that are more associated with a specific fear, ultimately creating a dysfunctional participation with their present surroundings.

Maladaptive fear may also inhibit someone from making appropriate decisions that then lead to less opportune responses because they are still anticipating danger (see the "Thought Field Therapy" section). Maladaptive fear affects physiological processes and cognitive functions in parts of the brain associated with "goal-oriented" behaviors. In contrast, tapping therapy enables and influences positive, change-driven, and goal-oriented psychological events. It is considered a psychological therapy because it can help to release fear and anxiety in a person's "emotional" psyche and may release limitations associated with one's beliefs or fears from the past.

Tapping therapy works with the body's energy system and is simply the *tapping* of your own acupuncture points with your fingers and can be accomplished on the face and on various points on the body. Tapping releases the "toxic" energy buildup of negative emotions, stress, unprocessed feelings, and similar energetic blocks that can eventually lead to unwanted physical pain. EFTs have also been shown to successfully remove negative emotions, such as fear, and reduce or eliminate pain and perceived pain severity. In addition, improvements in psychological awareness have been noted to help one implement and achieve positive goals.

Studies of Energy Psychology

An American psychotherapist, Roger Callahan, discovered and named for himself Callahan Techniques as the first to help to establish energy psychology over the past 4 decades. In 1979, he realized this energetic phenomenon during one of his psychology sessions with a client who had a water phobia since she was a child and was now past the age of 40. Dr. Callahan had been treating his client for more than a year using various psychotherapy techniques, such as cognitive therapy, hypnosis, relaxation therapy, rational emotive therapy, systematic desensitization, and biofeedback. Callahan had been interested in meridian points and the location of these energy points in the human body. During a particular session, his client was experiencing her fear of water and complained that she felt very sick to her stomach—and in that moment—Callahan asked her to tap a point under the eye, which is on the stomach meridian. In just a moment to remember, a few seconds of tapping achieved an end to his client's lifelong phobia, leaving her permanently free of it.

Callahan began extensive research into emotions and their links to specific meridian points. He developed TFT as a self-practice of releasing specific emotions by stimulating a combination of meridian points.

In 1995, Gary Craig, one of Callahan's students, evolved this energy psychology as an easy, systematic way of using Callahan's principles and called it "EFT". EFT involves muscle testing for weakness (somewhat akin to applied kinesiology), using a specific sequence of meridians. EFT was also considered "self-help" because people could administer it on themselves. In the 1990s, the clinical psychologist Fred Gallo coined the term "energy psychology" to describe all of these techniques, including Callahan's and Craig's techniques collectively.

Thought Field Therapy

TFT (originally associated with the Callahan Techniques) is different from other healing modalities for pain in mainstream medicine and contributed to forming EFT. By tapping precisely (however long you want or need to for reduced pain) on specific points on the body, there is an experience of relief of pain symptoms. These points include locations below the eyes, collar bone, index finger, and adjacent to the outside of the eyes. Similar to acupuncture or acupressure, TFT uses a meridian system. This treatment seems to be one of the least expensive, least intrusive, and most helpful energy medicine modalities, likewise for the newer EFT modality. EFTs are derived from TFT. We next will touch upon how individual thoughts can affect the experience of pain.

THOUGHTS AS ENERGY

New brain imaging techniques demonstrate how the occurrence of mental thoughts may be construed as specific measurements of energy during the creation of the thought. Mental thought then exhibits physical movements and behaviors and instructs the central nervous system—which is partially automated through reflex—to perform, regulate, and communicate by means of electrical energy.

In thermodynamic terms, a thought can convert the potential energy of an idea or thought to the kinetic energy of movement directed to fulfill the thought-idea harnessed to physiological responses in the neural, endocrine, and immune systems.

TFT helps to put words and thoughts into more appropriate actions and responses by unblocking conditioned personal beliefs in aspects of life, such as success, relationships, and connections with the "inner self." This treatment also alleviates overall pain perception. This new perception of pain can be freeing and used as a life skill for processing future emotional disturbances and balancing belief patterns. Negative thoughts automatically induce an effect of "limitation" and "limiting beliefs." Assessing the root of the energy-related problem, whether it is physical or emotional, unblocks the energy to return to a more natural flow in the body.

Some examples of emotional stressors (that are "bottled up" or "stuck" energy) include negative emotions, phobias, anger, guilt, grief, trauma, addictions, depression, and PTSD. These emotional "feelings" can affect performance at work and overall success in life, such as wealth, sports, and relationships. In the deepest form of conscious abilities, beliefs have an effect on thoughts and thus actions. For example, when under negative influences, individuals may not seem like their "true selves" because they are under a certain amount of pain and overall "energy" becomes easily depleted, making it more difficult to extend and apply cognitive abilities.

Chronic pain is one such prevalent problem in the United States. TFT has caught the attention of physicians when diagnosing and treating patients. One who has achieved very successful results is Dr. Robert Pasahow. Dr. Pasahow has conducted numerous studies with patients who suffer from chronic pain, and he and his patients have found a reduction in pain using TFT. In a study conducted in 2009 using only TFT, there was a major reduction in chronic pain and tinnitus (Pasahow, 2009). Dr. Pasahow has also completed studies with patients who have undergone intensive surgery, such as cervical and lumbar surgery; herniated, bulging and ruptured discs; spinal stenosis; carpal tunnel syndrome; radiculopathy; pinched nerves; and muscular strain and sprain syndromes. There has been a reduction of pain in patients after a short period time using TFT. Patients treated in an outpatient psychology private practice were seen to reduce musculoskeletal, nerve, and spinal pain in 10 of 12 cases (Pasahow, 2009).

Negative thoughts may have a negative effect on the body, as now scientifically demonstrated. A new, groundbreaking anatomical discovery made in 2015 by researchers at the University of Virginia School of Medicine (Louveau, Smirnov, Keyes, et al., 2015) has demonstrated that the brain is directly connected to the immune system by vessels previously thought not to exist. These previously unknown vessels are a part of the larger lymphatic system that had been keenly mapped out in every textbook over previous decades.

This research opens the door to discovering new treatments for many neurological disorders, including autism and Alzheimer's disease, dementia, multiple sclerosis, and Parkinson's disease. This discovery will change how researchers, scientists, and doctors fundamentally look at the central nervous system's anatomical connections and relations to the immune system.

Positive and motivationally driven thoughts can also have an impact on the immune system and the overall function of the body. For example, as seen with studies conducted at the HeartMath Institute on thoughts and feelings, the brain is connected to the immune system through energetic, hormonal, and neural processes. Now new studies in basic anatomy have shown the physical connection. The immune system is directly vulnerable to positive and negative thoughts that can inhibit or promote overall immune function.

Applying Thought Field Therapy

TFT sessions are similar to psychological interventions because they are solely based on the assessment of individuals, their levels of pain, and their emotional readiness for change. There are additional factors, such as complexity, intensity, and duration of the related symptoms and problems associated with life events. TFT is readily and easily available to anyone and can be learned by non–mental health practitioners and new graduate students. Health professionals have previously learned basic TFT methods in 2-day workshops, and patients have been able to learn in the comfort from their homes, using self-assessment tools with a combination of text, pictures, and videos. There are possible approaches by other practitioners, such as audiologists, who can provide these treatments, with only initial moderate supervision by TFT clinicians.

HEALING WITH THE HANDS, "QIGONG," AND T'AI CHI

Qigong (chi kung) is composed of two Chinese words. Qi is pronounced "chee" and is usually translated to mean the life force or vital energy that flows through all things in the universe. The second word, gong, pronounced "gung," means accomplishment or skill that is cultivated through steady practice. Together, qigong (chi kung) means cultivating energy with distinct intentions. Energy healing by qigong experts reveals that by using pure intention while administering energy with the hands can very well be accomplished (see Chapter 16).

What does hand healing feel like when it is being administered by a practitioner, as in reiki or qigong? Franz Anton Mesmer, an 18th-century doctor from Vienna, used "animal magnetism" by passages of his hands as early as 1773 to heal people suffering from various ailments ("mesmerism"). Mesmer went on to publish *Memoir on the Discovery of Animal Magnetism* when he discovered that similar energies in the body's electromagnetic field could be processed through the hands and described these feelings around the body as the influences of two magnets. *Mesmerism* led to a distinguished line of "magnetic healers" during the 19th century, which includes the founders of both osteopathic medicine and chiropractic medicine. In the early 20th century, mesmerism became formally known as the practice of "hypnotism," with many established medical and psychological therapeutic uses in the present day (see Section II).

Patients who practice qiqong mixed with t'ai chi found reduced levels of pain, stress, anxiety, depression, sleep quality, and therefore the techniques promoted relaxation, improved immune response and blood pressure, and a positive increased impact on quality of life (Abbott & Lavretsky, 2013; Martinez et al., 2015; Vincent, Hill, Kruk, Cha, & Bauer, 2010; Wang et al., 2010). Patients who underwent qigong treatment in a substance abuse group (narcotic addicts) were reported to have fewer withdrawal symptoms than the control group (Li, Chin & Mo, 2002).

When patients with Parkinson's disease mixed qigong and t'ai chi treatments, they had a reduction of overall balance impairments, improved functional capacity, slower function decline, and reduction in the number of falls (Abbott et al., 2013).

Patients who had experienced traumatic brain injury had a positive increase in mood and self-esteem, as well as reduced anxiety compared with an exercise control group (Blake & Batson, 2009).

T'ai chi and qiqong are relatively safe treatments that are low-to-moderate intensity. Researchers have found an overall increase in blood levels of endorphins and baroreflex sensitivity and reduced levels of inflammatory markers, such as adrenocorticotropic hormone and cortisol (Lavretsky et al., 2011; Ryu et al., 1996; Sato, Makita, Uchida, Ishihara, & Masuda, 2010).

QIGONG ENERGY AND CELLS

Studies have been performed on cell cultures and a qigong expert's ability to protect or grow brain cells and other types of cells under laboratory conditions. Specialists concur that biofield-energetic therapies can be difficult to measure with cultured cells because they are highly variable and are affected easily. In addition, the overall environments of the laboratories supplying valid cells depend on the expert's immediate ability to induce healing energy and the ability to focus. Researchers from the University of Oklahoma (working with an international group of like-minded researchers from various universities, including Harvard Medical School) found that qigong was a strong protective force against cell death caused by oxidative stress (Yan et al., 2004).

Qigong also has the ability to deeply affect cells, whether it is their own survival and death, and alter gene expression. A study conducted with small-cell lung cancer found cancer cells died and inhibited proliferation in others (Yan et al., 2012).

These findings suggest that qigong treatment may have anticancer effects through modulating gene expression in a way that facilitates cancer cell apoptosis while repressing proliferation, metastasis, and glucose metabolism (Yan et al., 2012). Qigong promotes the death of cancer cells and reduces *metastasis*, and thus rids energy that does not suit the organism or body any longer. Additional basic science and clinical research and applications are provided in Section III.

REFERENCES

Abbott, R. & Lavretsky, H. (2013). Tai chi and qigong for the treatment and prevention of mental disorders. *Psychiatr Clin North Am, 36*(1), 109–119.

Applewhite, R. (2004). The effectiveness of a conductive patch and a conductive bed pad in reducing induced human body voltage via the application of earth ground. *European Biology and Bioelectromagnetics, 1*, 23–40.

Baumann, O. & Mattingley, J. B. (2010). Medial parietal cortex encodes perceived heading direction in humans. *The Journal of Neuroscience, 30*(39), 12897–12901. http://www.jneurosci.org/content/30/39/12897.full.

Behrmann, M., Geng, J. J., & Shomstein, S. (2004). Parietal cortex and attention. *Current Opinion in Neurobiology, 14*, 212–217. http://home.gwu.edu/~shom/ACL/pubs/ParietalCON.pdf.

Blake, H. & Batson, M. (2009). Exercise intervention in brain injury: A pilot randomized study of Tai Chi Qigong. *Clinical Rehabilitation, 23*(7), 589–598. http://www.ncbi.nlm.nih.gov/pubmed/19237436.

Chang, N., Van Hoff, H., Bockx, E., Hoogmartens, M. J., Mulier, J. C., De Dijcker, F. J., et al. (1982). The effect of electric currents on ATP generation, protein synthesis, and membrane transport in rat skin. *Clinical Orthopaedics and Related Research, 171*, 264–272.

Chevalier, G. & Mori, K. (2007). The effect of earthing on human physiology. *Subtle Energies Energy Med, 18*(3), 11–34.

Chevalier, G., Sinatra, S. T., Oschman, J. L., Sokal, K., & Sokal, P. (2012). Earthing: Health implications of reconnecting the human body to the earth's surface electrons. *Journal of Environmental Public Health, 2012*, 291541. http://www.ncbi.nlm.nih.gov/pmc/articles/PMC3265077/.

Chevalier, G., Sinatra, S. T., Oschman, J. L., & Delany, R. M. (2013). Earthing (Grounding) the human body reduces blood viscosity—A major factor in cardiovascular disease. *Journal of Alternative and Complementary Medicine, 19*(2), 102–110. http://www.ncbi.nlm.nih.gov/pmc/articles/PMC3576907/.

Claunch, J., Chan, S. T., Nixon, E. E., Qiu, W. Q., Sporko, T., Dunn, J. P., et al. (2013). Commonality and specificity of acupuncture action at three acupoints as evidenced by fMRI. *American Journal of Chinese Medicine, 40*(4), 695–712. http://www.ncbi.nlm.nih.gov/pmc/articles/PMC3754829/.

Ghaly, M. & Teplitz, D. (2004). The biologic effects of grounding the human body during sleep as measured by cortisol levels and subjective reporting of sleep, pain, and stress. *Journal of Alternative and Complementary Medicine, 10*(5), 767–776. http://www.ncbi.nlm.nih.gov/pubmed/15650465.

Just, A. (1903). *Return to nature!.* http://www.soilandhealth.org/02/0201hyglibcat/020162.just.pdf.

Koopman, J. S., Vrinten, D. H., & van Wijck, A. J. (2009). Efficacy of microcurrent therapy in the treatment of chronic nonspecific back pain: A pilot study. *Clinical Journal of Pain, 25*(6), 495–499. http://www.ncbi.nlm.nih.gov/pubmed/19542797.

Krikorian, R., Shidler, M. D., Nash, T. A., Kalt, W., Vinqvist-Tymchuk, M. R., Shukitt-Hale, B., et al. (2011). Blueberry supplementation improves memory in older adults. *Journal of Agricultural and Food Chemistry, 58*(7), 3996–4000. http://www.ncbi.nlm.nih.gov/pmc/articles/PMC2850944/.

Lavretsky, H., Alstein, L. L., Olmstead, R. E., Ercoli, L. M., Riparetti-Brown, M., Cyr, N. S., et al. (2011). Complementary use of tai chi chih augments escitalopram treatment of geriatric depression: A randomized controlled trial. *The American Journal of Geriatric Psychiatry, 19*(10), 839–850.

Li, M., Chen, K., & Mo, Z. (2002). Use of qigong therapy in the detoxification of heroin addicts. *Alternative Therapies in Health and Medicine, 8*(1), 50–54. http://www.ncbi.nlm.nih.gov/pubmed/11795622.

Louveau, A., Smirnov, I., Keyes, T. J., et al. (2015). Structural and functional features of central nervous system lymphatic vessels. *Nature, 523*(7560), 337–341.

Martinez, N., Martorell, C., Espinosa, L., Marasigan, V., Domènech, S., & Inzitari, M. (2015). Impact of Qigong on quality of life, pain and depressive symptoms in older adults admitted to an intermediate care rehabilitation unit: A randomized controlled trial. *Aging Clinical and Experimental Research, 27*(2), 125–130. http://www.ncbi.nlm.nih.gov/pubmed/24927783.

Mölle, M. & Born, J. (2011). Slow oscillations orchestrating fast oscillations and memory consolidation. *Programmed Brain Research, 193*, 93–110. http://www.ncbi.nlm.nih.gov/pubmed/21854958.

Mölle, M., Marshall, L., Gais, S., & Born, J. (2002). Grouping of spindle activity during slow oscillations in human non-rapid eye movement sleep. *The Journal of Neuroscience, 22*(24), 10941–10947. http://www.jneurosci.org/content/22/24/10941.full.pdf.

Ober, C., Sinatra, S. T., & Zucker, M. (2010a). *Earthing: The most important health discovery ever?* (pp. 6–63). Laguna Beach, CA: Basic Health Publications.

Ober, C., Sinatra, S. T., & Zucker, M. (2010b). *Earthing: The most important health discovery ever?* (pp. 172–199). Laguna Beach, CA: Basic Health Publications.

Oschman, J. & Rosch, P. J. (Eds.), (2015). *Bioelectromagnetic and subtle energy medicine* (2nd ed., p. 429). New York: CRC Press. Chapter 38.

Oschman, J. L., Chevalier, G., & Brown, R. (2015). The effects of grounding (earthing) on inflammation, the immune response, wound healing, and prevention and treatment of chronic inflammatory and autoimmune diseases. *Journal of Inflammatory Research, 8,* 83–96.

Partridge, R. (2011). *Treasures of Tutankhamun gallery.* http://www.bbc.co.uk/history/ancient/egyptians/ tutankhamun_gallery_03.shtml.

Pasahow, R. (2009). Energy psychology and thought field therapy in the treatment of tinnitus. *International Tinnitus Journal, 15*(2), 130–133. http://www.tinnitusjournal.com/imagebank/pdf/ v15n2a05.pdf.

Ryu, H., Lee, H. S., Shin, Y. S., Chung, S. M., Lee, M. S., Kim, H. M., et al. (1996). Acute effect of qigong training on stress hormonal levels in man. *American Journal of Chinese Medicine, 24*(8874677), 193–198.

Sato, S., Makita, S., Uchida, R., Ishihara, S., & Masuda, M. (2010). Effect of Tai Chi training on barore-flex sensitivity and heart rate variability in patients with coronary heart disease. *International Heart Journal, 51*(4), 238–241.

Seaton, K. E. & Micozzi, M. S. (1998). Is cortisol the aging hormone? *Journal of Advancement in Medicine, 11*(2), 73–94.

Sokal, K. & Sokal, P. (2011). Earthing the human body influences physiologic processes. *Journal of Alternative and Complementary Medicine, 17*(4), 301–308. http://www.ncbi.nlm.nih.gov/ pubmed/21469913/.

Squire, L. R., Stark, C. E., & Clark, R. E. (2004). The medial temporal lobe. *Annual Review Neuroscience, 27,* 279–306. http://www.ncbi.nlm.nih.gov/pubmed/15217334.

Vincent, A., Hill, J., Kruk, K. M., Cha, S. S., & Bauer, B. A. (2010). External qigong for chronic pain. *American Journal of Chinese Medicine, 38*(4), 695–703. http://www.ncbi.nlm.nih.gov/pubmed/20626055.

Williams, E. & Heckman, S. (1993). The local diurnal variation of cloud electrification and the global di-urnal variation of negative charge on the Earth. *Journal of Geophysical Research, 98,* 5221–5234. http:// onlinelibrary.wiley.com/doi/10.1029/92JD02642/abstract.

Yan, X., Li, F., Dozmorov, I., Frank, M. B., Dao, M., Centola, M., et al. (2012). External Qi of Yan Xin Qigong induces cell death and gene expression alterations promoting apoptosis and inhibiting proliferation, migration and glucose metabolism in small-cell lung cancer cells. *Molecular Cellular Biochemistry, 363*(1–2), 245–255. http://www.ncbi.nlm.nih.gov/pmc/articles/PMC3567610/.

Yan, X., Shen, H., Zaharia, M., Wang, J., Wolf, D., Li, F., et al. (2004). Involvement of phosphatidylinosi-tol 3-kinase and insulin-like growth factor-I in YXLST-mediated neuroprotection. *Brain Research, 1006*(2), 198–206. http://www.ncbi.nlm.nih.gov/pubmed/15051523.

Suggested Readings can be found on the companion website, http://www.micozzipainconditions.com.

Chapter 4

Brain Biology and Neuroscience

The brain is a fascinating system of neural networks composed of precise chemical and electrical reactions that influence neural firings to make consciousness possible, at least at one level. Scientists are still struggling to understand the brain's abilities to change itself over time (plasticity), heal, and experience "consciousness" itself. Consciousness is considered to be awareness of external and internal stimuli and the ability to experience and feel while maintaining executive functions and control over the mind. Consciousness includes the ability to hone in on intuitive energetic processes. Every occurrence of thought, prevention of certain negative thoughts, initiation of thought, and the intention of the thought can be observed. Observation of thought can be practiced, thereby increasing one's authority and oversight over thoughts, sensations, and feelings.

One practical method of being observant of thoughts is through mindfulness and meditation (see Chapter 5). Mindfulness is that state of being situated in the present moment during daily tasks and all moments throughout the day. Mindfulness and meditation are powerful neurological enhancers that are actually able to increase the amount of gray matter in the brain. The brain is made up mostly of white matter—which consists of axons connecting different parts of gray matter to each other. Gray matter is more complex than white matter and contains cell bodies, dendrites, and axon terminals of neurons that perform chemical and electrical synapses, which are essentially "communications" with other neurons. Every time an electrical impulse, or action potential, goes down the axon of a neuron, a tiny electric field surrounds that cell. Gray matter consists of mostly unmyelinated axons and glial cells that transport nutrients and energy to the cells and neurons. Glial cells may influence neuronal intelligence by enhancing overall function and communication. Most myelinated (or white fatty, proteinated) axons are found in white matter, where it serves as insulation, improving transmission of neuronal signals. Gray matter processes information in an advanced and analytical manner, whereas white matter coordinates communications.

The mind is also in control of most of automatic life activities through the autonomic nervous system. This system does not require conscious thought to control functions such as breathing, heartbeat, and digestion and to influence the millions of functions cells undergo every second. However, mental states do affect heartbeat rhythm, and that in turn affects the body and brain as a whole. This process occurs in somewhat of a cycle until the mind can exercise awareness of specific mental states (stress, negative emotions) causing the onset of irregular or unstable heartbeats and elicit an appropriate breathing technique or shift in mindset. Perhaps the ability to have the perfect "automation" for emotional and mental intelligence in pain perception and management would change civilization as we know it. Conscious coping strategies and regulation of specific genes that may enhance pain and contribute to the offset of physical or emotional pain would greatly influence how we treat and monitor individuals who suffer from pain. Emotional intelligence programs placed in some school systems are yet to be brought into mainstream education.

Consciousness plays a deep role in the exercise and realization of human abilities on Earth and within the perceived universe. "Right" thoughts can help to create the right circumstances, and thoughts help to create experiences in lives every day. Many fundamental physicists have stated that there cannot be a universe without the mind entering into it. Without conscious thought, there would be no universe. This powerful statement is interesting to "keep in mind" as we examine how powerful every thought can be, especially because humans have an estimated 20,000 to 70,000 thoughts per day.

The human brain weighs approximately 3 pounds, yet it has a number of nerve cells or neurons and many more support cells that are comparable to astronomical numbers of stars in a galaxy. The brain consists of approximately 86 billion neurons that communicate via neurotransmitters within the brain. The neurons are clustered in parts of the brain called "modules", such as in the cortex, the "white matter" outer layer of the brain, which also includes the four lobes and the subcortical modules. The left and right hemispheres also have a band of fibers that connects the two hemispheres together, called the "corpus callosum". This hook-up of two hemispheres serves to connect more distant neurons and combine both sides and strengths of the brain into a "whole-flowing electrical current." The corpus callosum of a woman is more dense than that of a man and can help to explain why women's brains may be more symmetrical and why the two hemispheres can work in more synchronicity. Men's brains are usually a bit larger in the right frontal lobe, as well as the left occipital lobe, located in the back of the head.

BIOPSYCHOSOCIAL APPROACH TO PAIN

The ability to feel occasional pain is a standard biologic component of survival in the world and allows detection that something is wrong, direction of attention towards the location immediately, and appropriate behavioral responses (see "Adapting With Pain" in Chapter 5). The biopsychosocial approach further examines a person's biological, psychological, and social predispositions that form a subjective experience of pain. Each individual is an essential contributor to his or her own intuitive, normalized, and societal belief about the meanings of pain. These biological, psychological, and social notions govern overall health, behavior, as well as depth and density of pain experienced. Biology, gender, and social experiences shape the depths and characterization of individual experiences of pain intensity. Studies have shown that women often suffer and perceive higher pain intensity than men, and men usually report lower pain intensity than women (Horn, Alappattu, Gay, & Bishop, 2014; Paller, Campbell, Edwards, & Dobs, 2009; Wiesenfeld-Hallin, 2005).

Certain genes can affect pain intensity. Interleukin-1α gene polymorphism rs1800587 is associated with increased pain intensity and decreased pressure pain thresholds in patients with lumbar radicular pain (Schistad, Jacobsen, Røe, & Gjerstad, 2014). Patients obtained for the study were residents of Norway, and studies were performed at the University of Oslo, where evaluation of pain management continues to be an ongoing national program. Genetic predisposition can influence the experience, behavioral response, and sensation of pain (Fitzgibbon & Loeser, 2010). In addition to biology, social experiences can truly be traumatic and painful, such as when a loved one is lost, natural disasters occur, or mental and emotional abuse are inflicted.

LEARNING PAIN

Each active sensory mechanism to which humans are tuned (sound or vocal, sight, "vibes" from another person, intention, and other sensory modalities) can collectively bring about a personalized reaction based on individual sets of psychological, biological, and social principles. Reactions to pain can be found among the first observations humans make. Perceptions and beliefs are first shaped as a child and are influenced as people grow older. Learning proper coping mechanisms and understanding what pain is are part of handling traumatic and painful situations. Neuroplasticity, the brain's ability to change neural networks and enhance the growth of neurons and neurotransmitters, is able to reshape these reactions, perceptions, and beliefs. Other factors include psychological mindset and influences from culture and family life. Ongoing painful experiences, such as chronic emotional pain, can elicit psychological disorders, illness, and mental illnesses when coping skills (and neural nutrients) are depleted during high levels of stress. Painful experiences may eventually lead to psychological and psychiatric disorders, including posttraumatic stress disorder (PTSD), depression, disease, addiction, and disability (Institute of Medicine, 1987).

Professional fields of care, such as nursing, medicine, licensed clinical mental health counseling, clinical social work, clinical psychology, and health psychology, all include an appropriate role in regulating pain and stress. Clinical applications may include medications and unnatural approaches that conflict with natural, holistic remedies and programs. For example, successful and unsuccessful pain management for recovering addicts use pain prescriptions and medications, which become a systemic problem for primary care physicians, public health and safety, and patients who may abuse pain medications (Prater, Zylstra, & Miller, 2002).

Psychiatric prescription drugs can also serve as pain modifiers. Two major types of antidepressants, tricyclics and selective serotonin reuptake inhibitors (SSRIs), may have different roles in the treatment of pain; however, they act in brain pathways that regulate mood and the perception of pain.

CONGENITAL ANALGESIA

Congenital analgesia is a rare genetic disorder in which the individual is born unable to feel pain. Although some people may find this condition to be appealing, it is life threatening because pain serves as a warning against and about injury. Researchers are trying to reproduce this condition by genetically altering mice so that they can study the genetic contributions to pain perception. New research shows that pain has a key location in the brain—specifically the dorsal posterior insula. Researchers were able to show that the dorsal posterior insula has a fundamental role in human pain (Segerdahl, Mezue, Okell, Farrar, & Tracey, 2015). Although studies in the past had verified that this part of the brain "lights up" during painful stimulus studies, none had been specific to pain. The identity of this major pain location may help people to understand and address pain disorders, such as congenital analgesia.

The ability to feel pain depends on this inward perception of pain itself. Thus, although diverting the brain's attention away from pain may help, so may increasing clinical attention. Researchers may be able to change genetic instructions to alter pain perception. Researchers may now have the ability to alter pain sensitivity by increasing or reducing pain perception by using nondrug mediations, such as electrical currents focused on the pain center of the brain.

DARK ENERGY AND THE BRAIN

The default mode network (DMN) of the brain is when the mind is at rest, sometimes with wandering or aimless thinking, considered mainly to be free from uniform and undisturbed thought. Thinking about the future and past, as well as while fast asleep, results in internal modes of cognition—when the mind is not focused on a specific external task. During times of rest and "nothingness," the brain is actually having meaningful activity and observable communications between and among distinct brain regions. These interacting brain regions in proximity to one another include the medial prefrontal cortex and posterior cingulate cortex. Other regions that participate in the interactions are the inferior parietal lobe (IPL), lateral temporal cortex (LTC), and hippocampal formation (HF).

The DMN affects people who have abnormal streams of thinking and consciousness very differently. People who suffer from depression, borderline personality disorder, autism, schizophrenia, and Alzheimer's disease have inconsistent and unstable DMNs, and the instability of these regions further supports that these people suffer from incoherence of the mind. The DMN imbricates brain areas seen in these brain disorders, suggesting there may be damage to this intricate network during times of stillness or rest. For example, brain areas in Alzheimer's disease that have atrophied overlap areas in DMN. Borderline personality disorder is shown to have severe alterations in DMN connectivity and reduced efficiency in the abilities to focus and change between DMN and task-related modes (Kluetsch et al., 2012). Depression shows reduced activity in one brain region of

DMN and regions involved with emotion, whereas schizophrenia shows overall increased levels of signaling in all DMN regions (Mingoia et al., 2012; Sheline et al., 2009). A large fraction of the overall activity of the mind when at this DMN resting state—essentially the DMN's baseline—ranges from 60% to 80% of all energy used by the brain and occurs in circuits unrelated to external events. When focused on an external cognitive activity, such as reading or writing, the baseline increases only by less than 5%.

> ## A DIFFERENT VIEW
>
> Dark energy or dark matter, in astrophysics, is thought to have provided ongoing changes in the rate of expansion of the universe's more than 15 billion years. Dark energy makes up approximately 68% of all the mass of the universe and is still currently being examined by physicists. Specifically, astrophysicists are still learning about how the expansion rate is being affected by this dark force. It is interesting to speculate as to how neurologically and cosmologically these topics may overlap, reflecting the essential philosophers' views of the macro (universe) and micro (mind). Or, given some fundamental physicists' view of consciousness and the cosmos, is it the other way around? In addition (as we learned from earlier chapters), the visible universe, including the sun, the Earth, the planets, and everything in the galaxies, are made up of protons, neutrons, and electrons bundled together into atoms. This ordinary matter, which is also called "baryonic matter", makes up less than 5% of the mass of the universe. It can be demonstrated here a fundamental parallel of both the physical matter of the universe and the creative and physical, external actions of the brain (reading, writing, singing), comprising less than of 5% energy—versus the "dark" unseen space in the universe (68%) and "dark" resting state of the mind (estimated at approximately 60%–80%).

PAIN PERCEPTION

Pain perception, or nociception (from the Latin word for "hurt"), is the process by which a painful stimulus is relayed from the site of stimulation to the central nervous system (CNS). When something causes pain, nociceptors are the initial response. Contact with a pain stimulus can be mechanical, such as cuts, pressure on the skin, and punctures, as well as falls, chemical injuries, or burns. Reception of the pain starts in the peripheral nerves found immediately underneath layers of the skin (deeper wounds are often perceived as less painful). From the peripheral nerve cell, transmission is completed to signal the CNS and usually involves more than one neuron in its messaging system within the CNS. Lastly, reception has a two-step process—mainly because the brain receives information from the messages following the CNS for a second time and further processes information for deliberate, intentional action. This response can be seen when white blood cells are sent through the circulatory system to the specific location of pain within the body. Nociception uses different neural pathways than normal perception (like light touch, pressure, and temperature). The normal somatic receptors are neurons that fire when stimulation does not cause pain, and these receptors eventually may trigger a mental or emotional reaction based on the touch or sensation.

Pain perception is affected by brain structure. The presence of less gray matter in specific regions of the brain is associated with higher-intensity pain levels compared with people with more gray matter in those regions. Participants with higher pain intensity ratings had less gray matter in brain regions that contribute to internal thoughts and control of attention in one recent study (Emerson et al., 2014). Participants who rated higher pain intensity had less gray matter in the posterior cingulate cortex, parts of the posterior parietal cortex, and the precuneus.

Most of these locations are the same regions that make up the DMN—the posterior cingulate cortex, precuneus, and areas of the posterior parietal cortex. The posterior cingulate cortex and precuneus are part of this DMN, the set of connected brain regions associated with free-flowing thoughts. These high pain intensity areas may be competing with the DMN's "brain energy." In essence, increased DMN activity may generate less pain, and DMN activity influences the overall pain experience of the individual (Loggia et al., 2013). Furthermore, chronic pain patients suffer from the repercussions of pain and experience harm in other brain regions not related to pain (Apkarian et al., 2004). The continued evaluation of the role of DMN in clinical pain shows promise for uncovering the underlying causes in chronic pain perception (Becker, Vogt, & Ibinson, 2015; Loggia et al., 2013).

THINKING ON PAIN

Meditation has been shown to increase gray matter, as stated earlier. The increases have been shown to occur in the concentration and focus zones of the brain known as the "orbitofrontal cortex". In addition, meditation increases gray-matter density in the hippocampus, important for learning and memory, and in structures tied to self-awareness, compassion, and introspection. To increase gray matter also means to increase energetic processes and neuronal communications within the mind and influence greater control and affirmative direction of thoughts, as well as actions. In addition, several meditations (concentration, loving-kindness, choiceless awareness) are found to decrease DMN, or mind wandering, and deactivate the main two brain regions in DMN—the medial prefrontal and posterior cingulate cortices (Brewer et al., 2011).

Pain perception varies widely, depending on individual physiology, and deep, lively experiences of life, family, and situational circumstances and events, as well as our surrounding culture where we live. Pain perception is formed based on beliefs, expectations, and pain thresholds, influenced by what has been felt in the past, and whether the same experience of pain is continued when faced with similar circumstances.

Depending on symptoms, natural therapies performed at pain control clinics may include acupuncture, electrical stimulation, massage, exercise, hypnosis, relaxation therapy, thought distraction, and Thought Field Therapy. Studies have shown even invert placebo can help by diverting the brain's attention and reducing the overall effect of pain perception, even to the similar effect of analgesic drugs. All these topics are discussed in remaining sections of the book.

AMYGDALA AND THE FEAR AND ANXIETY RESPONSE

The amygdala (Greek for "almond") are two tiny almond-shaped clusters of nuclei located near the upper region of the brainstem. This "primitive" part of the brain is key in emotional regulation, such as fear and anger, and forms part of the ancient key survival mechanism for humans and animals. When this part of the brain is "overused," people can create and develop deep-rooted emotional habits. Studies show people with emotional distress usually have enlarged amygdalae compared with people who meditate or use mindfulness often. For example, during a Loving-Kindness meditation study, there was a deactivation of the amygdala (Brewer et al., 2011). When the amygdala is used more frequently, it can enlarge and be a used as a primary mechanism of how to engage and interpret emotions and pain. Overuse of the amygdala reinforces a feedback loop of the mind-body signal and an already previously routed path to regulate or deal with pain and emotions.

Activation of the amygdala in the brain can occur in two fundamental ways. One is the slow pathway in which sensory information is able to enter the cortex first and then proceed to the amygdala. The second is the fast pathway in which information is sent to the amygdala before it gets processed in the rest of the brain. The amygdala has the ability to capture signals not yet received or processed by the conscious brain and reflexively motion the body into a fight, flight, or freeze responses. The latter method can trigger your sympathetic nervous system into action and potentially cause unnecessary stress, anxiety, and panic. Essentially you can feel stressed or anxious without realizing why because, within a fraction of a second, the amygdala can trigger norepinephrine to spark electrical impulses (nerve firings) throughout the sympathetic nervous system and to activate adrenal glands. The adrenal glands are located on top of the kidneys (ad-renal) and release epinephrine and norepinephrine (also called adrenaline and nonadrenaline). These hormones increase blood pressure, heart rate, blood sugar, and increased awareness as we are filled with energy. The inner part of the adrenal glands, called the "medulla", helps to trigger the fight-or-flight or freeze response. The adrenal glands are part of the endocrine system, which is also responsible for important hormones, such as serotonin and dopamine, to be released in the body (see also Chapter 6). All these reactions occur unconsciously (Fig. 4.1).

Bringing Pain to Conscious Awareness

Afferent pain-receptive nerves, those that bring signals to the cortex, comprise at least two kinds of fibers: a fast, relatively thick, myelinated "Aβ" fiber that carries messages quickly with intense pain, and a small, unmyelinated, slow "C" fiber that carries the longer-term throbbing and chronic pain. These large-diameter Aβ fibers are non-nociceptive (do not transmit pain stimuli) and inhibit the effects of firing by

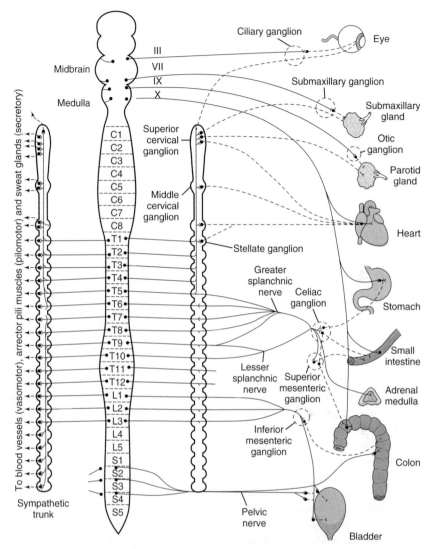

FIG. 4.1 | Autonomic nervous system and cranial nerves.

Aβ and C fibers. When you cut your hand, high potassium concentrations released from the inside of the damaged cells, and prostaglandins, histamines, and bradykinin from immune cells infiltrate the area during inflammation, or the inflammatory response. Substance P is also released from nearby nerve fibers. All of these substances cause action potentials in the nociceptor neurons. In addition, the original signal for this kind of pain is conducted rapidly by the A δ-type nociceptors. The pain is followed by a light, pulsed, prolonged, dull ache, which results from slower C fibers. Using chemical anesthetics, scientists can block one type of neuron and separate the two types of pain (Sung, Kirby, McDonald, et al., 2000; Dubin & Patapoutian, 2010).

PAIN PATHWAYS

Pain pathway mediations consist of three distinct spinal cord routes, including the neospinothalamic, paleospinothalamic, and archispinothalamic tracts. The first-order neurons are located in the dorsal root ganglion (DRG) for all three pathways and conduct impulses from cutaneous receptors and proprioceptors to the spinal cord and brain. The DRG contains the cell bodies of sensory neurons that bring information from the periphery to the spinal cord. Each pain tract originates in different spinal cord regions and ascends to terminate in different areas in the brain and CNS.

People given placebos for pain control often report that the pain ceases or diminishes (Dunlop et al., 2012; Leucht, Arbter, Engel, Kissling, & Davis, 2009; Tuttle et al., 2015). These descending pathways originate in the somatosensory cortex and relay information to the thalamus and the hypothalamus. Thalamic neurons descend to the midbrain. There, they synapse on ascending pathways in the medulla and spinal cord and inhibit ascending nerve signals. This effect produces pain relief (analgesia). Some of this relief comes from the stimulation of natural pain-relieving opiate neurotransmitters called "endorphins", "dynorphins", and "enkephalins".

Pain signals can set off autonomic nervous system pathways as they pass through the medulla, causing increased heart rate and blood pressure, rapid breathing, and sweating. The extent of these reactions depends on the intensity of pain, and they can be depressed by brain centers in the cortex through various descending pathways. As ascending pain pathways travel through the spinal cord and the mid pons, middle medulla, and caudal medulla, they can be set off by neuropathic pain, which is damage to peripheral nerves, spinal cord, or the brain itself. As in general pain, placebo responses have been increasingly reported for neuropathic pain, whereas regular drug treatments produce no change, raising many questions about continued use and regulation of prescription pain drugs (Tuttle et al., 2015).

Depending on the type of damage, the reactions of the brain's descending pathways may be limited. The influences of the descending pathways might also be responsible for psychogenic pain (pain perception with no physical cause). Thoughts and emotions can affect both ascending and descending pain pathways and affect the gate-control mechanism. Anger, guilt, and depression may open the gate, and thoughts and feelings of happiness and calmness may close the gate. Other factors, such as age, gender, memory, and fatigue, can influence pain. For example, in regards to memory, how pain has been experienced in the past can influence neural responses elicited by the limbic system.

PAIN AND THE HEART: RHYTHM AND PULSE

The heart, like the brain, has a very powerful electromagnetic field and generates the largest field in the entire body (see Chapter 10). The heart potential recorded on an electrocardiogram (ECG) is approximately 60 times greater in amplitude than the brain's electromagnetic field measured on an electroencephalograph. This electrical potential is supposedly one way people interact with each other people energetically and can sense or feel good or bad "vibes." With the right equipment, these interaction fields can be measured several feet away from two people.

When the heartbeat is erratic and not aligned, the entire body is put under a different kind of stress that may or may not rise to the level of conscious awareness in that moment. Thoughts and feelings have a direct effect on the heart's natural rhythm and rate, or beats per minute. The heartbeat, once thought to be like that of a metronome, actually fluctuates in a coherent rhythm. Recent research shows that this beat variation—also known as the "heart rate variability"—is very in tune with emotions and thoughts. Research conducted at Harvard University suggests that a drummer's imperfect rhythm may be a natural "off-beat" mathematical pattern. Indeed, the drummer and his patterns were correlated and followed a unique pattern that was likely to be repeated during the specific sequence or time that the musical instrument was played. For example, slower and faster beats in beginning segments often repeated themselves in later segments, suggesting that the human rhythm is more in sync than previously thought (Hennig, Fleischmann, & Geisel, 2012). These patterns could be replicated across different timescales that range from seconds to minutes. There is also reason to believe that there are internal rhythms produced by the brain, or biorhythms, as in the neurons of a musician's brain. These rhythmic deviations were played and shown through the hand, foot, or vocal cords, suggesting that there are similar alignments with general music. Anger, frustration, stress, and anxiety give rise to heart patterns that appear erratic and irregular, and positive emotions do the opposite. When people experience feelings such as love and joy, the heart's pattern is smooth and harmonious. The heart is greatly affected by our emotional state and our thoughts, which inevitably have a role in pain sensation and perception, as discussed earlier.

THE BRAIN ON WATER

Water is symbolized as rebirth and spiritual cleansing. Interpretations of "staying in the flow" in performance athletes can also be reflected in the neurological benefits of water. People often find themselves attracted to the beach, swimming pools, lakes, and creeks—which are naturally found to increase mindfulness and meditative state. There is a fascination with water that goes beyond the psychological and behavioral—water is part of us, it is in every cell of the body, and we need water more than any other substance on Earth to survive. The heart, brain, and the human body account for the same percentage of water (75%) that is found on Earth. Drinking water and staying hydrated is also important for cellular and central nervous processes in the body, as well as stabilizing mood, increasing contentedness and positive emotions, and decreasing confusion or "brain fog" (Pross et al., 2014).

Physiologically, when we are near or in water, our brains and bodies change. When we are removed from high-stressed environments, such as work, and into nature and water, we activate different portions of our brains, allowing feelings of connectedness and room for inspirational thought. The sound, feel, and smell of nature and water have calming affects and reduces stress and anxiety (Alvarsson, Wiens, & Nilsson, 2010; Levine, 1984; Pearson & Craig, 2014; Thoma et al., 2013).

Swimming is a low-impact aerobic exercise that stretches and exercises many muscles without stressing your joints. Naturally people benefit from immersion in water or hydrotherapy. Hydrotherapy has been found to be best at reducing general pain and knee joint pain with patients who have hemophilia (Mazloum, Rahnama, & Khayambashi, 2014; Mooventhan & Nivethitha, 2014). Winter swimming during the months of October to January significantly produced feelings of general well-bring, while pain, tension, fatigue, and mood-negative states decreased drastically (Huttunen, Kokko, & Ylijukuri, 2004). All swimmers reported less pain in rheumatism, fibromyalgia, and asthma and reported that winter swimming had relieved the pains. Cold showers have antidepressive effects attributed to the presence of high-density cold receptors in skin. These receptors send electrical impulses from peripheral nerve endings to the brain.

Patients with debilitating neurological diseases, such as multiple sclerosis, which is a chronic demyelinating neurological disease, have benefited from hydrotherapy exercise. Hydrotherapy in multiple sclerosis patients has been found to reduce pain and improve spasms, overall disability, fatigue, depression, and autonomy (Castro-Sánchez et al., 2011).

Nature contains negative ions, which are located in the air we breathe and are especially abundant near mountains, oceans, waterfalls, and large bodies of water. They are naturally occurring, found in soil, and can be created by solar radiation, waterfalls (impact of water creates new ions), snowstorms, and winds and thus understandably are less in number in urban areas. Negative ions have been reported to affect a range of psychological functions, including enhanced cognition, decreased pain and stress, and increased alertness (Andrade, Fernandes, Verghese, & Andrade, 1992; Nakane, Asami, Yamada, & Ohira, 2002). In contrast to positive ions, negative ions are believed to produce biochemical reactions that increase mood-enhancing chemicals, such as serotonin, which act as an antidepressive and help to boost our motivation and energy. In addition, in mixture with bright light, negative ions have been shown to be a successful treatment with patients who suffer from chronic depression (Goel, Terman, Terman, Macchi, & Stewart, 2005). Light has many benefits, including light-responsive proteins that are being introduced to cells, including brain cells of live animals. Ontogenetics is a new, innovative technology that is a combination of genetics and optics that has given scientists a chance to truly design and control genes and neurons with light. It includes the discovery and insertion into cells of genes that confer light responsiveness and deliver light deep within an organism. Scientists are able to turn neurons on or off with absolute precision, as well as modification of the DNA in neurons—which is beyond biological understanding and fascinating of neuroscience's relationship with photon and optic mechanisms. Even a few milliseconds off in the timing of a neuron's firing can sometimes completely reverse the effect of its signal on the rest of the nervous system and thus inhibit normal brain function, as seen with mental illness and clinical disorders. In a recent study, scientists were able to reduce and inhibit pain and reduce (or completely inhibit) fear perception (Daou et al., 2013; Gu et al., 2015; Iyer et al., 2013). Our subjective well-being (SWB) is measured around nature and water and has proven itself to enhance mood and positive emotions, such as happiness (Lyubomirsky & Layous, 2013; MacKerron & Mourato, 2012). The happiness level goes above the happiness baseline set by scientists. This happiness "baseline" is determined by genetics, the amount of time, and our choices in events and circumstances that make us happy. Beyond our own genetic predisposition of the happiness "set point" determined at birth, happiness affects our genes throughout our lives (Fredrickson et al., 2013).

MINDFULNESS MEDIATION AND NEUROPLASTICITY

We conclude this chapter and section of the book with an introduction to the next chapter and section, with a discussion of neuroplasticity and mental states and the ability to influence them. It has long been known that people who meditate and practice mindfulness "rewire" the ways in which they see the world. Current neuroscience research shows that the fabric of the mind itself becomes literally rewired. It is possible to intentionally alter the flow of mental experience and enhance perceptions and "better" beliefs that alter not just the "mind" but the brain itself. This fundamental change of the perceived world has been demonstrated to help with health, as well as well-being, perception, and behavior. The simple depth and clarity of focus allow the mind—the regulation of the flow of energy and information—to be fundamentally transformed. By inhibiting old emotional reactions and realizing power over old habits, neural firing patterns can be changed in the brain immediately.

Creating new automatic emotional reactions can reduce pain and mental suffering and enhance growth of the internally experienced world toward achieving an improved or optimal mindset. Shifts in focus of attention—the way the mind is used to channel the flow of energy and information through the various circuits of the brain—change patterns of activity in the brain (and thus affects the heart). With repetition, mindfulness practices can create intentional states of brain activation that may ultimately become character traits and change expression of genetic dispositions of the individual.

The property of neuroplasticity allows people who want to change their habits through self-observation and mindful practice to have the ability to disengage from once-normal behavior ingrained in unconscious or subconscious pathways. New pathways create space to eliminate old perceptions of pain and emotional reactions from the "education" of prior emotional experiences. On average, the mind is usually experiencing busy thoughts, automatic reactivity, and habitual responses. More specifically, these responses may include self-defeating thought patterns, negative autobiographical narratives, and reckless, maladaptive patterns of emotional reactivity. After mindfulness and meditation training and practice, awareness of these behaviors, thoughts, and feelings becomes increased. In neuroplasticity terms, new patterns of repeated neural circuit activation strengthen the synaptic connections associated with those states that then lead to synaptic strengthening and synaptic growth. New habits and practices enhance neural plasticity to alter synaptic connections in a way that transforms a temporary state into a more long-lasting trait of the individual. The developmental trajectory from effort-full state to effort-less trait can be seen as a fundamental component of how mindfulness can alter in-grained patterns of mental disorders, depression, addiction, and psychopathology. The next chapter provides the clinical background, research, and practice to achieve benefits of neuroplasticity through meditation and mindfulness.

REFERENCES

Alvarsson, J. J., Wiens, S., & Nilsson, M. E. (2010). Stress recovery during exposure to nature sound and environmental noise. *International Journal of Environmental Research and Public Health*, *7*(3), 1036–1046. http://www.ncbi.nlm.nih.gov/pmc/articles/PMC2872309/.

Andrade, A. C., Fernandes, C., Verghese, L., & Andrade, C. (1992). Effect of negative ion atmospheric loading on cognitive performance in human volunteers. *Indian Journal of Psychiatry*, *34*(3), 253–259. http://www.ncbi.nlm.nih.gov/pmc/articles/PMC2982078/.

Apkarian, A. V., Sosa, Y., Sonty, S., Levy, R. M., Harden, R. N., Parrish, T. B., et al. (2004). Chronic back pain is associated with decreased prefrontal and thalamic gray matter density. *Journal of Neuroscience*, *24*(46), 10410–10415. http://www.jneurosci.org/content/24/46/10410. abstract?ijkey=ac1c436ec1b0717c7fbfec82582a8cd9447e0031&keytype2=tf_ipsecsha.

Becker, C., Vogt, K., & Ibinson, J. (2015). The insula's functional connectivity to the default mode network is uniquely altered by pain perception. *The Journal of Pain*, *16*(4), S54. http://www.jpain.org/article/S1526-5900%2815%2900269-2/abstract.

Brewer, J. A., Worhunsky, P. D., Gray, J. R., Tang, Y. Y., Weber, J., & Kober, H. (2011). Meditation experience is associated with differences in default mode network activity and connectivity. *Proceedings of the National Academy of Sciences of the United States of America*, *108*(50), 20254–20259. http://www.pnas.org/content/108/50/20254.long.

Castro-Sánchez, A. M., Mataran-Penarrocha, G. A., Lara-Palomo, I., Saavedra-Hernandez, M., Arroyo-Morales, M., & Moreno-Lorenzo, C. (2011). Hydrotherapy for the treatment of pain in people with multiple sclerosis: A randomized controlled trial. *Evidence-Based Complementary and Alternative Medicine*, *2012*, 473963. http://www.ncbi.nlm.nih.gov/pmc/articles/PMC3138085/.

Daou, I., Tuttle, A. H., Longo, G., Wieskopf, J. S., Bonin, R. P., Ase, A. R., et al. (2013). Remote optogenetic activation and sensitization of pain pathways in freely moving mice. *Journal of Neuroscience*, *33*(47), 18631–18640. http://www.jneurosci.org/content/33/47/18631.short.

Dubin, A. E., & Patapoutian, A. (2010). Nociceptors: the sensors of the pain pathway. *Journal of Clinical Investigation*, *120*(11), 3760–3772. http://doi.org/10.1172/JCI42843.

Dunlop, B. W., Thase, M. E., Wun, C. C., Fayyad, R., Guico-Pabia, C. J., Musgnung, J., et al. (2012). A meta-analysis of factors impacting detection of antidepressant efficacy in clinical trials: The importance of academic sites. *Neuropsychopharmacology*, *37*, 2830–2836. http://www.nature.com/npp/journal/v37/n13/full/npp2012153a.html.

Emerson, N. M., Zeidan, F., Lobanov, O. V., Hadsel, M. S., Martucci, K. T., Quevedo, A. S., et al. (2014). Pain sensitivity is inversely related to regional grey matter density in the brain. *Pain*, *155*(3), 566–573. http://journals.lww.com/pain/pages/articleviewer.aspx?year=2014&issue=03000&article=00015&type=abstract.

Fitzgibbon, D. R. & Loeser, J. D. (2010). *Cancer pain: Assessment, diagnosis, and management* (Chapter 19; pp. 221). Philadelphia: Wolters luwer/Lippincott Williams and Wilkins.

Fredrickson, B. L., Grewenb, K. M., Coffeya, K. A., Algoea, S. B., Firestinea, A. M., Arevaloc, J. M. G., et al. (2013). A functional genomic perspective on human well-being. *Proceedings of the National Academy of Sciences of the United States of America*, *110*(33), 13684–13689. http://www.pnas.org/content/110/33/13684.full.

Goel, N., Terman, M., Terman, J. S., Macchi, M. M., & Stewart, M. (2005). Controlled trial of bright light and negative air ions for chronic depression. *Psychological Medicine*, *35*(7), 945–955. http://www.ncbi.nlm.nih.gov/pubmed/16045061.

Gu, L., Uhelski, M. L., Anand, S., Romero-Ortega, M., Kim, Y. T., Fuchs, P. N., et al. (2015). Pain inhibition by optogenetic activation of specific anterior cingulate cortical neurons. *PLoS One, 10*(2), e0117746. http://journals.plos.org/plosone/article?id=10.1371/journal.pone.0117746.

Hennig, H., Fleischmann, R., & Geisel, T. (2012). Musical rhythms: The science of being slightly off. *Physics Today, 65,* 65–65. http://scitation.aip.org/content/aip/magazine/physicstoday/article/65/7/10.1063/PT.3.1650.

Horn, M. E., Alappattu, M. J., Gay, C. W., & Bishop, M. (2014). Fear of severe pain mediates sex differences in pain sensitivity responses to thermal stimuli. *Pain Research and Treatment, 2014,* 897953. http://www.ncbi.nlm.nih.gov/pmc/articles/PMC3913346/.

Huttunen, P., Kokko, L., & Ylijukuri, V. (2004). Winter swimming improves general well-being. *International Journal of Circumpolar Health, 63*(2), 140–144. http://www.ncbi.nlm.nih.gov/pubmed/15253480.

Institute of Medicine. (1987). Psychiatric aspects of chronic pain. In M. Osterweis, A. Kleinman, & D. Mechanic (Eds.), *Pain and disability: clinical, behavioral, and public policy perspectives.* Washington DC: National Academies Press. http://www.ncbi.nlm.nih.gov/books/NBK219250/.

Iyer, S. M., Montgomery, K. L., Towne, C., Lee, S. Y., Ramakrishnan, C., Deisseroth, K., et al. (2013). Virally mediated optogenetic excitation and inhibition of pain in freely moving nontransgenic mice. *Nature Biotechnology, 32*(3), 274–278. http://www.nature.com/nbt/journal/v32/n3/full/nbt.2834.html.

Kluetsch, R. C., Schmahl, C., Niedtfeld, I., Densmore, M., Calhoun, V. D., Daniels, J., et al. (2012). Alterations in default mode network connectivity during pain processing in borderline personality disorder. *Archives of General Psychiatry, 69*(10), 993–1002. http://www.ncbi.nlm.nih.gov/pmc/articles/PMC4429518/.

Leucht, S., Arbter, D., Engel, R. R., Kissling, W., & Davis, J. M. (2009). How effective are second-generation antipsychotic drugs? A meta-analysis of placebo-controlled trials. *Molecular Psychiatry, 14,* 429–447. http://www.nature.com/mp/journal/v14/n4/full/4002136a.html.

Levine, B. A. (1984). Use of hydrotherapy in reduction of anxiety. *Psychological Reports, 5*(2), 526. https://www.researchgate.net/publication/16681230_Use_of_hydrotherapy_in_reduction_of_anxiety.

Loggia, M. L., Kim, J., Gollub, R. L., Vangel, M. G., Kirsch, I., Kong, J., et al. (2013). Default mode network connectivity encodes clinical pain: An arterial spin labeling study. *Pain, 154,* 24–33. http://scholar.harvard.edu/files/loggia/files/default_mode_network_connectivity_encodes_clinical.8.pdf.

Lyubomirsky, S. & Layous, K. (2013). How do simple positive activities increase well-being? *Current Directions in Psychological Science, 22*(1), 57–62. http://sonjalyubomirsky.com/files/2012/09/Lyubomirsky-Layous-20132.pdf.

MacKerron, G. & Mourato, S. (2012). Happiness is greater in natural environments. *Global Environmental Change, 23*(5), 992–1000. http://www.parisschoolofeconomics.eu/IMG/pdf/Mackerron_paper.pdf.

Mazloum, V., Rahnama, N., & Khayambashi, K. (2014). Effects of therapeutic exercise and hydrotherapy on pain severity and knee range of motion in patients with hemophilia: A randomized controlled trial. *International Journal of Preventive Medicine, 5*(1), 83–88. http://www.ncbi.nlm.nih.gov/pmc/articles/PMC3915478/.

Mingoia, G., Wagner, G., Langbein, K., Maitra, R., Smesny, S., Dietzek, M., et al. (2012). Default mode network activity in schizophrenia studied at resting state using probabilistic ICA. *Schizophrenia Research, 138*(2-3), 143–149. http://www.ncbi.nlm.nih.gov/pubmed/22578721.

Mooventhan, A. & Nivethitha, L. (2014). Scientific evidence-based effects of hydrotherapy on various systems of the body. *North American Journal of Medical Sciences, 6*(5), 199–209. http://www.ncbi.nlm.nih.gov/pmc/articles/PMC4049052/.

Nakane, H., Asami, O., Yamada, Y., & Ohira, H. (2002). Effect of negative air ions on computer operation, anxiety and salivary chromogranin A-like immunoreactivity. *International Journal of Psychophysiology, 46*(1), 85–89. http://www.ncbi.nlm.nih.gov/pubmed/12374649.

Paller, C. J., Campbell, C. M., Edwards, R. R., & Dobs, A. S. (2009). Sex-based differences in pain perception and treatment. *Pain Medicine, 10*(2), 289–299. http://www.ncbi.nlm.nih.gov/pmc/articles/PMC2745644/.

Pearson, D. G. & Craig, T. (2014). The great outdoors? Exploring the mental health benefits of natural environments. *Frontiers in Psychology, 5,* 1178. http://www.ncbi.nlm.nih.gov/pmc/articles/PMC4204431/.

Prater, C. D., Zylstra, R. G., & Miller, K. E. (2002). Successful pain management for the recovering addicted patient. *The Primary Care Companion to the Journal of Clinical Psychiatry, 4*(4), 125–131. http://www.ncbi.nlm.nih.gov/pmc/articles/PMC315480/.

Pross, N., Demazieres, A., Girard, N., Barnouin, R., Metzger, D., Klein, A., et al. (2014). Effects of changes in water intake on mood of high and low drinkers. *PLoS One, 9*(4), e94754. http://www.ncbi.nlm.nih.gov/pmc/articles/PMC3984246/.

Schistad, E. I., Jacobsen, L. M., Røe, C., & Gjerstad, J. (2014). The interleukin-1α gene C > T polymorphism rs1800587 is associated with increased pain intensity and decreased pressure pain thresholds in patients with lumbar radicular pain. *The Clinical Journal of Pain, 30*(10), 869–874. http://www.ncbi.nlm.nih.gov/pubmed/24300227.

Segerdahl, A. R., Mezue, M., Okell, T. W., Farrar, J. T., & Tracey, L. (2015). The dorsal posterior insula subserves a fundamental role in human pain. *Nature Neuroscience, 18*(4), 499–500. http://www.ncbi.nlm.nih.gov/pubmed/25751532.

Sheline, Y. I., Barch, D. M., Price, J. L., Rundle, M. M., Vaishnavi, S. N., Snyder, A. Z., et al. (2009). The default mode network and self-referential processes in depression. *Proceedings of the National Academy of Sciences of the United States of America, 106*(6), 1942–1947. http://www.ncbi.nlm.nih.gov/pmc/articles/PMC2631078/.

Sung, K. W., Kirby, M., McDonald, M. P., Lovinger, D. M., & Delpire, E. (2000). Abnormal GABAA receptor-mediated currents in dorsal root ganglion neurons isolated from Na-K-2Cl cotransporter null mice. *Journal of Neuroscience, 20*(20), 7531–7538.

Thoma, M. V., La Marca, R., Bronnimann, R., Finkel, L., Ehlert, U., & Nater, U. M. (2013). The effect of music on the human stress response. *PLoS One, 8*(8), e70156. http://www.ncbi.nlm.nih.gov/pmc/articles/PMC3734071/.

Tuttle, A. H., Tohyama, S., Ramsay, T., Kimmelman, J., Schweinhardt, P., Bennett, G. J., et al. (2015). Increasing placebo responses over time in U.S. clinical trials of neuropathic pain. *Pain, 156*(12), 2616–2626. http://journals.lww.com/pain/Citation/2015/12000/Increasing_placebo_responses_over_time_in_U_S_.27.aspx.

Wiesenfeld-Hallin, Z. (2005). Sex differences in pain perception. *Gender Medicine, 2*(3), 137–145. http://www.ncbi.nlm.nih.gov/pubmed/16290886.

Suggested Readings can be found on the companion website, http://www.micozzipainconditions.com.

Section II

MIND-BODY MEDICINE

Chapter 5

Mind, Meditation, and Mindfulness

To live with chronic pain is the experience of many. Accepting such adversity and suffering is necessary because it is commonly understood that there are no entirely sufficient treatments for everyone (although we propose some advancements in matching the right treatments to the right individual in Appendix I [pp. 572–579]). The Buddha said that we are all suffering. In the case of the chronic pain, patient suffering is a manifestation of daily living. The Buddha also said that we all have attachments and cling to something. We may come to realize that the daily problems we encounter are due to attachment, or holding on to something. Part of the problem may be "holding on to pain," which is a common experience among many pain patients. Also common to both ancient Chinese and Greek philosophy is the experience of being in a deep and fast flowing river clinging to a stone to not lose control and drown. This kind of stone or weight can symbolize pain, which may somehow make the patient feel safe, clinging to pain because it seems like life itself is attached to and somehow depends upon it. Perhaps this image may be of help as you read about the various experiences of pain in the mind and in meditation and mindfulness.

Section II and this chapter explore why and how actions that take place primarily, or solely, in the mind may mediate the experience of pain and how and why mental practices of meditation and mindfulness can be so effective. Pain is complex. The International Association for the Study of Pain (IASP) defines pain as "an unpleasant sensory and emotional experience associated with actual or potential tissue damage, or described in terms of such damage" (IASP, 1994). This description is accepted as a standard definition of pain by clinical practitioners and pain researchers worldwide. It indicates that pain is always a subjective experience, including both sensory and affective dimensions. On the one hand, tactile tissue or nerve damage is not a necessary condition to experience pain. Pain can be also present without actual nociceptive processing. The individual's experience of pain serves as both a necessary and sufficient condition for the presence of pain. When a patient expresses that he or she is in pain, health professionals need to acknowledge the experience, regardless of other information or lack of information (e.g., lack of "physical" evidence). Also important is the context in which the afflicted individual experiences pain. Various psychological, social, and cultural factors interact with the underlying brain mechanisms involved in pain processing (see Chapter 4). The mental state of the individual and the circumstances in which pain is experienced contribute significantly to the neurobiological aspects of pain. Accordingly, pain may be seen as a biopsychosocial phenomenon in both pain treatment and research. To engage fully with patients, it is important to understand the various factors that interact and contribute to pain conditions.

ANATOMY OF PAIN

The complexity of pain is demonstrated on the anatomical level by the complicated and highly distributed neural components involved in pain processing. The 17th-century French philosopher René Descartes is known not only for the infamous "mind-body" division but also for his concept of pain as a hard-wired system passively transmitting the noxious stimulus through sensory channels to the pineal gland, which he considered "le siège de l'âme" ("the seat of the soul;" Descartes & Timmermans, 1649/2010). Today new, noninvasive brain imaging technologies demonstrate that the conscious experience of pain is the result of cortical activity. There are two main pathways: ascending and descending pain processing. Ascending input originating in the peripheral nerves projects to the dorsal horn of the spinal cord and via the brainstem to a large and distributed network of brain regions. In contrast, descending pain processing can either facilitate or inhibit the noxious information processing via this network.

ADAPTING WITH PAIN

Pain researchers now characterize pain as part of an adaptive "salience detection system" defined as a system involved in detecting, orienting attention towards, and reacting to the occurrence of salient sensory events (Legrain, Iannetti, Plaghki, & Mouraux, 2011). The fundamental role of the nociceptive system is to detect salient changes and facilitate appropriate responses in accordance with the homeostatic principle as part of adaptation to the environment (see Chapter 6). The descending pain modulatory system is considered to act as a bidirectional central control of nociception that can either inhibit or facilitate nociceptive processing. In terms of adaptive survival the former can be advantageous in "fight-or-flight" situations, whereas the latter can be useful in situations in which attention and care to injured tissue is needed. The problem occurs when either hypoalgesia or hyperalgesia (IASP, 1994) becomes a chronic state. Some hypoalgesic patients risk serious tissue damage due to reduced cortical processing of noxious input. Conversely, one of the biggest challenges in pain management is to help patients whose hyperalgesic states remain "switched on" long after normal and expected healing time, as is often the case in chronic pain conditions. Like pain itself, pain modulation is a multidimensional process. The descending pain modulatory system is believed to project from cortical regions, the anterior cingulate cortex (ACC), and via the periaqueductal gray matter (PAG) in the midbrain through the rostral ventromedial medulla (RVM) to the spinal cord. Other areas, such as the amygdala, thalamus, and hypothalamus, may also be involved. However, evidence suggests that the prefrontal regions serve as the main regulators of top-down pain modulation, especially the ventrolateral prefrontal cortex (VLPFC) and dorsolateral prefrontal cortex (DLPFC).

ADAPTING TO PAIN

Cognitive processes influence pain. The major cognitive processes relate to attention, coping, and expectations, which will be discussed in turn. This perspective stresses the importance of context. A number of psychological and social factors mediate and modulate the experience of pain. Psychosocial context surrounding the pain patient is often a major contributor to the subjective experience of pain and to neurobiological pain mechanisms. In research studies, expectations about pain have been shown to account for between 25% and 80% of the variance in pain intensity scores (see Benedetti, 2009; Meissner et al., 2011; and Price, Finniss, & Benedetti, 2008). The desire for pain relief has also been demonstrated as a critical motivational factor. This desire is related to wanting something, either wanting something to happen (e.g., pain relief) or wanting to avoid something from happening (e.g., augmentation or persistence of pain). These desires and apprehensions lead to the role of anxiety in pain experience so that pain processing becomes more palpable (potentially to the point of palpitations) yet more complex. It is not known exactly how anxiety and pain interact, but it is well established that these two factors mutually affect one another. As a core example of negative affect, anxiety is a pronociceptive mechanism, which increases pain sensitivity at a neurophysiological level. Patients who have a high degree of anxiety are thereby more sensitive to pain signals. It may be the case that anxiety enhances pain, and pain may also generate or exacerbate anxiety.

THE FULL CATASTROPHE

This cybernetic reciprocal link between pain and anxiety can lead to further negative emotional affect and pain catastrophizing thoughts, fueling a vicious cycle, particularly for chronic pain patients. The Pain Catastrophizing Scale (PCS) developed by Sullivan, Bishop, and Pivik (1995) is often used both in clinical practice and in pain research to investigate the possible presence and influence of exaggerated negative mental activity during pain perception or anticipation of pain (Keefe, Brown, Wallston, & Caldwell, 1989; Sullivan, Stanish, Waite, Sullivan, & Tripp, 1998). Studies have established comparable links for depression (Gormsen, Rosenberg, Bach, & Jensen, 2010) and stress (Logan et al., 2001). Coping efficacy, sense of control, and personality have also been shown to influence pain processing (Folkman & Lazarus, 1988).

APPROACHES TO TREATMENT

Conceptualization and treatments for pain have developed over time and across geographical regions. Cultural and social factors provide foundations for both expression and treatment of pain. Cultural contexts shape perceptions and experiences of pain and pain behavior, as well as pain treatment strategies (Jegindø, 2012). The social and cultural context that surrounds the person in pain affects pain descriptions and expressions, the words (and sounds) used to express pain, and the medical assessment of pain. The immediate social environment, especially family history, plays an important role in how pain is experienced, and even how pain will be continue to be experienced in the future. The prevalence of pain disorders is significantly higher in patients whose parents have a history of pain disorder, as well as affective disorders, such as depression and anxiety (Hudson, Goldenberg, Pope, Keck, & Schlesinger, 1992). Parental behavior and other mental factors may influence pain in children and adolescents. Similarly, the interactions among pain patients and their spouses often contribute to the dynamics of actual pain experience and verbal and nonverbal pain communications (Gauthier, Thibault, & Sullivan, 2011). A critical aspect of the patient context includes the set of cultural beliefs and norms that shape both pain response and pain treatment. For instance, cultural and religious beliefs may produce certain expectations and assumptions about the causes of pain, and tolerance for pain, in addition to diseases in general. In some cultures and religious traditions, illness is interpreted in terms of sin, black magic, bad karma, or impurity. Likewise, treatment strategies and outcomes are likely to be affected by such beliefs (Jegindø, 2012).

DIMENSIONS OF PAIN MANAGEMENT

Distraction is one of the most effective and well-documented pain modulators. Several behavioral and neuroimaging studies have confirmed the effectiveness of distraction. Drawing attention away from the painful stimulus by attention to a nonpainful sensory stimulus or a cognitively demanding task can help to relieve pain by reducing attention to the nociceptive input (see Buhle & Wager, 2010). This modulation relates to the salience detection mechanism, which helps to orient attention. In some situations, the appropriate response may require a shift in attention from one sensory stimulus to another stimulus that is more salient in terms of adaptive survival.

The effect of emotional pain regulation, or coping, is modulation that occurs when affective states are able to influence pain processing. Emotional stress, negative affect, and anxiety increase pain sensitivity, whereas positive affect and positive arousal decrease pain sensitivity. The context of the painful event and the subject's conscious or unconscious interpretations of this context have major influences on pain regulation. Sense of control and acceptance both decrease pain sensitivity and serve as adaptive coping strategies.

Likewise using a coping strategy known as reappraisal helps to reduce the level or salience of pain as a sensory input, which would otherwise be interpreted as life (or tissue) threatening and detected as such by the relevant brain regions. Pain may be re-evaluated through reappraisal mechanisms as guided by the prefrontal brain regions (Ochsner & Gross, 2005). Adding meaning and positive beliefs also generate positive reappraisal effects. A familiar and potent example of this reappraisal effect is childbirth. Most women consider it to be an exceedingly painful experience. However, framed in the context of delivering a child, the painful event is often reinterpreted due to the highly meaningful and (now typically) non–life-threatening context, driven primarily by positive affect and expectations.

Placebo and Nocebo Effects

Expectations about the outcome of a treatment, the progression of an illness, or even experimental conditions, are all known to contribute to major variances in pain outcome measures. Expectations form an important part of the psychosocial context of pain experiences and research, as well as pain treatment. They can be induced by the power of suggestion (see Chapter 7) or by operant conditioning and be either conscious or unconscious to the subject. The psychosocial context of a research study, or a treatment, also depends on external aspects, such as the physical properties of the environment. For example, the way a clinic waiting room or a surgical operating room typically looks, the scientific objects that are present, and the profession-specific uniforms worn by the health care staff are features of the environment that influence expectations, as well as context-dependent behaviors and procedures carried out. Patients expect physicians, nurses, and experimental research scientists to do and say certain things. What they choose to (or not) do and say, and how they do and say it, can all have major impacts on patient expectations and, therefore, on their brains and their experiences of pain.

Fabrizio Benedetti, a placebo and nocebo researcher, is known for stressing that placebos literally change the patient's brain (Benedetti, Carlino, & Pollo, 2011). He explains that placebo treatments are based on the administration of an inert substance, or sham physical treatments, such as sham surgery or acupuncture, but placebos, as such, are not inert. They consist of potent "words and rituals, symbols, and meanings, and all these elements are active in shaping the patient's brain" (Benedetti, et al, 2011). Together with verbal suggestions of clinical benefit and/or conditioning, "inert" substances have real and significant neurobiological, behavioral, and subjective effects. The placebo effect is also the result of a learning process based on Bayesian mechanisms. The magnitude of placebo analgesia thus depends on previous experiences of analgesic effects.

Over the past few decades, placebo and nocebo studies have established highly significant roles for positive and negative expectations on neural pain processing and modulation. Nocebo effects are the opposite of placebo effects, wherein expectations of a negative outcome lead to worsening of a symptom or a clinical condition. A series of studies by Colloca and colleagues from Benedetti's laboratory have shown how words can be harmful and painful. Negative verbal suggestions can lead to increased anxiety and increased pain sensitivity (Colloca & Finniss, 2012).

Molecules of Pain

In the late 1970s, Levine et al. demonstrated that the opioid antagonist, naloxone, could block both opioid and placebo analgesia (Levine, Gordon, & Fields, 1978). Since then it has been accepted that at least some types of placebo analgesia are opioidergic. In other words, positive expectations can engage the body's own natural painkiller molecules. Experiments using open/hidden paradigms and protocols have further emphasized the critical role of both positive and negative expectations in neuromodulation. In 1995, Benedetti et al. showed that the analgesic effect of the drug proglumide occurs in a placebo context only when expectations are given to patients and not when the drug is given without the patient's knowledge in a hidden infusion (Benedetti, Mayberg, Wager, Stohler, & Zubieta, 2005). The analgesic effects of an old prescription drug, Darvon, and of the popular over-the-counter drug acetaminophen have also been show to be based largely on placebo (although the toxic side effects of both drugs are very real and can be very painful indeed). Similarly, even morphine and other potent opioid analgesics have been found to be significantly less effective in hidden trials when patients are completely unaware that a painkiller has been administered. By contrast, an open injection of saline thought to be morphine (a placebo trial) can be just as effective as a hidden infusion of 6 to 8 mg morphine (Levine, Gordon, Smith, & Fields, 1981). Disruption of postsurgical morphine delivery dramatically increased pain levels, except when disconnection of the infusion was unknown to the patient. These clinical perspectives are important for treatment because they illustrate the importance of interactions and relationships with patients. So-called placebo effects fundamentally change the neural basis for patients' current and future experiences of both pain symptoms and the effectiveness of health care to manage pain. Words and actions influence the experience of pain and can both ease or augment pain.

BEHAVIORAL AND COGNITIVE COUNSELING THERAPIES

Psychotherapy and psychological approaches for treating pain provide some of the most noninvasive treatments. Mainstream medicine struggles with appropriate diagnosis and treatment of pain. There are now available more integrated approaches, including modalities from other disciplines, to help develop more appropriate safe and effective treatment methods. They provide a more "whole" understanding of patients' suffering.

Chronic pain is different from other medical symptoms or problems and is a complex condition that may include one or more physical, psychological, or neurological factors. Thus it becomes more complex to diagnose a particular pain case. A primary care practitioner may guide a patient through a series of questions to identify pain locations and symptoms.

The following are some categories of questions for the patient:
- What kind of pain problem
- Location of pain
- Pain scale
- Pain worse during what part of the day

Once identified, a practitioner may assist by providing strategies for overcoming chronic pain. Some treatments include mind-body modalities, attention diversion, reality testing, positive self-coping statements, and mindful breathing. Potential analgesics may be recommended after appropriate education on dosage to prevent abuse of medication. Overall, individual goal setting is extremely significant because every circumstance is unique.

COGNITIVE-BEHAVIORAL THERAPY AND THE BRAIN

Patients with chronic pain show reduced gray matter in areas of experience and transmission of pain. However, cognitive-behavioral therapy (CBT) provide patients with appropriate recovery in correlation with gray-matter density, showing that loss of gray-matter density is not the cause but the consequence of long-term chronic pain (Naylor, Naud, Keefe, & Helzer, 2010; Rodriguez-Raecke, Niemeier, Ihle, Ruether, & May, 2009). Physicians who are treating patients with chronic pain and noninvasive treatments can be comfortable referring them to CBT.

MINDFULNESS MEDITATION

Teaching mindfulness meditation to chronic pain patients entails being with them in the moment. The most important role for the mindfulness teacher is to really be present. The practitioner cannot completely remove pain and neither can the patients. With judicious effort, meditative and mindfulness practice exercises can target fundamental issues of living with pain and managing chronic pain. Practice is essential but cannot be done solely with a textbook (although we recommend McCown, Reibel & Micozzi, 2017). Knowledge and shared experience about working with chronic pain patients may well be necessary.

Origins of Meditation

The origins of meditation are ancient, but the science of their physiological effects is very recent as the concept of meditation has been introduced into the realm of modern Western medicine. The Cartesian split between the mind and body in the early 17th century resulted in science emphasizing the body and medicine going in the "scientific" direction of studying the material aspects of the body. However, perceiving the reality of mind and body requires understanding that the two are not separate (they have always been together) and have an interactive influence on each other. Meditation is said to realign the mind and body and integrate consciousness with the physical body, creating more harmonious interactions.

Similar to the word medicine, the word meditation suggests something to do with healing. In 1983, David Bohm, physicist and author of *Wholeness and Implicate Order,* looked at wholeness as a property of the physical material world. He points out the root in Latin means "to cure" but that its deepest root means "to measure." But what does medicine or meditation have to do with measuring? The ancient Greeks said, "Man is the measure of all things." According to Jon Kabat-Zinn, PhD, Director of the Stress Reduction Clinic at the University of Massachusetts Medical Center:

"It has to do with the platonic notion that every shape, every being, everything has its right inward measure. In other words, a tree has its own quality of wholeness that gives it particular properties. A human being has an individual right inward measure, when everything is balanced and physiologically homeostatic—that's the totality of the individual at that point in time" (McCown et al., 2017).

Medicine can be seen as the science and the art of restoring right inward measure when it is thrown off balance. From the meditative perspective and from the perspective of the new mind-body medicine, as well as traditional Ayurvedic and Chinese medicines, health does not have a finite or static destination. Health is a dynamic energy flow that changes over a lifetime, with influences toward both health or illness coexisting together.

Some meditative practices have come to the West through traditional Asian spiritual practices, particularly those of India, China, and Japan. Others can be traced to other ancient cultures of the world, and there is a strong early-American tradition of deliberate, mindful experience of man and nature, as with the New England transcendentalists Emerson and Thoreau (McCown & Micozzi, 2012).

Many Western meditators practice a contemplative, "mindful," form of meditation, as well as other active forms of meditation, such as the Chinese martial art, t'ai chi, the Japanese martial art aikido, and the walking meditations of Zen Buddhism. Yoga as a devotional, spiritual, meditative practice also has its more active form in the Hatha-Yoga, or physical yoga, popular in the West (see Chapter 19).

MEDITATION FOR HEALTH

Until recently, the primary purpose of meditation has been religious or spiritual in nature. However, during the past 25 years, meditation has been shown to be a healthful means of reducing stress on both mind and body. Many studies have found that various practices of meditation appear to produce beneficial physical and psychological changes. Meditation is self-directed and results in relaxing and calming the mind and body. Methods of meditation include focusing on a single thought or word for a specific time. Some forms of meditation focus on a physical experience, such as breathing or a specific sound or mantra. All forms of meditation have the common objective of stilling the restlessness of the mind so that mental focus can be directed inwardly. As a health practice, meditation is used to calm mental activity; endless, restless thoughts; and stressful ways of reacting to circumstances and environment. As long as accumulated impressions linger in the inner recesses of the mind, nagging for attention (what we believe relates to your emotional boundary type—see Appendix I [pp. 572–579]), it remains difficult to experience an inner state of peace, calm, and health. Fast-paced Western society, filled with external stimuli, has conditioned us to push our minds and bodies to the point of exhaustion, often to the detriment of our own well-being. To be still, to experience the peace and contentment that lies within, we must free ourselves from this preoccupation with external materialism. Meditation is the process of calming and releasing these distractions from the mind for the purpose of opening up and awakening to our true inner natures.

ASIAN TECHNIQUES AND TRANSCENDENTAL MEDITATION

In the mid-1960s, a popular trend in meditation called "transcendental meditation" (TM) began to emerge. The Vedic philosophy and practice was brought from India and adapted to the United States by its founder, Maharishi Mahesh Yogi. The Maharishi had eliminated ancient yogic elements that he considered unnecessary or unpalatable in a contemporary environment. Intentionally omitting more difficult or challenging physical postures, exercises, and procedures, his reformed version became more readily accepted and practiced by Westerners. On Maharishi's first visit to America in 1959, a San Francisco newspaper heralded TM as a "non-medicinal tranquilizer" and praised it as a promising cure for insomnia. TM soon began to ride a crest of popularity, with almost half a million Americans learning the technique by 1975. It was embraced by many celebrities of that day, such as the Beatles; since then, it has been notable for creating a few celebrities. It is believed that more than 2 million people currently practice TM in the United States and millions more practicing worldwide (who have been encouraged to become avid celebrity book-buyers).

PRACTICING TRANSCENDENTAL MEDITATION

TM is relatively simple in application. A student is given a mantra (a word or sound) to repeat silently over and over again while sitting in a comfortable position. The purpose of repeating the sound or word is to prevent distracting thoughts from entering the mind. Students are instructed to be passive, and if thoughts other than the mantra come to mind, to note them and return the attention to the mantra. TM is generally practiced in the morning and in the evening for approximately 20 minutes.

HEALTH BENEFITS

In 1968, Harvard's Herbert Benson (see also Chapter 6) was asked by Maharishi International University in Fairfield, Iowa, to test TM practitioners on their ability to lower their own blood pressures. Benson initially refused to participate but was later persuaded to do so. Benson's studies and other research showed that TM was associated with reduced health care costs, increased longevity, and better quality of life. He found reduced anxiety, lowered blood pressure, and reduced serum cholesterol levels. Meditation has been used as a viable treatment of posttraumatic stress disorder in Vietnam War veterans and for reduction in chronic pain.

WESTERN TECHNIQUES AND MINDFULNESS MEDITATION

The term mindfulness was coined by our colleague Jon Kabat-Zinn, PhD, known for his work using mindfulness meditation to help medical patients with chronic pain and stress-related disorders (McCown et al., 2017). As with other mind-body therapies, mindfulness meditation can induce deep states of relaxation, at times directly improve physical symptoms, and help patients to lead fuller and more satisfying lives. Asian forms of modern TM involve focusing on a sound, phrase, or prayer to minimize distraction, but the practice of mindfulness can be seen to do the opposite. In mindfulness meditation, "distractions" emanating from the outside environment are not ignored but focused on. This form of meditation practice can be traced originally from the Buddhist tradition and is approximately 2500 years old. The method was developed as a means of cultivating greater awareness and wisdom, with the aim of helping people to live each moment of their lives as fully as possible. There is also a distinctively Western and American tradition of mindful contemplation and thought that extends back to Founding Fathers George Washington, John Adams, and Thomas Jefferson in the 18th century and to leading American philosophers during the early 19th century, Ralph Waldo Emerson and Henry David Thoreau, and other icons of American letters (McCown & Micozzi, 2012).

Mindfulness is about more than feeling relaxed or stress free. Its true aim is to nurture an inner balance of mind that allows an individual to face life situations with greater clarity, stability, and understanding and to respond more effectively from that sense of clarity. An integral part of mindfulness practice is to accept and welcome the stress, pain, anger, frustration, disappointment, and insecurity when those feelings are present. Kabat-Zinn believes that acknowledgment is paramount. Whether pleasant or unpleasant, admission is the first step toward transforming that reality. Kabat-Zinn founded the Stress Reduction Clinic at the University of Massachusetts Medical Center in Worcester, where he is an associate professor of medicine. Established in 1995, the Center for Mindfulness in Medicine is an outgrowth of the clinic. Since the clinic was founded, thousands of medical patients have gone through his mindfulness meditation programs, almost all referred by their physicians. The Center for Mindfulness has published dozens of research studies on mindfulness-based stress reduction (MBSR). Unlike standard medical and psychological approaches, the clinic does not categorize and treat patients differently depending on their illnesses. Their 8-week course offer the same training program in mindfulness and stress reduction to everyone. They emphasize what is "right" with their patients, rather than what is "wrong" with them, focusing on mobilizing their inner strengths and changing their behaviors in new and innovative ways. Facilitators maintain that their programs are not held out as some kind of magical cure when other approaches failed; rather, they provide a sensible and straightforward way for people to experience and understand the mind-body connection firsthand, using that knowledge to better cope with their illnesses.

In the practice of mindfulness the patient begins by using one-pointed attention to cultivate calmness and stability. When thoughts and feelings arise, it is important not to ignore or suppress them or analyze or judge them by their content; rather, the thoughts are observed intentionally and nonjudgmentally, moment by moment, as events in the field of awareness. This inclusive noting of thoughts that come and go in the mind can lead to a detachment from them, allowing a deeper perspective about the stresses of life to emerge. By observing the thoughts from this vantage point, one gains a new frame of reference. In this way, valuable insight can be allowed to surface. The key to mindfulness is not the particular topic of attention but the quality of awareness brought into each moment. Observing the thought processes, without intellectualizing them and without judgment, creates greater clarity. The goal of mindfulness is to become more aware, more in touch with life and its happenings at the time it is actually happening in the present. Acceptance does not mean passivity or resignation. Accepting what each moment offers provides the opportunity to experience life more completely. In this manner any situation can be handled with greater confidence and clarity. One way to envision how mindfulness works is to think of the mind as the surface of a lake or ocean. Many people think the goal of meditation is to stop the waves so that the water will be flat, peaceful, and tranquil. The spirit of mindfulness practice is to experience the waves.

HEALTH BENEFITS

The consistent practice of mindfulness meditation has been shown to decrease the subjective experience of pain and stress in a variety of research settings. A 65% improvement in pain symptoms and an approximate 60% improvement in sleep and fatigue levels occurred from before to after meditation in a 77 patients with fibromyalgia. Another study used electroencephalographic (EEG) recordings to differentiate between two types of meditation, concentration and mindfulness, and a normal relaxation control condition. They found significant differences between readings at numerous cortical sites, suggesting that concentration and mindfulness meditations may be unique forms of consciousness and not merely degrees of a state of relaxation. In a study using mindfulness of movement as a coping strategy for multiple sclerosis, patients attended six individual one-on-one sessions of mindfulness training and balance improved significantly.

Eighty cancer patients were followed up for 6 months after attending a mindfulness meditation group for 1.5 hours each week for 7 weeks. They were also asked to practice meditation at home on a daily basis. Results showed significantly lower mood disturbances and fewer symptoms of stress at the 6-month follow-up for both male and female patients. However, the greatest improvement occurred on subscales measuring depression, anxiety, and anger. Results of various mindfulness meditation techniques are consistent with other meditation-based interventions.

Nurses are often known to make mindfulness practice part of their continuing education. They find that this technique often prevents compassion fatigue and burnout, enhances health, and increases awareness of holism within the self.

Mindfulness Therapy for Pain

For most patients who suffer from some form of chronic pain condition, their symptoms cannot be explained by well-defined medical or surgical conditions. Pain conditions characterized by such symptoms have been termed *bodily distress syndrome* (BDS). The presence of BDS requires the presence of functional somatic symptoms from at least three out of four bodily systems: the cardiopulmonary, gastrointestinal, musculoskeletal, or general symptoms, in addition to moderate-to-severe impairment in daily living, of at least 6 months of duration. The BDS classification was developed from empirical research and may provide a unifying basis for functional somatic syndromes, such as fibromyalgia, chronic fatigue syndrome, irritable bowel syndrome, and chronic whiplash and somatization disorder (Fink & Schroder, 2010). These conditions belong to the same family of disorders, and BDS may be useful as a nonstigmatizing designation for this group of closely related conditions that are currently divided and haphazardly distributed among medical and psychiatric disorders.

In clinical applications of mindfulness therapy, primarily in the context of chronic pain, co-occurrence of negative affect and pain is well recognized. An impaired ability to evaluate and categorize painful sensations could indicate a deficiency in the cognitive regulation of pain perception in patients suffering from chronic pain. This dysfunction may be due to changes in the parietal and prefrontal brain cortices, areas that sustained mindfulness training may improve (Hölzel et al., 2008). Impairments of sensory processing may also lead to repetitive overloading, which may in turn lead to fear of movement and unhealthy coping strategies. Patients often describe that they alternate between trying to ignore, being completely overwhelmed, or incapacitated by the pain and other somatic symptoms. Patients often describe an inability to detect and react to bodily sensations as a state of stress in the body of which they are not able to maintain awareness. Mindfulness training may improve stress and emotional regulation and train patients to notice when bodily sensations, thoughts, and emotions arise, as well as helping them to embrace these sensations with friendly, nonjudgmental awareness. Mindfulness training may enable one to better notice the selective mental processes or automatic filtering processes that regulate the flow of energy and information, and awareness.

A new study demonstrated that MBSR was effective in reducing pain and improving quality of life in patients with chronic low back pain after only eight sessions (the standard approach to group MBSR; Banth & Ardebil, 2015). Of course, anxiety and depression often accompany chronic pain. A group of chronic pain patients who completed the Mindfulness Meditation Training Program demonstrated significant improvement in anxiety, depression, pain, and global impression of positive results during a 1-year observation period (Rod, 2015). The standard MBSR program, which is evaluated in research studies, consists of eight weekly sessions. However, one can gain many of the benefits of meditation in daily life without signing up for formal classes (or even entering a Buddhist Monastery). Micozzi's book, *New World Mindfulness,* from Inner Traditions/ Healing Arts Press and co-author Don McCown provides practical guidance for patients to achieve mindfulness every day in the middle of their busy lives (McCown & Micozzi, 2012).

MINDFUL MENTAL PROCESSING OF PAIN

The ways in which patients perceive pain is an important factor in determining how they react. If they think "this pain is ruining my life," it may well do just that. Many people, not just chronic pain patients, speculate about situations or events that have gone wrong in their lives. Psychotherapy can examine new and old conflicts and the reasons why patients repeat the same undesirable reaction patterns. CBT works with the thoughts that lead to disability, low self-esteem, and disorder-driven behavior. When patients experience a high degree of pain and/or other symptoms, it may be difficult to find a cause, particularly in the case of chronic (idiopathic) pain. Symptoms may persist even when they learn to change their thought patterns and their behaviors. Mindfulness can be particularly helpful because it can increase acceptance of symptoms that are impossible or difficult to change.

Accepting life, just as it is right now, often involves approaching feelings of denial, anger, and sorrow. Patients may be deluded, thinking how great their lives were before the pain occurred, and/or dejected, thinking how they may never get better. There is no need to turn these internal conversations into a debate. The role of the mindfulness teacher is to listen and offer connection. The mindfulness teacher also has to care for the entire group and may need to schedule an individual meeting. When the connection is sufficiently strong and the time is right, it may become useful to start questioning such delusions or dejection, and often mindfulness participants actually begin to accomplish that questioning by themselves. Such insights often come with practice. Many patients have misconceptions about pain and physical symptoms that interfere with healing and can lead to destructive behaviors. Mindfulness keeps asking about their thoughts, feelings, and behavior related to the symptoms. It takes a "friendly," accepting approach to noticing symptoms and to viewing ideas about pain as just passing thoughts, not permanent truths. Attempting to divide symptoms into physical and psychological categories is an obsolete approach, as we see in the chapters of this section. Intensity of pain also varies over time. Negative thinking makes pain worse (e.g., catastrophizing pain and thinking it will never get better or thinking it will definitely get worse from now on). The mind cannot concentrate for an indefinitely long period of time, nor can it concentrate on pain all the time. If one really focuses attention and concentration on the pain, the attention moves nonetheless, just as it does when one tries to keep the concentration focused on breathing. It may help patients to place a hand where it hurts and have them say to themselves, "I'm taking care of this."

The mind is inherently critical and judgmental. Negative thinking affects the body. We are all prone to negative thinking when tired, sad, or experiencing pain and other symptoms. If a person has offended us, the mind has already prepared a long series of thoughts about how terrible it all is. A tone of voice, a movement, and we are in pain. It does not take much for the mind to have a whole narrative story or "novel" ready. Becoming conscious of the negative thoughts that are influencing and even controlling one's life is an important step toward improving one's well-being. The most difficult part of mindfulness may be the practice of not taking thoughts too seriously. We are used to "existing" in our thoughts, and frequently we do not discover the other, bigger, and more interesting reality. When life is difficult, it is almost second nature to think that "something is wrong." We often run into self-blame when we feel lonely, sad, ashamed, or angry. Pain and suffering become amplified when thinking goes off onto such a track, and pain or other difficulties are experienced as a personal failure. The task is to guide patients to take responsibility for the original pain, to allow them to feel it—and then to let it pass. They need to work on their tendencies either to ignore or to amplify the pain.

OPEN AND SHUT EXPERIENCES OF MINDFULNESS

During meditation, people may discover emotions, thoughts, or tensions previously unknown to them. Patients should be instructed not to try to explain to themselves why a certain feeling overwhelms them. Many people believe they have to find an explanation for their emotions or tensions. That attitude will frequently only trigger even more thoughts. As with all experiences in mindfulness, negative feelings and sensations should be seen, held, and acknowledged. Through mindfulness, patients can practice not holding on and not fueling pain with the added burdens of fear, anger, and sadness. Instead, practice letting the feeling pass. Practice letting go.

At certain points, most people feel the need to shut out the world. Reality can be so hard that patients cannot afford to confront it. It can be difficult to endure when we or loved ones face difficulties. The technique of "shutting out" is as old or older than the technique of opening up. When meditating, practice imagining awareness as a door that can be opened or closed. Instruct patients to work on their limits and to keep the hinges well lubricated. The door should not be held wide open all the time. Each person needs to feel when enough is enough and when to close the door again. The task is to be awake the whole time and conscious when opening and closing the door. Chronic pain patients often catastrophize about their conditions; for example, thinking that pain will definitely get worse, that it will never end, or that there is nothing they can do to reduce pain. It may be useful to examine and ultimately challenge such thoughts to break the vicious cycle. A patient was once given a letter and was told she could open the letter only when very sad or very happy. She opened the letter when she was very sad, and the letter said, "It won't last." The only thing that is constant is change.

What Mindfulness Practice Brings to Pain Treatment

Chronic pain patients have typically experienced and undergone the travails of various treatments through the mainstream health care system and through alternative treatments. The word mindfulness implies to "remember." Remembering the body, the mind (intelligence), and the heart (kindness) forms a triad that seems obvious and trivial. Teaching how to feel whole, physically present, mentally clear, and emotionally balanced may indeed be integral parts of treatment. Because pain patients start with a problem in the body, learning how to be present in the body, instead of trying to escape from it, is a very practical and useful skill of mindfulness. Medical assessment is also important to ensure that the patients receive the right diagnosis as the basis for the right treatment(s). Mindfulness may very well be the right treatment when the body is distressed and/or in pain to a level where the person is no longer functioning. Chronic pain patients are suffering, and mindfulness entails working with the very stress and pain that cause the suffering. For many chronic pain patients, the physical suffering is so omnipresent that it cannot be ignored. When pain patients enter the clinic, they often have a therapeutic expectation looking to have their body "fixed," rather than examine what it means for them to be suffering and to work with this reality. Tools typically offered by mainstream medicine, including psychiatry, are intended to "fix" or attack the symptoms, not to release suffering or promote well-being. Treatment includes helping patients to recognize that pain is a multidimensional and complex phenomenon. The brain can produce a conscious experience of pain so vivid and intense that patients feel certain that "something is seriously wrong with me." Even intense and disabling pain experiences may not be due to physical injuries. Patients should be reassured that pain is a very common human phenomenon, not an indication or further verification of their own judgments of themselves as someone in whom there is "something wrong." Chronic pain patients need to work with other aspects of their pain experiences, in particular with their relationships to the pain. This step is where mindfulness practice can be a particularly good tool in their daily battles with pain. How to engage individuals with chronic pain conditions in the work of observing and embracing a painful and/or fatigued body; how to inspire them to use what is now known from modern medical science; and how to engage in their everyday lives is an ever evolving process are all goals in which mindfulness can make real contributions.

WHAT MINDFULNESS PRACTITIONERS BRING TO PAIN TREATMENT

Practitioners must also bring certain attributes and qualities to mindfulness practice. Mindfulness work is all about "relationality"—relationship to the patients, to what they share or do, and to your own practice. It is ultimately about facilitating a change in patients' relationships to themselves and to the issues with which they are struggling. Success as a mindfulness practitioner also depends on the ability to trust the practice, patient, and group. Practitioners cannot assume they know what it is like to be in pain, fatigued, and anxious all the time. In case one does know, they still do not know what it is like for the particular patients they are teaching. But you do not have to know. What you have to do is engage with the patients, give safe directions, and know what is called for moment by moment.

Mindfulness teachers may think they can know who is "getting it" and who is not during meditation group practices. They may locate the wisdom, desire, and trouble within different participants in the group. It is important to remind oneself that in actuality, we cannot know in the beginning. Sometimes people that we think are easy to move seem stuck. We never know. During the first class or two, participants sometimes consider the teaching unclear, and as a teacher, you may therefore spend a lot of effort trying to refine your points. As discussed earlier, words can be extremely influential in modulating pain within clinical settings. They are part of the psychosocial context surrounding the treatment and hence constitute a key factor in practitioner-patient relationships. Naturally, practitioner-patient communication includes nonverbal cues, such as body language, eye contact, and tone. Indeed, all of these "nonspecific" factors are likely to contribute to clinical outcomes. Further studies of the role of language and psychosocial factors in mindfulness therapy are warranted. Meantime, the essential ingredient remains the ability to engage people. The only way to accomplish this engagement is by being genuine to yourself and patients. Being in a meditation group is a real privilege and pleasure. Do not push, do not pretend, and do not be afraid. Be still, listen, learn, and trust that something much larger than yourself will take care of the process. Teachers must take good care of their own practices too and learn from their patients.

DOSE AND SCHEDULE

Many MBSR participants say they do not experience any difference during the first weeks. However, by the end of an 8-week course, they are surprised to find that they have either completely stopped or are using considerably less pain medications. Practicing mindfulness daily involves learning to focus on and examine their pain in a friendly and nonjudgmental way. Most patients find that the sensation of pain tends to move or change in quality and/or intensity over time. This experience is worth directly examining with patients throughout the course of mindfulness sessions because this perspective helps them to recognize that pain is not "a constant." It allows patients to acknowledge and experience that pain is dependent on several factors and thus becomes manageable—at least to some degree and at least in some moments. The context in which pain occurs changes pain processing and experience. The patients should try to examine their thoughts and feelings that surround their actual sensations of pain. Your patients may discover that pain is much more than just the physical sensation of pain. In addition, they can learn to experience pain as "just pain" without its surplus burdens. Potentially such practices may alter the patient's appraisal of the pain and facilitate more adaptive coping, as discussed earlier.

Managing Pain and Recovery

Pain management and rehabilitation following stress and chronic pain follow the same principles as rehabilitation after a broken limb or a sports injury. Correct and regular rehabilitation results in fewer complications and fewer relapses. Breaking from rehabilitation principles (forcing rehabilitation and ignoring warning signs) results in an irregular process, with large oscillations in outcome, which often prevent patients from becoming well. Life consists of good days and bad days. Many people are not conscious, when they are facing pain or illness, that their moods still continue to swing down and up, just at lower levels. Often when pain patients are in a better mood, they think they better get going and go out and do something. However, they can overstrain themselves, end up feeling even worse, and may have started over a vicious cycle. The appropriate alternative is for patients to mindfully examine how bad they feel on bad days and to accept it, then slowly practice their way up from there, one step at a time, like slowly but deliberately climbing a staircase.

Mindfulness practice offers great insights into how we are feeling (including feeling pain) and into the ways we are living our lives. Any undesirable pattern of behavior can be difficult to change. Every day and every moment offer an opportunity to change. Will we continue along the same lines or will we try something new? Every single moment can be a new beginning. Meditative and mindfulness therapies may help show the way.

REFERENCES

Banth, S. & Ardebil, M. D. (2015). Effectiveness of mindfulness meditation on pain and quality of life of patients with chronic low back pain. *International Journal of Yoga, 8*(2), 128–133.

Benedetti, F. (2009). *Placebo effects: Understanding the mechanisms in health and disease.* Oxford, New York: Oxford University Press.

Benedetti, F., Carlino, E., & Pollo, A. (2011). How placebos change the patient's brain. *Neuropsychopharmacology: Official Publication of the American College of Neuropsychopharmacology, 36,* 339–354.

Benedetti, F., Mayberg, H. S., Wager, T. D., Stohler, C. S., & Zubieta, J. K. (2005). Neurobiological mechanisms of the placebo effect. *Journal of Neuroscience: The Official Journal of the Society for Neuroscience, 25*, 10390–10402.

Buhle, J. & Wager, T. D. (2010). Performance-dependent inhibition of pain by an executive working memory task. *Pain, 149*, 19–26.

Colloca, L. & Finniss, D. (2012). Nocebo effects, patient-clinician communication, and therapeutic outcomes. *JAMA, 307*, 567–568.

Descartes, R. & Timmermans, B. (1649/2010). *Les passions de l'âme* (Réimpression ed.). Paris: LGF.

Fink, P. & Schroder, A. (2010). One single diagnosis, bodily distress syndrome, succeeded to capture ten diagnostic categories of functional somatic syndromes and somatoform disorders. *Journal of Psychosomatic Research, 68*, 415–426.

Folkman, S. & Lazarus, R. S. (1988). The relationship between coping and emotion: Implications for theory and research. *Social Science and Medicine, 26*, 309–317.

Gauthier, N., Thibault, P., & Sullivan, M. J. (2011). Catastrophizers with chronic pain display more pain behaviour when in a relationship with a low catastrophizing spouse. *Pain Research & Management: The Journal of the Canadian Pain Society, 16*, 293–299.

Gormsen, L., Rosenberg, R., Bach, F. W., & Jensen, T. S. (2010). Depression, anxiety, health-related quality of life and pain in patients with chronic fibromyalgia and neuropathic pain. *European Journal of Pain, 14*(127), e121–e128.

Hölzel, B. K., Ott, U., Gard, T., Hempel, H., Weygandt, M., Morgen, K., et al. (2008). Investigation of mindfulness meditation practitioners with voxel-based morphometry. *Social Cognitive and Affective Neuroscience, 3*, 55–61.

Hudson, J. I., Goldenberg, D. L., Pope, H. G., Jr., Keck, P. E., Jr., & Schlesinger, L. (1992). Comorbidity of fibromyalgia with medical and psychiatric disorders. *The American Journal of Medicine, 92*, 363–367.

IASP. (1994). Classification of chronic pain. Descriptions of chronic pain syndromes and definitions of pain terms (Taskforce). (2nd ed.). Seattle, WA: IASP Press.

Jegindø, E. E. (2012). *Pain and coping in the religious mind.* Aarhus, Denmark: Aarhus University.

Keefe, F. J., Brown, G. K., Wallston, K. A., & Caldwell, D. S. (1989). Coping with rheumatoid arthritis pain: Catastrophizing as a maladaptive strategy. *Pain, 37*, 51–56.

Legrain, V., Iannetti, G. D., Plaghki, L., & Mouraux, A. (2011). The pain matrix reloaded: A salience detection system for the body. *Progress in Neurobiology, 93*, 111–124.

Levine, J. D., Gordon, N. C., & Fields, H. L. (1978). The mechanism of placebo analgesia. *Lancet, 2*, 654–657.

Levine, J. D., Gordon, N. C., Smith, R., & Fields, H. L. (1981). Analgesic responses to morphine and placebo in individuals with postoperative pain. *Pain, 10*, 379–389.

Logan, H., Lutgendorf, S., Rainville, P., Sheffield, D., Iverson, K., & Lubaroff, D. (2001). Effects of stress and relaxation on capsaicin-induced pain. *The Journal of Pain: Official Journal of the American Pain Society, 2*, 160–170.

McCown, D. & Micozzi, M. S. (2012). *New world mindfulness.* Rochester, VT: Inner Traditions.

McCown, D., Reibel, D., & Micozzi, M. S. (2017). *Teaching mindfulness.* (2nd ed.). New York: Springer.

Meissner, K., Bingel, U., Colloca, L., Wager, T. D., Watson, A., & Flaten, M. A. (2011). The placebo effect: Advances from different methodological approaches. *The Journal of Neuroscience: The Official Journal of the Society for Neuroscience, 31*, 16117–16124.

Naylor, M. R., Naud, S., Keefe, F. J., & Helzer, J. E. (2010). *Therapeutic interactive voice response (TIVR) to reduce analgesic medication use for chronic pain management.* http://www.ncbi.nlm.nih.gov/pmc/articles/PMC3045626/.

Ochsner, K. N. & Gross, J. J. (2005). The cognitive control of emotion. *Trends in Cognitive Sciences, 9*, 242–249.

Price, D. D., Finniss, D. G., & Benedetti, F. (2008). A comprehensive review of the placebo effect: Recent advances and current thought. *Annual Review of Psychology, 59*, 565–590.

Rod, K. (2015). Observing the effects of mindfulness-based meditation on anxiety and depression in chronic pain patients. *Psychiatria Danubina, 27*(Suppl. 1), S209–S211.

Rodriguez-Raecke, R., Niemeier, A., Ihle, K., Ruether, W., & May, A. (2009). *Brain gray matter decrease in chronic pain is the consequence and not the cause of pain.* http://www.ncbi.nlm.nih.gov/pubmed/19889986.

Sullivan, M. J. L., Bishop, S. R., & Pivik, J. (1995). The pain catastrophizing scale: Development and validation. *Psychological Assessment, 7,* 524–532.

Sullivan, M. J., Stanish, W., Waite, H., Sullivan, M., & Tripp, D. A. (1998). Catastrophizing, pain, and disability in patients with soft-tissue injuries. *Pain, 77,* 253–260.

Suggested Readings can be found on the companion website, http://www.micozzipainconditions.com.

Chapter 6

Stress Management, Relaxation, and Biofeedback Therapies

The concept and term *stress* was brought into popular usage for health and medicine during the mid-20th century by Dr. Hans Selye, Director of the Institute of Experimental Medicine and Surgery at the University of Montreal, Quebec, Canada. He adapted and interpreted the term stress from mechanical engineering to human health as "the rate of wear and tear on the body." Different perspectives continue to be applied to the role of stress in health and medicine, whether stress is a factor or *the* factor causing wear and tear on the body, and whether it is the resulting damage. Selye described the physiologic stress response as the "general adaptation syndrome" (GAS), which implies that this response is, or once was, a normative biological mechanism for adapting or adjusting to short-term changes in the environment. GAS may be seen as an early phase of adaptation that occurs in the individual as we outline in Box 6.1.

GAS has three phases: an immediate *alarm* reaction, a phase of *resistance*, and a phase of *exhaustion*. A stress cause, or stressor, mobilizes GAS by activating the sympathetic portion of the autonomic nervous system (primarily based on the epinephrine or adrenalin hormones (see Fig. 4.1).

These hormones bring about physiological changes in the body, originally described as the "fight-or-flight response" (Szabo, Tache & Somogyi, 2012). Through these changes, emotional states may actually become embodied throughout one's being (Jawer & Micozzi, 2009).

THE PROBLEM OF STRESS

Stress with its various colloquial and medical meanings has continued to receive widespread publicity in the media over the years. We have also heard the cliché that "stress" was the epidemic of the 1980s, and then the 1990s, and now the 21st century. Back in 1979, futurist Alvin Toffler, in his book *Future Shock,* posited that humans had already reached their maximum capacity for tolerating change and stress. If Toffler was correct, we may need an entirely new term to describe the experiences of the 21st century thus far! Another dissonant development is that stress is almost ignored in medical practice and treatments while it preoccupies the concerns of the average patient. It has become apparent that stress is a cause of common medical

BOX 6.1 *Adaptation and Time Dimensions*

1. Individual adaptation
   A. Homeostatic (seconds to months)
      For example, at high altitude (low partial pressure oxygen), increase respiratory rate in seconds; increase hematocrit and red blood cell count over weeks; "thicken" blood.
   B. Ontogenetic (during the growth period)
      For example, at high altitude, increase lung capacity during growth and development; over a lifetime.
2. Population adaptation
   A. Cultural
      Environmental determinism posits that environmental factors influence cultural practices (decades to centuries).
      For example, chewing of coca leaf at high altitude to prevent "thicker" blood from clotting.
   B. Genetic adaptation to environment
      Shifts in gene frequency (thousands to millions of years), such as hemoglobin polymorphisms, lactose tolerance, phenylthiocarbamide (PTC) taste sensitivity (ability to taste bitter compounds from plants).
   C. Genetic adaption to cultural/agricultural practices
      With exposure to agriculture and animal domestication: gluten sensitivity, lactose tolerance/intolerance, "thrifty" gene, metabolic syndrome.
      Cultural adaptions occur more quickly than genetic adaptions and can fill the gap in time for human populations, allowing them to adapt more rapidly and ultimately be more successful in their environments.

conditions such as high blood pressure (BP), and common chronic diseases such as cardiovascular diseases, diabetes, and many cancers. But the academic-government-industrial medical complex continues to talk about myths such as cholesterol, saturated fats, and salt as the "causes" of chronic diseases, although there has never been any real evidence to support them.

Meanwhile, stress has become a buzzword that has acquired a highly negative connotation. While the mainstream medical establishment has been slow to catch on, we have nonetheless been the recipients of much advice over many years from management consultants, New Age gurus, "natural-know-it-alls," "Johnny-come-lately" physicians, and many other sources, about different approaches to controlling stress. All the alarmist and negative publicity has stimulated further anxiety and concern in many people's minds—a fear of stress itself, which cybernetically leads to more stress. Having been made aware, everyone now wants to manage stress, and many (perhaps too many) cater to this growing market. This rapidly growing industry consists of various self-styled experts, consultants, and therapists. Vitamin regimens, herbal supplements, energy beverages, fitness programs, relaxation techniques, "life coaching" (put me in, coach), and personal development courses are all being offered in the quest for stress management.

All sorts of experts, both those with no or limited health qualifications, and those who are self-appointed, are convinced that their particular product or service can banish stress for good. In the land of the blind, the one-eyed man is king. Part of the problem is that so-called experts have been working without complete knowledge or understanding of what we have called the "spiritual anatomy of emotion," which lies at the heart of the experience of stress, for good or ill (Jawer & Micozzi, 2009). The fact remains that there are no magic cures and no silver bullets. Malign stress is essentially a result of interactions among a negative environment, unhealthful lifestyles, and self-defeating attitudes and beliefs. Therefore, contrary to the beliefs of the stress management consultants, no one particular technique, method, program, or regimen of vitamins or herbs can eliminate long-term stress for everyone equally effectively. For guidance on how to match the right stress reduction approaches to the right patients, please see the interactive tools provided in Appendix I, pp. 572–579.

A growing movement, in part due to its simplicity, and in light of its effectiveness, is "Mindfulness-Based" meditation, and mindfulness-based stress reduction (MBSR) among the mindfulness-based interventions (MBI) (McCown & Micozzi, 2017). There is a large, rapidly growing international program of practices, teachers, and participants bringing wonderful new insights into how everyone can live *with* whatever stress exists in their lives. These mindfulness approaches are the single most effective and accessible approaches to stress management, as they can be practiced by everyone, everywhere (McCown & Micozzi, 2017).

WHAT CONSTITUTES STRESS

Stress is most often seen or perceived as outside pressures and problems that encroach on busy, demanding lives: deadlines, excessive work, noise, traffic, pollution, problems with family or friends, and allowing excessive demands to be made by others. The limited time element is also crucial. Stress includes the unconscious response to such demands. Ultimately, stress is not just "those things out there," but rather what happens inside our minds and bodies as we react unconsciously to those situations or people that we experience as stressful. Normally, we experience some degree of stress in everything we do and everything that happens to us. Research shows that within reasonable limits, and depending upon psychometric character and personality types, some stress ("eustress," or positive stress) is helpful in bringing about adaptive changes in the way our minds and bodies work.

In addition to the immediate and short-term effects, stress may also have an adaptive value in the individual during the ontogenetic growth period (see Box 6.1). Joseph Chilton Pearce wrote, "Stress is the way intelligence grows" (Pearce, 1992). He explains that, under stress, the brain immediately grows massive numbers of new connecting links among brain neurons that enable learning. While the stressed-adapted mind/brain grows in ability and the unstressed mind lags behind, the overstressed mind/brain can collapse into physiological shock. Essential to this balance and to maintaining an optimal level of stress is *relaxation*.

Measuring Stress

Part of the problem of coming to terms with stress in medical practice has been the unavailability or neglect of tools for measuring stress. When the stress response is minor, we may not notice any symptoms. The greater the stimulation, the more symptoms we notice. From the 1960s, Holmes and Rahe's scale of life changes provided a guide to the amount of stress that may be attached to major life events, such as marriage, relocation, emigration, loss of a job, death of a spouse, or birth of a child. These significant life events, whether we judge them as positive, negative, or neutral, can quickly overload our ability to cope. In *The Human Zoo*, Desmond Morris wrote in 1995 that modern humans are engaged in the "Stimulus Struggle": "If we abandon it, or tackle it badly, we are in serious trouble." We are trying to maintain the optimal level of stimulation—not the maximum—but rather the level that is most beneficial, somewhere between understimulation and overstimulation.

Stress becomes a health problem when it reaches excessive levels, or when the demands exceed our ability to respond or to cope effectively. When we are under excessive, prolonged stress and no longer able to cope or adjust, the "stress" becomes "distress." Imbalances then develop that lead to stress-induced symptoms, illnesses, and diseases. The physical body "engine" begins to "rev" at high speed, totally absorbing restricted, unproductive energy. Over extended periods, this "wear and tear" begins to take its toll, and disorders and diseases creep into the body.

CHANGE AND CONTROLLING STRESS

One way we can learn to begin controlling responses to stress is by changing the way that we think. Stress management includes developing the ability to assert control over our behaviors. When we become aware of our ability to control attitudes and behaviors, we naturally begin to assert control over life situations that were once deemed stressful. It is not the stress itself that is harmful but our reactions that create havoc in the body, mind, and spirit.

The greatest stressor that most people experience daily is change. The only thing constant in life today is change. Challenges, frustrations, conflicting demands, and periodic losses, grievances, and suffering are among the many subconscious responses to change. These life events are inevitable and continually require adaption to new situations and circumstances. If you do not adapt to change by altering attitudes, then both mind and body may suffer. When changes take place in your environment, career, and personal relationships, it becomes essential to learn how to behave, think, and feel differently to cope effectively with new situations and circumstances.

We all continuously adjust to changing conditions, like a heating, ventilation, and air-conditioning system (HVAC) controlled by a thermostat. As the weather outside changes, the thermostat turns on the heater or air conditioner unit and turns it down or up, which begins to bring the interior temperature back to a specified normal level of comfort. The greater the changes outside, the harder the boiler, furnace, or air compressor has to work to keep up. If the external temperature moves into extreme ranges, the system will be pushed to the limit. If it exceeds its specified limits, it will eventually break down and burn out.

So too with the human body, which continuously reacts to whatever is happening around or inside it. You can respond physically, mentally, and emotionally to even the most minute changes. This process is occurring constantly, whether you are consciously aware of it or not.

SUBJECTIVITY, PERSONALITY, AND PSYCHOMETRIC TYPES

Stress is a very subjective condition. No two people respond to life's ups and downs in the same way. We know people who can remain cool, calm, and collected under the most trying circumstances, and we know others who are unable to cope when faced with even minor situations. The differences may result from different upbringings, past understandings, present experiences, attitudes, belief structures, family values, perceptions, and coping skills developed over years and generations, as well as youth and aging. For example, spending money shopping is extremely stressful for some people. For others, it is a joyful experience—and a way of actually adapting or responding to stress. A fighter pilot like Chuck Yeager can handle flying experimental aircraft traveling faster than the speed of sound without experiencing stress but is stressed when confined to a desk. A typical government bureaucrat (from the French word for desk, "bureau") builds a lifelong cushy comfort zone sitting in an office (what pilots call "desk jockeys") but would be stressed beyond belief behind the stick of an aircraft.

Some people have a higher stress tolerance than others. We know that Type A personalities are naturally "high-strung" and react strongly to stress. Type B personalities are more "easy-going" and can better tolerate more stress. Back in the 1950s, researchers found that these behavior patterns affect health. In fact, they found that Type A personalities are more likely to develop coronary heart disease than are Type B personalities.

We also now recognize there are Type C personalities. They actually deny their feelings of stress. Outwardly, they appear cool, relaxed, and totally in control of their surroundings and themselves. But by ignoring their stress, they wind up heightening their risk of developing all the major health problems mentioned above. (Of course, there is one other "type." The type of boss who says, "I don't get heart attacks, I give them.") All of this can make stress hard to pin down. We believe that the psychometric "personality boundary type" developed by the late Dr. Ernst Hartmann at Tufts University, Boston, Massachusetts, is the single best way to determine the disorders that stress may cause in you, and which mind-body therapies will work best for you in managing these stress-related disorders. Our simple psychometric profile can be found in Jawer and Micozzi (2015) and in Appendix I (pp. 572–579).

We also have a good tool for measuring stress as mentioned in the Life Change Index. This tool counts and scores major life changes that occur during the course of a lifetime and can be found online. A higher score, reflecting more major life changes, means running a greater risk of a heart attack and other diseases during the ensuing period. Interestingly, this index measures "major life changes," not just "negative life changes." The body experiences stress as stress. It does not distinguish between a wedding and a divorce or between a new job versus a layoff. We might interpret a given change as "good" or "bad," but our health does not.

But we also have another tool for diagnosing stress: our own feelings. Some people are very good at judging whether they feel stress. In fact, in a recent study in the United Kingdom, researchers simply asked men and women if they experienced high stress. If the subjects said yes, the researchers discovered that this response accurately predicted future heart health (Anderson et al., 2013).

Sometimes, when doctors or scientists struggle to measure or understand stress in people, they might just try asking them!

Overall, humans are largely creatures of habit. We do not respond well to change, positive or negative. Even the most unique characters among us are somewhat "wired" for conformity. For example, when you see someone laugh or smile, most of us tend to return the smile and sentiment. Or when your partner—or even your pet—yawns, chances are, you will too. So, naturally, when you work with stressed-out colleagues, you feel stress too.

YOUR BRAIN ON STRESS

This interconnectedness observed among humans is unique among large animals who live at the top of the food chain (along with canines). Humans typically work in groups or teams rather than alone. As social animals, human brains are biologically wired to relate to others, whether laughing, yawning, or panicking. Anxiety almost appears to spread like a virus. Crossover stress occurs between spouses and among coworkers, and stress can also spill over from the workplace to the home and vice versa.

According to the American Institute of Stress in New York, during the past decade, workplace stress led to $300 billion in annual health care costs as a result of missed work alone. During the same time period, the Organizational Science and Human Factors Branch of the National Institute for Occupational Safety and Health (NIOSH) claimed that stressed workers incurred health care costs nearly 50% higher, an average of $600 more per person, than other employees.

MIRRORING REALITY

The brain has "mirror neurons." These highly evolved brain cells react by mimicking the actions and emotions of others. Italian scientists (who would seem to have plenty of opportunity to observe such actions and emotions in everyday life) first identified mirror neurons in the 1990s. They learned about these special neurons while studying macaque monkeys. These specific groups of neurons in the brain light up whenever the monkeys perform, or even just observe, specific types of movements. Mirror neurons in monkeys and humans are located near motor neurons, so reflected behaviors directly affect movements, speech, and even emotions. It seems like the old saying "monkey see, monkey do" applies to humans too. This kind of mirror reflection is one reason why stress is highly contagious. Researchers have observed the contagious nature of stress for a long time, but now we understand something about how and why it happens.

Humans process stress in a core of the ancient "reptilian" brain. We cannot consciously control this part of the brain, and it simply cannot rationalize the stresses of the modern world. No wonder stress factors into five out of six of the leading causes of death. Even government agencies like the Centers for Disease Control and Prevention (CDC) now recognize that stress kills more people than traffic accidents or smoking—although the government is increasingly obsessed with antitobacco campaigns (while many are encouraging smoking of another dangerous plant, marijuana) while virtually ignoring the stress that is killing us. Of course, the real problem for more and more people is that the government itself is the biggest cause of stress in our lives (Box 6.2).

Effects of Distress and Treating Pain

When different individuals experience *distress,* the symptoms they develop are also different; different people appear to channel excessive stress into different parts of the body. The long-term effects of different responses include physical illnesses, such as *chronic backaches, headaches,* high BP, ulcers, or other chronic disorders. Decades of research have linked stress, either directly or indirectly, to coronary heart disease, cancer, strokes, lung ailments, accidental injuries, cirrhosis of the liver, immune system deficiencies, suicide, violence, and homicide. Stress is often a component of chronic illness, as a precursor of disease and/or as an outcome. People who manage stress are more resilient, experience fewer symptoms, and experience an improved quality of life.

BOX 6.2 *Stress Dump*

When someone dumps emotional stress on you, instead of latching onto it, take a step back and reframe the narrative to reality. Someone else's irrational stress is not your emergency. Use your more evolved rational brain instead of allowing your reptilian brain to call the shots. This approach can be equated to using logic over emotion. Logic can be associated with the prefrontal cortex where "executive functions" like planning and decision making also take place, whereas emotional responses can be found in the amygdala. The amygdala is associated with the processing of fear, negative emotions, emotional behaviors, and emotional responses.

Stress Management and Relaxation

Harvard cardiologist Herbert Benson began investigating the benefits of stress and relaxation in the late 1960s and continues to delve into the effects of stress on various disease-specific populations. Benson's group has examined the stress phenomenon and its effect on cardiovascular diseases and neurodegenerative diseases (Esch, Stefano, Fricchione, & Benson, 2002). They found that stress has a major impact on the circulatory and nervous systems, playing a significant role in susceptibility, progress, and outcome of both cardiovascular and neurodegenerative diseases. However, they also found that some amounts of stress (eustress) can actually improve performance and thus can be beneficial in certain cases.

Testing the effect of cognitive-behavioral techniques (including meditation; see Chapter 5) on hypertension, for example, no single technique appears to be more effective than any other in treating high BP or essential hypertension. But when prescribed in the absence of other behavioral interventions, cognitive-behavioral techniques were not as effective as standard antihypertensive pharmacotherapy. The key, of course, is matching the specific technique to the individual personality boundary type, or emotional type (see Appendix I, pp. 572–579). They all have the potential to work when properly matched, while none may work well, or work at all, if matched to the wrong person.

A new study from Sweden adds another illness to the list, and it is not one you might normally consider. Sweden, which generally has good health care and high-quality medical research, conducted a study on how stress affects women's health and considered factors like divorce, life strain, and health issues involving family matters. Researchers in Sweden can sometimes include the entire population of the country in their studies. Although the national population is nowhere near the size of the United States, when they include everyone in the country, it makes for a large, high-quality study. This particular recent study did not actually take into account the entire population of Sweden, but it did include 800 middle-aged women (a good-sized sample) over a period of 4 decades. The study found that the cognitive effects of stressful events are not short lived. In fact, stress in middle age makes a person more susceptible to developing to chronic dementia or Alzheimer's disease decades later. It is possible that chronic stress, through its effects on certain hormones, can change the workings of brain circuitry. That, in turn, may leave people more susceptible to the impact of Alzheimer's-type brain changes at older ages (Johansson et al., 2013). Of course, cognitive processing is a major factor in managing pain.

Relaxation Response

Initially believing that benefits of meditation and relaxation could potentially lower high BP, which reacts quickly to stress, Benson researched a variety of psychological and physiological effects that appear common to many mind and body practices. In the 1970s, he first identified the relaxation response, which elicited a similar response common to meditation, prayer, autogenic training, and some forms of hypnosis (see Chapter 7). His research indicated that excessive stress could cause or aggravate hypertension and its related pathologic outcomes, including atherosclerosis, heart attack, and stroke. He then examined the nature of the relaxation response, showing that physiological changes as remarkable as those seen in the "fight-or-flight" response also occur during true relaxation, including lowering of oxygen consumption, metabolism, heart rate, and BP, as well as increased production of alpha brain waves. A marked decrease in blood lactate was also found. Blood lactate has often been linked with anxiety.

BENSON RELAXATION RESPONSE

According to Benson, following these guidelines can help patients achieve the relaxation response:

Do Try This at Home
1. Try to find 10 to 20 min in daily routine; before breakfast is generally a good time.
2. Sit comfortably.
3. For the period of practice, try to arrange things to have no distractions (i.e., turn on the answering machine, turn phone to "silent" or to airplane mode, ask someone to watch the children).
4. Time by glancing periodically at a clock or watch (but do not set an alarm). Commit to a specific length of practice.

Expanding on these guidelines, several approaches can be used to elicit the relaxation response; Benson suggests the following:

Step 1: Pick a focus word or short phrase that is firmly rooted in a personal belief system. For example, a nonreligious individual might choose a neutral word such as "one," "peace," or "love." A Christian person wanting to use a prayer could pick the opening words of Psalm 23, "The Lord is My Shepherd"; a Jewish person could choose "Shalom."

Step 2: Sit quietly in a comfortable position.

Step 3: Close eyes.

Step 4: Relax muscles.

Step 5: Breathe slowly and naturally, repeating focus word or phrase silently with exhalations

Step 6: Throughout, assume a passive attitude. Do not worry about how well it is going. When other thoughts come to mind, simply state, "Oh, well," and gently return to the repetition.

Step 7: Continue for 10 to 20 min. Open eyes to check the time, but do not use an alarm. When finished, sit quietly for a minute or so, at first with eyes closed and later with eyes open. Then do not stand for 1 or 2 min.

Step 8: Practice the technique once or twice a day.

Benson's subsequent research into the relaxation response covered several efficient techniques of relaxation training, including transcendental meditation, Zen and yoga, autogenic training, progressive relaxation, hypnosis, and sentic cycles (Table 6.1). He found that these methods had four common elements: a quiet environment, an object to focus the mind, a passive attitude, and a comfortable position. Some practices are more effective than others, and some are easier to learn and practice than others (Benson, 1993).

TABLE 6.1 *Relaxation Response*

Technique	Oxygen Consumption	Respiratory Rate	Heart Rate	Alpha Waves	Blood Pressure	Muscle Tension
Transcendental meditation	Decreases	Decreases	Decreases	Increase	Decreases*	(Not measured)
Zen and yoga	Decreases	Decreases	Decreases	Increase	Decreases*	—
Autogenic training	(Not measured)	Decreases	Decreases	Increase	Inconclusive	Decreases
Progressive relaxation	(Not measured)	(Not measured)	(Not measured)	(Not measured)	Inconclusive	Decreases
Hypnosis with suggested deep relaxation	Decreases	Decreases	Decreases	(Not measured)	Inconclusive	(Not measured)

*In patients with elevated blood pressure.

TREATING PAIN, INFLAMMATION, AND RELATED CONDITIONS

Benson's group also found that patients with chronic pain who meditated regularly had a net reduction in general health care costs, suggesting that the effects of relaxation techniques are cost-effective. Drug-resistant epileptic patients who practiced Benson's relaxation response for 20 minutes each day experienced decreased frequency of seizures, increasingly significant between 6 and 12 months of continued practice. Duration of seizures also declined over the 12 months. The value of Benson's technique for patients with heart failure was evidenced in a study in nearly 60 veterans who received relaxation response training. Approximately half the group reported physical improvements that went beyond disease management and into pain, lifestyle changes, and improved relationships.

Dr. Benson and his team of researchers have recently discovered that relaxation actually causes the genes in cells to switch to a different mode (Pakhomova, Gregory, Semenov, & Pakhomov, 2013). In other words, relaxing or meditating can regulate genes to kick in to counteract the toxic effects of stress. (This effect may finally explain the long-observed profound control that experienced yogis develop over all their vital functions, for example; see Chapter 18.) The researchers noted four specific types of gene responses. The first involved genes related to mitochondria, which generate energy and water for all cells. This response resulted in better mood, energy, and sleep in the subjects who meditated. The second gene response was seen in genes linked to insulin. This effect also boosts energy in the cells by regulating all-important blood sugar metabolism. So responses one and two together influence the most basic energy processes of the body: oxygen and water through cellular respiration in the mitochondria, and carbohydrate metabolism for utilization of calories.

Third, the researchers found that people who meditated had less activity in genes that turn on the inflammatory response. In other words, their immune systems were better modulated, or balanced. An unbalanced immune system and chronic inflammation may very well be a primary cause of persistent chronic problems such as heart disease and cancer. Finally, meditation also influenced genes related to telomeres in cells. Telomeres cap off the ends of chromosomes and protect the genetic material (DNA) of cells in nuclei, especially during cell division and multiplication. Normally, cells continually divide and multiply to replace older, worn-out cells with newer, healthy cells. This factor means they are directly related to longevity. Meditation can extend life span (as has been well observed in the aforesaid yogis, or meditators, for over a century).

And just 10 to 20 minutes per day can have profound benefits.

EXERCISE FOR STRESS REDUCTION

Michael Sacks, MD, professor of psychiatry at Cornell University Medical College, originally found that various forms of exercise can be powerful methods of relaxation effective for dealing with the stress of daily life. Researchers have found in various studies that exercise can decrease anxiety and depression, improve an individual's self-image, and buffer people from the effects of stress. Not every study has shown the precise benefits researchers were seeking, but taken as a whole, the research strongly supports the common experience that exercise can elevate mood and *reduce anxiety and stress* (Sacks, 1993).

Although most research has largely focused on the physical benefits of exercise, any exercise can help people feel more focused and relaxed as long as the activity is enjoyable to them. Regular exercise does seem to affect one aspect in particular: the ability to withstand stress. Exercise and physical fitness can act as a buffer against stress so that stressful events have a less negative impact on psychological and physical health.

BIOFEEDBACK THERAPIES

Biofeedback (BF) therapies emerged in the 1960s and 1970s, when advances in psychological and medical research converged with developments in biomedical technology. Improved electronic instruments could convey information to patients about their nervous systems and their muscles in the form of audio and visual signals that patients could understand. The term BF became the general term to define the procedures and treatments that make use of these instruments as articulated in the book *Beyond Biofeedback* (Green & Green, 1977). The very same year that Elmer Green and his wife published this seminal book, Micozzi met them in Laguna de Bay, Luzon, Philippines, at a special World Health Organization (WHO) conference on Filipino Faith Healers. Micozzi had just traveled to Southeast Asia under a Henry Luce Foundation Fellowship and was literally blown off course by a typhoon and delayed in his journey. Micozzi ended up at this conference, sponsored by the Caliraya Foundation as his first introduction to mind-body healing. Also present was Alan Landsberg, producer of a new television series called *In Search Of,* hosted by the late Leonard Nimoy (Mr. Spock on *Star Trek*). Micozzi realized this topic was of great popular interest and pushed the boundaries of our concepts of health and healing.

BF therapy uses special instruments, devices, and methods to expand the body's natural internal feedback systems. By observing a monitoring device, patients can learn by trial and error to adjust their thinking and other mental processes to control bodily processes previously once thought to be entirely involuntary, such as BP, temperature, gastrointestinal functioning, and brain wave activity. Of course, Indian yogis have been demonstrating that so-called involuntary physiologic processes are subject to voluntary control (see Chapter 18).

BF can be used on almost any bodily process that can be measured accurately. BF-assisted relaxation training is associated with decreased medical care costs, decreased numbers of claims and costs to insurers in claims payments, reduction in medication and physician use, reduction in hospital stays and rehospitalization, reduction of mortality and morbidity, and enhanced quality of life.

BF is more useful for some clinical problems than for others, and for some individuals depending upon their mind-body psychometric type, as we discovered and presented in our book, *Your Emotional Type: Inner Traditions* (Jawer & Micozzi, 2012). It has also become an integral part of the treatment of many disorders, including anxiety, asthma, *headaches*, and *muscle pain* disorders.

BF can be successful in helping patients learn to regulate many physical conditions by putting them in better contact with specific parts of their bodies.

THE PATIENT IS IN CONTROL

The general goal of BF therapy is to lower body tension and change negative biological patterns, which we find are related to emotional type boundaries, to reduce symptoms. While many people can and do reach goals of relaxation without the use of BF, and BF may not be necessary, it can usually still add something useful to any treatment. A major reason why many patients find BF training appealing is that, as with behavioral approaches in general, it puts the patient in charge, giving each individual a sense of mastery and self-reliance over their illness. Such an attitude can play a critical role in shortening recovery time, reducing disease incidence, and lowering health care costs for almost any medical condition. In terms of psychometric evaluation, many patients with "thick" boundaries find that getting real data and information back from their bodies helps them make their problem (and treatment) more concrete and realize it is not "all in your head" (see Appendix I, pp. 572–579).

HOW BIOFEEDBACK WORKS FOR PAIN

BF is a mind-body therapy based on classic behavioral psychology operant learning. Reflexes are developed to respond to stimuli, through feedback, in ways that are helpful and healthy in responding to stress. A BF client receives information about his or her specific physiological function(s) and, with practice, through simple empirical trial and error, learns to control responses to stress. BF requires monitoring and displaying accurate and meaningful information from a body site in an easily read and recognizable form. "Correct" or desired responses and reactions are reinforced by sound or visual feedback, facilitating learning. With the guidance of a health practitioner and regular practice, the client can repeatedly and reliably control one or more physiologic responses.

For example, *headache, muscle pain,* and *tension* may be measured with surface sensors from the forehead. The output is converted to visual or auditory signals that are made available to the patient, such as a sound that fluctuates depending on the level of tension. Being able to observe and learn which muscles are tense or relaxed allows the patient to voluntarily respond to self-regulate these physiological processes. Undesirable internal states are associated with increased levels of sound or light. Reinforcement of desirable internal states is provided for desired responses, such as relaxed muscles (Box 6.3).

BOX 6.3 *Factors Involved in Biofeedback Approaches*

1. A monitoring instrument is utilized.
2. The person observes and receives information.
3. Desired responses are reinforced (operant conditioning).
4. Repetition is necessary for optimal results.

There are three broad categories of BF treatment:

1. Stress reduction in which lower arousal is reinforced.
2. Muscle retraining, in conditions where muscle tone is lower than desired.
3. Brain wave training, for disorders in which electroencephalogram (EEG) patterns are associated with specific problems of attention and concentration.

FIVE FORMS OF BIOFEEDBACK THERAPY

1. *Electromyographic biofeedback.* Electromyographic (EMG) feedback measures muscular tension. Sensors are attached to the skin to detect electrical activity related to muscle tension in that area. The biofeedback instrument amplifies and converts this activity into useful information, displaying the various degrees of muscle tension. This form of biofeedback therapy is most often used for tension *headaches,* physical rehabilitation, *chronic pain,* incontinence, and general relaxation purposes.

2. *Thermal biofeedback therapy.* Thermal biofeedback therapy is used to measure skin temperature as an index of *blood flow changes* from the constriction and dilation of blood vessels. Low skin temperature usually means decreased blood flow in that area. A temperature-sensitive probe is taped to the skin, often on a finger. The instrument converts information into feedback that can be seen and heard and can be used to reduce or increase blood flow to the hands and feet. Thermal biofeedback is often used for *migraine headache* and *anxiety disorders* and to promote general relaxation.

3. *Electrodermal activity therapy.* Electrodermal activity therapy is used to measure changes in sweat activity too minimal to feel. Two sensors are attached to the palm side of the fingers or hand to measure sweat activity. They produce a tiny electrical current that measures skin conductance on the basis of the amount of moisture present. Increased sweat can mean arousal of part of the autonomic nervous system. Electrodermal activity therapy can be used to measure the sweat output stemming from stressful thoughts or rapid deep breathing. It is most often used for *anxiety* and sweating.

4. *Finger pulse therapy.* Finger pulse therapy measures pulse rate and force. A sensor is attached to a finger and helps measure heart activity as a sign of arousal of part of the autonomic nervous system. It is most often used for *anxiety* and some cardiac arrhythmias.

5. *Breathing biofeedback therapy.* Breathing biofeedback therapy measures breathing rate, volume, rhythm, and location. Sensors are placed around the chest and abdomen to measure airflow from the mouth and nose. The feedback is usually visual, and patients learn to take deeper, slower, lower, and more regular breaths using abdominal muscles. This simple form of biofeedback is most often used for *anxiety.*

Electromyography (EMG), thermal, skin conductance, BP, brain wave, and heart rate are the most common types of feedback. The EMG measures levels of skeletal muscle contraction and the raw data is converted to an auditory signal. For disorders in which excess muscle tension and overarousal are associated with symptoms and lowered responsiveness, surface muscle tension monitoring (SEMG) is most appropriate. However, when the objective is to increase motor muscular activity, needles are often inserted.

Thermal biofeedback (TBF) provides information about the temperature of the skin, which is directly related to blood flow in the small arteries underlying the area where the sensor is placed. The most common placement is on the palmer surface of the index or middle finger of either hand, with occasional placement on the underside of the toes. Skin conductance feedback monitors the activity of the sweat glands directly beneath the sensors.

Brain wave (EEG) feedback, also called "neuro-feedback", involves monitoring brain wave activity of certain areas of the brain underlying the areas where electrodes are placed.

Heart rate and BP feedback provide information about regulation of the cardiovascular system. A newer form of BF is heart rate variability, which helps the patient learn to control heart rate oscillation (variability). Lower heart rate variability has been linked to cardiovascular disease (see Section I).

Similar behavioral techniques have been applied to individuals who demonstrate orthostatic intolerance (blood rushes to the feet upon standing) after exposure to zero or low gravity in outer space. Normally, when a person stands up, gravity draws blood down through the blood vessels, as in a standing column of fluid, to the legs and away from the head. Automatic reflexes normally adjust the flow of blood through the different blood vessels so that blood supply is maintained to the head and upper body in the standing position. Without exposure to gravity, as in outer space, over time these automatic reflexes are attenuated or extinguished. Pilots have been trained with BP BF to increase BP under supine and head-up tilt conditions. Autogenic therapy and BF were applied to control motion sickness in otherwise healthy and well-conditioned astronauts. The protocol trained multiple physiological responses simultaneously for a total of 6 hours. Transfer of the responses learned in the laboratory were made to a variety of stimulus conditions, such as rotary chair, flight, and space shuttle flights—mission accomplished. Back on Earth, BF is often combined with symptom monitoring by the practitioner, relaxation therapy (RT), patient education, psychotherapy, and medical pharmacotherapy (Box 6.4).

BOX 6.4 *A Typical Biofeedback Session*

In a normal biofeedback session, electrodes are attached to the area being monitored. These electrodes feed the information to a small monitoring box that registers the results by a sound tone that varies in pitch or on a visual meter that varies in brightness as the function being monitored decreases or increases. A biofeedback therapist leads the patient in mental exercises to help the patient reach the desired result. Through trial and error, patients gradually train themselves to control the inner mechanism involved. Training for some disorders requires 8 to 10 sessions; however, a single session can often provide symptomatic relief. Patients with long-term or severe pain may require longer therapy. The aim of the treatment is to teach patients to regulate their own inner mental and bodily processes eventually without the help of a machine.

RELAXATION THERAPIES

When the primary objective is to lower arousal, relaxation is an integral part of therapy. Relaxation is of two basic types: active or passive. Active relaxation is defined as producing lower arousal by voluntarily tensing and releasing tension from specific muscle groups and learning to differentiate between tension and relaxation to consciously lower tension. This approach could also be referred to as "applied relaxation" and "progressive relaxation." Passive relaxation consists of deep breathing or using words, phrases, or visualization and imagery (see Chapter 18). For example, autogenic relaxation (as may also be the case in hypnosis) uses specific phrases dealing with sensations of heaviness in the muscles and warmth in the hands, such as "my legs are getting heavier" or "my hands are getting warmer." A key to effective relaxation (as in meditation) is repetition of phrases or behavior (such as breathing) on a daily basis until a reliable relaxation response can be produced quickly when needed.

Home practice of relaxation with or without portable feedback devices is critical to learning and long-term maintenance of newly acquired skills. Generalization of the relaxation response to conditions of daily living allows the patient to use relaxation to counter the effects of stressful situations. The experience of decreasing the severity of a stress response or blocking the response with relaxation (rather than relying on medication) increases confidence in the ability to use the technique. Different relaxation techniques have specific effects, and the provider guides the patient in differentiating among various responses and matching each signal to a strategy: breathing, passive or active relaxation, or imagery.

"Doing" Relaxation

Patients record symptoms and this information is reviewed with the practitioner at each session. Reliable symptom monitoring before, during, and following treatment is necessary to first establish the baseline, then monitor the progress of treatment, and finally determine the outcome. Symptom monitoring both informs treatment and serves as a source of reinforcement of progress. A pretreatment baseline can be easily established if the patient tracks frequency, duration, and severity of symptoms and medication use prior to the initiation of BF. The patient also becomes fully engaged in the therapeutic process.

Patient education provides easy-to-understand explanations of the rationale for BF based on physiological principles. For example, feedback for disorders of excess muscle tension and tension-type headaches is logical and quickly grasped. The relation between a high-pitched or high-frequency sound and high muscle tension is intuitively obvious. Other symptom-feedback pairs are less obvious and require greater effort to make the required tasks comprehensible to patients. For example, a patient with a *migraine headache* who is going to learn to warm her hands with TBF might be told the following:

"When you are in a stressful situation, your body gets ready to react. This reaction includes tensing your muscles, increasing your pulse rate, and sending blood to your muscles. Thus blood is diverted away from internal organs, like your digestive system, and your hands and feet. When there is less warm blood in your fingers, they get cold. With feedback, you will learn to warm your hands consciously. This is part of learning how to decrease responses to stress, which seem to be related to your headaches."

BLOOD FLOW AND PAIN RESPONSES

Increases in pulse rate over the long term can have consequential effects on the body and cardiovascular system. New research shows that meditation and yoga reduces mild to moderate high BP. Thirty years ago, researchers in Europe studied BP treatment guidelines. They found that half the world's population would be considered at risk by the age of 24 years when using the 120/80 standard BP threshold, and 90% by the age of 49 years. These numbers account for more than three quarters of the world's entire adult population, and they represented quite a prime market for drug companies over the last 30 years.

In a recent clinical trial, University of Pennsylvania researchers studied 120 participants with mild to moderate high BP. Patients were 50 years old, on average, and their average systolic BP was 134 mm Hg. The researchers gave the participants three treatment options: yoga, diet, and yoga-diet combined. Then, they divided the participants into three groups. One group practiced yoga two or three times a week in a studio. The second group began a walking regimen and received nutritional counseling. The third group practiced yoga and received dietary counseling. Men and women who practiced yoga reduced their (systolic) BP by 5 to 6 mm Hg after 12 weeks, and they reduced both their systolic and diastolic numbers at 24 weeks. The lead researcher said, "It's not a huge decrease in blood pressure; it's not a drug effect; but it is significant." And for those experiencing early, mild to moderate elevations in BP, lifestyle modifications like yoga can help keep you off drugs.

Interestingly, the University of Pennsylvania researchers presented these findings at the 2013 American Society of Hypertension Scientific Sessions (Lenzer, 2012). This same group rejected my (Micozzi) study on stress and high BP 40 years ago. That study examined the effects of stress on schoolchildren in Southeast Asia. Eventually, the study did get published elsewhere in the *American Journal of Public Health*, but at the time, the American Society of Hypertension was not so open-minded. The very first study connecting yoga with lower BP also appeared 40 years ago in the British journal *Lancet*. However, the medical community is slow to embrace alternative approaches and usually does so only after drug approaches are demonstrated to be wasteful or harmful.

The mind influences blood flow by communicating with the small muscles and arteries and adjusting the blood vessels' tone, size, dimensions, and flow. Different mental states, imagery, BF, relaxation, and meditation all influence this kind of blood flow. While blood flow to the head, which influences migraine pain, may be consciously influenced, there are also direct influences on the brain. Regarding the application of EEG feedback for enhanced concentration, the explanation for its effects may be as follows. Certain brain wave patterns are associated with sleep, others with attention and good concentration, and others with lack of attention or daydreaming. Patients can learn to generate brain waves that are associated with good concentration and paying attention, instead of being distracted or unfocused.

Coping with Mood in Pain Conditions

Clinical depression is often prominent in patients with chronic *headaches* or other *pain* syndromes. In women, chronic severe headache and disability were found to be associated with depression. A neuro-psycho-chemical association is common to both pain and negative emotion. Cognitive-behavioral therapy (CBT) is commonly used in conjunction with BF in anxiety and mood disorders. CBT explores negative and irrational thoughts that contribute to mood symptoms and teaches the patient to counter these thoughts with more realistic approaches to situations. Therefore, the therapy emphasizes generating more positive thinking patterns and acquiring effective coping skills.

An intensive treatment protocol is recommended for patients who have long-standing moderate or severe symptoms, who are poorly motivated, and whose lives are focused on pain. When pain or disability is severe, the practitioner may request that the patient return to the physician for medication to facilitate the relaxation process. As symptoms improve, the need for some types of pain medication, particularly analgesics or antianxiety agents, may decrease. With steadily decreasing symptoms that require medication, the patient is encouraged to talk to the physician about lessening the dosage of pain drugs. The joint management of patients by physicians and mind-body practitioners is becoming more the norm than the exception.

Specific Chronic Pain Conditions

Research on exactly how BF and relaxation works is somewhat inconclusive. Some studies link its benefits directly to physiological changes that the patient learns to make voluntarily (specific). Other experiments find benefits even for patients who do not make the desired changes in the physiological measures (general). The following discussions will consider both general and specific effects in the treatment of various pain conditions.

Headache

Treatment is helpful for *tension-type* and *migraine headaches, posttraumatic headache,* and headache from overuse of medications. Patients are trained to specifically decrease tension levels and to produce a general relaxation response. Surface sensors placed on the forehead detect a wide range of muscular activities, and responding to grimacing, frowning, and teeth clenching helps patients regulate muscle tension and decrease pain. The relaxation process is then generalized to stressful situations where patients feel muscle pain or tension or notice the early signs of headache.

The most common treatment for nondrug therapy of migraine headache is TBF accompanied by RT. The results of temperature BF and relaxation are comparable to use of the drug propranolol, and superior to simply waiting (letting time heal) and to placebo. Long-term management of headache by relaxation therapy is effective when patients learn to generalize the relaxation response to stressful situations and continue to use the adaptive coping techniques learned during therapy.

Posttraumatic Headache and Headache Due to High Levels of Drug Consumption

These pain conditions pose special therapeutic challenges. Over half of sufferers report at least moderate improvement in the number of headaches, and nearly all show increased ability to relax and cope with the pain. In general, the longer the duration of posttraumatic pain, the poorer the response. Headache patients who use high doses of multiple classes of pain medications are also challenging. Withdrawal of pain medication can be accomplished on an outpatient basis and should precede treatment in this group. However, the active involvement of the therapist is critically important to success, rather than just passively writing prescriptions for pain medications.

Children and the elderly are appropriate candidates for relaxation therapies. Children do not necessarily learn BF skills faster than adults, but children's success rates are higher than adults, perhaps because most children do not present with the companion depressive features so common in adults who struggle with daily pain. Younger patients are often intrigued by the equipment, comfortable with video game–type technology, and adapt to treatment settings quite easily. In contrast, older persons often require additional sessions and learning may be somewhat slower. Nonetheless, EMG BF has been found to help decrease total headache activity and increase headache-free days in older persons.

Musculoskeletal Pain

Patients with chronic pain often report a myriad of psychological and physical symptoms. In addition to pain, patients suffer from sleep disturbances, vague sensations of discomfort, anxiety, and depression. Therefore, successful treatment must include interventions for each problem of mind and body. Chronic *low back pain* requires a combined approach of BF with other modalities such as physical therapy, exercise, correction of gait and posture, massage, and possibly shoe prosthetics.

BF is useful in training general relaxation and in correcting specific muscle tension problems. It is important to monitor tension when in postures other than reclining in a chair because muscles automatically relax when the head is supported by a headrest. Poor posture, bracing, insomnia, and depression are often contributory or perpetuating factors in long-term pain. EMG BF is provided while in the sitting or standing positions. In addition, CBT may be necessary to modify moods, thoughts, and behaviors as with other chronic pain conditions. Follow-up sessions are strongly recommended because continued relaxation practice is key in maintaining improvement. Relapse can occur after having learned the basic skills, particularly if lifestyle and posture have not changed.

Older people remain good candidates for treatment for chronic pain as with headache. Mind-body therapies for older adults with pain from *osteoarthritis* (OA) work as well as they do in younger adults for achieving 50% reduction in symptoms after biofeedback, progressive muscle relaxation, or guided imagery.

Fibromyalgia-Chronic Fatigue Syndrome

Fibromyalgia-chronic fatigue syndrome (FM-CFS) is a complex psycho-physiological disorder manifested by muscle pain, tender points, and sleep disturbance. Many sufferers also report headache, fatigue, memory problems, anxiety, and depression. Environmental conditions such as changes in weather, noise level, and anything that interrupts sleep often exacerbate the pain and discomfort. This chronic illness is severely distressing and physical symptoms are intensified by chronic stress. A patient who is already anxious is more aware of body pain, and then becomes more anxious when feeling pain, provides an example of an unhealthy, stressful BF loop. This pathologic manifestation suggests that the processes associated with this condition may also be alleviated with positive BF.

Management of fibromyalgia (FM) syndrome is guided by a step-wise treatment. The first step is making the right diagnosis, which is usually followed by beginning low-dose tricyclic antidepressants (TCAs) to address depression and break the cycle of pain and sleep disturbance, and physical therapy and/or CBT. An important early goal is to restore sleep, which is also accomplished by TCAs. The cognitive component is of major importance, since more intense pain due to low mood state may be misinterpreted as worsening of the syndrome. There is good evidence for the efficacy of both CBT and BF in fibromyalgia. Mind-body therapy in fibromyalgia may still be effective in increasing function, even if not specifically decreasing pain. Change in the *perception of pain* is accomplished in both normal subjects and in FM and chronic pain patients after training with feedback. A study of 30 patients with *fibromyalgia* syndrome who received BF showed statistically significant improvements in mental clarity, mood, and sleep (Mueller, Donaldson, Nelson, & Layman, 2001).

Temporomandibular Joint Disorders and Neck Pain

Psychological-behavioral approaches should be used together with medical-dental treatments for temporomandibular joint (TMJ) pain conditions at the time of initiation of care and not as a last resort. Tension levels may not always be significantly higher in TMJ patients. Factors besides actual muscle tension must be considered in treatment.

Treatment of *chronic neck pain* should ideally include patient education, relaxation, BF, and CBT. Patients receive explanations of the transmission of the pain signal, increase awareness of and reduce neck-bracing responses, and learn the muscular relaxation response. CBT is used to decrease the habitual negative moods and thoughts that impact the pain experience, including the maladaptive muscle contractions.

Osteoarthritis and Rheumatoid Arthritis

These conditions differ biologically and in the role of inflammation but share the disability associated with both pain and emotional distress. Similar to other pain conditions, older adults with arthritis pain do as well as younger adults with the application of BF, guided imagery, and progressive relaxation. In one study, 92 patients with the painful *rheumatoid* condition of systemic lupus erythematosus (SLE) were assigned randomly to receive BF-assisted treatment or usual medical care. Those who received BF had significantly greater improvements in *pain* and *psychological functioning*. At 9-month follow-up, the BF group continued to exhibit relative benefit compared with controls (Greco, Rudy, & Manzi, 2004).

ANXIETY AND DEPRESSION WITH PAIN CONDITIONS

Anxiety and mood disorders are common psychiatric conditions and frequent *companions of chronic pain*. Anxiety disorder may present as *cognitive* symptoms such as fear of losing control, dying, or going crazy, or as *somatic* symptoms such as racing heart, sweating, or shortness of breath. In addition to chronic pain, appropriate candidates for BF include patients with clinical psychiatric illnesses who can learn to modify specific physiological or psychological responses associated with their disorders. In school-age children, some students can readily be identified as "anxious" (although not diagnosed with a specific disorder by a mental health provider). Significant reductions in situational and baseline anxiety can be achieved at this early age with BF.

Learning *facial relaxation* with BF promotes lower nervous system activity and can be effective in managing both the somatic and cognitive components of anxiety. Generalized anxiety disorder can also be treated in diagnosed adults. In anxiety, the effects of BF may be nonspecific.

With *phobias*, RT is integral to systematic desensitization therapy. Gradual exposure to the phobic stimulus is combined with guided relaxation. Psychophysiological approaches including BF and RT are suggested as a first step in management and followed by medication if necessary. BF can shorten the time required to learn relaxation under conditions of exposure to the phobic stimulus.

Syncope (fainting) can also be symptomatic of simple phobia. For example, the sight of blood or injury can result in loss of consciousness in susceptible individuals. EMG and TBF can be combined with systematic desensitization to treat long-standing blood/injury phobia. With therapy, individuals learn to identify prefainting cues and use BF and RT to block fainting when confronted with the phobic stimulus. Neuro-feedback has also been used to treat anxiety disorders, particularly generalized anxiety and phobias. EMG feedback, with enhancement of alpha-wave brain activity, produces decreases in anxiety.

Patients with *posttraumatic stress disorder* (PTSD), another of the anxiety disorders, always require therapy beyond BF and relaxation. Some of the instigating causes of chronic pain are traumatic events, like military combat, personal assaults, motor vehicle accidents, or serious work injury. Victims should be evaluated for the presence of PTSD before BF is initiated.

Phantom limb pain following traumatic amputation of a limb has been treated with BF to reduce pain and to modify reorganization of nervous system pain pathways in the brain that occur over time as a result of the chronic pain. Chronic pain is partially a learned behavior. Repeated episodes of experiencing pain alter neuronal arrangements in the somatic and sensory cortex areas and memory areas of the brain. Applications of operant conditioning and BF may be used to help eliminate pain memories.

BF has not traditionally been recommended for patients with *major depressive disorder* or *dysthymia*, although there are no contraindications or reports of worsening of depression after BF. Depressed, chronic pain patients commonly experience a sense of helplessness regarding pain and the limitations imposed by pain. BF is based on the principle of gaining a sense of control over maladaptive physiology and responses. The experience of success can be translated into a sense of self-control. During the course of therapy, this major nonspecific effect of BF (i.e., developing a sense of control over physiological responses to stress) can facilitate the learning of pain control methods. Assessment of mood is important for the use of BF for any chronic pain condition. Even if the severity of the mood disorder does not require psychiatric intervention, the nonspecific effects of BF may be mobilized and directed toward improvement in both pain and mood (Box 6.5).

PAIN AND SLEEP DISORDERS

Sleep disorders invariably accompany chronic pain as a contributing cause or result in a self-reinforcing negative feedback loop. Categories of disturbed sleep that can be addressed by BF include both primary insomnia (one of the dyssomnias) and secondary insomnia related to chronic pain. Patients with recurrent pain report

---

BOX 6.5 *Pain, Inflammation, Depression, and Breast Cancer*

Michael H. Antoni of the University of Miami in Coral Gables, Florida, said that depression is common during cancer treatment and after. Women who took a stress management course after being diagnosed with breast cancer continued to receive the benefits, even *after* the course ended. Breast cancer patients who completed the 10-week stress management program early after diagnosis had higher mood and quality-of-life scores compared to others who did not take the course.

Cognitive-behavioral stress management techniques, muscle relaxation, and deep breathing helped these woman become more productive with positive thinking about their lives. Cortisol, a hormone released during stress, can be better regulated through these treatments and thus helps depression and inflammation.

The study included women who had breast cancer surgery between 1998 and 2005 and who were randomly assigned to a 1-day breast cancer education seminar or a 10-week group-based stress management behavioral therapy program with guided sessions on coping skills, identifying sources of stress and modifying stress response, anger management, muscle relaxation, and breathing exercises.

In 2013, the authors followed up and were able to reassess 51 women in the stress management group and 49 in the comparison group, 8 to 15 years after the original stress management program. This follow-up was second to a previous follow-up, and *again,* those in the stress management reported better quality of life and physical and emotional well-being.

difficulties in initiating and maintaining sleep. The results of a poor night's sleep are daytime fatigue and problems functioning. In addition to disordered sleep as a consequence of pain and mood disorders, sleep deprivation, particularly resulting from sleep interruptions (not simply fewer total hours), increases awareness of pain and may disrupt pain inhibitory mechanisms in the brain. Another vicious feedback loop is when pain interrupts sleep, in turn, aggravating the pain.

Sleep hygiene is always important and should be tried first. These recommendations are relatively simple and provide a step, at home, that encourages the patient to begin taking responsibility for healthful sleep (instead of relying on dangerous prescribed pain and sleep medications). Effective mind-body therapies for sleep disorders include progressive relaxation, CBT, and stimulus control. However, BF alone is not recommended for treatment of sleep disorders in either primary insomnia or sleep disturbance in chronic pain patients.

Progressive relaxation facilitates improvements in shortening the time required for the onset of sleep, but evidence to date does not favor the use of BF alone. Stimulus control therapy is used to address situations when pain has a learned association to the bed or bedtime. Contemplating going to bed produces anxiety or stress over not being able to sleep instead of being associated with relaxation and drowsiness. Pain patients are encouraged to remove any stressful stimuli from the bedroom and recondition bedtime as a time for relaxation and mental quietude.

BF relaxation techniques have been used with success to treat problems such as *insomnia, chronic fatigue,* and *body pain*. Results showed that BF alone was not superior to standard medical care, but those who received BF had significantly improved *anxiety* and *depression* (Norton, Chelvanayagam, Wilson-Barnett, Redfern, & Kamm, 2003).

PAIN TREATMENT: GENERAL AND SPECIFIC

There is strong scientific evidence for BF as treatment for several chronic pain disorders, particularly tension-type and migraine headaches. The effects of BF may be specific, nonspecific, or both. Nonspecific positive effects are produced by gaining confidence, improving concentration, and developing more effective coping strategies. The primary effects of BF are learning to gain control of your individual physiological processes, such as brain waves or muscle tension. Such effects may also be very specific. BF actively involves the patient directly in the therapeutic process.

The immediacy and accuracy of the BF information provided to the patient are critical, but the relationship between the practitioner and the patient remains important. People with stress-related pain and mood disorders acquire maladaptive response patterns that lead to dysfunctional coping and oversensitivity to stress. Even neutral stimuli may be perceived as threats so that, over time, risk of suffering pain manifestations over psychological conflicts increases. Patients who react in a maladaptive manner clearly need new coping skills. However, skills may not be enough. The ability to self-regulate requires more than simply learning a technique.

Self-regulation requires a conceptual shift. Patients must come to realize that controlling physiological and psychological responses is possible. As they learn to self-regulate, sensory information is processed differently. For example, pain is interpreted directly as a message from the body. Pain is not necessarily viewed as an inevitable prelude to an incapacitating migraine, specifically, or to a global indictment on everything that ever went wrong in life. A healthier response to the pain message involves learning skills, in part, but also making cognitive adjustments and positive psychological responses. Although the practitioner begins with a framework and a standard treatment package in mind, the therapy should be flexible enough to be modified for each patient as an individual (discussed in Appendix I, pp. 572–579).

PRACTITIONERS AND PRACTICE SETTINGS

BF and RT are therapy techniques provided by various mental health professionals. They do not represent medical practice specialties or subspecialties, so the patient will not necessarily be looking for a "BF therapist," but rather a health practitioner who utilizes BF. BF does not belong to any particular field of health care. In addition to being a mind-body technique of complementary or alternative medicine, it is used in many health care disciplines, including internal medicine, dentistry, physical therapy and rehabilitation, psychology and psychiatry, and pain management. It is best, but not always possible, for the same practitioner to provide both psychotherapy and BF. When a clinical psychologist, clinical counselor, social worker, or psychiatric nurse is also trained in BF, single treatment sessions can integrate psychotherapy, hypnosis, or imagery with BF. For example, one might spend the first half of a 1-hour session in psychotherapy and the other half practicing BF. On the other hand, a session might start with guided imagery-assisted BF to create an atmosphere of trust between patient and practitioner followed by psychotherapy. An experienced therapist can also help manage lack of motivation or uncertainty.

REFERENCES

Andersen, K., Farahmand, B., Ahlbom, A., Held, C., Ljunghall, S., Michaëlsson, K., & Sundström, J. (2013). Risk of arrhythmias in 52,755 long-distance cross-country skiers: a cohort study. *European Heart Journal, 34*(47), 3624–3631.

Benson, H. R. (1993). The relaxation response. In D. Goleman & J. Gurin (Eds.), *Mind-body medicine.* New York: Consumer Report Books.

Esch, T., Stefano, G. B., Fricchione, G. L., & Benson, H. (2002). The role of stress in neurodegenerative diseases and mental disorders. *Neuro Endocrinology Letters, 23*(3), 199–208.

Greco, C. M., Rudy, T. E., & Manzi, S. (2004). Effects of a stress-reduction program on psychological function, pain, and physical function of systemic lupus erythematosus patients: A randomized controlled trial. *Arthritis & Rheumatism, 51*, 625–634. http://dx.doi.org/10.1002/art.20533.

Green, E., & Green, A. (1977). *Beyond biofeedback.* New York: Delta.

Jawer, M. & Micozzi, M. S. (2009). *The spiritual anatomy of emotion: How feelings link the brain, the body, and the sixth sense.* https://books.google.com/books?id=m6Nu1Oxby_IC.

Jawer, M. & Micozzi, M. S. (2012). Your emotional type. Rochester, VT: Healing Arts Press.

Jawer, M. & Micozzi, M. S. (2015). *Fundamentals of complementary and alternative medicine.* (5th ed.). St Louis: Elsevier.

Johansson, L., Guo, X., Hällström, T., Norton, M. C., Waern, M., Östling, S., et al. (2013). Common psychosocial stressors in middle-aged women related to longstanding distress and increased risk of Alzheimer's disease: A 38-year longitudinal population study. *BMJ Open, 3,* e003142.

Lenzer, J. (2012). Cochrane review finds no proved benefit in drug treatment for patients with mild hypertension. *BMJ, 345,* e5511.

McCown, D. & Micozzi, M. (2017). *Teaching mindfulness* (2nd ed.). New York: Springer Publishers.

Mueller, H. H., Donaldson, C. C. S., Nelson, D. V., & Layman, M. (2001). Treatment of fibromyalgia incorporating EEG-Driven stimulation: a clinical outcomes study. *Journal Clinical Psychology, 57*(7), 933–952. http://citeseerx.ist.psu.edu/viewdoc/download?doi=10.1.1.519.9069&rep=rep1&type=pdf.

Norton, C., Chelvanayagam, S., Wilson-Barnett, J., Redfern, S., & Kamm, M. A. (2003). Randomized controlled trial of biofeedback for fecal incontinence. *Gastroenterology, 125*(5), 1320–1329.

Pakhomova, O. N., Gregory, B. W., Semenov, I., & Pakhomov, A. G. (2013). Two modes of cell death caused by exposure to nanosecond pulsed electric field. *PLoS One, 8*(7), e70278 http://dx.doi.org/10.1371/journal.pone.0070278.

Pearce, J. C. (1992). Magical child. *Plum, 1977,* 30–31.

Sacks, M. (1993). Exercise for stress control. In D. Goleman & J. Gurin (Eds.), *Mindbody medicine.* New York: Consumer Reports Books.

Szabo, S., Tache, Y., & Somogyi, A. (2012). The legacy of Hans Selye and the origins of stress research: A retrospective 75 years after his landmark brief "letter" to the Editor[#] of Nature. *Stress, 15*(5), 472–478. http://selyeinstitute.org/wp-content/uploads/2013/06/TheLegacuyofHansSelyearticle.pdf.

Suggested Readings can be found on the companion website, http://www.micozzipainconditions.com.

Chapter 7

Mental Imagery, Visualization, and Hypnosis

Since the time that human societies first began contemplating the nature of human experiences, both moral and natural philosophers tried to define and explain the interior processes of the mind. Those personal experiences are not conventionally accessible and visible to others because they do not have established physical referents. Philosophers speculated at length on the nature of mental imagery as part of human experience. In ancient Greece, Aristotle long ago asked the question, "Is thought possible without imagery?"

In the 20th century scientists still found these phenomena difficult to verify or measure. Behavioral psychologists of the 1920s went so far as to say that mental images simply did not exist. These early-stage ideas included the imageless thought debate. William Wundt, the first person to ever call himself a psychologist, founded the first formal laboratory for psychological research in Leipzig, Germany. Wundt proposed three basic elements of consciousness, including thoughts and feelings. He also proposed that studying images would also mean studying thought because he believed images coexist with thought. Evidence supporting the idea that imagery was *not* required for thinking came from observations by Sir Francis Galton (nephew of Charles Darwin) during the late 19th century that people who had difficulty forming visual images were still capable of thinking. The later dominance of behaviorism between the 1920s and 1950s took imagery-based research out of mainstream psychology.

Since the cognitive science evolution of the 1960s, psychologists have done more work exploring and categorizing mental imagery and inner processes. Contemporary psychologists distinguish several types of imagery. The most common of which people routinely experience as memory. When trying to remember (recollect or recall) a place one used to live, the furniture in a former residence or old house, or what the seats of an old car feel like, one immediately and necessarily conjures up a visual image in the mind—or the "mind's eye." People often refer to

Acknowledgments to Michael Jawer and Denise Rodgers for prior contributions in Micozzi, M.S. (ed.), (2016). *Fundamentals of commentary and alternative medicine* (5th ed.). St Louis: Elsevier Health Sciences/ Saunders; and Michael Weintraub and Roberta Temmes for prior contributions in Micozzi, M.S. (ed.), (1999). *Medical guides to complementary and alternative medicine*, Churchill-Livingstone/Elsevier.

this experience as forming a mental picture. Some believe and describe that they do not actually "see" or visualize the scene but simply have a strong sense or feeling about the scene and "know" what it looked and felt like.

IMAGERY PROCESSING

The term "imagery" can be used to refer to mental processes and also to describe a wide array of procedures used in therapy to encourage changes in attitudes, behaviors, or physiologic reactions (as with biofeedback in Chapter 6). As a mental process, imagery is often defined as any thought representing a sensory quality or re-creating a sensation in perception. In addition to the visual (seeing), it includes all the other senses: aural (sound, hearing), tactile (touch), olfactory (smell), proprioceptive (position or orientation), and kinesthetic (movement). Imagery is often synonymous with visualization.

However, visualization refers only to "seeing" or visualizing something in the mind's eye, whereas imagery can use one sense or a combination of senses to produce an image. In this "sense," imagery goes beyond visualization to essentially "imaging" any sensory perception. Mental scanning was developed by Kosslyn as a technique to support the depictive theory of imagery in which people create mental images and then scan them in their minds. He was one of the first to introduce theories in both imagery and perception (i.e., perceptual images that we see with our own eyes). To demonstrate that we use the same spatial mechanisms in the brain in imagery as we do with perception, Kosslyn performed an experiment. He asked participants to memorize a picture of an object in their mind and to focus on one particular part of the object.

Participants were then asked to look for another part of the object and to press one of two buttons (yes or no) as to whether they previously found this object in the original picture or if they could not find the "new" object. Kosslyn wanted to observe whether or not participants took longer to find other objects located farther away from the initial object. If not, people would be scanning across the entire object as a "whole." Kosslyn took on further experiments and continued research in imagery for more than a decade. He eventually gave new insights and formed the conclusion that imagery, like perception, is served by a spatial mechanism and that these mechanisms are shared with perception (Box 7.1).

BRAIN, PERCEPTION, AND IMAGERY
IMAGERY NEURONS IN THE BRAIN

Single recordings of neurons in the brain are rare—but have been accomplished. These studies show what individual neurons in the brain "light up" when using perceptual vision (receiving information through the eyes) versus using imagination. Kreiman and Koch discovered that when a person uses perceptual vision of an object, neurons respond similarly to when mentally imaging the same object (Kreiman, Koch, & Fried, 2000).

BOX 7.1 *Ancient and Modern Methods of Loci*

Imagery appears to have attracted attention during the first mnemonic encounters in Greece. The method of loci is a unique memory retrieval system in which things that are remembered are placed at different locations in a mental image of a spatial layout. Mnemonics, which are patterns of letters, ideas, or associations that assist in remembering something, were discovered by the Greek poet and sophos (wise man) Simonides (c.556–c.468 BCE). According to legend, Simonides was briefly asked by the gods to go outside from a banquet located in Thessaly, where he recited a poem. While he was briefly outside of the hall conversing to the gods, the roof collapsed, crushing humans beyond physical recognition. Later, he was able to identify corpses whose damaged features were impossible to recognize, by using his memory of the location of people situated around a banqueting table when he had initially left the party. Thus, the method of loci was initiated (in Latin, "locus" is a location, "loci" is the plural). Simonides stated that people must select places and form mental images of the objects they wish to remember and store those images so that the order of the objects will preserve the order of things (Blakeslee, Macknik, & Martinez-Conde, 2011).

It has been said that this occasion was the origin of the mnemonic technique known as the method of loci, described by Roman rhetoricians and orators, such as Cato, Cicero, and Quintilian (CE c. 35–c. 95). The mythical ancient Greek musician and poet Apollo, god of knowledge and of medicine, was said to have laid out the groundwork for the modernized "peg system." This approach is a form of linking any number of items to a particular digit. Rhyming the words are essential for the peg system—such as won for one, hive for five, and so forth. The last step would be associating the "number word" with a vivid visual image. These elements are more easily remembered if one can tap into the emotional body and have great interactions among them. A rule of short-term memory is that the average individual can memorize up to seven digits (e.g., the old phone numbers), and anything more is too much for the short-term memory capacity to hold.

Ganis, Thompson, and Kosslyn (2004) used functional magnetic resonance imaging (fMRI) for detecting areas of activity in the brain. Brain scans that show activation in the frontal lobe for perception and imagery are almost identical. There was slightly more activity in performing perceptual tasks in the part of the brain that serves as the location of the visual receiving area. As light enters the eyes into the retina, impulses then travel along the optic nerve to reach the visual cortex in the occipital lobe.

CREATING IMAGES AND THE SUBCONSCIOUS

Creating images with the mind, and in the mind, offers a path to communicating with the subconscious and unconscious (deeper-than-conscious) aspects of the mind. For example, this occurrence of such communication becomes apparent when considering the dream state. Dreams communicate mainly in images, which are then consciously interpreted to make a story. Although Sigmund Freud had made a name for himself as a psychotherapist with his book, *The Interpretation of Dreams,* one essentially interprets one's own dreams long before they get reported to the therapist.

The unconscious serves up various vivid images, and the conscious aspects of the mind automatically work to string them into some kind of coherent story or narrative (assuming they can be remembered at all). Dreams occur during the fifth stage of sleep, which is called "rapid eye movement" (REM). REM sleep occurs more frequently and deeply as the morning approaches. Interestingly, the body behaves as if it were awake during REM sleep—typically, the brain produces the same beta waves as it does when awake and demonstrates psychologic, physiologic, and biochemical activity. REM sleep also involves theta waves. These work in the hippocampal region of the brain and improve short-term memory processes (Baars & Gage, 2010).

Sleep Deprivation and the Brain

When one does not get enough sleep, the prefrontal cortex (responsible for problem solving and alertness) decreases in performance. This area of the brain is in charge of processing working memory needed to eventually retain information in the long term and for proper mental functioning on both simple and complex tasks. It can perhaps be compared with the "random access memory" in your personal computer. Long-term memory is affected when not getting enough hours of sleep the prior night. For example, every night it is important to get adequate sleep, in contrast to "catching up" on sleep on the weekends (even if one "sleeps in" on the weekends). For the complete process of new information to be formed and retained, it needs to be done within 24 hours. Information composed of short-term memory (also known as "working memory"; like random access memory on your personal computer) needs to be moved to long-term memory (like your computer hard drive) in order to be retained.

COMMUNICATIVE QUALITY OF IMAGERY

This communicative quality of imagery is important because feelings and behaviors are primarily motivated by subconscious and unconscious factors. Insofar as imagery often involves directed concentration, imagery can also be regarded as a form of guided meditation or relaxation (see Chapters 5 and 6). Many practices discussed in this section of the book use a component of imagery. Psychotherapy, hypnosis, and biofeedback all use various elements of this process, and it comes into play during mindfulness, meditation, and yoga practices. Any therapy that relies on the mental imagination (another word for imagery) to stimulate, communicate, solve problems, or evoke a heightened, altered awareness or sensitivity may be considered a form of imagery. Numerous early studies indicated that mental imagery brings about significant physiologic and biochemical changes. These findings helped encourage the development of imagery as a health care resource. It has been established that imagery demonstrates the capacity to do the following:

- Influence oxygen supply in tissues (Olness & Gardner, 1988),
- Bring about changes in cardiovascular (Barber, 1969), vascular, or thermal regulation (Green & Green, 1977),
- Effect the pupillary and cochlear reflexes,
- Change heart rate and galvanic skin responses (Jordan & Lenington, 1979),
- Stimulate salivation (Barber, 1984; White, 1978).

Communication with the unconscious had previously been the domain of hypnosis (see later in this chapter). Hypnosis originated in the 18th century when Franz Anton Mesmer demonstrated the ability to influence what he called "animal magnetism," borrowing a term from contemporary studies in electricity and magnetism (see Section III). These practices were continued throughout the 19th century by a variety of "magnetic healers" who emphasized the power of "mind over matter" for healing purposes without the need for physical interventions on the body. Nowadays hypnotism consists of two basic components: (1) the use of a technique to induce a state of consciousness that allows greater access to the deeper parts of the mind and (2) a method for communicating with those deeper parts of the mind. This kind communication involves making suggestions (the "power of suggestion") to the inner depths of the mind. The hypnotist suggests ideas or behaviors desired for betterment. But first, one must be placed under a state of hypnosis (as explained further in this chapter). Several different techniques are used to induce the necessary state of consciousness, and some may be quite similar to more common relaxation techniques and to meditation.

Imagery as Therapy

Imagery is essentially a way of thinking that accesses sensory capabilities and functions in the absence of sensory input. It can be considered as one of the brain's higher-order encoding systems. The system with which we are most familiar is the sequential information processing system. This system underlies linear, analytic, and conscious verbal thinking typically associated with the left hemisphere of the brain. For example, medical and scientific professionals must come up through an educational system in which they become highly educated and are highly rewarded for their abilities using this mode of information processing.

However, imagery is the language used by a simultaneous information-processing mode, which underlies the holistic, synthetic, pattern thinking of the unconscious mind—typically associated with the right hemisphere of the brain.

CASE STUDY

A real-life example shared by our colleague, Dr. Marty Rossman, an international expert and early pioneer on guided imagery, brings out the importance of this relational pattern. A 60-year-old woman with metastatic cancer and chronic pain was having difficulty creating mental images of her immune system vigorously fighting her tumor. As famously demonstrated at the Simonton Center, cancer patients typically form images of their own immune system cells (white blood cells) eating the cancer or fighting the cancer in some other way.

Her imagery consisted of a few relatively inert immune cells sitting on her image of the tumor, which she described as a "blob." Numerous therapeutic interventions failed to increase the activity she imagined. Then she was asked to allow her mind to form an image for anything that interfered with her ability to more actively visualize her healing. An image of a large chasm came to her mind. Across the chasm, she saw her husband and grown children waving for her to come over. She began to cry at this image, the first emotion evidenced in many sessions. She explained that her family was emotionally distant and estranged from each other in varying degrees and she had not been able to overcome it. In her imagery she wanted to build a bridge over to them (she was an engineer by training). She imagined building a bridge and walking across into the welcoming arms of her embracing family. She determined to ask her family to meet together with a family therapist, something they had never done. After a short series of deeply moving sessions, the family members bonded in ways they never had before. Subsequently, her healing imagery became very vigorous and active, as did her participation in other aspects of her treatment, including nutrition, exercise, and an experimental clinical trial of monoclonal antibodies.

The use of guided imagery allowed the woman in this case to access, experience, and overcome an emotional barrier to her being more participatory in her care. Her mental ability to form an image had not only cognitive but also emotional information. This simultaneous processing brought that information to her in a nonlinear but meaningful way that led to action.

Language for Healing Pain

Imagery is a language of the arts and is also a language of emotions. Emotions reveal what is important to us. They can be either potent motivators or barriers to changing lifestyle and habits. Emotions motivate us to action. They also produce characteristic physiologic changes in the body, including varying patterns of muscle tension, blood flow, respiration, metabolism, and neurologically and immunologically active peptide secretions (as with biofeedback and relaxation therapy in Chapter 6).

Modern research in the field of psychoneuroimmunology points to the emotions as key modulators of neurologically active peptides secreted by the brain, gut, and immune systems. Imagery relates to cognition, emotion, and physiology and can be considered as a code or connection among mind-body interactions.

Imaging provides a rapid route to insight and motivation. Imagery also has direct physiologic consequences and effects. In the absence of competing sensory cues, the body responds to imagery as it would to a genuine external experience. Imagery has been shown in numerous research studies to be able to affect almost all major physiologic systems of the body, including respiration, heart rate, blood pressure, metabolic rates in cells, gastrointestinal mobility and secretion, sexual function, and immune response. Imagery can improve memory in many ways, including the three main components discussed in this chapter: visualizing interactive images, organization in the method of loci, and associating items with nouns.

Imagery is a natural part of the way we think. It can almost always be helpful in a virtually unlimited number of situations for people with chronic pain. For simplicity, it may be helpful to consider the following three major categories for chronic pain:

1. Relaxation and stress reduction—easy to teach, easy to learn, and almost universally helpful (see Chapter 6).
2. Visualization, or directed imagery, in which clients are encouraged to imagine desired outcomes in a relaxed state of mind. This approach can be compared with cognitive-behavioral therapy, in which the client is encouraged to go out with a new frame of mind and build a fund of positive new experiences as a reservoir of good, or better, feelings about life. With directed imagery, one actually imagines these positive experiences occurring, and the mind and body begin to benefit from positive feelings before they actually occur in "reality." But to the mind, and the body's responses, the fund of positive feelings is real.

   This approach also affords a sense of participation and control in one's own healing, which is of significant value in itself. It may well relieve or reduce pain symptoms, stimulate healing responses in the body or behaviors, and/or provide effective motivation for making positive life changes. Guided imagery works directly on the brain's perception of pain.

3. Receptive, or insight-oriented, imagery, in which the images formed are invited into awareness and explored ("interpreted") to gather more information about a pain symptom, underlying illness, mood, situation, or solution. This approach is more like traditional psychotherapy, or psychoanalysis without all the rigid Freudian interpretations, but instead focusing on current experiences and feelings (e.g., instead of past feelings, for example, about mother).

   There are considerations by the practitioner in choosing approaches as to whether imagery will be most effective as a (a) self-care technique, (b) in a group or class, or (c) as part of an individual counseling or therapy relationship. Self-help books and tapes are an inexpensive option if patients are capable of using these techniques on their own. However, effectively dealing with highly charged emotional issues often requires the assistance of a competent professional imagery guide.

   In practice, patients and practitioners often explore all of the above-mentioned options and choose the one(s) best suited for a given individual, as well as the unique individual nature of the problem, coping responses, approaches to healing, and the amount of time, energy, and funds willing or able to be invested in the process.

TREATMENT TECHNIQUES AND SETTINGS

A ubiquitous guided imagery technique used for any situation involves guiding through some abdominal breathing, a simple body scan, and/or progressive muscle relaxation. Then the client is invited to imagine being situated in a "beautiful, safe place they love." This approach provides a simple and relatively nonthreatening introduction to the effects of imagery. Depending on the patient and practitioner, the location might be termed a "healing place" or "powerful place" rather than a "safe place," but safety always remains a critical factor. It may be a place that the patient knows and has been before, either in real life or only in the imagination, or a new place that comes to mind. When guided with an interactive approach, patients are invited to describe the places in which they imagine themselves to be, while staying there in the mind. The guide asks what the patient sees, hears, and feels there and allows the patient to respond.

Questions such as "What time of day does it seem to be?" and "What is the weather like?" help to focus on the senses and deepen the subjective reality of the imagery.

As simple as this technique may be, it illustrates the utility of the interactive approach. One may be taught to suggest that patients imagine themselves at a beautiful beach with warm sun and sand and blue-green waves breaking on the shore. This setting works well for many people, but it may be that the patient had been particularly affected by watching the movie *Jaws*. There is nothing to be gained by not simply guiding interactively and suggesting specific images. When invited to go to a place that is beautiful, safe, and relaxing, the patient will always pick a place that fulfills those criteria, without having to be told a specific kind of setting.

HEALING IMAGES

Imagery consists of more than just visualization. Although vision is a dominant sense for humans, it is only one of five. For many there may also be "sounds of healing" that you may imagine (as common in shamanic healing in traditional cultures), or a fragrance that accompanies it, or body sensations of warmth, coolness, tingling, or others that accompany one's individual healing imagery. You can be encouraged to explore all the senses in creating and elaborating your personal healing imagery. fMRI has shown that as people imagine different senses, different areas of the cerebral cortex are activated in the brain. Recruiting different senses and more cortical areas of the brain is likely to make the imagery more subjectively real and more powerfully stimulating of the subcortical responses that mediate healing and immune system functions.

Together with physiologic healing imagery, some imagery of the actual outcome desired is also useful. Ideal model imagery focuses on what it will be like to experience full recovery from chronic pain or another condition. Patients imagine doing what they love doing, with the people whom they love, and then to imagine themselves enjoying significant landmark events and goals, such as family weddings, births, graduations, and other significant life events. Ideal model imagery is not always easy and may bring up significant barriers to investing hopes in recovery— which then allows one to work with those potential interfering barriers. Ideal model imagery can bring up grief, which can be simply acknowledged and processed as much or as little as needed until the desired goal is an intended direction without the grief.

CHRONIC PAIN AND RELATED CONDITIONS

Visualization can be a powerful tool for combating chronic pain, cancer, infections, and other illnesses—when the imagery is guided by a practitioner with expertise and ethics. However, visualizing certain outcomes under the wrong conditions may actually lead to declines in motivation and achievement because visualizers seem to "feel" like they have already achieved their objectives. For example, among the current proliferation of so-called management consultants and "gurus," it has been observed that by "jumping the gun," they can easily make everyone "feel good" in the workplace before they have actually accomplished anything. This ham-handed approach actually takes away productivity and undermines resolving real problems by providing people the psychic rewards before achieving any real results. This facile approach also seems typical for children today in school, sports, and other kinds of performance.

Competent practitioners, by combining the benefits of optimism with the pragmatic survival skills of realism, can create a healthy balance without undue emphasis on unrealistic expectations or imaginary feelings. Being able to also visualize the worst-case scenario actually reduces anxiety levels. When you can assess how bad things can possibly get, you usually discover ways that you could cope (and usually that things never get that bad at all).

A related component of healing imagery that is useful to understand is what is called "nocebo" effect. The placebo effect is many things—but one interpretation has been the healing power of intention and expectation (tapping into the body's own potent self-healing potential). In contrast, the nocebo effect relates to poor patient expectations that lead to poorer health outcomes. This component is especially important if the patient has heard or experienced negative messages about prognosis form his or her doctors (thus the nocebo or "nonhealing" vs. the placebo, or healing, response), whether communicated intentionally or unintentionally. For example, when patients in a clinical drug trial are informed about all the possible "side effects" of a treatment, they may actually experience them—even if they are given the placebo rather than the actual drug. In fact, many patients actually drop out of studies due to the nocebo effect—11% of the placebo group in a fibromyalgia study. In statin (cholesterol) drug trials, nocebo-related dropout rates ranged from 4% to 26% (Häuser, Hansen, & Enck, 2012). Of course, many doctors and patients now recognize that these statin drugs to lower cholesterol are useless and harmful, and the whole story about cholesterol and heart disease is a medical myth.

Many patients will say something like, "I will never forget the look on my doctor's face when he told me I would just have to learn to live with my pain," or "there is really nothing we can do." A doctor's choice of words also makes an important difference. Dr. Bernard Lown, a pioneer of nonsurgical treatments for heart disease, originated of the concept of "avoidable care." Dr. Lown stated, "Words are the most powerful tool a doctor possesses, but words, like a two-edged sword, can maim as well as heal."

For example, when given pain-reliving injections prior to surgery, patients felt better when told it would make the procedure go better (Häuser et al., 2012), but they felt worse when warned that the injection would hurt. In these days of risk management and informed consent, patients are recited a long litany of everything that could possibly go wrong and all the negative side effects they might feel. And simply telling them makes them feel worse. Thus informing patients about side effects increases the likelihood that they will actually experience them—which has a net negative effect on quality of care. This problem, of course, poses an ethical dilemma. For everyone's peace of mind, though, your hospital or medical center probably now has a paid professional "medical ethicist" on staff—yet another medical subspecialty that has been minted due to our overspecialized mainstream health care system and the abdication of many doctors to attend to their own ethics of practice.

In a healing situation, we do not really want doctors to be just like regular people; we want them to be potent and powerful healers and helpers, somewhat like an ideal parent to a child. Verbal and nonverbal cues from doctors can create anxiety, depression, or even a kind of posttraumatic stress syndrome with intrusive thinking, sleep disturbance, excessive vigilance, and anxiety. This situation is especially difficult to treat and often requires much attention to neutralize or negate. Imagery of being in the doctor's office, with a calendar on the wall, with a future date that is meaningful to the patient, imagining the doctor reviewing their tests and giving them good news and being pleased (or just thoughtful) often influences the illness. It provides an image that the patient can substitute for an alarming one they may have unconsciously adopted and provides a way to respond in a more internally effective manner.

Dose Response

Practitioners do not know how to determine the "dose response" of healing imagery even when they observe it is having an effect. Most studies have used protocols of 20 minutes 2 to 3 times a day. Studies indicate that the more people perform the practices the more they benefit, whether due to the practice itself or because intensive practice simply serves as a marker of the intention to treat and to heal, the determination to help, and belief that it will succeed. Patients are encouraged to think frequently about their healing imagery, even for a few seconds, and especially whenever they do anything they hope or think will help their healing, like taking medications, vitamins, herbs, or other treatments. At the same time, patients are encouraged to take time during the day to relax, shift attention, and focus on nothing but the healing process, however it is imagined. Using interactive dialogue can help to personalize healing imagery and practices in ways that are individualized and likely to produce the most powerful healing imagery for each individual. Patients who will be more susceptible to imagery and imagery-based healing can be assesses using the interactive tools described in Appendix I (pp. 572–579).

Interactive Imagery Technique: The Healer Within

This interactive technique can be used with an image that represents anything the client or guide wants to know more about. In many ways it is essentially an insight psychotherapy technique. It can be used to explore (1) an image of a symptom, whether physical, emotional, or behavioral; (2) an image that represents the pain; (3) an image for resistance to or interference with healing that arises anywhere in the process. The selection of focus is highly dependent on the clinical situation and orientation of the patient. None of these techniques should be forced but only offered at appropriate times as possibilities.

The point is not to analyze the images but to communicate with them as if they are alive—which they are. Not to say that they have an existence apart from the individual but that the images represent personal complexes of thoughts, beliefs, attitudes, feelings, sensations, and values that at times can function as relatively autonomous aspects of the personality. Visualizing having conversations with an imaginary figure that is both wise and loving can be helpful.

An inner healer is defined and characterized by the qualities of wisdom and compassion (and can be characterized in analytic psychotherapy terms as an ego ideal). As the client is invited to imagine a figure that has these qualities, an exploration of whatever image arises can be meaningful and helpful. An inner healer can provide a way to access the patient's own wisdom and compassion. These attributes offer useful qualities in most circumstances and especially in many situations that arise in the treatment of chronic pain.

Evocative Imagery

The use of evocative imagery helps to shift moods and mental states at will, thus making new behaviors and insights more accessible. Through the structured use of memory, fantasy, and sensory recruitment, clients are encouraged to identify a personal quality or qualities that would serve especially well in current situations. Evocative imagery helps to access inner strengths to help to make best use of treatments and healing abilities (Box 7.2).

BOX 7.2 *What's the Buzz About Grounding?*

Grounding: Moving From Insight to Action

Grounding is a process by which the insights evoked by imagery are turned into actions, and the new awareness and motivation is focused into a specific plan for attitudinal, emotional, or behavioral change. This process of adding the will to the imagination involves clarification of insights, brainstorming, choosing the best option, affirmations, action planning, imagery rehearsal, and constant reformulating ("rebooting") the plan until it actually succeeds. It is often the "missing link" in image therapy, connecting the new awareness to specific action. Imagery can be used to enhance this process, by providing creative options for action and allowing troubleshooting and practice through rehearsal. This process can actually help to change dietary and exercise habits and reduce pain and stress by resolving problems that one was previously unable to resolve.

When having an "out of body" experience, one may find it to an unpleasant state or feel a "buzzing" (dissonant energy) that comes from the lack of connection within oneself. Buzzing (dissonance) can occur from situations like being on the laptop for hours without a break or from working without being fully in the present moment. A buzzing feeling can be an uneasy energy within oneself. For example, being ungrounded can feel as if there is a buzzing sensation in or toward the top of the head, or it can mean that you are not thinking clearly and feel high-strung, or it can mean feeling nervous, temperamental, and unstable. By connecting to yourself and your own awareness of yourself, insights come through more easily. For instance, strong concentration on mental images will help you to connect to yourself, more deeply inspiring powerful change.

Interactive Guided Imagery

Guided imagery (GI) is a term variously used to describe a range of techniques from simple visualization and direct imagery-based suggestion to metaphor and storytelling. Guided imagery is used to help to teach psychophysiologic relaxation, relieve pain symptoms, stimulate healing responses in the body, and help people to tolerate painful and uncomfortable procedures and treatments.

"Interactive guided imagery" as a term is registered by the Academy for Guided Imagery to represent a particular approach to using therapeutic imagery. In this approach, imagery is evoked from the patient by a guide without suggesting specific imagery—the practitioner and client interact to discover appropriate imagery. This approach provides clients with ways to draw on their own inner resources to support healing, to make appropriate adaptations to changes in health, and to find creative solutions to challenges that they previously thought were insoluble. It encourages clients to access their own strengths and resources and tends to lead toward greater autonomy and self-efficacy.

The key to the effectiveness of interactive guided imagery is the interactive communications component that it incorporates. For example, by working interactively instead of just passively reading an imagery script, the interactive imagery guide ensures that the experience has personal meaning for the client and that it proceeds at a pace determined by the client's needs and abilities. Both the content and the direction are set by the client, and it is the client who actually begins to guide the entire process toward the resources needed to support healing, change, and positive therapeutic results. Whenever possible, the interactive imagery guide uses nonjudgmental, content-free language because it encourages clients to tap their own inner resources to find solutions for solving their own problems.

CASE STUDY

A 27-year-old patient with pain was invited to allow an image to come to mind that could represent his disease. Rather than encountering an image that was frightening, a benign spirit image appeared. The patient was encouraged to imagine that he could communicate with the image and that it could communicate with him in a way he could understand. When he asked the image what it wanted from him, it said, to his surprise, "You are a spiritual being but there is no room for me in your life. Make room for me to live or I will have to return with you to the world of the spirits." He cried and talked at length about his own spiritual seeking as an adolescent and young adult. He had become very involved in a lucrative business years before his diagnosis, and it consumed all his waking hours. He had already been divorced and lost many friends to his obsession with the business. He changed his priorities and went through a successful treatment. A much more balanced life followed, including more time with friends, a spiritual practice, and philanthropic activities, all initiated rather directly from that process. (Shared by Dr. Rossman.)

If this particular image were suggested to other pain patients, none of them might be able to relate. By evoking the patient's own imagery, he was empowered to become aware of important unconscious needs that he related to his pain and healing. Another term for interactive guided imagery is one that practitioners and spiritual teachers use. The term "higher self" is used when a person receives a "download" of information and when there are extreme moments of enlightenment. You are usually asked to "ask" what your "higher self" thinks about something or to try to connect or tap into an intelligence that is a part of you but may not be a part of your "everyday thinking."

Treatment of Chronic Pain and Related Conditions

Imagery can be used to contribute to the healing of physical problems and has been used extensively in the area of chronic pain management. In one method the individual allows an image for his or her pain to emerge. For example, an individual may create an image that characterizes the area of pain, and then create a second image to counteract the pain. After images are formed, the individual uses a relaxation or meditation technique to open access to the levels where his or her self-healing power resides and to imagine the healing image. This process may be repeated as often as necessary, allowing changes in the healing image that might either spontaneously appear or be appropriate if the image associated with the pain were to change. Similarly, by repeatedly imagining oneself as having already achieved a desired goal, the deeper mind gradually accepts this new image and works to bring it into reality.

Of the various mind and body modalities, the practice of guided imagery appears to be widely used and accepted among many nursing departments. A community-based nursing study was conducted in Sydney, Australia, where people with advanced cancer experiencing anxiety and depression were randomly assigned to one of four treatment conditions: (1) progressive muscle relaxation training, (2) guided imagery training, (3) both treatments, and (4) control group. Patients were tested for anxiety, depression, and quality of life. There was no significant improvement for anxiety, but there were significant positive changes for depression and quality of life. Nurses at a community hospital in Pennsylvania found that offering their patients guided imagery compact discs (CDs) can be effective in a variety of ways. They report that guided imagery (1) helps patients to relieve pain and anxiety before and after surgery, (2) helps patients to relax and sleep better during evening hours, (3) helps to lower blood pressure, and (4) reduces the need for breathing and respiratory devices. Nurses also report that the CDs are often more effective than sedation for easing confusion in older patients. Each bedside contains a packet of CDs and a CD player with earphones. Each CD focuses on a major component of a successful hospital stay (e.g., health and healing, comfort, peaceful rest, courage, serenity). In addition, all the staff nurses, therapists, social workers, and managers are trained in the use of the CDs and use them for their personal benefit.

Differences in pain control were examined at Kent State's College of Nursing, where patients were randomly assigned to treatment and control groups. Those who received guided imagery had decreased pain during the last 2 days of the 4-day trial (Lewandowski, 2004). An early study was conducted to compare the effectiveness of various types of guided imagery for preoperative patients. Three outcomes were examined: intraoperative blood loss, length of hospital stay, and use of postoperative pain medication. A large number of surgical patients were randomly assigned to five groups. Each of the four experimental groups were provided with a guided imagery audiotape created by four different therapists. The control group received an audiotape with a "whooshing" noise with no meaningful physiological effect. Results showed that three of the four audiotapes produced no significant benefits on any of the medical outcomes examined. By contrast, the guided imagery audiotape produced by Belleruth Naparstek, a highly regarded therapist and imagery practitioner, produced highly significant results in two outcomes, blood loss and length of stay. Naparstek's tape was much more sophisticated than the others. Her imagery had been scored with specially composed music designed to highlight and accompany each image, with an emphasis on spiritual connectedness. Naparstek included visualizations of positive outcomes, faster wound healing, less pain, and no nausea.

Cleveland Clinic researchers measured 130 colorectal surgery patients for anxiety levels, pain perceptions, and narcotic medication requirements. The treatment group listened to guided imagery tapes for 3 days before their surgery, during anesthesia induction, intraoperatively, after anesthesia, and for 6 days after surgery; the controls received routine perioperative care. Patients in the guided imagery group experienced considerably less preoperative and postoperative anxiety and pain, and they required 50% less narcotic medication after surgery than did controls.

GI represents one of the approaches that relies on the power of the mind guided by a professional to form images in the "mind's eye" that literally overcome pain. One of the most common and problematic orthopedic surgical procedures nowadays is knee replacement surgery, ostensibly done to reduce pain and improve function. Studies show that only approximately one in three knee replacement surgeries performed are appropriate. GI is now being recommended as a natural therapy for pain relief following orthopedic surgery. New research shows GI is a useful treatment for most patients, and they show high levels of participation and satisfaction when offered for pain following surgery (Draucker, Jacobson, Myerscough, Umberger, & Sanata, 2015).

FINDING PRACTITIONERS

Many use GI in their work, though they may have learned only to lead someone through noninteractive scripts. The quality of training and competence with this intervention is quite variable. Because there is potential for doing harm when these techniques are used inappropriately or without adequate skills, standards of practice and quality control are important.

The Academy for Guided Imagery is a postgraduate training institution founded in 1989 to bring quality standards to the training and certification of imagery practitioners. Quality assurance is largely based on direct observation of clinical work in small group and individual supervision sessions during the training program. Each candidate is observed by four to six different faculty members during their 52 hours of supervision.

In addition, there are important personal qualities that the guide brings to the therapeutic experience, including a nonjudgmental attitude, patience, and trust in the client's own abilities. There is a consistent emphasis on the client's own resources and solutions. Repetitive inner focus provides inner sources for solutions and strengths. The belief that the client has more internal resources than they had imagined helps to prevent transference to the therapist. This approach provides greater opportunities for effective self-care, an enhanced sense of self-control, and the rapid development of independence.

HYPNOSIS

Hypnosis has earned a secure place in the practice of modern medicine against pain and related conditions. It has had a long and somewhat questionable history, so this therapeutic development may seem unlikely. Despite its somewhat mysterious quality and its regular (or irregular) use at times in some decidedly unscientific places, health practitioners maintain a continued interest in its use for pain. Communication with the unconscious had been the domain of hypnosis until the development of therapeutic applications of imaging, relaxation, and other techniques, as discussed in the chapters in this Section. Hypnosis ultimately earned a well-deserved place in modern medicine because it has been observed to accomplish truly remarkable results, although its "mechanism of action" has never been established. It is one of the highly effective, noninvasive treatment options available for pain, provided the patient is susceptible to hypnosis, which is based upon personality type (see Appendix I, pp. 572–579). It is completely noninvasive and harnesses the body's own power to heal itself.

Hypnosis had its formal beginning during the late 18th century when Franz Anton Mesmer demonstrated the ability to influence what he called "animal magnetism," borrowing a term from contemporary studies in electricity and magnetism (Goldsmith, 1934). Since these origins, dating back to the late 1700s, it certainly took time for hypnosis to gain the respect it merits. These practices were continued throughout the 19th century by a variety of "magnetic healers" who emphasized the power of "mind over matter" for healing purposes without the need for physical interventions on the body. Hypnosis finally found its way into mainstream medical practice in the 1950s. In 1955, the British Medical Association endorsed it. Then a few years later—in 1958—both the American and Canadian Medical Associations followed suit.

Since then, interest in hypnosis has grown, and its practice has found numerous clinical applications, including pain management. The technique is important for various psychological and medical conditions and has also been used successfully to treat anxiety, phobias, and to help people to quit smoking. The technique has also found important applications in the treatment of such varied disorders as migraine headaches, irritable bowel syndrome (IBS), and sleep disorders, as well as in the relief of chronic and acute pain.

Many people do not realize that hypnosis is a promising tool for many pain disorders and related conditions, not only based on numerous anecdotal accounts. Several controlled studies of its effects have appeared. With the advent of sophisticated brain imaging techniques, such as magnetic resonance imaging (MRI) and positron emission tomography (PET) scanning, it has been possible for the first time to understand some of the brain, as well as physiologic, changes that accompany a hypnotic state.

There are many new scientific studies on the benefits of hypnosis. There are abundant reviews and reports published in the medical literature describing the benefits of hypnotherapy for a wide variety of medical conditions. The following are examples:

- One study published in April 2012 showed that hypnosis can help ringing, buzzing, and hissing in the ears associated with tinnitus (Yazici et al., 2012).
- Another study showed significant blood sugar–lowering benefits in patients with type 2 diabetes who used hypnosis along with acupressure (Bay & Bay, 2011).
- According to a review by the University of Maryland Medical Center in Baltimore, hypnosis may help the functioning of the body's immune system and also provide relaxation benefits of other mind-body practices, such as easing stress and anxiety (Ehrlich, 2011).
- Two specific studies showed impressive benefits of hypnosis for IBS. In one study, 40% of patients in the hypnosis group experienced significant relief—compared with only 12% in the control group. In the other study, 85% of IBS patients who used hypnosis reported that they still felt the benefits 7 years later.
- Thrusting hypnosis further into the realm of modern scientific technology, some high-tech imaging techniques are now available that demonstrate its effects on the brain. MRIs and PET scans in particular have made it possible for researchers to see the actual metabolic changes that occur during hypnosis. Hypnosis is very much "for real."

How Hypnosis Works

Like many other functions of the human brain, the precise physiologic mechanisms of hypnosis still are not fully understood. On a superficial level, hypnosis patients appear to be asleep, but their electroencephalogram (EEG) brain wave patterns resemble wakefulness. The difference between "normal" wakefulness and the hypnotic state appears to reside in the locations where the brain wave activity occurs. Neurologic studies using EEGs in hypnotized individuals have shown a shift of brain wave activity to different regions of the brain. For example, imagining colors ("imaging") while hypnotized results in measurable increases in blood flow to the visual cortex—the area of the brain that is normally stimulated during actual sight.

By most accounts, hypnosis is characterized by increased mental focus and concentration, a "belle indifference" (a French-like indifference) to the external environment and heightened receptiveness to suggestion. Most people describe feeling a pleasantly altered state of consciousness (but not sleep), an air of calm, and a general feeling of well-being. Hypnosis works best when the hypnotized subject is able to thoroughly discontinue conscious "censoring" of information, in other words, to suspend their disbelief (which most people have a lot of practice doing simply from watching movies—or just observing the evening news from Washington, DC). However, a large percentage of patients benefit from even "light" levels of hypnosis.

You have no doubt seen hypnosis depicted by swinging a pocket watch in front of a person's face. Along with the phrase "You're getting very sleepy…" However, you will not often see either of these techniques used in real life (nor see many pocket watches) anymore. There is no uniform method for inducing hypnosis, but there are three common elements in most applications of clinical hypnosis:

- Absorption in the words or images presented by the hypnotherapist.
- Dissociation from the client's ordinary critical faculties.
- Responsiveness to the suggestions presented by the hypnotherapist ("power of suggestion").

A hypnotherapist either leads patients through relaxation, mental images, and suggestions, or he or she teaches patients to perform the techniques themselves. Many hypnotherapists provide guided audiotapes for their patients so that they can practice the therapy at home on their own. The images presented are specifically tailored to the particular individual's needs and may use one or all of the five (or six) senses.

A hypnosis session typically incorporates the following five steps or phases:

1. *Preparation.* The client is placed in a comfortable, secure environment. Usually sitting in a quiet room. Distractions and interruptions are minimized.
2. *Induction.* The client is guided to a state of relaxation by deep breathing, progressive muscle relaxation, and/or the use of imagery.
3. *Deepening.* The hypnotic state is deepened through repetition and reinforcement. Conscious thinking is minimized.
4. *Purpose.* The specific goal of hypnosis therapy is addressed. Hypnotic suggestions are given to modify perceptions or behaviors. For example, in the case of pain management, the client may be asked to transform the perception of pain to a numbness or tingling sensation. For example, for certain types of pains associated with fibromyalgia-chronic fatigue syndrome (FM-CFS), the "pain" may become interpreted as a less unpleasant paresthesia, such as tingling, warming, or "buzzing"—which may well be a more accurate way of describing what is happening with the central processing centers of sensations in the brain.

5. *Awakening*. The client is gradually brought out of the hypnotic state. During this stage, the therapeutic suggestions presented during step 4 are repeated and reinforced as the level of hypnosis lightens. Then the hypnotherapist offers some final suggestions, such as, "And you will awake refreshed and relaxed."

A hypnosis session will usually produce immediate positive results. Patients also generally report a sense of well-being and calm, although they are often uncertain about how deeply they were "under." They often comment on how they were completely aware of what was going on, with a curious unconcern about their surroundings (belle indifference), and whether they engaged in something that was embarrassing. Subsequent sessions usually produce "deeper" levels of hypnosis because patients are usually less apprehensive about the technique and feel safer. A typical hypnosis session takes between 30 minutes to 1 hour. There are no studies or guidelines setting an optimal frequency for hypnosis sessions, but weekly sessions are probably realistic for most people. Between sessions most patients are encouraged to practice "self-hypnosis." The self-hypnosis method is not quite as effective as guided therapy with a skilled hypnotist but relies on the patient's own skills at achieving a hypnotic state by applying breathing techniques and imagery learned during regular sessions.

POWER OF SUGGESTION FOR PAIN

Hypnotism nowadays consists of two basic components: (1) the use of a technique to induce a state of consciousness that allows greater access to the deeper parts of the mind and (2) a method for communicating with those deeper parts of the mind. This kind communication involves making suggestions (the power of suggestion) to the inner depths of the mind. The hypnotists suggest items or behaviors desired for betterment of health, work, or daily living. Several different techniques are used to induce the necessary state of consciousness, and some may be quite similar to more common relaxation techniques and meditation techniques.

This chapter deals primarily with the use of hypnosis in the management of pain. The long noted anxiety-relieving properties of hypnosis are intimately associated with its pain-relieving effects and are also discussed. Reference will be made to contemporary prospective, controlled studies, the foundation of clinical research, in validating therapeutic applications. However, this original application of "mind-body" therapies involving the use of mental imagery has been used for well over 2 centuries, long before the modern controlled clinical trial research model. Hypnosis still has much to teach about using "mysterious" mind-body therapies that are effective, even while so-called mechanisms of action still remain to be elucidated. Thus we continue with a look back on the fascinating history of hypnosis and its evolution as a modern therapeutic technique. The mind-body knew something all along.

THE LONG HISTORY OF HYPNOSIS (OR, "YOU ARE GETTING SLEEPY...")

The origins of hypnosis as a distinctive medical practice are found in the colorful career of the Austrian physician Franz Anton Mesmer (1734–1815), a charismatic but controversial figure. Mesmer used trancelike states and the power of suggestion in treating patients, using what he termed "animal magnetism," and in turn giving rise to the term "mesmerism." Mesmer did not ask questions but made suggestions. He developed a large elite European continental clientele who often experienced improvement in their pain and other symptoms using mesmerism.

However, his ideas were judged as progressively radical even in light of the interests of 18th-century natural science in vitalism. Mesmer developed theories involving animal magnetism, astrology, and the effects of planetary tides on the body's "gravitational forces." Controversy surrounding Mesmer's work led him to leave Austria for France, following in the footsteps of the fated Marie Antoinette, who had joined the royal court of the Bourbons in Paris. The French medical and scientific establishment ultimately recommended a commission to be assembled in Paris by King Louis XVI to evaluate Memser's work. This assembly included such luminaries as the chemist Antoine Lavoisier (who was soon to lose his head, together with King Louis and Marie Antoinette) and Joseph Guillotine (the inventor of the humane execution apparatus, who brought about these decapitations, soon to become popular in revolutionary France), as well as the American ambassador of the new United States to France, Benjamin Franklin. The panel initially designed experiments that would have provided a fair scientific evaluation, but it soon degenerated into arguments about mechanisms of action—which have currently not been resolved to this day—and the result was not kind to Mesmer. They ultimately labeled him a fraud and concluded that any apparent benefit of his technique was the work of the "imagination."

However, Mesmer had discovered the true power of mental imagery and suggestion in modifying somatic symptoms, such as pain. One of his students, Dr. Charles D'Elson, commented after the Louis XVI committee report:

If Mesmer has no other secret than that he has been able to make the imagination exert an influence upon health, would he not still be a wonder doctor? If treatment by the use of the imagination is the best treatment, why do we not make use of it?

This good question still resonates today in the era of so-called "health care reform" and in the era of so-called "evidence-based" medicine.

Interest in mesmerism was rekindled in the 1840s when British surgeons used hypnotic techniques in their clinical practices for anesthesia before the development of chemical anesthetics. It was as that time the term "hypnotism," from the Greek hypnos (sleep), was coined by the English surgeon James Braid. He realized that hypnosis was not a result of external forces but of the subject's ability to summon his or her own powers of focus and concentration (Graci & Sexton-Radek, 2006). An influential 19th-century practitioner of early hypnosis for surgical anesthesia was the Scottish surgeon James Esdaile. In the era even before chemical anesthetics, such as nitrous oxide and ether, Esdaile used hypnosis as the sole method of anesthesia in more than

(Continued)

300 major operations, receiving widespread notice in Europe and the United States. With a relatively low mortality rate for these surgical procedures, Esdaile's efforts lent respectability to the clinical practice of hypnosis. Then, chemical anesthetic agents began to be used, following Morton's experiments at Massachusetts General Hospital, shortly thereafter. They quickly supplanted hypnosis for surgical anesthesia because they were easier to use and took less time to administer, although far more dangerous.

Later, during the 19th century, hypnosis was revived in France through the interest of those in the newly developing fields of psychiatry and psychology. At that time, neuropathologists were searching for anatomic-pathologic causes of disorders, such as schizophrenia (dementia precox), mania, and hysteria (for which we have yet to identify specific pathologic brain tissue abnormalities to this day). Meanwhile, medicine assumed that other mental diseases (that we now know are caused by pathologic processes), such as general paresis of the insane (tertiary syphilis of the brain), were actually primary mental disorders. For example, Sigmund Freud started out as a neuropathologist looking for the organic brain lesions of schizophrenia, which neither he nor anyone else has yet found; he gave up in frustration to become one of the founders of psychiatry to study the nonphysical dimensions of mental illness. Likewise the eminent French neurologist Jean Martin Charcot thought that the hypnotic state was a "pathological" condition akin to hysteria. (His observations, in turn, of tertiary syphilis patients with "general paresis of the insane," stumbling around on damaged but painless leg joints, lead to the pathognomonic attribution of "Charcot joint.") Sigmund Freud, in a further turn, later retraced Mesmer's journey from Austria to France, and met with Charcot at the Hospital Salpetriere in Paris where he became fascinated with hypnosis as a tool to explore the subconscious mind in the diagnosis and treatment of neuroses. However, Freud later abandoned the technique, striking a blow to its credibility and role in psychiatry and psychology in the succeeding years.

Interest in hypnosis by the medical community again waned. Later, amid the dislocation, suffering, and trauma of WWII and subsequent conflicts of the mid-20th century, hypnosis was again shown effective for the treatment of posttraumatic stress disorder (PTSD) and for pain relief (Graci & Sexton-Radek, 2006). Hypnosis eventually found its way back into mainstream medical practice with an endorsement by the British Medical Association in 1955 and by the American Medical Association and the Canadian Medical Association in 1958, where the former professor of one of us (Micozzi) at the University of Pennsylvania, Martine Orne, MD, had led the effort. Since then, interest in hypnosis has been growing, and the practice is finding numerous clinical applications. There has recently been a steady stream of clinical research, putting hypnosis on a solid scientific footing.

PHYSIOLOGY OF HYPNOSIS

Physiologically hypnosis resembles other forms of deep relaxation (see Chapter 6; and Fig. 4.1). It decreases nervous system activity, decreases oxygen consumption, and lowers blood pressure and heart rate. It can also increase or decrease certain types of brain wave activity. Hypnotherapy's effects and effectiveness lie in the complex connections between the mind and the body. It is now understood how illness affects emotional states and, conversely, that emotional states affect physical state. For example, stress, an emotional reaction, can make pain (or heart disease, for that matter) worse. And heart disease or pain, as physical conditions, can cause depression, as well as manifesting physical pain. Hypnosis carries these connections another logical step by using the power of the mind to bring about changes in the body. No one is quite sure how hypnosis works, but with more sophisticated brain imaging techniques, and research in psychoneuroimmunology, scientists are beginning to see where and how the brain "thinks" in various emotional-mental states of hypnosis, meditation, prayer, and how these mental states influence physiology throughout the body (Fig. 7.1)

HYPNOTIC SUSCEPTIBILITY

It is widely acknowledged that there is considerable variability in individual susceptibility to hypnosis ("hypnotizability" or "hypnotic suggestibility"). More recently, we have observed that there is individual variability in susceptibility to other natural mind-body approaches as well (see Appendix I, pp. 572–579). The large majority of patients can be hypnotized to some degree. Perhaps 10% cannot be hypnotized at all and another 10% are particularly susceptible. Women are more hypnotizable than men; children are more receptive than adults. The Drs. Speigel, father and son, at Stanford University developed and applied "hypnotic susceptibility scales" to provide a biostatistical basis for evaluating receptivity to hypnosis without implying any particular underlying mechanism of action. This kind of approach can in

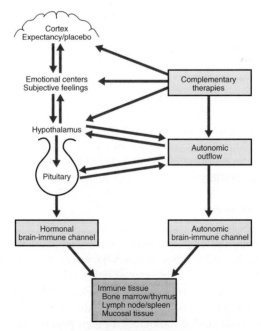

FIG. 7.1 | Brain-immune pathways of mind-body medicine.

turn provide a basis for the improved, individualized application of other complementary and alternative medical modalities and mind-body therapies, in which the
mechanism(s) of action is controversial, obscure, or remains "foreign" in the view
of the contemporary biomedical paradigm. There is no longer any question that the
anatomic, neurologic, hormonal, and immunologic connections exist (see Fig. 7.1)

We discuss details on how to find the individual approaches that will work best
for each individual patient based on their psychometric type (or to which individuals are most "susceptible") in Appendix I (pp. 572–579).

THE HYPNOTIC STATE

Although the precise physiologic mechanisms of hypnosis (as with many functions
of the human brain) are not fully understood, superficially it can be seen as resembling a sleep-like state (thus the Greek *hypnos,* or sleep). Hypnosis is characterized
by waking EEG brainwave patterns. Neurologic studies using EEGs in hypnotized
individuals have shown a shift of brain wave activity to different regions of the
brain. Hypnotic imagination of color perception results in measurable increases
in blood flow to the visual cortex, which is normally stimulated during actual sight
and vision.

By most accounts, hypnosis is characterized by increased mental focus and concentration, an indifference to the external environment, and heightened receptiveness or susceptibility to suggestion ("suggestibility"). Most individuals describe a
pleasantly altered state of consciousness (but not sleep), an air of calmness, and
a general feeling of well-being while under hypnosis. When properly performed,
hypnosis is almost always accompanied by reduced perception of anxiety and stress.

Facilitation of suggestibility appears to develop from an inclination by the hypnotized subject to suspend conscious cortical "censoring" of received information
(in the "higher" centers of the cortex of the brain). Hypnosis has been likened to
a state of "highly focused attention with a constriction in peripheral awareness"
(Spiegel, 2007). There is controversy about how deep a level of hypnosis is required
for its therapeutic effects to take hold. Most recent studies suggest that deep hypnosis is not necessary and a large percentage of patients with pain benefit from even
"light" levels of hypnosis. A smaller percentage of patients will be able to achieve
complete hypnotic anesthesia.

PRACTICING HYPNOSIS

There is no uniform method of hypnotic induction. However, there are elements
common to most applications of clinical hypnosis. Hypnosis has the three major
components discussed earlier: absorption (in the words or images presented by the
hypnotherapist), dissociation (from your ordinary critical faculties), and responsiveness. A hypnotherapist either leads patients through relaxation, mental images,
and suggestions, or teaches patients to perform the techniques themselves. Many
hypnotherapists provide guided audiotapes for their patients so that they can practice the therapy at home. The images presented are specifically tailored to the particular patient's needs and may use one or all of the senses.

TYPICAL HYPNOSIS SESSION

The hypnosis session usually incorporates several components.

1. *Preparation.* The patient is placed in a comfortable, secure environment, usually sitting in a quiet room. Distractions and interruptions are minimized.
2. *Induction.* The patient is guided to a state of relaxation by deep breathing, progressive muscle relaxation, and the use of imagery.
3. *Deepening.* The hypnotic state is deepened through repetition and reinforcement. Conscious thinking is minimized.
4. *Purpose.* The specific goal of the hypnotherapy session is addressed. Hypnotic suggestions are used to modify perceptions or behavior (Montgomery, David, Winkel, Silverstein, & Bovbjerg, 2002). In the case of pain management, the subject may be asked to transform the perception of pain to a numbness or tingling sensation.
5. *Awakening.* The patient is gradually brought out of the hypnotic state. This stage affords an opportunity to repeat and reinforce therapeutic suggestions as the level of hypnosis lightens. Final suggestions are offered to bring about a feeling of relaxation combined with energy and vitality on awakening.

The hypnosis session usually produces immediate positive results. The subject will report a sense of well-being and calmness. Although often uncertain about their depth of hypnosis, patients often comment on their awareness of what was going on, but with a curious unconcern about their surroundings. Subsequent sessions usually produce "deeper" levels of hypnosis because the patient is less apprehensive about the technique and feels safer. Evidence of the secondary benefits of hypnosis in pain management is typically assessed at clinical follow-up.

Although a typical hypnosis session will take 30 to 60 minutes, there are no studies or guidelines about the optimal frequency of hypnosis sessions, and practitioners must adapt to the practical realities of time constraints and scheduling limitations. A weekly session at the outset may be feasible for some caregivers. Between sessions the patient is encouraged to practice "self-hypnosis." This method, although not quite as effective as guided therapy with a skilled hypnotist, uses the patients' own skills at achieving a hypnotic state. Patients are also instructed to apply breathing techniques and imagery learned during regular sessions. Self-hypnosis is a useful adjunct in hypnotherapy, which can be used often and when needed by the patient.

PAIN AND RELATED CONDITIONS

ANXIETY AND PHOBIAS

Hypnosis can be used to establish a new pattern of reaction and to reset emotional boundaries around anxiety-producing environments and thoughts to specific anxiety-causing activities, such as stage fright, airplane flight, and other phobias. Typically the hypnotherapist helps the patient to reverse a conditioned physiologic response, such as hyperventilation or nausea. This method can also be used to help to calm athletes who are preparing to compete. Hypnotherapy can be used to quell most any fear, whether associated with examinations, public speaking, or social interactions.

HEADACHE AND PAIN MANAGEMENT

Hypnosis can also be effective in reducing the fear and anxiety that accompanies pain. Because it is observed that anxiety can increase pain, hypnotherapy helps a patient to gain control over the fear and anxiety, thereby reducing the pain (see Chapter 5). Many controlled studies have demonstrated that hypnosis is also an effective way to reduce migraine headache attacks in children and teenagers. In one experiment, 30 schoolchildren were randomly assigned a placebo or the drug propranolol (a blood pressure–lowering agent used for migraine) or taught self-hypnosis. Only the children who used the self-hypnosis techniques had a significant decrease in severity and frequency of headaches (Olness & Gardner, 1988). A study of chronically ill patients reported a more than 100% increase in pain tolerance among highly hypnotizable subjects compared with a control group who did not receive hypnosis (De Benedittis, Panerai, & Villamira, 1989).

Researchers at Virginia Polytechnic Institute found that during a hypnotic state aimed at bringing about pain control, the prefrontal cortex of the brain directed other areas of the brain to reduce or eliminate their awareness of pain (Gordon, 2004). A technique used for surgery in people with little or no tolerance for chemical anesthesia is called "spinal anesthesia illusion", developed by Philip Ament, a dentist and psychologist from Buffalo, New York. In this method, a deep state of relaxation is induced by having the patient count mentally or focus on a specific image. The patient is given the suggestion that he or she will feel a growing numbness begin to spread from the navel to the toes as he or she counts to higher and higher numbers. After the patient feels numb, the surgery can proceed. After the surgery, the therapist gives the patient suggestions that lead to the gradual return of normal sensations.

Nearly 20 years ago, Price, Milling, Kirsch, Duff, Montgomery, et al. (1999), at the Mount Sinai Medical School, set out to organize and tabulate the extant medical literature on the subject of hypnosis and pain management (Montgomery, DuHamel, & Redd, 2000). The field to that point had been in a state of disarray, with numerous anecdotal and uncontrolled reports leaving the medical community uncertain of the clinical benefits. Montgomery's group undertook a meta-analysis of nearly 20 previously published trials including almost 1000 patients. The studies included both clinical patients as well as experimental pain groups of healthy volunteers (i.e., focal pressure). The patients included those with pain due to burn injuries, cancer, headaches, coronary disease, and invasive radiologic procedures.

The results of the analysis revealed significant benefits for hypnotic interventions in the treatment of pain. Effects were more pronounced in highly "hypnotizable" subjects (~10%). However, "midrange patients," making up the largest group in terms of hypnotic susceptibility (~80%), also had significant pain relief from the hypnosis intervention. This finding supports the clinical experience that a deep level of hypnosis is not required to achieve clinical benefit. Furthermore, the technique has little downside risk.

OPERATIVE PAIN AND SURGERY

Montgomery's group (2000) also reported an analysis of hypnosis for general surgical patients. Twenty published studies with more than 1600 patients were reviewed. Hypnosis was typically administered in the form of a relaxing induction phase followed by suggestions aimed at modifying postoperative side effects, such as pain, nausea, or distress. Most of the interventions consisted of live sessions administered by a health care professional, whereas the remainder used audiotapes.

There were broad benefits from hypnosis for a number of clinical outcomes. Nearly 90% of patients in the hypnosis groups benefited in comparison with patients receiving standard care. Positive effects included improved levels of anxiety and depression, pain, pain medication use, and physiologic indicators (i.e., blood pressure, heart rate, and catecholamine levels). Benefits were similar among live and audiotape patient groups.

Labor and Childbirth

Hypnosis has been used for more than a century in the management of childbirth pain (Cyna, McAuliffe, & Andrew, 2004). A noninvasive method to assist in childbirth pain is of great importance to obstetric and anesthesia practitioners, particularly when epidural anesthesia is impractical or contraindicated. There have been a number of reports on the effectiveness of hypnosis in obstetric analgesia.

Cyna et al. (2004) undertook a meta-analysis to assess the role of hypnosis in the pain of childbirth. The results of the analysis revealed a significant benefit of the hypnosis intervention. Parturient women who received hypnosis rated their labor pain less severe than did controls and required less pharmacologic analgesia during labor. Martin published a randomized, controlled trial on obstetrical hypnosis in 42 teenage patients. The treatment patients received a four-session sequence of hypnotic focused relaxation and imagery. Suggestions were directed at the patients' ability to manage stress and discomfort. The treatment patients had a significantly lower length of stay, fewer complications, and required less conventional anesthesia during labor and postpartum than did controls. It is believed that Lamaze and other popular breathing techniques used during labor and delivery may actually work by inducing a hypnotic state. Women who have used hypnosis before delivery tend to have a shorter labor and more comfortable delivery than other pregnant women. There are even reports of cesarean sections performed with hypnosis as the sole anesthesia. Women are taught to take advantage of their body's natural anesthetic abilities to make childbirth a less painful, more positive experience.

Dental Pain and Procedures

Hypnosis has been used successfully for pain management in dentistry.

Some people have learned to tolerate dental work (e.g., drilling, extraction, periodontal surgery) using hypnosis as the sole anesthesia. Even when an anesthetic is used, hypnotherapy can also be used to reduce fear and anxiety, control bleeding and salivation, and lessen postoperative discomfort. Used with children, hypnosis can decrease the chances of developing a dental phobia.

Ghoneim, Block, Davis, Marchman, & Sarasin (2000) conducted a prospective, randomized study of 60 patients scheduled for third molar extraction. The intervention group received an audiotape incorporating hypnotic induction and suggestions designed to alleviate pain and enhance healing. The treatment group listened to the tape daily in the week preceding oral surgery. Patients receiving hypnotherapy reported less anxiety before their scheduled procedure. However, there was no decrease in the consumption of analgesics, and the benefit of the intervention was unclear. Other groups have discerned greater benefit from hypnosis in dental surgery patients, including a diminished requirement for postoperative analgesics (Enqvist & Fisher, 1997; Enqvist, von Konow, & Bystedt,1995).

FINDING A PRACTITIONER

Hypnotherapy is generally provided by a licensed mental health practitioner, such as a psychiatrist or psychologist, or a dentist who is also trained in the clinical practice of hypnosis. A state of trust and confidence should exist between hypnotist and subject. The patient often requires reassurance, particularly at the first session, that there will be no loss of control or inappropriate suggestions. Medical hypnosis should be distinguished from the "stage" variety, with which many patients are most familiar and which is performed for purposes of entertainment.

Although hypnotherapy is generally provided by a licensed mental health practitioner, such as a psychiatrist or psychologist, other kinds of practitioners are also trained in the clinical practice of hypnosis. The American Society of Clinical Hypnosis (http://www.asch.net; 1-630-980-4740) is a resource that can help to locate a hypnotherapist in your area.

Most patients—even the most open-minded ones—usually need some reassurance, especially at the first session, that they will not be surrendering control or be subjected to inappropriate suggestions. Good practitioners ease the mind of these worries and allow relaxation in a safe, comfortable environment—which after all is an essential part of effective hypnotherapy.

REFERENCES

Baars, J. & Gage, N. M. (2010). *Consciousness and attention.* http://neurocognitiva.org/wp-content/uploads/2014/04/Baars-2010-Cap-8-Consciousness-and-Attention.pdf.

Barber, T. X. (1969). *A scientific approach.* New York: Van Nostrand.

Barber, T. X. (1984). Changing "unchangeable" bodily processes by hypnotic suggestions: A new look at hypnosis, imaging and the mind/body problem. *Advances, 1*(2), 7.

Bay, R. & Bay, F. (2011). Combined therapy using acupressure therapy, hypnotherapy, and transcendental meditation versus placebo in type 2 diabetes. *Journal of Acupuncture and Meridian Studies, 4,* 183–186. http://www.ncbi.nlm.nih.gov/pubmed/21981869.

Blakeslee, S., Macknik, S., & Martinez-Conde, S. (2011). *Sleights of mind: What the neuroscience of magic reveals about our brains.* Great Britain: Clays, Bungay, Suffolk.

Cyna, A. M., McAuliffe, G. L., & Andrew, M. I. (2004). Hypnosis for pain relief in labor and childbirth: A systematic review. *British Journal of Anesthesia, 93*(4), 505–511.

De Benedittis, G., Panerai, A. A., & Villamira, M. A. (1989). Effects of hypnotic analgesia and hypnotizability on experimental ischemic pain. *International Journal of Clinical and Experimental Hypnosis, 37,* 55–69.

Draucker, C. B., Jacobson, A. F., Umberger, W. A., Myerscough, R. P., & Sanata, J. D. (2015). Acceptability of a guided imagery intervention for persons undergoing a total knee replacement. *Orthopedic Nursing, 34*(6), 356–364.

Ehrlich, S. D. (2011). *Hypnotherapy.* http://umm.edu/health/medical/altmed/treatment/hypnotherapy.

Enqvist, B., von Konow, L., & Bystedt, H. (1995). Stress reduction, preoperatie hypnosis and perioperative suggestions in maxillo-facial surgery. *Stress Medicine, 11*, 229–233.

Enqvist, B. & Fisher, K. (1997). Preoperative hypnotic techniques reduce consumption of analgesics after surgical removal of third mandibular molars: A brief communication. *International Journal of Clinical and Experimental Hypnosis, 45*, 102–108.

Ganis, G., Thompson, W. L., & Kosslyn, S. M. (2004). Brain areas underlying visual mental imagery and visual perception: An fMRI study. *Cognitive Brain Research, 20*, 226–241. http://www.ncbi.nlm.nih.gov/pubmed/15183394.

Ghoneim, M. M., Block, R. I., Sarasin, D. S., Davis, C. S., & Marchman, J. N. (2000). Tape-recorded hypnosis instructions as adjuvant in the care of patients scheduled for third molar surgery. *Anesthesia and Analgesia, 90*, 64–68.

Goldsmith, M. (1934). *Franz anton mesmer: A history of mesmerism.* (p. 155). Garden City, NY: Doubleday, Doran, and Company, Inc.

Gordon, D. (2004). *The fresh face of hypnosis: An old practice finds new uses.* Better Homes & Gardens.

Graci, G. & Sexton-Radek, K. (2006). Treating sleep disorders using cognitive behavior therapy and hypnosis. In R. A. Chapman (Ed.), *Clinical use of hypnosis in cognitive behavior: A practitioner's casebook* (p. 296). New York, NY: Springer Publications.

Green, E. & Green, A. (1977). *Beyond biofeedback.* New York: Delta.

Häuser, W., Hansen, E., & Enck, P. (2012). Nocebo phenomena in medicine: Their relevance in everyday clinical practice. *Deutsches Ärzteblatt International, 109*, 459–465. http://www.ncbi.nlm.nih.gov/pubmed/22833756.

Jordan, C. S. & Lenington, K. T. (1979). Psychological correlates of eidetic imagery and induced anxiety. *Journal Mental Imagery, 3*, 31.

Kreiman, G., Koch, C., & Fried, I. (2000). Imagery neurons in the human brain. *Nature, 408*, 357–361. http://www.ncbi.nlm.nih.gov/pubmed/11099042.

Lewandowski, W. A. (July 2004). Patterning of pain and power with guided imagery. *Nursing Science Quarterly, 17*(3 233-241). http://dx.doi.org/10.1177/0894318404266322.

Montgomery, G. H., David, D., Winkel, G., Silverstein, J. H., & Bovbjerg, D. H. (2002). The effectiveness of adjunctive hypnosis with surgical patients: A meta-analysis. *Anesthesia and Analgesia, 94*, 1639–1645.

Montgomery, G. H., DuHamel, K. N., & Redd, W. H. (2000). A meta-analysis of hypnotically induced analgesia: How effective is hypnosis? *The International Journal of Clinical and Experimental Hypnosis, 48*(2), 138–153.

Olness, K. & Gardner, G. G. (1988). *Hypnosis and hypnotherapy with children* (2nd ed.). Philadelphia: Saunders.

Price, D. D., Milling, L. S., Kirsch, I., Duff, A., Montgomery, G. H., & Nicholls, S. S. (1999). An analysis of factors that contribute to the magnitude of placebo analgesia in an experimental paradigm. *Pain, 83*(2), 147–156.

Spiegel, D. (2007). The mind prepared: Hypnosis hypnosis in surgery. *Journal of National Cancer Institute, 99*, 1280–1281.

White, K. D. (1978). Salivation: The significance of imagery in its voluntary control. *Psychophysiology, 15*(3), 196.

Yazici, Z. M., Sayin, I., Gökkuş, G., Alatas, E., Kaya, H., & Kayhan, F. T. (2012). Effectiveness of Ericksonian hypnosis in tinnitus therapy: Preliminary results. *B-ENT, 8*, 7–12. http://www.ncbi.nlm.nih.gov/pubmed/22545384.

Suggested Readings can be found on the companion website, http://www.micozzipainconditions.com.

Chapter 8

Mental and Spiritual Healing, and Spiritually Based Rapid Healing

MENTAL HEALING

The idea that consciousness can affect the physical body is a time-honored concept with a respected historical base, as well as grounding in fundamental physics (see Chapter 4). The observation that "there is a measure of consciousness through-out the body" is present in 2400-year-old Hippocratic writings. Before the ancient Greeks, the ancient Persians (Zoroastrian) also expounded on this concept. They believed that a person's mind can intervene, not just in his or her own body, but also in that of another individual located at a distance far away. The great Muslim physician Abu Ali ibn Sina (Avicenna in Latinized form, AD 980–1037) later postulated that the faculty of imagination could enable humans to make themselves ill or to restore health (Amri, Abu-Asab, & Micozzi, 2013).

The attitudes of the ancient Greek, Persian, and Islamic physicians toward the interaction among minds and bodies eventually gave rise to two very different types of healing: local and nonlocal. The Greeks believed that the action of the mind on the body was a "local" event in the here and now. The Persians, however, viewed the mind-body relationship as "nonlocal." They held that the mind (as consciousness) was not localized or confined to the body but extended beyond the body. These views are also consonant with the ancient Ayurvedic teachings of the Hindu Civilization in India (see Chapter 19). This belief implied that the mind was capable of affecting any physical body, local or nonlocal. A modern example is when someone prays for the benefit of another (see Power of Prayer section).

IMPLICATIONS OF NONLOCALITY

Fundamental physicists have for many decades recognized the concept of non-locality. These developments rest partially on an idea in physics called "Bell's theorem," introduced in 1964 by Irish physicist John Stewart Bell and supported by subsequent experiments (Mayor & Micozzi, 2011; see also Chapter 9). Bell showed that when distant objects have once been in contact, any change in one thereafter causes an immediate change in the other, even were they to be separated to the opposite ends of the universe. It is important to realize that nonlocality is not just a theoretical idea of the theory of relativity in fundamental physics, but that its proof rests on the results of actual experiments that have been done on "quantum entanglement" (see Chapters 4 and 9).

An idea prevalent in contemporary science is that the mind and consciousness are entirely local phenomenon and specifically localized to the mind and confined to the present moment in time. From this perspective, nonlocal healing cannot occur in principle because the mind is bounded by the "here and now." Research studies examining distant mental influences challenge these modern-day assumptions. Dozens of experiments conducted over the past 4 decades suggest that the mind can bring about changes in nonlocal physical bodies, even when shielded from all sensory and electromagnetic influences. This observation suggests that what we have called "mind" and "consciousness" may not be located at fixed points in space (Braud, 1992; Jahn & Dunn, 1987).

Some physicists believe that nonlocality applies not just to the domain of electrons and other subatomic particles but also to our familiar world consisting of dense matter. A growing number of physicists think that nonlocality may apply to the mind. Physicist Nick Herbert, in his book *Quantum Reality,* stated "Bell's theorem requires our quantum knowledge to be nonlocal, instantly linked to everything it has previously touched" (Herbert, 1987; see Chapter 9).

For the Western model of medicine, the implications of a nonlocal concept are profound and include the following:

1. Nonlocal models of the mind could be helpful in understanding the actual dynamics of the healing process. They may help to explain why in some patients a cure suddenly appears unexpectedly, "spontaneously," or a healing appears to be influenced by events occurring nonlocally.
2. Nonlocal manifestations of consciousness complicate traditional experimental designs, which cannot account for them (see Chapter 9) and require innovative research methods, because the mental state of the healer may influence the experiment's outcome, even under "blinded," "controlled" conditions (Solfvin, 1984).

Nonlocality assumptions give rise to the idea that consciousness could prevail after the death of the body/brain, which suggests that some aspect of the psyche is not bound only to specific points in space or time. This idea, in turn, leads toward a nonlocal model of consciousness, which allows for the possibility of distant healing exchange.

This nonlocal model of consciousness implies that at some level of the psyche, no fundamental separations exist among individual minds. Nobel laureate quantum physicist Erwin Schroedinger suggested that at some level, and in some sense, there may be unity and oneness of all minds (Schroedinger, 1969). In the nonlocal model, distance is not fundamental but is completely overcome. In other words, because of the unification of consciousness of the mind (as with quantum entanglement of particle physics), the healer and the patient are not separated by physical distance.

For 40 years, psychologist Lawrence LeShan investigated the local and nonlocal effects of prayer and mental healing. He taught these techniques to more than 400 people and ultimately became a healer himself. He maintained that healing influences were observed to have occurred 15% to 20% of the time but could never be predicted in advance of any specific healing (LeShan, 1966). LeShan found that mental-spiritual healing methods can be categorized into the following two main types:

- *Type I (nonlocal).* The healer enters a prayerful, altered state of consciousness in which he or she views himself or herself and the patient as a single entity. There is no physical contact or any attempt to offer anything of a physical nature to the person in need, only the desire or intention to connect and unite. These healers emphasize the importance of empathy, love, and caring in this process. When the healing takes place, it does so in the context of unity, compassion, and love. This type of healing is considered a natural process and merely speeds up the normal healing processes.
- *Type II (local).* The healer does touch the patient and may imagine some "flow of energy" through his or her hands to the area of the patient receiving the healing. Feelings of heat are common in both the healer and patient. In this mode, unlike type I, the healer holds the intention for healing.

Research into the origins of consciousness and how it relates to the physical brain had been practically nonexistent. Although hypotheses purporting to explain consciousness do exist, there is no agreement among researchers as to its nature, local, or nonlocal (see Chapters 4 and 9).

SPIRITUALITY AND HEALING

Throughout the ages, mystical traditions have valued spiritual qualities of humans beyond the physical, emphasizing transcendence of one over the other. In the background of most mystical traditions is the idea that the body is somehow at odds with the spirit. A war wages, and one must fight the war to achieve an enlightened status. Still other theologians postulate that the greatest spiritual achievement of all may lie in the realization that the spiritual and the physical are one and that perhaps the ultimate spiritual goal is not to transcend anything but to realize the integration and oneness of being. Such a truth would seem to obviate the need for Western Transcendentalism, or for Eastern Transcendental Meditation, once realized.

A new quality of spiritual awakening has been emerging worldwide over the past 40 years. This innovative approach encourages people to develop faith in their own capacity to create their own reality in partnership with a "G-d-force within." In many cultures, both Eastern and Western, prayer-based spiritual healing is an integral part of modern religious practices, including the "charismatic" practices of Christianity and Roman Catholicism.

The premise of creating our own reality is, in essence, a spiritual one. This concept is sometimes contrary to many fundamental religious positions that embrace G-d as an external being, because spirituality also emphasizes a "G-d-within" reality, or duality. Transcending some boundaries and limitations of specific religions, a spiritual practice honors a relation between the individual and the G-d-force as a kind of partnership.

When people consider the possibility that they create their own realities, the question that invariably arises is, "Through what source? What is the source of this power of creation that runs through my being?" The answer to this question is found not externally but internally. This internal source seeking to understand our own nature is considered divinity in action, incarnated in each person.

The blending of spirituality with the tenets of natural, alternative, and complementary therapies provides individuals with one means of understanding how they contribute to the creation of their illness and to their healing. This understanding does not come from a place of self-blame and does not view illness as a result of the will of G-d but rather is an attempt to understand a spiritual purpose for suffering in a physical body. The relationship that is cultivated ultimately transcends the human value system of punishment versus reward, and it grows into a relationship based on principles of co-creation and co-responsibility. Therefore, the journey of healing for patients as well as the journey of life is freed of a burden of feeling victimized by fate, circumstances, or the deity, and patients are free to have faith and hope not only in G-d but in themselves as well.

Research in the last 40 years has made an indelible mark on the way health care professionals think about the role of spirituality and religion in physical, mental, and social health. Hundreds of studies have explored the relations between body and spirit. Most studies have been cross-sectional, but some have also been longitudinal. Many studies now document an association between religious involvement and lower anxiety, fewer psychotic symptoms, less substance abuse, and better coping mechanisms. A comprehensive review found that 478 of 742 quantitative studies (67%) reported a statistically significant relationship between religious involvement and better mental health and greater social support. The review also found that almost 80% of those who are devoutly religious have significantly greater feelings of well-being, hope, and optimism compared with those who are less religious (Koenig, McCullough, & Larson, 2001).

At Duke University, studies were conducted examining the effects of religiousness on the course of depression in 850 hospitalized patients over the age of 60 years. Results showed that religious coping predicted lower levels of depressive symptoms at baseline and at 6 months following discharge (Koenig et al., 1992).

Koenig's studies and others have shown that spirituality and religiosity are clearly associated with longer survival, healthier behaviors, and less distress and are believed to have an effect on coping (Pargament, Smith, Koenig, & Perez, 1998; Tix & Frazier, 1997), anxiety (Koenig, Ford, George, Blazer, & Meador, 1993), success in aging (Crowther, Parker, Achenbaun, Larimore, & Koenig, 2002), end-of-life issues (Daaleman & VandeCreek, 2000), and cortisol levels in patients with human immunodeficiency virus infection and acquired immunodeficiency syndrome (Ironson et al., 2002).

POWER OF PRAYER

The use of prayer in healing may have begun in human prehistory and continues to this day as an underlying tenet in almost all religions. The records of many of the great religious traditions, including the mystical traditions of Christianity, Daoism, Hinduism, Buddhism, and Islam, give the strong impression that enlightenment comes when one begins to explore the dynamic qualities of interrelation and interconnection among the self and the source of all being.

The word prayer comes from the Latin *precarious,* "obtained by begging," and *precari,* "to entreat"—to ask earnestly, beseech, or implore. This definition suggests two of the most common forms of prayer: petition, asking something for one's self, and intercession, asking something for others.

Prayer is a genuinely nonlocal event, not confined to a specific place in space nor to a specific moment in time. Prayer reaches outside the here and now; it operates at a distance and outside the present moment. Prayer is initiated by mental action and intention, which implies that some aspect of the psyche also is genuinely nonlocal. Nonlocality implies infinitude in space and time, because a limited nonlocality is a contradiction in terms. In Western terms, this infinite aspect of the psyche has been referenced as the soul. Empirical evidence for the power of prayer, therefore, may be seen as indirect evidence for existence of the soul.

Scientific attempts to assess the effects of prayer and spiritual practices on health began in the nineteenth century with a treatise by the early statistician Sir Francis Galton (a nephew of Charles Darwin), "Statistical Inquiries into the Efficacy of Prayer" (Galton, 1872). Galton initially used these new methods to study human growth but believed that statistical analysis could be brought to any topic even when the "mechanism of action" was unknown, such as in the example of prayer. This application also helps make the point that useful statistical, psychometric profiles can be brought to the study and application of any mind-body therapy, such as hypnosis, where there is no known "mechanism" for how, when, and why it is observed to work for whom (see Chapter 7, and Appendix I, pp. 572–579).

Galton assessed the longevity of people who were frequently prayed for, such as clergy, monarchs, and heads of state. He concluded that there was no demonstrable effect of prayer on longevity. By current scientific standards, Galton's study was flawed. He was successful, however, in promoting the idea that prayer is subject to empirical scrutiny. Galton acknowledged that praying could make a person feel better. In the end, he maintained that although his attempts to prove the efficacy of prayer had failed, he could see no good reason to abandon prayer (reminiscent of Pascal's wager).

Those who practice healing with prayer claim uniformly that the effects are not diminished with distance. Therefore, it falls within the nonlocal perspective discussed earlier. Claims about the effectiveness of prayer do not rely on anecdote or single case studies. Numerous controlled studies have validated the nonlocal nature of prayer. Much of this evidence suggests that praying individuals, or people involved in compassionate imagery or mental intent, whether or not it is called "prayer," can purposefully affect the physiology of distant people without the awareness of the receiver.

The medical community has already begun to acknowledge the importance of exploring the associations among spirituality and medicine. Many medical schools have long offered courses in religion, spirituality, and health. According to a 1994 survey, 98% of hospitalized patients ascribed to a belief in God or some higher power, and 96% acknowledged personal use of prayer to aid in the healing process. In addition, 77% of 203 hospitalized family practice patients believed that their physicians should consider their spiritual needs. In contrast, only 32% of the patients' family physicians actually discussed spirituality with their patients (King & Bushwick, 1994).

Anecdotal accounts of the power of prayer are legendary, and countless books on the subject are available. However, literature of scientific value remains limited.

A now-famous prayer study involving humans was published in 1988 by Randolph Byrd, a staff cardiologist at University of California, San Francisco, School of Medicine. Byrd randomly assigned 393 patients in the coronary care unit either to a group receiving intercessory prayer or to a control group receiving no prayer. Intercessory prayer was offered through interventions outside the hospital. They were not instructed how often to pray but were told to pray as they saw fit. In this double-blind study, the prayed-for patients did better on several counts. Although the results were not statistically significant, there were fewer deaths in the prayer group. These patients were less likely to require intubation and ventilator support. They required fewer potent drugs. They experienced a lower incidence of pulmonary edema and they required cardiopulmonary resuscitation less often (Byrd, 1988).

In 1999, W.E. Harris attempted to replicate Byrd's findings at the Mid America Heart Institute in Kansas City. Although the study did not produce statistically significant results, the researchers reported that patients received significant benefit from intercessory prayer, as reflected by a coronary care unit outcome measure (Harris et al., 1999). Critics have charged that performing controlled studies on prayer is impossible because extraneous prayer for the control group cannot be eliminated. According to such critics, if available methods cannot be used to study something, it should not be studied. This antiscience attitude was famously documented in Thomas Kuhn's (1970) classic treatise *The Structure of Scientific Revolutions*, which points out that the prevailing scientific paradigm is always limited by the questions that can be asked based only upon the scientific tools and methods that are available or considered acceptable.

Other studies have been conducted to assess the effect of intercessory prayer on the treatment of alcohol abuse and dependence (Walker, Tonigan, Miller, Corner, & Kahlich, 1997), the well-being of kidney dialysis patients (Matthews, Conti, & Sireci, 2001), and feelings of self-esteem (O'Laoire, 1997). A prospective study of 40 patients with class II or III rheumatoid arthritis compared the effects of direct-contact intercessory prayer with distance intercessory prayer. Persons receiving direct-contact prayer showed significant overall improvement at the 1-year follow-up. The group receiving distant prayer showed no additional benefits (Matthews, Marlowe, & MacNutt, 2000).

The benefits of spiritual healing were examined in 120 patients with chronic pain at the Department of Complementary Medicine, University of Exeter, United Kingdom. Patients were randomly assigned to face-to-face healing or simulated face-to-face healing for 30 minutes per week for 8 weeks or to distant healing or no healing for the same time. Although subjects in both healing groups reported significantly more "unusual experiences" during the sessions, the clinical relevance of was unclear. It was concluded that a specific effect of face-to-face or distant healing on chronic pain could not be demonstrated over eight treatment sessions in these patients (Abbot et al., 2002).

Research problems are difficult to overcome in evaluating the power of prayer, but Byrd's initial prayer study broke significant ground in medical research. Many questions still remain unanswered, and further study is warranted to define the effects of intercessory prayer on quantitative and qualitative outcomes and to identify end points that best measure efficacy. While validated evidence continues to build concerning the efficacy of prayer, Dossey (1993) raised serious questions in the wake of these early experiments. Evidence shows that mental activity can be used to influence people nonlocally, at a distance, without their knowledge. Experiments on prayer also show that it can be used to great effect without the subject's awareness. There is a question as to whether it is ethical to use these techniques if recipients are unaware that they are being used. This question becomes even more compelling as one considers the possibility that prayer, or any other form of mind-to-mind communication, may also be used at a distance to harm people without their knowledge. Institutional review committees that oversee the design of experiments involving humans to ensure their safety have rarely had to consider these types of ethical questions.

DISTANT HEALING

A set of studies was performed to examine the effects of a healer's use of distance healing on cells in a cell culture, where we don't have to contend with the same ethical challenges (to date). This healer explained that he uses intention to focus his mind and channel "Divine love through his heart" to perform healing. This claim and similar energy medicine practices are often called "distant healing" because the practitioners do not place their hands on the patient or subject. Practitioners of this form of healing believe that the distance does not matter. Most, however, do their work within a foot or two of their patients. This particular healer usually placed his hands within inches of the person on whom he was working. He also performed diagnosis by placing his hands near the person but without touching the person. The approach of this healer is typical of the so-called "laying on of hands" practiced in many cultures and accepted and associated traditionally with healing in Western medicine as well as Judeo-Christian tradition.

A strong placebo effect that results from belief and expectation generated during the encounter is an explanation often given for any benefit seen from energy medicine of this kind (see Chapter 9). The investigators intended to minimize this effect by using cells grown in laboratory culture. The healer came to the laboratories one morning per week throughout much of two sequential winters. The researchers wanted to understand how he "communicated" with cells in the laboratory and influenced them with his "intention" in a positive and healthful way. This study would not involve diagnosis or even a human subject. By working with cultured cells in a laboratory setting, the investigators increased their experimental and control parameters by comparing the effects of the healer to no treatment or to sham treatment, by comparing treatments at different doses and time periods, and by examining the effects of various other environmentally controlled conditions, including the effects of expectation with blinding.

The healer was asked to alter the calcium flux of the cells in such a way as to increase the concentration of calcium ions inside the cells. Any change in cellular calcium was measured by placing the cells in a scintillation counter before and after the healer's "treatments." A demonstration of significant effect would provide powerful evidence that something, some form of energy presumably, flowed from the healer to the cells and changed their biochemistry in a targeted, intentional, and specific way.

The studies used Jurkat cells, an immortalized line of T lymphocytes derived from human immune system cells. They had been established as an immortalized line in the late 1970s, available for purchase, and easy to grow and maintain in the laboratory. They have been used extensively to study mechanisms of action for human immunodeficiency virus and anticancer agents. There is a vast amount of literature on Jurkat cells because they are a favorite choice for cellular immunobiologists interested in understanding cellular mechanisms of the immune system.

The materials and methods were quite simple. Jurkat cells were grown in tissue culture dishes to near confluence. On the day of the experiment, the cells were suspended in a balanced salt solution, "loaded" with calcium-sensitive dye (fura-2) and placed inside a square cuvette tube. Due to activity of the dye, the amount of light emitted by the cells is proportional to the amount of free calcium ions inside the cell. When the light is measured spectrofluorometrically, this technique provides an accurate and objective measure of the amount of free calcium inside the cells.

The healer was asked to increase the internal concentration of calcium ions inside the cell. He told the investigators that he would need 15 minutes of relative quiet while he placed his hands near the cuvette of cells and concentrated on his intention. The experiments were repeated in six independent trials occurring on different days. Internal cellular calcium concentrations were significantly increased by 30% to 35% ($p < 0.05$, Student's t-test) compared with controls run in parallel. Varying the distances between 3 and 30 inches did not seem to have an effect on the outcome (Kiang, Ives, & Jonas, 2005).

Three independent attempts were made by the healer to affect calcium concentrations in this cell system from approximately 10 miles distance. He tried first with internal visualization, then with a photograph of the cells to focus his attention, and finally with a video camera display of a "live" version of the cells. None of these tests produced any noticeable change in the calcium concentrations. A few uncontrolled tests were run in which the healer's hands were kept behind his back rather than "aiming" toward the cuvette tube of cells. This position seemed to interfere with his ability to affect calcium concentration. The researchers documented a "linger effect" in which cells put on the table where the healer had focused his intention, but after he had left, showed an increase in calcium concentration similar to that of the cells that had been directly subjected to his intention. This linger effect disappeared over time, and within 24 hours cells placed in this manner had a calcium concentration no different from that of controls.

Finally, the investigators attempted to block the healer's "energy" or intention by placing a grounded copper Faraday cage around the cuvette tube containing cells. The healer, although still within 30 inches of the cells, had to keep his hands outside of the wire enclosure surrounding the cells. There was no significant difference in effect on the internal calcium concentration. It was still raised by the healer's 15-minute "treatment." This observation suggests that, whatever is this energy, it is not blocked by a Faraday cage the way an electric or electromagnetic field would be blocked.

Spiritually Based Rapid Healing

There are other ethical questions to consider when studying the phenomenon of "Deliberately-Caused Bodily Damage" (DCBD), where believers intentionally injure themselves to observe the effects of spiritual belief, and to practice, on remarkably rapid healing. These practices have been observed throughout South and Southeast Asia as well in the Middle East. A particularly well-studied example of rapid healing appears among Sufi Healers.

Sufism is a devotional branch of Islam, with various orders that date back to the Middle Ages or earlier (some say even pre-Islamic) and has many followers today throughout the Middle East, in the West, and globally. These orders are perhaps best known to Western observers for the "Whirling Dervishes" derived from the old Persian word *darwish*, for a supplicant—"one who goes door-to-door"—now referring to a Sufi aspirant. The term is also used for a mystical "holy man" (a term not used in orthodox Islam) by which each order is led. Members of this particular "Dervish" order, the Naqshbandi, are geographically found in North Africa, the Arabian Peninsula, Turkey, Afghanistan, and into Southeast Asia. Sufism also crosses ethnic lines among Muslims ranging from North African Berbers, to Arabs, Turks, and Persians. One origin of the word Sufi means "thread," like a mystical woolen thread or pathway leading to the divine, but as an internal search for the divine. It may also have connections with the Greek word for wisdom, *sophia*. There are some similarities to the traditional, devotional forms of yoga in India (see Chapters 18 and 19), which of course predate Islam. The orthodox practices of Islam at various times in history were not accepted as outward practice by various Sufi orders. Some Sufi orders are also notable for their practice of DCBD as a devotional practice. Under such circumstances, remarkable healing has been observed. Sufism has at times been criticized by orthodox Islam for using such metaphors as being "drunk on divine love," or for referring to sexual intercourse to describe a sublime, transcendent love of the divine. (Here one may discern a pattern connected to Tantra yoga, see Chapter 19.)

Such states of consciousness may be colloquially described as "feeling no pain," for reasons that will become apparent in the next section of this chapter.

A School of Sufism

The Sufi Islamic school of mysticism in Baghdad, Iraq, is one of the largest Sufi schools in the Middle East (Hussein, Fatoohi, Al-Dargazelli, & Almuchtar, 1994, a-c; Hussein, Fatoohi, Hall, & Al-Dargazelli, 1997). Followers (dervishes) of this Sufi school have demonstrated instantaneous healing of DCBD. For example, dervishes have inserted a variety of sharp instruments (e.g., spikes, skewers) into the body, hammered daggers into the skull bone and clavicle, and chewed and swallowed glass and sharp razor blades without harm to the body and with complete control over pain, bleeding, and infection, as well as rapid wound healing within 4 to 10 seconds. The Tariqa Kasnazaniyah School of Sufism has described extraordinary phenomena of instantaneous healing of wounds from DCBD. This Sufi school's name, Tariqa Kasnazaniyah, can be attributed to three of its senior scholars, that is, Imam Ali bin Abi Talib; Shaikh Abd al-Quadir al-Gaylani; and Shaikh Abd al-Karim al-Kasnazan. Linguistically and historically, *Al-Kasnazan* is a Kurdish (Eastern Turkey and Syria, and Northern Iraq and Iran) word that means "no one knows" (similar to a meaning taken for Zen). It was first associated with Shaikh Abd al Karim, as a title when he spent 4 years in seclusion, meditating and worshiping Allah (God) in the Qara Dagh (Black mountains in Kurdistan, Iraq).

No One Knows

During that period of isolation, Shaikh Abd al Karim experienced the sublime joy and love of drawing nearer to Allah. Following his period of isolation, dedication, and worship, the Prophet Muhammad gave him the blessing of a great secret. This revelation was said to be the extraordinary ability to tolerate, without harm, strong electrical shocks, immunity against snakes and scorpions, rapid healing form being stabbed or shot, protection against being burned, as well as healing of clinical conditions such as cancers, heart disease, infertility, depression, and psychosis. During his absence, when anyone would ask about the shaikh, the answer was "Kasnazan," meaning that no one knew where he was. With the passage of time, this word turned into a title for that revered shaikh and his path. Thus, the expression "Al-Tariqa" has the added meaning of the way of the secret that no one knows of the glorious Quran, the course of the Prophet, and his pious companions. Al-Kasnazania became a family title associated with his descendants as well as a name of Tariqa. After reviewing early and updated research, this chapter introduces new clinical applications of Tariqa Kasnazaniyah Sufi spiritual healing without DCBD.

Early Research

Researchers reported that such extraordinary abilities are accessible to anyone and are not restricted to only a few talented individuals who have spent years in special training. These unusual healing phenomena have also been reproduced under controlled laboratory conditions and are not similar to hypnosis (Hall, Don,

Hussein, White, & Hostoffer, 2001). Similar DCBD phenomena have been observed in various parts of the world in a variety of religious and nonreligious contexts (Don & Moura, 2000; Hussein et al., 1997). For example, trance surgeons in Brazil have employed sharp instruments to cut, pierce, or inject substances into a patient's body for therapeutic purposes. Laboratory electroencephalographic (EEG) investigation of trance surgeons has shown that this "state of spirit possession" of the healers was associated with a hyperaroused brain state (waves in the 30- to 50-Hz band) (Don & Moura, 2000). In the United States, little scientific attention has been given to the investigation of these claims of rapid healing. In fact, claims of extraordinary healing abilities have been met with scorn and challenged by so-called skeptic groups such as the Committee for the Scientific Investigation of Claims of the Paranormal. These groups offer monetary incentives to discredit such claims in unscientific and dangerous settings (Mulacz, 1998; Posner, 1998; see Dossey, 1989; Fatoohi, 1999; and Fatoohi & Al-Dargazelli, 1999, for a response), sometimes employing the services of career magicians who make their living as illusionists, not scientists.

"OTHERS-HEALING" PHENOMENON

Followers of the Tariqa Kasnazaniyah School of Sufism describe the ability to accomplish DCBD healing as an "others-healing" phenomenon within the context of healing energies (Hussein et al., 1994, a-c). This "higher energy" is alleged to be instantly transferable, mediated through a spiritual link from the current shaikh of the Sufi school and through the chain of masters to Muhammad and ultimately to Allah (Hussein et al., 1997). As noted in the Quran, "The Prophet is closer to the Believers than their own selves" (33:6). This Sufi "higher energy" might be characterized as a "biophysical" phenomenon.

When becoming aware of DCBD phenomena, the first question to naturally arise is: How might Western scientists empirically investigate such unusual claims of healing? From a scientific perspective, this process would demand a series of systematic observations of the Sufi rapid wound healing phenomenon in both field and laboratory settings. Of course, the first question that needs to be addressed was whether this phenomenon is real. This would require field trips to directly observe, video record, and possibly even experience DCBD healing. If these initial observations showed the phenomenon to be genuine, then the question would become, "Can the phenomenon be explained by traditional paradigms, such as hypnosis or the placebo effect?"

SUGGESTIBILITY

A Cleveland clinical psychologist, Dr. Howard Hall, conducted research in hypnosis and psychoneuroimmunology (Hall, 1982, 1989; Hall, Minnes, & Olness, 1993; Hall, Minnes, Tosi, & Olness, 1992; Hall, Mumma, Longo, & Dixon, 1992; Hall, Papas, Tosi, & Olness, 1996) as well as clinical work in hypnosis for over 25 years. It was of interest to him to compare this rapid healing with hypnotic phenomena during a visit to Iraq for field observations and direct experience of DCBD healing (Box 8.1). It was his impression following the visit that what had been seen

BOX 8.1 *How Sufism Explains Rapid Healing*

Sufism can form a unified theory for mechanistic, mind-body, and spiritual healing. Traditional Islamic theology recognizes that Allah created a world that can apparently operate under mechanistic and Newtonian principles. As noted in the Quran (6:95–99), Allah created order in this world, causing seeds to sprout, the sun to rise and set, and the rain to fall. "Such is the judgment and ordering of (Him) the exalted in Power, the Omniscient" (6:96).

This view is consistent with the mechanistic Newtonian view of the world and humans. Thus, there is no rejection of mechanistic views in traditional Islamic philosophy. Sufi philosophy goes further, noting that mechanistic views can also be explained within a vitalistic perspective. From this point of view, Sufism can predict the biophysical aspects of Sufi healing phenomena in ways that Newtonian models cannot.

Sufi Shaikh Gaylani explains it as follows:

The belief of the followers of the Book and the Sunna of the Messenger of Allah (Salla Allah ta'ala 'alayhi wa sallam) is that the sword does not cut because of its nature, but it is rather Allah ('Azza wa Jall) who cuts with it, that the fire does not burn because of its nature, but it is rather Allah ('Azza wa Jall) who burns with it, that food does not satisfy hunger because of its nature, but it is rather Allah ('Azza wa Jall) who satisfies hunger with it and that water does not quench thirst because of its nature, but it is rather Allah ('Azza wa Jall) who quenches thirst with it. The same applies to things of all kinds; it is Allah ('Azza wa Jall) who uses them to produce their effects and they are only instruments in His hand with which He does whatever He wills (Al-Kasnazani & Al-Husseini, 1998).

Thus, according to this belief, most of the time, the world operates by mechanistic laws allowed by Allah, but mediation by a Sufi shaikh, based on the shaikh's nearness to Allah and through Allah, would allow for fire not to burn or a knife not to cut, so that mechanistic laws are suspended. The Quran is clear in several verses that what are called natural laws can be suspended by Allah. For example, 2:117 says, "when He (Allah) decreeth a matter, he saith to it: 'Be,' and it is."

The goal of the Sufi and all spiritual paths is nearness to G-d. In Sufism, this goal is pursued by following the Sufi path, practicing remembrances, and engaging in jihad or struggling against the lower self or *nafs* that keeps humans distant from G-d. Islam and Sufism are about surrendering to the will of G-d by following this path. Once this nearness to God has been achieved, alterations of mechanistic laws may occur in this belief. This nearness to Allah is the explanation for "miracles" performed within religious contexts in ancient times and today.

Rapid wound healing is a very impressive phenomenon to observe and experience. Islam and Sufism teach that one's heart is the center of one's being, and it becomes diseased (5:52) and hardened (6:43) from wrongful acts (sins). Sufism, however, offers healing for the heart, as noted in the Quran: "O mankind! There hath come to you a direction from your Lord and a healing for the (diseases) in your hearts—and for those who believe a guidance and a Mercy" (10:57). Thus, when the heart has been purified through remembrances, and jihad, the nearness and true healing will occur.

and experienced represented a phenomenon that went beyond classical Newtonian mechanics and argued for explanations for DCBD healing involving psychological factors that influence healing, such as the placebo effect, hypnosis, or altered states of consciousness (Hall, 2000).

The next question in systematic observation was, "Can this unusual healing phenomenon be exported to the United States and observed within a traditional medical setting?" If the phenomenon could be brought to the United States, what measures should be employed to help understand the underlying processes of DCBD healing, particularly if it represents a new paradigm as defined by Kuhn (1970), for example, in describing the structure of scientific revolutions? After Dr. Hall and colleagues found that DCBD healing could be transported to the United States, he then undertook a series of structured observations of the phenomenon to explore possible underlying mechanisms, using both traditional and novel instruments and measures.

Laboratory Studies

These systematic observations laid the foundation for more traditional follow-up laboratory studies that can be conducted with randomized control groups, or what Kuhn (1970) might refer to as the puzzle-solving process of "normal science." (Kuhn does caution, however, that anomalous observations that do not fit within existing paradigms can result in a crisis and lead to the revolutionary process of a paradigm shift.) The ultimate interest may lie in the more important area of the translational application of this research to the healing of clinical conditions. Normal science, in general, has long been criticized for its typical lack of interest in translating basic science into practical applications (Shapley & Roy, 1985). Translating anomalous findings into practical use is an exciting venture and opportunity to expand our views of health and healing.

Field Investigations

In 1998, with an invitation from the shaikh of the Tariqa Kasnazaniyah School of Sufism in Baghdad and support from the Kairos Foundation, Dr. Hall traveled alone to Baghdad to meet with the spiritual leader of this group, Shaikh Muhammad Al-Kasnazani, and witnessed a group demonstration of DCBD healing at their major school (Hall, 2000). At this meeting, which was professionally videotaped, there was an opportunity to examine firsthand the objects that were employed during the DCBD demonstrations, such as knives, razor blades, and glass, and observe them being inserted into various parts of the body. What Hall witnessed and recorded is consistent with the extraordinary claims made by this group about rapid wound healing and lack of apparent pain.

Although there was no evidence of a ruse, some skeptics might question whether the observer had somehow been deluded, even with video footage. Thus, Hall requested permission, while at this demonstration, to experience DCBD healing by having his cheek pierced (Hall, 2000). After witnessing several demonstrations of DCBD healing, an assistant asked him to face the shaikh to ask permission to allow the healing energy for rapid wound healing. The shaikh nodded, indicating that Hall had his permission. What was most striking was that he did not feel any different or in an altered state, and his cheek was not numb. The assistant then inserted a metal ice pick through the inside of his left cheek to the outside. It felt like a poke, but with no pain. Hall walked around the group circle with the ice pick in his cheek, introspecting on how it was not hurting, bleeding, or numb. He could feel the weight of the object and noticed a metal taste but felt no discomfort. Again, consistent with the reports, his cheek healed rapidly in minutes, with only a couple of drops of blood shed. This personal experience was compelling, despite his considerable doubt and dislike of pain. Nonetheless, Hall still imagined that skeptics would question whether such practices could be demonstrated outside this religious context and exported to the West.

BIOMEDICAL PERSPECTIVES

A demonstration of such rapid wound healing was clearly needed within a Western medical setting, given the scientific implications of such healing. If such spiritually based healing approaches are genuine, they hold much promise for addressing some of today's most serious medical issues.

The investigation of such unusual healing phenomena in the West raises many questions. What should be measured within a scientific context? Would standard measures of brain and immune activity be associated with changes in rapid wound healing, or should standard measures, such as EEG activity, be used in less standard ways? Would high-frequency EEG activity need to be examined for hyperaroused brain states? Would new approaches be needed to detect "fields of consciousness," such as the examination of changes in the output of a random event generator (REG)?

CASE STUDY

With the support of the Kairos Foundation of Wilmette, Illinois, a Sufi practitioner was invited from the Middle East to a local radiology facility in Cleveland, Ohio, on July 1, 1999. He had permission from the shaikh of the Kasnazaniyah Sufi School to perform a demonstration of rapid wound healing after insertion of an unsterilized metal skewer, 0.38 cm thick and approximately 13 cm long, while being videotaped by a film crew in the presence of scientists and health care professionals (Hall et al., 2001). This was apparently the first demonstration by a practitioner from this Sufi school in the United States. The practitioner consented to sign a release of liability for the medical facility and personnel against claims from possible injuries. Emergency medical technicians were present. The major goal of this demonstration was to observe the authenticity of rapid wound healing following a deliberately caused injury within a medical setting.

The demonstration was conducted with radiological, immunological, and EEG evaluations, as well as a Zener noise diode REG, similar to equipment employed at Princeton University by Dr. Robert Jahn and colleagues. Based on previous studies in Brazil with healer mediums engaged in quasi-surgical practices, it was hypothesized that DCBD healing would be accompanied by alterations in brain waves and effects on REGs. The alterations in brain waves found in the Brazilian healer mediums showed statistically significant enhancement of broadband 40-Hz brain rhythms (Don & Moura, 2000). A statistically significant deviation from random behavior in REGs was found in a test run covertly, while the Brazilian healer mediums were in a trance. This methodology was developed by Robert Jahn and associates at the Princeton Engineering Anomalies Research (PEAR) Laboratory (Nelson, Bradish, Dobyns, Dunne, & Jahn, 1996, 1998). Such energy fields have been considered to be theoretically associated with rapid wound healing (Don & Moura, 2000).

Nineteen-channel EEGs were recorded during baseline resting conditions, while the dervish inserted the skewer through his cheek, and immediately after removal of the instrument. An REG device, plugged into the serial port of a computer, was run in the background without informing the dervish. The distribution of binary digits was tested for possible significant deviations from random behavior. Data were acquired before and after the self-insertion, as well as during the self-insertion. Before insertion of the skewer and about 1 hour after the piercing, blood was collected from the practitioner and from three volunteers (used as control subjects) for an immunological analysis of the percent change in white blood cell CD4, CD8, and total T-cell counts.

Results

Radiological images were made while the skewer was inserted. Computed axial tomographic images through the lower mandibular region showed artifact from dental metal. In addition, a horizontally oriented metallic bar elevated the left lateral soft tissues just anterior to the muscles of mastication. There was no associated underlying mass. A single frontal fluoroscopic image showed the presence of EEG leads over the maxilla and mandibular regions. A transverse piece of metal was superimposed, extending from the soft tissues on the right through to the left without interval break.

Because of movement and scalp muscle artifacts throughout the experimental self-insertion condition, it was impossible to assess the EEG for the hypothesized 40-Hz brain rhythms. The frequency spectrum of scalp muscle discharge overlaps the 40-Hz EEG frequency band of interest.

The REG output during baseline periods did not differ significantly from random behavior. However, during the self-insertion condition, there was a trend toward significant nonrandomness. The chi-square test result was 3.052, df = 1, and P was approximately 0.07.

Field of Consciousness

The behavior of the REG was in the predicted direction of nonrandomness. This finding has been interpreted by the PEAR laboratory as being associated with states of heightened attention and emotion. Further, the PEAR group has proposed that a "field of consciousness" is associated with such nonrandomness. Unfortunately, the 40-Hz brain wave hypothesis was not testable because of the excessive amount of scalp artifacts and thus awaits further exploration. The presence of increased theta rhythms after the insertion condition (and a slight decrease in average alpha power) suggests a mild hypoaroused altered state of consciousness. The Sufi practitioner performing this feat was doing so for the first time. With further practice or with testing of more experienced subjects, it may be feasible to obtain EEG data without large amounts of scalp artifacts. Because the subject reported no perceived pain during the self-insertion, preliminary relaxation exercises might eliminate all or most of the artifact. This circumstance would enable us to test the 40-Hz hypothesis definitively. Clearly, further work is indicated.

The immunologic analysis did not reveal any major difference between the Sufi practitioner and the control subjects. These data suggest that the variation found in the practitioner was not different from that of normal controls. The radiological film documented that the skewer had actually penetrated both cheeks, which addresses the arguments of skeptic groups that such practices are the result of "fakery." After the removal of the skewer, there was a slight trickle of blood, which stopped with application of pressure to the cheek, using clean gauze. The physicians and scientists present documented that the wound healed rapidly within a few moments. The practitioner also reported that there was no pain associated with the insertion or removal of the metal skewer. This demonstration was conducted outside the traditional religious context, where chanting, drumming, and head movements (which would compromise some scientific measurements) are generally part of the ceremony when it is performed in the Middle East. Thus, our case study argues against the view that a religious context, with its accompanying state of consciousness, is important to the successful outcome of such a demonstration. This case study also demonstrated that DCBD healing could be done when a large distance separated the dervish from the master (from Baghdad to Cleveland). This condition would suggest a robust phenomenon independent of the distance separating the source and the scene where the DCBD phenomenon occurs.

It should also be noted that the skewer stayed in the dervish's cheeks for more than 35 minutes, longer than the few minutes I had observed during my field observations at the major school of Tariqa Kasnazaniyah. Thus, this case study argues against the necessity of a brief piercing for a successful outcome of rapid healing following DCBD. Further, the dervish in this demonstration reported that there was no pain associated with the piercing, minimal bleeding, and no postprocedural infection. Finally, about a half hour after the completion of the demonstration, the dervish had dinner with seven other people who had witnessed the DCBD event.

EXPERIENCE OF RAPID WOUND HEALING

After witnessing rapid wound healing in the Middle East and experiencing it there, Hall was initiated into the Sufi order with the ritualistic handshake, which took about 2 to 3 minutes. After a subsequent visit with the shaikh in the United Kingdom in June 2000, he was given a license to perform DCBD rapid healing.

Hall first requested permission from the shaikh in Baghdad to perform a cheek piercing on himself in May at the 2001 World Congress on Complementary Therapies in Medicine in Washington, DC, chaired by Micozzi. After lecturing on

DCBD rapid healing, Hall informed the audience he needed to take an earlier flight home because of a family medical emergency in Cleveland. Skipping a break, he went directly into the cheek piercing for the first time on his own, with his mind on the family medical crisis back home. As instructed, he began to focus on connecting with the shaikh, asking mentally for spiritual energy for rapid wound healing before the piercing. This process took about a minute. One physician in the audience was particularly skeptical, so Hall invited him to stand next to him for the piercing. Please note that this occasion was about 4 months before September 11, 2001, so Hall had been able to bring a meat skewer from his kitchen drawer (to be used for the demonstration) in his carry-on luggage through airport security.

After a 1-minute mental connection with the energy from the shaikh, and with much nervousness, he pushed a very dull skewer through his left cheek while quite worried about the medical situation at home. The most difficult aspect of this experience was getting this dull object through the cheek. Eventually it went through with no pain. The skeptical medical colleague was very quiet after that. Hall pulled it out and there were a couple of drops of blood, which he blotted with a tissue until the bleeding stopped. From there, he had a friend take him directly to the airport.

The second time Hall demonstrated DCBD healing on himself (his third experience with DCBD healing including Baghdad) was at the Fifth World Congress on Qigong in November 2002. Because this event was after September 11, 2001, he had to shop locally at the destination for a better piercing instrument. This demonstration was preceded by a video interview by some of the leading scientists in the field of energy healing attending the conference. The video camera was then set on a stand by his left cheek. He again focused on connecting with the energy of the shaikh for rapid wound healing. He did not feel different but had faith that the connection was there, despite the distance in space. Again, he found that pushing the metal pick through his cheek was very difficult. After some effort *(jihad)*, both physical and mental, it went through. He also spoke on camera about how he was feeling, with the object through his cheek. After the interview, he pulled out the pick and padded a tissue against his cheek to absorb the few drops of blood. The wound closing was also documented on film for the first time. Hall had cut himself shaving early in the morning of the previous day, before flying to the conference. Immediately after the demonstration, the shaving cut was more noticeable than the piercing. He was able to enjoy eating dinner after this demonstration.

BIOPHYSICAL PERSPECTIVES

The day after the demonstration, Hall had the opportunity to meet and to be evaluated by Dr. Konstantin Korotkov, professor of physics at St. Petersburg State Technical University in Russia. Dr. Korotkov used his gas discharge visualization (GDV) technique, which measures human energy fields, as did the earlier Kirlian photography (Korotkov, 2002, 2004; Korotkov, Bundzen, Bronnikov, & Lognikova, 2005). Dr. Korotkov first took a baseline measure of Hall's energy field from his fingers and displayed the results on a screen to the audience. He then asked Hall to invoke the Sufi energy. He again took about a minute and requested energy distantly from the shaikh for this demonstration. It should be noted that he had not planned this energy reading or obtained prior permission from the shaikh for this energy demonstration. After about 1 minute, Hall was ready for the second (after-energy) measure. Dr. Korotkov outwardly expressed surprise at how quickly Hall had invoked energy. This time when Korotkov took the energy reading from Hall's hand, the computer malfunctioned, and another one had to be brought in. After the new computer was in place, the GDV reading revealed a major increase in Hall's energy field after the 1 minute energy invocation.

Hall's fourth experience with DCBD healing occurred in response to a request by National Geographic Television and Film (Washington, DC) to participate in a program to be aired for the cable network series "Is It Real?," titled "Superhuman Powers," in 2005. This demonstration was performed in collaboration with Gary Schwartz, PhD, at his Human Energy Systems Laboratory, Center for Frontier Medicine in Biofield Science, at the University of Arizona in Tucson (Hall & Schwartz, 2004). Again, Hall obtained distant permission from the shaikh to conduct another DCBD demonstration and also explored whether there were any changes in brain activity associated with this process or any changes in energy field or aura as indicated by the GDV measures. A 19-channel EEG, along with GDV recordings, was taken before and after Hall pierced his left cheek with a 5-inch ice pick while being filmed by National Geographic. This demonstration took about 90 minutes to complete, as he again connected with the current shaikh and other masters who are part of this Sufi school's chain of shaikhs (i.e., silsila).

During the demonstration, Hall's mind did reach a more relaxed state as measured by EEG recordings. There was, however, no anomalous neurological activity, such as seizure, sleep, or hyperaroused brain patterns. Pre- versus post-piercing changes on GDV measures did show, for the first time ever, a selective decrease in the energy field where the cheek was pierced, revealing a gaping hole in the "aura" in that area. As with prior experiences with DCBD healing, there were a few drops of blood after the ice pick was removed, but the wound healed very quickly and was not noticeable after a few minutes. Again, even with these additional scientific measures, traditional paradigms offer little insight to account for the rapid wound healing phenomenon.

Such an observation was consistent with the results of the demonstration involving the Sufi practitioner from the Middle East, described earlier in the case report, which also failed to find any correlations between DCBD healing and any of the blood tests or imaging studies. The only hints of associations were the GDV energy measures and the trend of the REG output, which also suggested some change in the energy field. Work in this area might take us beyond Newton's classical mechanics to quantum mechanics and quantum physics to account for possible subtle energy constructs. Our colleague Eric Leskowitz (2005) proposes a multidimensional model of wound healing, incorporating energy concepts to help shift our current paradigm of wound healing beyond the physical and psychological dimensions or, as he describes it, from biology to spirit as well as to biophysical aspects of healing (see Chapter 9).

CURRENT RESEARCH

Recent research on Sufi rapid wound healing was done in collaboration with Jay Gunkelman, Erik Peper, Tom Collura, and a Sufi living in Europe. For this project, they measured the impact of Sufi rapid healing from a skewer going from inside the bottom of the mouth to the outside of the throat, with EEG analysis. The most interesting finding was that the Sufi demonstrated an extreme state of relaxation despite having a skewer through his throat, and he was able to selectively disengage a broad-based brain network that may be related to attention.

CLINICAL APPLICATIONS OF SUFI SPIRITUAL HEALING WITHOUT DCBD

Al-Shaikh Muhammad Al-Kasnazani has granted spiritual healing for a variety of medical conditions. To receive this spiritual healing, the person is invited to become spiritually connected to the shaikh by taking *bay'a,* a brief ceremony that pledges allegiance to Allah, the Prophet Muhammad, and the chain of shaikhs down to the present master. The other major part of bay'a is also having one repent for one's shortcomings. Although bay'a may appear to be very simple, it entails many spiritual aspects. A male who wants to take bay'a puts his dominant hand in the right hand of the master or one of his caliphs or deputies. A female would hold the caliph's beads instead of his hand.

Bay'a is not restricted to men but is open to women and adolescents, as well as individuals from other religious paths. Some describe bay'a as being a spiritual touch from the disciple's soul connecting to that of the master, who is connected to the chain of masters who preceded the current master. Bay'a existed during the time of the prophet of Islam, it is written, and after his departure, Iman Ali inherited the spiritual touch as well as the succession of caliphs, down to the present master. Thus, this unbroken chain of spiritual healing remains intact today. Once bay'a is taken, the new Sufi is instructed in frequent meditation, or "remembrance," as it is known in Sufism. Much healing can result from such remembrances. Sometimes the shaikh will prescribe a specific Quran remembrance for a particular number of repetitions for a particular person.

REFERENCES

Abbot, N. C., Harkness, E. F., Stevinson, C., Marshall, F. P., Conn, D. A., & Ernst, E. (2002). Spiritual healing as a therapy for chronic pain: A randomized clinical trial. *Pain, 91*(1/2), 79.

Al-Kasnazani. (1998). *Purification of the mind (Jila'al-khatir).* Philadelphia: Alminar Books.

Amri, H., Abu-Asab, M., & Micozzi, M. S. (2013). *Avicenna's canon of medicine new translation.* Rochester, VT: Healing Arts Press.

Byrd, R. C. (1988). Positive therapeutic effects of intercessory prayer in a coronary care unit population. *Southern Medical Journal, 81*(7), 826.

Crowther, M. R., Parker, M. W., Achenbaun, W. A., Larimore, W. L., & Koenig, H. G. (2002). Rowe and Kahn's model of successful aging revisited: Positive spirituality—The forgotten factor. *Gerontologist, 42*(5), 613.

Daaleman, T. P. & VandeCreek, P. (2000). Placing religion and spirituality in end-of-life care. *Journal of American Medical Association, 284,* 2514.

Don, N. S. & Moura, G. (2000). Trance surgery in Brazil. *Alternative Therapies in Health and Medicine*, *6*(4), 39.

Dossey, L. (1989). *Recovering the soul: A scientific and spiritual approach*. New York: Bantam Books.

Dossey, L. (1993). *Healing words: The power of prayer and the practice of medicine*. San Francisco: Harper.

Fatoohi, L. (1999). Response to Peter Mulacz. *Journal of the Society for Psychical Research*, *63*(855), 179 (letter to the editor).

Fatoohi, L. & Al-Dargazelli, S. (1999). *History testifies to the infallibility of the Qur'an*. Kuala Lumpur, Malaysia: AS Noordem.

Galton, F. (1872). Statistical inquiries into the efficacy of prayer. *Fortnightly Review*, *12*, 11225.

Hall, H. R. (1982). Hypnosis and the immune system: A review with implications for cancer and the psychology of healing. *American Journal of Clinical Hypnosis*, *25*(2-3), 92.

Hall, H. R. (1989). Research in the area of voluntary immunomodulation: Complexities, consistencies and future research considerations. *International Journal of Neuroscience*, *47*(1–2), 81.

Hall, H. (2000). Deliberately caused bodily damage: Metahypnotic phenomena? *Journal of the Society for Psychical Research*, *64*(861), 211.

Hall, H., Don, N. S., Hussein, J. N., White, E., & Hostoffer, R. (2001). The scientific study of unusual rapid wound healing: A case report. *Advances in Mind-Body Medicine*, *17*, 203.

Hall, H., Minnes, L., & Olness, K. (1993). The psychophysiology of voluntary immunomodulation. *The International Journal of Neuroscience*, *69*(1–4), 221.

Hall, H. R., Minnes, L., Tosi, M., & Olness, K. (1992a). Voluntary modulation of neutrophil adhesiveness using a cyberphysiologic strategy. *International Journal of Neurosciences*, *63*(3–4), 287.

Hall, H. R., Mumma, G. H., Longo, S., & Dixon, R. (1992b). Voluntary immunomodulation: A preliminary study. *International Journal of Neurosciences*, *63*(3–4), 275.

Hall, H., Papas, A., Tosi, M., & Olness, K. (1996). Directional changes in neutrophil adherence following passive resting versus active imagery. *International Journal of Neurosciences*, *85*(3–4), 185.

Hall, H. & Schwartz, G. (2004). Rapid wound healing: A Sufi perspective. *Seminars in Integrative Medicine*, *2*(3), 116.

Harris, W. S., Gowda, M., Kolb, J. W., Strychacz, C. P., Vacek, J. L., Jones, P. G., et al. (1999). A randomized, controlled trial of the effects of remote, intercessory prayer on outcomes in patients admitted to the coronary care unit. *Archives of Internal Medicine*, *159*(19), 2272.

Herbert, N. (1987). *Quantum reality*. Garden City, NY: Anchor/Doubleday.

Hussein, J. N., Fatoohi, L. J., Al-Dargazelli, S., & Almuchtar, N. (1994a). Deliberately caused bodily damage phenomena: Mind, body, energy or what? Part 1. *International Journal of Alternative and Complementary Medicine*, *12*(9), 9.

Hussein, J. N., Fatoohi, L. J., Al-Dargazelli, S., & Almuchtar, N. (1994b). Deliberately caused bodily damage phenomena: Mind, body, energy or what? Part 2. *International Journal of Alternative and Complementary Medicine*, *12*(10), 21.

Hussein, J. N., Fatoohi, L. J., Al-Dargazelli, S., & Almuchtar, N. (1994c). Deliberately caused bodily damage phenomena: Mind, body, energy or what? Part 3. *International Journal of Alternative and Complementary Medicine*, *12*(11), 25.

Hussein, J. N., Fatoohi, L. J., Hall, H., & Al-Dargazelli, S. (1997). Deliberately caused bodily damage phenomena. *Journal of the Society for Psychical Research*, *62*, 97.

Ironson, G., Solomon, G. F., Balbin, E. G., O'Cleirigh, C., George, A., Kumar, M., et al. (2002). The ironson woods spirituality/religious index is associated with long survival, health behaviors less stress, and low cortisol in people with HIV/AIDS. *Annals of Behavioral Medicine*, *24*(1), 34.

Jahn, R. G. & Dunn, B. J. (1987). *Precognitive remote perception*. In *Margins of reality: The role of consciousness in the physical world* (p. 149). New York: Harcourt Brace.

Kiang, J. G., Ives, J. A., & Jonas, W. B. (2005). External bioenergy-induced increases in intracellular free calcium concentrations are mediated by Na^+/Ca^{2+} exchanger and L-type calcium channel. *Molecular and Cellular Biochemistry*, *271*(1–2), 51.

King, D. E., & Bushwick, B. (1994). Beliefs and attitudes of hospital inpatients about faith healing and prayer. *Journal of Family Practice*, *39*, 349.

Koenig, H. G., Cohen, H. J., Blazer, D. G., Pieper, C., Meador, K. G., Shelp, F., et al. (1992). Religious coping and depression in elderly hospitalized medically ill men. *American Journal of Psychiatry*, *149*, 1693.

Koenig, H. G., Ford, S., George, L. K., Blazer, D. G., & Meador, K. G. (1993). Religion and anxiety disorder: An examination and comparison of associations in young, middle-aged, and elderly adults. *Journal of Anxiety Disorders, 7*, 321.

Koenig, H. G., McCullough, M., & Larson, D. B. (2001). *Handbook of religion and health: A century of research reviewed.* New York: Oxford University Press.

Korotkov, K. (2002). *Human energy field: Study with GDV bioelectrography.* Fair Lawn, NJ: Backbone Publishing.

Korotkov, K. (2004). *Measuring energy fields: State-of-the-science.* Fair Lawn, NJ: Backbone Publishing.

Korotkov, K. G., Bundzen, P. V., Bronnikov, V. M., & Lognikova, L. U. (2005). Bioelectrographic correlates of the direct vision phenomenon. *Journal of Alternative and Complementary Medicine, 11*(5), 885.

Kuhn, T. S. (1970). *The structure of scientific revolutions* (2nd ed.). Chicago: University of Chicago Press.

Leskowitz, E. (2005). From biology to spirit: The multidimensional model of wound healing. *Seminars in Integrative Medicine, 3*(1), 21.

Matthews, D. A., Conti, J. M., & Sireci, S. G. (2001). The effects of intercessory prayer, positive visualization, and expectancy on the well-being of kidney dialysis patients, Alternative Therapies. *Health and Medicine, 7*(5), 42.

Matthews, D. A., Marlowe, S. M., & MacNutt, F. S. (2000). Effects of intercessory prayer on patients with rheumatoid arthritis. *Southern Medical Journal, 93*(12), 1177.

Mayor, D. & Micozzi, M. S. (2011). *Energy medicine.* London: Elsevier Health Sciences.

Mulacz, W. P. (1998). Deliberately caused bodily damage (DCBD) phenomena: A different perspective. *Journal of the Society for Psychical Research, 62*, 434.

Nelson, R. D., Bradish, G. J., Dobyns, Y. H., Dunne, B. J., & Jahn, R. G. (1996). Field REG anomalies in group situations. *Journal of Scientific Exploration, 10*(1), 111.

Nelson, R. D., Bradish, G. J., Dobyns, Y. H., Dunne, B. J., & Jahn, R. G. (1998). Field REG II: Consciousness field effects—Replications and explorations. *Journal of Scientific Exploration, 12*(3), 425.

Pargament, K. I., Smith, B. W., Koenig, H. G., & Perez, L. (1998). Patterns of positive and negative religious coping with major life stressors. *Journal for the Scientific Study of Religion, 37*, 710.

Posner, G. (1998). *Taking a stab at a paranormal claim.* http://www.csicop.org/sb/9509/posner.html.

Schroedinger, E. (1969). *What is life? and mind and matter.* London: Cambridge University Press.

Shapley, D. & Roy, R. (1985). *Lost at the frontier: U.S. science and technology policy adrift.* Philadelphia: ISI Press.

Solfvin, J. (1984). Mental healing. In S. Krippner (Ed.), *Advances in parapsychological research*, vol. 4. Jefferson, NC: McFarland.

Tix, A. P. & Frazier, P. A. (1997). The use of religious coping during stressful life events: Main effects, moderation, and meditation. *Journal of Consulting and Clinical Psychology, 66*, 411.

Walker, S. R., Tonigan, J. S., Miller, W. R., Corner, S., & Kahlich, L. (1997). Intercessory prayer in the treatment of alcohol abuse and dependence: A pilot investigation, alternative therapies. *Health and Medicine, 3*(6), 79.

Suggested Readings can be found on the companion website, http://www.micozzipainconditions.com.

Section III

ENERGY HEALING, HAND-MEDIATED, AND BIOPHYSICAL APPROACHES

Section II addressed mind-body techniques that work with the mind to affect both the mind and body for treating pain. Section III addresses energy, bodywork, and manual and physical manipulations of the body that help the body and have profound effects on the mind for treating pain.

Chapter 9

Energy Medicine and Therapeutic Touch

In introductory physics courses, energy is defined as the ability to do work. Energy has two basic forms, potential and kinetic. Potential energy is stored and has the latent ability to do work. Kinetic energy is, simply put, movement, from the motions of air or water molecules to propagation of sound waves, to splitting neutrons into atomic nuclei. Underlying these standard descriptions are several subtleties that have been investigated and understood to the extent that they can harness the awesome power of atomic energy—which is not subtle at all.

In terms of another microscopic energy, cellular energy, medical science has a stochastic model whereby a cellular receptor binds an agent (micronutrient, phytochemical, or drug) often releasing potential energy that was stored in the characteristic shape of the cell receptor itself. The change in receptor configuration releases stored energy and helps propel or allow the movement of molecules and atoms across the cellular membrane. This process consumes potential energy stored in the molecule adenosine triphosphate (ATP), the universal "battery" that provides energy in the biology of cellular reactions and actions. ATP provides a vehicle for storing energy (battery) by means of chemical bonds. This energy is captured during cellular respiration, which combines oxygen with carbohydrates and yields carbon dioxide as a by-product along with water for cellular hydration, and energy. Chemically, this reaction is combustion, which "burns" hydrocarbon and carbohydrate "fuel" by combining it with oxygen to create energy "fire" and releases combustion byproducts of carbon dioxide and water vapor. In the case of a wood fire (or internal combustion engine), the energy is heat, and the carbon dioxide and water vapor are given off as exhaust gases. In the cells, the energy is captured in the chemical bonds of ATP molecules and the water "by-product" is retained in liquid form within the cells, which actually provides the majority of the water for cellular hydration. This kind of cellular respiration occurs in the mitochondria. The role of physiologic respiration through the lungs (breathing) is to provide oxygen from the air to the cells for cellular respiration and to remove the carbon dioxide by-product and release it back into

Acknowledgment to John Ives and Wayne Jonas for prior contributions in Micozzi, M.S. (Ed.), (2016) *Fundamentals of complementary and alternative medicine* (5th ed.). St Louis: Elsevier Health Sciences/ Saunders; and Eric Leskowitz for prior contribution in Mayor, D. F. & Micozzi, M. S. (Eds.), (2011). *Energy medicine east and west*. Edinburgh: Churchill Livingstone.

the air after transport from the cells back to the lungs. The neural signal for breathing comes from the buildup of carbon dioxide in the blood rather than lack of oxygen.

It is this kind of energy on which the pharmaceutical industry and much of allopathic medicine have focused their efforts. However, increasingly "energetic" discussions about "hydration" focus on fluids and electrolyte intakes but typically ignore the elegant role of cellular hydration generated by cellular respiration. In the biomedical model, this cellular space is where endogenous molecules such as pharmaceutical agents ultimately interact with the physical body. These agents are seen to cause and modulate cellular responses through interactions with a class of biomolecules called "receptors." Sometimes the agent is harvested and acquired from natural sources (materia medica), and sometimes it is synthesized in a laboratory. Nearly always it is seen to interact with a naturally occurring receptor type that is associated with some tissue or organ, or groups of tissues or organs. All of these steps and their consequences involve the use of energy and its transformation from potential to kinetic and back again with some loss to heat and inefficiency at every step. There is increasing concern among molecular biologists that much of the toxicity of modern drugs results from their interference with cellular respiration as an unwanted side effect.

Our understanding of the nature of these biochemical reactions is that all life is dependent upon them and that life ceases when they stop. Health and healing involve these biochemical, energy-driven reactions. In this way, all healing can be considered as forms of energy medicine.

SUBTLETY OF VITAL ENERGY

The introduction describes a conventional view of energy in medicine. Beyond this contemporary biomedical model, it is also well known that different types and sources of energy may interact, which results in modulation or change in the energies involved. At this subtle interface, "energy medicine" takes place, and there are models for understanding this interface.

The "energy" in so-called energy medicine has the same nature as that described in conventional models. This subtle energy is not directly measurable. It does not appear to decrease in power with distance by the inverse square law that applies in Newtonian mechanics (as related to the concept of nonlocality (as described in Chapter 8). It is not insulated by the barriers that block conventional energy. This distinction in types of energies is important. Often these two very different concepts are used interchangeably and confusion results. Yet both types of "energy medicine" are placed in this single category, for example, by the National Center for Complementary and Alternative Medicine (NCCAM). This shortsightedness should not come as a surprise. Twenty years ago, shortly after leading members of Congress first legislated the funding to create what is now the NCCAM at the National Institutes of Health (NIH), managers at the NIH told Congress that NIH "does not believe in bioenergy" (Sen. Arlen Specter R/D-PA, personal communication). The author (Micozzi) suggested to Congress that the US Department of Energy may be a better place to study bioenergy, since NIH says they do not believe in it.

The intriguing and disputed energy medicines such as qigong, reiki, and Therapeutic Touch are thought to involve putative forms of energy (see Section IV). There have been questions about the efficacy of these energy medicine modalities. There are no unequivocal demonstrations of the involvement of either known or heretofore unknown forms of energy from the healer or between the healer and the patient. These modalities are based on philosophy, historical use, and cultural traditions (some more recent than they first appear) without definitive modern scientific explanation. They are thought to involve interactions between the "energy field" of the patient and the energy field or the intention of the healer. These ideas of intention and interactions with forms of energy can be related to the concept of the quantum enigma.

INVERSE SQUARE LAW VERSUS QUANTUM ENIGMA AND ENTANGLEMENT

Most forms of energy obey an inverse square law. That is, the effect or force decreases as an inverse square of the distance. Quantum effects do not show this drop-off with distance. Furthermore, all other energies exert their influence either at or below the speed of light. Quantum effects, however, like many phenomena in energy medicine, seem to happen immediately without any appreciable time delay. Thus, two of the anomalous aspects of energy medicine, independence of time and independence of distance, are also observed in quantum effects (Julsgaard, Kozhekin, & Polzik, 2001). This idea is one way to explain the exchange of healing information, or "subtle energy," between healer and patient from a distance (Bennett & DiVincenzo, 2000). Smith (1998) has postulated that the body functions as a macroscopic quantum system. This idea may also be applicable to related fields of energy medicine (Mayor & Micozzi, 2011). The data reported by Smith (2003) suggest that the acupuncture meridian system is made up of quantum domains and networks. The proposition has been made that consciousness and intention are connected, through quantum mechanical means, to the body's healing potentials (Jahn & Dunne, 1986). However, quantum effects have only been demonstrated on an extremely small scale. They have been thought by most physicists to not be applicable in domains larger than Planck's constant (e.g., photons and electrons) and that only traditional Newtonian mechanics applies to domains we experience in everyday life. Smith proposes that there is a hierarchical series of networks and domains in which quantum effects are transmitted to molecules through their quantum particles, and that molecules transfer this information to cells, and so on, until the intact organism is involved and influenced by quantum effects.

Quantum mechanics has had an "entanglement" with the idea of consciousness from the beginning of the recognition of quantum forces. It is the most rigorously tested theory in all of science but has been unable to escape the "subjective" effects of human observation, perception—and consciousness. No experiment ever performed has ever failed to agree completely with the theory (Rosenblum & Kuttner, 2008). So, what is the problem?

Quantum mechanics is applied in much of our daily lives, without our direct awareness or understanding, from computers to magnetic resonance imaging. However, there are aspects that remain counterintuitive and paradoxical. This enigma has been well illustrated with the behavior of light in what is called the "double-slit experiment." Light has a dual (and paradoxical) nature. It can behave as a wave (electromagnetic [EM] radiation) or as a particle (photon). Nobel Prizes have been awarded both for demonstrating that light is a wave and for demonstrating that light is a particle. Further, our conscious observation determines which of these properties of light is exhibited in any given moment. Nobody knows why, at this point in time, but the evidence has never been refuted. The more sophisticated the experiments and tests have become, the more entrenched and mysterious this phenomenon (Walborn, Terra Cunha, Padua, & Monken, 2003).

The double-slit interference experiment is outlined as follows. Light shines into the back of two open boxes with slits on the front side. On the wall opposite the slits, on the other side from the light source, is a projection screen. No light can reach this screen except the light that comes through the slits. If the slits are narrow enough and spaced properly, the waves of light come out through the slits. The light is made of waves with high points (peaks) and low points (valleys), and the waves can interact and interfere with each other analogous to waves on water. The light spreads out from the two slits, and the waves interact where they strike the screen. Where two peaks reach the screen at the same point, there is a light band. Where two valleys reach the screen at the same point, there is a shadow, because no light has reached this point. As demonstrated in physics courses, there emerges a series of light and dark stripes, or an "interference pattern." This pattern is considered definitive evidence for the wave nature of light.

In the next part, the experiment can be run so that only a single "packet" of light exists in both boxes. This experiment has been done many times. When this procedure is followed, the interference pattern is still generated, which demonstrates that light is a wave and that the wave of energy was distributed in both boxes. However, if there are photon detectors in both boxes, and we observe them while the experiment is running, only one of the detectors will react, and a photon (a quantum of light energy) will be found in only one box. Furthermore, the typical interference pattern will not appear because there is no longer a wave of light. The wave function is said to "collapse" and form the photon particle. No one has been able to adequately explain this undisputed observation, called "complementarity", and no physicist disputes this phenomenon. There is considerable controversy as to its interpretation. The majority of science simply ignores it and its implications. (To the extent that the mechanisms of much of complementary medicine become understood as based on this quantum enigma, it may someday be labeled "complementarity medicine.")

When this experiment is repeated many times, it always results in one of these two observations. If there is no photon detector, then we see the wave nature of light. If there are photon counters in both boxes that we observe, then we only see photons and no wave. Furthermore, the probability of finding the photon in one box or the other is exactly 50:50. This phenomenon caused Einstein to try to wish it away by famously stating, "God does not play dice."

This quantum enigma is where consciousness comes in. As strange as it sounds, the collapsing of the wave function is dependent not only on the presence of the instruments but also on our conscious awareness of them. This phenomenon is demonstrated elegantly in the established work by Walborn, Terra Cunha, Pádua, and Monken (2002) and Walborn et al. (2003) on a phenomenon called "quantum erasure".

Walborn et al. address another aspect of quantum physics called "entanglement". It appears that the universe, like Noah before the flood, makes most, if not all, things in pairs. Thus, it is possible to entangle two photons so that they have paired aspects of their quantum natures. Two photons thus entangled have a very strange property. Without any detectable form of energy transfer or communication and in a distance-independent manner, whatever is done to one photon immediately affects the other entangled photon, without time delay and no matter the distance separating them. This effect is not causal. Observation and the observer do not cause the effect. Rather, the effect is said to be a nonlocal connectivity or nonlocal correlation (Hyland, 2003).

This effect prompted another episode of cognitive dissonance for Einstein:

I cannot seriously believe in [quantum physics] because ... physics should represent a reality in time and space, free from spooky actions at a distance.

(Albert Einstein)

Light has a dual nature, and which of its two natures it demonstrates depends on how we look at it. When photons, and apparently other very small quanta, become entangled, they remain entangled regardless of the distance between them. Whatever happens to one is immediately reflected in the other without any time delay and with no detectable or explainable form of energy or information transfer. Some physicists (e.g., Rosenblum & Kuttner, 2008) conclude that these phenomena demonstrate interaction among consciousness and energy and matter that appears to go beyond currently understood principles of physics. There are ways to transfer information that are independent of distance and through means that physics has not yet definitively determined or explained. Consideration of quantum physics in a discussion of energy medicine provides a possible explanation for some of the empirical observations and anomalies typical of this therapy and helps to explain a role for consciousness and intention in healing. In energy medicine, quantum mechanics and physics may explain some of the anomalous observations that have been made in aspects of energy medicine such as distant healing (discussed in Chapter 8). Some of the enigmas of quantum entanglement and quantum tunneling have been demonstrated to operate in biological systems and establish the role of quantum phenomenon for sustaining life, and potentially healing (Box 9.1).

The universe begins to look more like a great thought than a great machine.

(Sir James Jeans)

BOX 9.1 *Quantum Effects Explain Enigma of Enzyme Function,*
         Photosynthesis and Animal Migration
         SCHRÖDINGER'S CAT (THAT GOT THE CANARY OR ROBIN)

"Schrodinger's cat" is the name given to a thought experiment, illustrating a profound paradox, proposed by Austrian fundamental physicist Erwin Schrödinger in 1935. He initially suggested the experiment as an absurdity to illustrate what he saw as the problem of the Copenhagen interpretation of quantum mechanics when applied to everyday experience, as discussed in this chapter. His scenario presented a cat that may be simultaneously both alive and dead, like the state known as a "quantum superposition", which arises from being linked to a random subatomic event that may or may not occur.

The thought experiment is also often featured in theoretical discussions of the interpretations of quantum mechanics. Schrödinger was the scientist who actually coined the term *Verschränkung,* a German word for *entanglement,* in the course of developing this thought experiment. In 1935, the experiment was meant to show that quantum superposition and entanglement, when projected to observable phenomenon, was too strange to be a serious reality (thus leading to Einstein's initial consternation). However, subsequent experimental observations during the 20th century have demonstrated the substance of these challenging concepts. Now in the 21st century, it seems that these kinds of quantum concepts can help explain the energetic aspects of living beings that were once considered ineffably mysterious up through the mid-19th century.

For centuries, philosophers had grappled with the question of what makes living beings or organisms "alive," as opposed to inanimate. Until the reductionist, mechanistic, positivistic paradigm took hold of biology and medicine during the late 19th century, serious scientists still sought the vital spark that accounted for life, a natural philosophy known as "vitalism." They wondered why the stuff of life is so different from inanimate material. They asked whether life follows the same laws and principles as inanimate objects, whether they have the same fundamental physics and chemistry, and what happens when an organism dies? These questions were a source of endless and timeless speculation.

These questions have been addressed by moral and natural philosophers and scientists and by the rest of humanity for as long as history has been recorded. Some archaeologists believe they have found evidence for such thinking among the earliest humans in prehistory. The consensus conventional thinking among virtually all human cultures, civilizations, and societies had always been that life was something special, animated by some kind of soul, spirit, *qi,* bioenergy, or vital spark not to be found among the nonliving. By the end of the 19th century, this theory of vitalism was thought to have been discredited by the discovery that living organisms are made from the same chemicals as the inanimate world (atoms and organic molecules of carbon, nitrogen, oxygen) and that they obey the same physical laws.

In the late 19th century, scientists concluded that life is simply a series of elegant and complex chemical reactions, based on the same principles of classic chemistry and physics that had already been harnessed during the Industrial Revolution in the West,

Continued

BOX 9.1 *Quantum Effects Explain Enigma of Enzyme Function, Photosynthesis and Animal Migration—cont'd*

to drive steam engines, to make steel from carbon, iron in blast furnaces, and other "mysteries" that had become commonplace after centuries of relative stasis. Suddenly after all the rules had been settled in the early 20th century, starting in the midst of World War I, a strange new science came to light that questioned all of the classic rules of science that had become familiar in everyday life.

Quantum mechanics is the science of very small particles and spaces. It has also been used to explain and predict cosmic events. Quantum science describes how fundamental particles can be in 1 or 2 million places at once, can pass through impenetrable barriers, or possess "impossible," instantaneous, interconnections that are maintained over vast times and distances. Perhaps most startling, our consciousness influences what we can observe of these particles, and even their existence. Most scientists had believed that quantum science could only be relevant to the subatomic fundamental particles of which atoms and molecules are composed.

In 1944 (during World War II), in his book called, *What is Life?*, Erwin Schrödinger, claimed that at least some aspects of life must be governed by quantum rather than classical rules. Of course, biologists and medical scientists steadfastly ignored Schrödinger's claims about the quantum nature of life. During the 20th century, biomedicine continued to consider life as nothing more than the workings of a very complex machine. Medicine had a great 100-year run with a biomedical paradigm based on 17th-century typological biology and Newtonian mechanics, or classical physics. Twenty-first century biology has finally turned to probing the dynamics of ever-smaller biological systems, and quantum effects have begun to emerge (McFadden, 2016).

Enzymes are proteins that act as catalysts for biochemical reactions and metabolic processes. Enzyme reactions also exhibit *quantum tunneling*. Their purpose is to vastly accelerate the speed of chemical reactions so that processes that would otherwise take thousands of years (by standard chemical laws of mass action and thermodynamics) actually take place continually within milliseconds inside all living cells. Exactly how they are able to speed chemical actions by such enormous rates, a trillion times faster, had remained another mystery of life. Research has now shown that several enzymes work by another strange fundamental property called "quantum tunneling". Enzymes feature a process where electrons and protons vanish from one position in a molecule to instantly reappear in another place, without ever having to travel through the molecular spaces in between, in a kind of quantum teleportation. Enzymes make every molecule in every cell, and every cell of every living creature. They appear to use quantum tunneling to keep beings alive.

The living system known as the "plant kingdom" preceded animal life on earth by hundreds of millions of years. Photosynthesis is essential to all life, plant metabolism, and to the carbon, oxygen, and water cycles of the Earth—and it appears to show quantum coherence. Photosynthesis maybe the most remarkable chemical reaction in the cosmos. Using solar energy, it converts light, together with air, water, and selected minerals into nutrients for grass, trees, grains, fruits, forests and, ultimately, foods for all animals who eat either the plants themselves, and/or other animals who eat the plants.

BOX 9.1 *Quantum Effects Explain Enigma of Enzyme Function, Photosynthesis and Animal Migration—cont'd*

The initiating event is the capture of a particle of light energy (photon) by a chlorophyll molecule in a plant cell. That light energy is gathered by an electrical particle that moves through a jungle of chlorophyll molecules to find its way to a biochemical factory called the "reaction center". There, that energy is used to fuse atoms together to form molecules. It has been a botanical paradox that the energy of these particles would be expected to simply get lost in the jungle of the plant cells. But the energy almost always arrives precisely in the right reaction center. In 2007, Fleming and colleagues, at the University of California at Berkeley, discovered that instead of just going by one random route or another (as would be expected from classical physics), the energy makes its way to the reaction center as a quantum wave that travels through all possible routes simultaneously to find the quickest way (McFadden, 2016).

Quantum entanglement also appears to be involved in the mystery of animal migration and navigation. Birds and other animals migrate and make their way around the world by using biological compasses to detect the Earth's magnetic field. How they work has been another one of science's biggest enduring enigmas of life. Studies with the European robin demonstrated that their navigational compass possesses several unusual features. It requires light and detects the angle of magnetic field lines relative to the Earth's surface, rather than direction. Scientists figured out that these features could only make sense if birds have a kind of chemical compass that uses quantum entanglement.

This phenomenon is so strange that even Einstein (who theorized black holes and warped space-time warps—which were eventually experimentally observed) could not believe it. He called it "spooky action at a distance," because quantum entanglement allows vastly distant particles to remain instantaneously connected. To demonstrate whether the scientists were right, the robin's compass should have been disrupted by high-frequency radio waves. The physicists teamed up with ornithologists to demonstrate that the bird's compass was indeed thrown off course by radio waves (which raises other questions about what is happening to migrating birds by the radio waves that now flood the atmosphere). It seems this "spooky action" is actually responsible for the mysterious migrations of billions of birds, and other animals, around the world every season of the year.

Schrödinger predicted that life navigates a narrow path between the classic and quantum worlds, called the "quantum edge." The old "vital spark" of life, discounted and disparaged for 150 years by modern biomedical scientists, is back on the "cutting edge."

MECHANISM OF ACTION

Accordingly, with the considerations mentioned earlier, no rational mechanism of action in the practice of energy medicine is typically available or readily comes to mind. The confounding of mechanism with empiricism in the study of healing has been an ongoing challenge in all of medicine. This idea of mechanism provides a distinction between veritable forms of energy medicine, such as magnetic therapy, and the putative forms such as healing touch or reiki (NCCAM, 2007).

Despite this gap in conventional understanding and knowledge, there is tremendous stress placed on understanding the mechanism of the biomedical model, which remains bounded by its own conventional 20th-century paradigm. It is difficult to find funding for basic mechanistic studies in energy medicine, which creates the circular conundrum that there is little or no funding for the kind of studies that would be required for further elucidation of mechanisms in energy medicine as required by mainstream medicine, which in turns controls the availability of research funding, and so on. For several years, the NCCAM dedicated over 60% of its budget to clinical research and 20% to applied research at clinical centers, with only the remaining funds allocated to basic research (http://nccam. nih.gov, 2007). The NCCAM had continued to move more toward clinical trials (although the methodology for such trials is frequently inappropriate) and to the further exclusion of basic and applied research. Thus, basic research on energy (both veritable and putative) medicine remains scarce.

Recent literature on forms of bioenergy—qi, ki, *prana*—and their biomedical applications has significantly increased, as demonstrated in this text, but the forms of energy involved in energy medicine remain inherently mysterious. There are examples in the English-language literature of attempts to characterize this energy (e.g., Ohnishi & Ohnishi, 2008), but these studies have not been replicated. A complete, criteria-based, systematic review of this field was provided in the book by Jonas and Crawford (2003a). An additional comprehensive survey was compiled by Benor (2004). Over the past 30 years, considerable work has been done on the measurement of external qi as physical energy. The majority of publications in this field are in Chinese and, therefore, not easily accessible to the Western scientific community. Among English-language references dealing with bioenergy is a book by Lu (1997). A more complete review by Zha (2001) is found in the Proceedings of the Historic Samueli Institute for Information Biology meetings in Hawaii. A thorough review of previous work on physical measurements of external qi is outside the scope of this chapter (see also Section IV). It appears that previous experiments were not done in a rigorously controlled manner and utilized instruments that are not current. The documented experiments reveal low levels of physical energy associated with external qi emission by qigong practitioners and healers (Hintz et al., 2003).

The lack of solid evidence or an accepted mechanistic explanation for the "energy" in energy medicine presents a large hurdle to acceptance by Western biomedicine. There is no universal agreement as to what is meant by the "energy" in energy medicine—or even what kind it might be. Terms such as "subtle energy," "qi energy," and "prana" are often used (see Mayor & Micozzi, 2011, for a survey). There does seem to be consensus that whatever it is, it is not the energy currently identified and described by traditional Western physics or Newtonian mechanics. For a concept of such "energy" to be of value and adopted within the scientific community, there should be consilience with accepted physics, chemistry, and biology. Any putative bioenergy involved in energy medicine should not only be internally consistent but also allow for consistency with the other known and accepted energies as well.

Energy/Endocrine Correspondences

Energy Center (Chakra)	Endocrine Gland	Emotional Function	Energy Sensation
Crown	Pineal	Bliss	Scalp tingling
Brown	Pituitary	Intuition	Inner "lightbulb"
Throat	Thyroid	Truth	Choking up
Heart	Thymus	Compassion	Broken heart
Solar plexus	Pancreas	Personal power	"Butterflies"
Genital	Gonads	Sexuality	Sexual arousal
Root	Adrenal	Survival	"Adrenaline rush"

- Endocrine/energy center correspondences were discovered in introspective traditions that did not allow dissection.
- Psycho-endocrinology: the emotional function of each energy center relates to physiological function of each corresponding endocrine gland.
- Everyday experiences of intensified life energy flow represent the palpable interface of subtle energy with gross physiology.

FIG. 9.1 | Energy and Endocrine Correspondences.

A cybernetic or systems analysis approach consistent with conventional descriptions of electromagnetic energies describing this system is shown in Fig. 9.1. This depiction provides a level of abstraction based on the concepts of (1) information sources, (2) a medium for carrying the signal, and (3) receivers. In this view, the underlying physical layer of information transfer is intentionally hidden to allow discussion of the transfer of bioinformation without any a priori decision about the physical mechanism(s) by which that transfer occurs (Hintz et al., 2003).

In this model, a bioenergy system may be characterized as one that comprises (1) a source that generates energy and modulates it in some manner so that it conveys information, (2) coupling mechanism(s) connecting the bioenergy source to a transfer medium, (3) transfer medium(s) through which the bioenergy flows, (4) coupling mechanism(s) connecting the transfer medium to a bioenergy sink, and (5) a terminal sink that includes a mechanism for the perception of information. The input and output coupling depends on properties of the source, the transfer medium, and the sink. The term "perception" rather than reception is used to imply some active process that uses some form of perceptual reasoning in processing the information based on its content (consciousness). The means by which information is transmitted and interacts with the system is not clear in the sense that physicists understand it. Feedback loops in biosystems are examples of information transfer.

In most, if not all, cases, the physical means by which the feedback is provided to the system either is understood or is assumed to involve interactions among actual physical objects and processes. For example, in the case of the placebo pill and a branding study, it is not self-evident how the information is transmitted but, de facto, it appears to be.

RESPONSES TO PAIN

In these studies, information is able to significantly influence a biological system and its responses to pain. Although we have some understanding of the biological consequences of energy medicine (Yan et al., 2008), the means by which it is accomplished, through the "energy," remains unknown. For example, qigong has been demonstrated to have antidepressive effects in patients. Although the psychological mechanisms underlying this effect have been described, the neurobiological mechanism remains unclear (Tsang & Fung, 2008). The same may be said of hypnosis, for which the clinical effects are now widely accepted (thanks in part to statistical and psychometric profiling of "susceptibility" to hypnotic "suggestion"), but the neurobiological mechanism has remained unclear since the time of Mesmer (see Chapters 5 and 7).

Further research is needed to elucidate the biology and consolidate its scientific base. There are examples in the field of veritable energy medicine, however, in which there is a good understanding of the energies and energy fields involved. For example, the magnetic fields employed in transcranial magnetic stimulation are well characterized (see Chapters 10 and 11). Even so, the biology and biological mechanisms at work and affected by the magnetic fields are only beginning to be understood (Lopez-Ibor, Lopez-Ibor, & Pastrana, 2008). Transcranial magnetic stimulation has been shown to be an effective alternative for the treatment of refractory neuropathic pain through epidural motor cortex stimulation, but the mechanisms at work remain poorly understood (Lazorthes, Sol, Fowo, Roux, & Verdié, 2007).

STANDARDS OF RESEARCH AND PRACTICE

It is facile to recommend that complementary and alternative medicine (CAM) be held to the same standards as conventional medical science. The complexity and intricacies of studying CAM have been widely discussed, as documented by the White House Commission on Complementary and Alternative Medicine Policy (2002). This reality particularly holds true for energy medicine. Studies are conducted in nearly all CAM disciplines that lend themselves to the hypothesis-driven paradigm, and the medical literature attests to that fact. Essentially, CAM scientific research follows the same standards used for conventional research, including (1) use of statistically significant numbers of subjects, specimens, or replications; (2) introduction of internal and experimental controls and the definition of response specificity; and (3) the requirement for reproducibility. The last is perhaps the most challenging. In several cases, experiments have shown positive results, but when repeated, sometimes in the same laboratory, do not replicate despite following the precautions of maintaining identical experimental conditions.

This challenge is illustrated in the work published by Yount et al. (2004). They investigated the effect of 30 minutes of qigong on the healthy growth of cultured human cells. A rigorous experimental design of randomization, blinding, and controls was followed. A pilot study included 8 independent experiments and a formal study included 28 independent experiments showing positive effects. However, the replication study of over 60 independent experiments showed no difference between the sham (untreated) and treated cells. This study represents an example of holding basic science research on energy medicine to the highest standard of experimental methodology.

This level of rigor is rarely achieved in energy laboratory research, however, nor is it achieved in much mainstream research. The basic and clinical research in the area of distant mental influence on living systems (DMILS) and energy medicine has been reviewed and the quality of the research is quite varied. Although a few simple research models met all quality criteria, such as in mental influence on random number generators or electrodermal activity, much basic research into DMILS, qigong, prayer, and other techniques has been of poor quality (Jonas & Crawford, 2003a). In setting up these evaluations, the reviewers established basic criteria that should be met for all such laboratory research (Jonas & Crawford, 2003b; Sparber, Crawford, & Jonas, 2003).

In basic scientific research, formulating the testable hypothesis is sometimes not the major challenge that lies in setting up and testing the practice itself. The example of Yount et al. (2004) followed the most rigorous methodological and experimental designs, but the practice under investigation was not a simple treatment with defined doses of a pharmaceutical compound or agonist-antagonist drug of a specific cell receptor. Instead, it was an unknown amount of energy of unknown characteristics emanating from the hands of a number of different qigong practitioners, with variable skill levels. Acupuncture, which is thought to be related, lends itself to use in animal models for in vivo and ex vivo evaluation of its effects. By applying electroacupuncture, researchers are able to control the amount of energy delivered. However, the challenge is the placement of the needles. Although in humans needles are placed based on meridian (or channel) maps, in animal experimental models, they must be placed so they will not be disturbed during normal grooming while still being located along a meridian location of relevance. In addition, 20-minute electroacupuncture sessions are often used because this method is what would be done in humans (Li et al., 2008), due to clinical limitations, but the time and dose parameters should ideally be adjusted to the animal's body size.

MIND-BODY THERAPIES

Mind-body–based therapies are often not considered energy medicine, especially when applied to oneself, although they are also considered in this light for the purposes of this book (see Section II). When the goal is to produce a change in an outside entity through meditation, for example, we can claim this result as a form of energy medicine. As such, it is very challenging to explore in a laboratory setting. There are several studies showing the effects of meditation on cell growth (Yu, Tsai, & Hwang, 2003), differentiation (Ventura, 2005), water pH, and temperature change, as well as on the development time of fruit fly larvae (Tiller, 1997). For these studies, the necessary level of methodological rigor has typically not been met. Independent replication has been especially problematic. On the other hand, some CAM applications, such as homeopathy, phytotherapy, and dietary supplements (Ayurveda or Traditional Chinese Medicine) are relatively easy to translate to the laboratory setting. These practices and their products of use can be considered like conventional interventions using pharmaceutical compounds, for which dose and time-course experiments can be designed.

Energy, Expectation, Intention, and Placebo

It would be reasonable to assume that subjects given a placebo for pain would get little to no relief. An early study reported at the 1979 Society for Neuroscience Conference showed evidence that the expectations (or intentions) of the physician significantly affected outcomes (Gracely et al., 1979). All subjects were given the same placebo, but half were given it by physicians who thought they were giving active medication. The patients of physicians who thought they were giving an active agent experienced a significant reduction in pain, whereas subjects in the other study group received no relief and their pain actually worsened.

The impact of expectation was further explored in a four-arm study carried out by Margo (1999). One group was given an "unbranded" placebo, another group was given a "branded" placebo, a third group was given unbranded aspirin, and the fourth group was given branded aspirin. There appears to be an analgesic effect just from the act of taking a pain pill, and this effect is significantly improved if the pill is branded. In this study, actual aspirin produced greater analgesia than the branded placebo, and branded aspirin worked better than unbranded aspirin for analgesia. The author interpreted these data to indicate that taking a pill has significant analgesic effect for patients with pain, whether or not the pill has any conventionally defined bioactive agent. Further, branding of the pain pill enhances the effect whether it is placebo or active. This finding was a demonstration of the power and efficacy of therapeutic expectation (a form of intention) (Kirsch, 1999).

Even the color of the pill apparently makes a difference in peoples' expectations. Hot colors, such as red, yellow, and pink, have a stimulatory effect while pills that are cool in color, such as blue or green, have a calming effect (Blackwell, Bloomfield, & Buncher, 1972). Less surprising is that the number of pills taken impacts healing rates even when the pills are inert placebos. Placebo healing rates rise with the number of pills taken per day. In patients with painful stomach ulcers, subjects who took four placebo pills per day recovered faster than those who took two per day (de Craen et al., 1999). In a similar vein, switching a placebo treatment from oral to subcutaneous injection had a greater likelihood of decreasing headache severity over the course of 2 hours (de Craen, Tijssen, de Gans, & Kleijnen, 2000). de Craen also showed that giving a treatment at the hospital compared to at home serves to increase the placebo effect, likely as a result of people's expectation of an effect.

We do not know the mechanism for energy medicine. There is legitimate debate as to whether there even is such a thing as "subtle energy." Some of the discussions taking place in the field and the literature around energy medicine shows there are at least three theories as to how the underlying mechanisms give rise to the observed effects of energy medicine: (1) a conventional energy explanation, (2) an explanation based on placebo effects, and (3) a quantum entanglement explanation. The actual mechanism of the well-established, clearly observed placebo effect is not addressed in this distinction. The quantum mechanics approach is the most novel and perhaps least understood of the theories, but it also best fits all the best data collected so far regarding all forms of energy medicine.

One mechanism that also might help explain the effects of energy medicine is the placebo effect as discussed earlier. In other words, whatever is happening takes place as the result of patients convincing themselves, or intending, that they are healing or being healed. Thus, they may feel less pain, have fewer complaints, and so on—but still "nothing really happened" between the healer and patient. However, this explanation is not really more satisfactory and also does not fit some of the best data. The placebo effect itself, while unquestionably real and clinically meaningful, is not well understood or well defined. Thus, invoking the placebo effect still begs the question of mechanism. Second, if patients actually experience healing or feel better, then something is "really" happening consciously. Thus, we are back to our first point of still not knowing the underlying mechanism while in fact having authentic healing. Thus, invoking the placebo effect may be equivalent to confessing that something really is happening with the patient but that we do not know how or whether it is coming from within or from without. In addition, the known mechanics of placebo, such as belief, expectancy, intention, and conditioning, do not account for some of the best-replicated data on these direct effects in living and nonliving systems and blinded distant effects (Jonas & Crawford, 2003a).

BIOFIELDS

The idea of a "vital force" has been a core aspect of traditional healing practices for millennia and has often been used to explain therapeutic practices in the West such as mesmerism, magnetic healing, and faith healing (see Section II). It has also been part of discussions in Western science since at least 1907 when Henri Bergson proposed it as an explanation for why organic molecules could not be synthesized at the time (Bergson, 1911). Part of this thinking held that electricity—the physics and engineering wonder of the time—was somehow connected with this vital force. Chinese and Indian healers had another idea that has lately been seen as equivalent, called "qi" and "prana". Clearly such an idea has been around a long time.

A modern expression of this idea is often called the "biofield hypothesis" (Rubik, 2002). For this discussion, the important aspect of the biofield hypothesis is its dependence on classical electromagnetic fields and forces. As Rubik points out, "The biofield is a useful construct consistent with bio-electromagnetics and the physics of nonlinear, dynamical, non-equilibrium living systems." Some aspects of energy medicine may be explained by the biofield. It is completely consistent with and even sufficient to explain magnetic therapy (see Chapters 10 and 11). There are at least two aspects of some forms of energy medicine that biofield hypothesis does not adequately explain. One is the apparent distance independence. The other is the apparent instantaneous state change (like quantum entanglement) that forms part of some forms of energy medicine. This factor is the second anomaly of subtle energy medicine: it often happens faster than classical mechanics can explain.

It is possible that these anomalies, and the very fundamental aspects of energy medicine, have their explanation and source in quantum physics. Others disagree with this idea (May, 2003). Still others feel that although it is not the whole explanation, some aspects of quantum physics may be relevant and may play a role in energy medicine (Dossey, 2003). If it is true that energy medicine often works through nonclassical and quantum forms of energy, it is now possible to visualize a future in which energy medicine uses a combination of classical and quantum energy fields and forces to target and regulate endogenous processes and fields within the body to affect health and healing.

If energy medicine and distant healing are fundamentally forms of information transfer, then quantum mechanics may provide the explanation and means for this process. In addition to explaining the transfer of healing energy between people, it may underlie the natural self-healing process itself. Rein (2004) proposed that this information flow within the body is necessary for health and that, when impeded, ill health and disease result. In this thinking, energy medicine is also the flow of information through quantum effects between healer and patient. In an analogous fashion, health is the free flow and transfer of information within the body and the interchange of information with the environment to augment this flow. Thus, the fields of information and quantum models continue to be important areas of focus for future research and practice. If testable theoretical models can be developed that explain data from both veritable and putative forms of energy medicine, a new paradigm of understanding in science and health care may emerge. Such a development is as important and revolutionary as molecular biological and biochemical models have been in the 20th century.

ENERGY THERAPIES

Reiki, healing touch (HT), qigong, and Therapeutic Touch (TT) are all "energy therapies" that use gentle hand techniques thought to help repattern the patient's energy field and accelerate healing of the body, mind, and spirit. They are all based on the belief that human beings have fields of energy (biofields) in constant interaction with other fields of energy from other humans and from the environment. The goal of energy therapies is to purposefully use the energetic interaction between the practitioner and the patient to restore harmony to the patient's energy system.

Most energy therapies are based on a holistic philosophy that places the patient within the context of that individual's life and an understanding of the dynamic interconnectedness with themselves and their environment (Cassidy, 1995). They are about often healing rather than cure (Engebretson & Wardell, 2007).

The most common contemporary touch therapies used in nursing practice are TT, HT, and reiki. The first two were developed by nurses, whereas reiki came from pre-WWII Japan. Although not directed toward nursing, reiki is used by many in hospital settings (Engebretson & Wardell, 2007; Kreiger, 1993; Mentgen, 2001). Controversy has accompanied the use of these therapies, even after their inclusion by the North American Nursing Diagnosis Association (NANDA). The controversy has not prevented their increasing popularity within the profession to promote health, reduce symptoms, and ameliorate treatment side effects. Practitioners use TT and HT to improve health and healing by addressing, in the words of the official NANDA diagnosis, a patient's "Disturbed Energy Field: disruption in the flow of energy surrounding a person's being that results in a disharmony of the body, mind, and/or spirit" (NANDA, 2008).

Like many other energy therapies, TT is not designed to treat specific diseases but instead to balance the energy field of the patient or, through a boosting of energy, improve the patient's feeling of energy. TT was developed by Dolores Krieger, PhD, RN, in the 1970s. She borrowed from and mixed together ancient shamanic traditions and techniques she learned from well-known healers of her time. Like acupuncture, qigong, and yoga, HT is based on the idea that illness and poor health represent an imbalance of personal bioenergetic forces and fields that exist around and through a person's body. Rebalancing and boosting these energies is done through a clear intention to support and harmonize the person with his or her innate energy balance. These practices typically begin with the practitioner performing some form of ritual that clears and focuses the intention to bring harmony and balance to the person who is in need.

In a typical TT session, the practitioner begins with a centering process to calm the mind, access a sense of compassion, and become fully present with the patient. The practitioner then focuses intention on the patient's highest good and places his or her hands lightly on the patient's body or slightly away from it, often making sweeping hand motions above the body.

Practice Exercise

Begin by placing your arms out in front of you, hands facing each other about 1 foot apart. Bring the hands close enough together to feel warmth but without making physical contact. Then begin to slowly move the hands farther apart and closer together, and notice any nonthermal sensations, especially when they are about a foot apart. Closing your eyes can help you tune in. Many people describe a tingling or bouncing feeling, almost magnetic in quality. This sensation is one that TT practitioners use to assess the status of the energy field of their patients.

Sufficient research on TT has been published in peer-reviewed journals to perform a meta-analysis of the combined results from separate studies. Two meta-analyses have determined that TT produces a moderately positive effect on psychological and physiological variables hypothesized to be influenced by TT, primarily anxiety and pain (Peters, 1999; Winstead-Fry & Kijek, 1999). A systematic review of the HT research published in 2000 included 19 randomized controlled trials involving 1122 patients (Astin, Harkness, & Ernst, 2000). The reviewers found that 11 studies (58%) reported statistically significant treatment effects. Another systematic review of the literature on wound healing and TT found only four studies that met the author's criteria for quality. Of these, two showed statistically significant effects, whereas the other two found no effect from TT. The evidence has been insufficient to conclude that TT works for wound healing (O'Mathuna & Ashford, 2003, 2012).

Applications for which TT and HT seem to work well include reducing anxiety, improving muscle relaxation, aiding in stress reduction, promoting relaxation, enhancing a sense of well-being, promoting wound healing, and reducing pain. In addition, no serious side effects have been associated with these healing modalities (Engebretson & Wardell, 2007). One review of touch therapies looked at studies with outcomes such as pain reduction, improvement of mood, reduction of anxiety, promotion of relaxation, improvement of functional status, improvement of health status, increase in well-being, wound healing, reduction of blood pressure, and increase in immune function. The authors found that studies were mixed in their quality and the degree of evidence supporting the effectiveness of touch therapies in influencing these outcomes (Warber, Gordon, Gillespie, Olson, & Assefi, 2003).

A 2008 systematic Cochrane Review of the literature on touch therapy for pain relief included studies of HT, TT, and reiki (So, Jiang, & Qin, 2008). The authors evaluated the literature to determine the effectiveness of these therapies for relieving both acute and chronic pain. They also looked for any adverse effects from these therapies. Randomized controlled trials and controlled clinical trials investigating the use of these therapies for treatment of pain that included a sham placebo or "no treatment" control group met the criteria for inclusion. A total of 24 studies, including 16 involving TT, 5 involving HT, and 3 involving reiki, met these criteria. On average, a small but significant average effect on pain relief (1 unit on a scale of 0 to 10) was found. The greatest effect was seen in the reiki studies and appeared to involve the more experienced practitioners. The authors state that the data were inconclusive with regard to which was more important, the level of experience or the modality of therapy. The authors concluded that the evidence supports the use of touch therapies for pain relief. Application of these therapies also decreased the use of analgesics in two studies. No statistically significant placebo effect was seen, and no adverse effects from these therapies were reported. The authors pointed out the need for higher-quality studies, especially of HT and reiki (So et al., 2008).

In one study involving a combination of HT and guided imagery (GI), 123 returning combat-exposed active duty military with significant posttraumatic stress disorder (PTSD) symptoms were randomized into a 1-month study receiving either HT + GI or treatment as usual (TAU) (Jain et al., 2012). The primary outcome measure was impact on PTSD symptoms and secondary outcome measures were depression, quality of life, and hostility. Analysis of outcomes indicated a statistically and clinically significant reduction in PTSD symptoms (effect size of 0.85 [Cohen's *d*]) and depression (effect size 0.70) for HT + GI compared to TAU. In addition, compared to TAU, HT + GI produced significant improvement in mental quality of life and cynicism. The authors concluded that participation in this complementary medicine intervention resulted in a clinically significant reduction in PTSD and related symptoms in a returning, combat-exposed active duty military population.

ENERGETIC TREATMENTS OF CHRONIC PAIN SYNDROMES

Recent advances in understanding the neuroanatomical model of pain have been based on imaging technology, central sensitization, molecular biology, neurotransmitter receptor activity (new drug development), and the like. A different model of pain etiology emerges when adopting an energy perspective, as can be shown by focusing on the specific energy dynamics of four common pain diagnoses: myofascial pain (MFP), fibromyalgia (FM), complex regional pain syndrome (CRPS), and phantom limb pain (PLP). The first two are characterized by specific point disturbances that correspond to acupoint imbalances. CRPS is related to a drain of emotional energy, and PLP to an imbalance in the underlying energetic matrix.

Myofascial Pain

The key clinical finding in MFP is the induction of pain by localized trigger points (TrPs) (Kwok, Cohen, & Cosic, 1998). TrPs appear to be randomly dispersed, according to the map of Western medicine, because they are found in anatomically heterogeneous tissues and locations. However, from an energy medicine perspective, they can be seen to function as key acupuncture points. In fact, the Western medicine treatment of MFP via trigger point injections has been likened to acupuncture (see Chapter 15). The trigger points are "inactivated" by injecting a range of substances such as steroid drugs, anesthetic medication, or a benign substance (even normal saline solution will work), and sometimes by simple "dry" needling. This procedure may be likened to acupuncture needling, although much less invasive. A smaller diameter needle is used in acupuncture than in TrP inactivation, and the practitioner's intention may be quite different. In using this technique, Western medicine may be stumbling upon the existence of qi in spite of itself.

The electromagnetic activity at acupoints and TrPs has been investigated (Myss, & Shealy, 1998; Schlebusch, Maric-Oehler, & Popp, 2005). An emerging consensus is that TrPs are characterized by extensive electromyographic activity. Energetically, MFP acupoints and TrPs can be described as having an excess of qi and therefore needing "reduction"' (in contrast to the tender points of fibromyalgia, which are deficient in qi). TrPs are generated when a physical injury causes a local or regional energy backlog, unless and until the emotional components are addressed so that the block can be released. The following case study, provided by Dr. Eric Leskowitz, illustrates how the emotional root of MFP can be addressed via energy therapy.

CASE STUDY

EMOTIONAL FREEDOM TECHNIQUE

Maria is a 35-year-old woman who received a mild concussion and cervical hyperextension injuries in a boating accident. Her neck and shoulder pain syndrome was largely myofascial, and responded only minimally to standard stress management training or physical therapy stretching or strengthening exercises. During a course of emotional freedom technique, or EFT (introduced in Section I), she was able to access memories of the event (remembering her subjective experience of the time she was outwardly unconscious) in a way that triggered a dramatic healing response. She described this recovery of memory as being psychologically crucial to restoring her sense of wholeness. Within minutes of completing the EFT process, she was able to demonstrate full range of motion in her neck and shoulder, and her pain level almost completely disappeared. This case is discussed in more detail in Bruyere (1994).

Fibromyalgia

The two key components of FM are primarily energetic in nature: (1) profound fatigue and (2) pathognomonic tender points. As with TrPs, the location of FM tender points is somewhat mystifying from the anatomical perspective. They were first linked to acupoints 40 years ago by Ronald Melzack, the pioneering pain psychologist of the Melzack-Wall Gate Control Theory of Pain (Kepner, 2002). Melzack found more than 70% correlation of tender points with acupuncture points. Work (Travell & Simons, 1983) suggests that tender points are more likely to be so-called extra points, lying off the major meridians, and the significance of this distinction is not clear (see Chapter 15).

The fatiguing life history that precedes the diagnosis of FM is often striking for the degree of cumulative stress and attendant symptomatology that builds up before medical attention is sought. FM patients often describe, matter-of-factly, how they have adapted to 80-hour workweeks, multiple surgeries, or mounting caregiver responsibilities, without even considering that these burdens are worthy of special comment. Yet from an energetic perspective, it seems likely that these cumulative stressors have totally depleted the patients' energy. Western medicine talks of adrenal exhaustion (Colbert, Hammerschlag, Aickin, & McNames, 2004) as the indicator of breakdown in the fight-or-flight response to stress. The parallel energetic process would be a breakdown in the center that regulates these survival issues, the root center, which is the foundation of the Ayurvedic chakra system cascade. In effect, energetic exhaustion leads to a collapse of this center, which falls into complete energetic and endocrine collapse. One well-known experimental finding suggests that the energy drain of insomnia may create the early symptoms of FM. Healthy volunteers who are deprived of the restorative phase of sleep known as slow wave sleep will reliably develop tender points, which then disappear when normal sleep cycles are restored.

Comprehensive treatment of FM addresses all these centers. One such approach is Jacob Teitelbaum's comprehensive FM treatment protocol, which addresses endocrine dysfunction at all levels and is one of the few FM treatments that has shown statistically significant benefit in double-blind, controlled experiments (Leskowitz, 2001a,b). His protocol involves supplementation or replacement of each endocrine gland hormonal product: dehydroepiandrosterone (DHEA) supplementation restores adrenal (root chakra) function; thyroxine restores thyroid (throat center) function; melatonin restores crown chakra (pineal) function, and so on, as the chakra-endocrine axis is reconstructed. While his model does not use subtle energy terminology, it calls to mind the chakra and endocrine parallels (see Chapters 18 and 19).

Complex Regional Pain Syndrome

From an energy medicine perspective, the pathophysiology of CRPS (formerly referred to as reflex sympathetic dystrophy, or RSD) is frequently acknowledged in the pain literature to involve a significant psychosomatic component. As Ochoa and others originally noted (Melzack, Stilwell, & Fox, 1977), the strong placebo responsiveness in CRPS speaks to the psychophysiological reactivity of these patients. Mainstream pain literature has explored the mind-body link in CRPS only via survey research instruments, showing the incidence of childhood trauma is 30%, for example (Birch, 2003). The role of physically insignificant traumas as precipitants has been widely noted but not fully explored. The physically insignificant initial traumas (sprained ankle, stubbed toe, injection of medication) may be revealed by in-depth psychodynamic interviews to be emotionally significant, even devastating, to the patient. By adopting a careful psychodynamically cued interview technique with CRPS patients, a significant degree of unaddressed emotional pain may be found in CRPS patients. The intensity of CRPS psychological symptoms does not approach that seen with PTSD, and it is more aptly described as suppressed dysphoric emotion, typically anger.

The energy model of CRPS proposes that the mildly injured body part becomes so identified (often consciously) with the emotional conflict that the patient chooses to ignore or at least withdraw attention from that part of the body. In other words, vital energy is withdrawn from a specific region as a psychological defense against experiencing the associated unpleasant emotions that are somatically embedded in that area. In time, the typical sequence of CRPS symptoms develops, initially as effects of autonomic disturbances (allodynia, vasomotor instability), but ultimately progressing to frank tissue damage (loss of hair, cornification of nails, and osteoporosis). These latter symptoms are all characterized by loss of tissue vitality and can be readily recognized as signs of chronic energy depletion. This "qi withdrawal" model may explain why energizing therapies like exercise can be so effective, particularly in younger and adolescent patients (Fries, Hesse, Hellhammer, & Hellhammer, 2005). Vigorous aerobic exercise re-establishes circulation in the affected areas, not only of blood but also presumably of qi. Contrast baths and sensitization gloves are a gentler step in opening the energy pathways. By allowing the patient to become comfortable with gentle stimulation and sensation in the area that has been blocked, attention is in effect returned to it. When patients are again emotionally balanced enough to "reinhabit" the affected body part, symptoms resolve. The tingling feelings patients often describe in the affected area during an energy treatment resemble the feelings of energy activation that students of the energy healing arts learn to detect. Physicians often explain them by referring to the nerves regrowing or healing themselves. In fact, it may be that the flow of qi, as a precondition for nerve regeneration, is what is actually perceived.

CASE STUDY

COMPLEX REGIONAL PAIN SYNDROME

The following three case studies, from Dr. Eric Leskowitz, highlight the imbalances in energy physiology that underlie several specific pain diagnoses and that may be etiologic.

Michelle presented as a 20-year-old college student who maintained a high level of function despite unremitting CRPS pain that spread initially from her left leg to include her right arm as well. The pain began at age 11, after she sprained her ankle during basketball practice. She was taken to the local emergency department and treated far more aggressively than she had been led to expect, including an intramuscular steroid injection by a doctor whose manner clearly communicated the doctor's disbelief in the legitimacy of Michelle's pain. Within minutes of that intervention, pain began at the injection site and spread in characteristic CRPS fashion over the following months. Michelle never expressed her rage and hurt at the offending doctor, yet it came to the surface readily during her initial evaluation. This case shows that the subjective meaning of the physical injury to the patient (not to mention the intention of the treating physician) is more important than the degree of actual tissue damage incurred.

Jean was another college student who developed CRPS gradually, without any clear precipitant that she could remember, either emotional or physical. Her progress in an inpatient pain program was slow, until the day after she had her first reiki treatment. That night, she had a dream in which she was visited by an angel who placed hands on her affected arm, creating sensations of heat and tingling, which led to complete recovery of function and sensation when she awoke the next morning. A few secondary gain factors included family pressure on her to return to home responsibilities after the current semester break ended. This case illustrates the difficulties of ascertaining a mechanism of action in CRPS, especially post hoc. Possible explanations run the spectrum from malingering to angelic intervention and include energy reactivation via reiki and vigorous placebo responsiveness.

Sherry was a 35-year-old bank manager with a history of CRPS. She responded well to a range of supportive functional activities. Her history of developing symptoms soon after the death of her beloved pet parakeet was intriguing. The parakeet developed a circulatory problem in its left leg, which eventually spread and killed it. Sherry's symptoms also began in the same location. When she remarked on this coincidence, she recounted several other examples of her extreme empathic identification with her pet. This case shows that unconscious emotional identification patterns (of the sort usually associated with conversion disorders) may impact qi dynamics and cause CRPS.

Phantom Limb Pain

PLP provides a challenge to the neuroanatomical model in light of its poor response to nociceptive-oriented treatments. The perceived phantom limb is generally theorized to be a cortically induced perception (in other words, a hallucination). PLP's responsiveness to certain energy therapies (Moldofsky, 1986) suggests that an energetic etiology is worth considering. There is no well-established and widely accepted method for visualizing energy fields, so field anomalies cannot be correlated with symptoms. Using the technique of Kirlian photography to image electrostatic fields around living organisms, some images appear to show that an EM field exists around a leaf even after its tip has been cut off. This "phantom leaf" effect (Teitelbaum et al., 2000) has been compared to phantom pain. The energy field seems to be a preexisting matrix around which the leaf (or limb) is structured, rather than an artifact of the electrical activity that can be measured in living tissue. Analogously, iron filings array themselves in alignment with invisible magnetic lines of force; the force does not arise from the filings but is separate and independent. It has been hypothesized (Ochoa & Verdugo, 1995) that phantom pain sensations are generated by imbalances in this invisible energy matrix as a result of the emotional trauma of amputation. The energetic rebalancing that comes with healing the preexisting psychological trauma should relieve the pain.

CASE STUDY

Phantom Limb Pain

These case studies were also from Dr. Eric Leskowitz regarding the use of therapeutic touch (TT). Joe was a 35-year-old cargo loader whose leg was crushed in a work injury, necessitating an above-knee amputation 5 years before. His chronic phantom pain was only marginally responsive to a regimen of selective serotonin reuptake inhibitor (SSRI) antidepressants and opiates (oxycodone). He did not benefit from cognitive-behavioral retraining, and was offered a trial of TT, about which he knew nothing. During the assessment phase, the same energy "presence" or magnetic push that was also felt around the remainder of his body also felt in the region of his missing leg. At the same moment, Joe (whose eyes were closed) reported that he could feel touching on his phantom leg. As sweeping of the surrounding energy field continued, he reported that pain sensations seemed to be draining out the bottom of his phantom foot. Surprisingly, he asked to stop the treatment before the pain could be completely alleviated, saying that he feared becoming pain-free because it would provide proof to him that his leg was in fact gone. His pain was serving a psychological function of defending him against the shock that would come with full acceptance of his loss. This case is discussed in more detail by Goldberg, Pachas, & Keith (1999).

Mary was a 73-year-old woman who had a below-the-knee amputation of her left leg to prevent the worsening of peripheral vascular disease–induced gangrene. She had expected to lose only a toe, not an entire limb. From the moment she awoke from surgery, she experienced severe phantom pain in the toe that was gangrenous.

No standard medications such as opiates, anticonvulsants, or antidepressants were helpful, but she responded almost immediately to TT. She felt the pain drain out of the bottom of her phantom foot and became pain-free for the first time in more than a year. She could amplify the effects of this treatment by visualizing a soothing blue light coating her painful limb. She eventually learned to perform TT on herself and reported that she could start each day with a TT session and remain quite comfortable throughout the day, unless her stress level rose above a certain threshold.

Regarding *Emotional Freedom Technique,* Jeri was a 65-year-old administrative assistant with a 7-year history of postamputation pain. She described the onset of phantom pain following a left below-knee amputation to save a limb with severely compromised circulation following surgery to repair the limb after a fall down some stairs. Pain was manageable, averaging 6 out of 10 on a regimen of Percocet (oxycodone and acetaminophen) and Ultram (tramadol). The original treatment plan to apply emotional freedom technique (EFT) desensitization to her memories of the fall was changed. Jeri said that the scariest part of her accident was the feeling of falling that recapitulated an experience she had at 9 years of age in a swimming accident when she fell into a pit of water at the beach. A round of EFT was performed in relation to that memory. After completing the EFT, Jeri found that she no longer had the swooning internal feeling that accompanied this old memory, and her leg pain markedly decreased. She went on to experience the first pain-free period in the 7 years since surgery.

THERAPEUTIC TOUCH FOR ACUTE AND CHRONIC PAIN

Burns and Thermal Injuries

Pain, anxiety, and impaired immune function are all known to follow significant burns to the skin and body surface. One study (Rosa, Rosa, Sarner, & Barrett, 1998) measured the impact of regular TT treatments on these three variables in patients in a hospital burn unit. Again using sham TT control intervention, this single-blinded randomized clinical trial determined that 5 days of regular TT caused statistically significant reductions in self-reported pain (McGill Pain Questionnaire Rating Index) and anxiety (Visual Analog Scale). Immune function was also altered, as reflected by a 13% decrease in $CD8^+$ cell concentration, although the clinical significance of this cellular change was not clear. The authors called for more studies to investigate the long-term effects of ongoing TT and to control more tightly for behavioral variables that might influence outcome.

Headache

One of the best-designed TT studies looked at the effects of TT on tension headache pain (Meehan, 1993). By using a sham TT intervention method, expectancy and placebo factors were taken into consideration. A matched group of 60 headache patients was studied, all of whom were naïve to prior TT treatments. Ninety percent of the members of the active treatment group experienced improvements in symptoms following TT, averaging a 70% decrease in degree of symptom intensity.

Of the control patients, 80% reported pain reduction that averaged 37% in degree. Both groups also practiced deep breathing, so the placebo group was actually receiving a treatment known to be helpful in itself for mild headache symptoms, while the treatment group actually received two treatments, TT plus breathing. This differential benefit was even more pronounced four hours after the initial treatment, again favoring TT over sham TT controls.

Peripheral Neuropathy

A clinical vignette highlights potential applications of TT to peripheral neuropathy, although formal research studies have not been conducted with this specific syndrome. Lillian was a 68-year-old woman who developed neuropathic pain in the distribution of her femoral nerve, which was accidentally injured during vascular surgery several years earlier. She obtained only slight relief with standard medications for neuropathic pain. In addition, her allodynia was so severe that she could not participate in any form of rehab that involved direct physical contact, including PT manipulation and tactile thermal desensitization. However, during the course of a TT treatment, she felt the sensitivity decrease to such an extent that she allowed the TT practitioner to touch her leg, the first time she had allowed another person to touch her. This decreased sensitivity opened the door to a range of other standard pain management approaches, which decreased her discomfort significantly. During psychotherapy, she was—again for the first time—able to express her rage and disappointment at the once-trusted surgeon who had damaged her nerve.

CASE STUDY

PERIPHERAL NEUROPATHY

Dan was a 39-year-old man with AIDS-related peripheral neuropathy. His bilateral foot pain had not responded to opiates, tricyclic antidepressants (TCAs), or anticonvulsants. His primary care nurse attempted to alleviate his attendant anxiety with a course of TT. Dan's anxiety level decreased, and his pain level went from a self-rating of "very bad" to "not much." Unfortunately, his pain returned the next day. He continued to respond favorably to each TT session, and the duration of pain relief lasted several hours.

Postoperative Pain

In a single-blind clinical trial that measured postoperative pain in 108 patients (Turner, Clark, Gauthier, & Williams, 1998), a single TT treatment reduced their need for analgesic medication, although reported pain levels were similar between patients who received genuine TT and those who received a sham TT control intervention. Presumably, the untreated patients used additional analgesics to make up for the differential impact of TT. Taking a cautious approach, TT may be best conceptualized as an adjunctive pain therapy, rather than as a primary treatment modality.

Old Controversies

Despite this promising list of neurologic and other medical and physiological processes shown to be affected by TT, the general view of this technique is often extreme skepticism. This attitude stems in part from a lack of awareness of the body of research data cited previously. There was also massive publicity given to a unique report—the *Journal of the American Medical Association*'s (*JAMA*) publication of an 11-year-old schoolgirl's science fair project titled "A Closer Look at Therapeutic Touch" (Rosa et al., 1998). This publication is important on many levels and is worth discussing in some detail.

The unique study of therapeutic touch in *JAMA* used a simple research protocol to test whether nurse practitioners of TT could reliably detect the presence of their client's so-called energy field. The nurses were blindfolded and then asked to guess over which of their outstretched hands the researcher was placing her own hand. In other words, they were asked to sense the energy field emanating from the experimenter's hand. Interestingly enough, the nurses were only accurate 40% of the time in their guesses, indicating that they performed even more poorly in their energy assessments than would be expected with random guessing. The authors then concluded that because there was no experimental validation of the energy fields that purportedly underlie TT therapy, there could be no clinical effectiveness of TT as a treatment intervention. The *JAMA* editors joined in, urging patients to refuse such treatments until scientific evidence of efficacy could be produced.

As a tide of rebuttal letters to *JAMA* (Freinkel, 1999) and editorial commentaries elsewhere (Achterberg, 1999; Leskowitz, 1999) pointed out, there were numerous crucial methodological flaws in the study. There were also logical fallacies in the conclusions reached. The degree of expertise of the TT volunteers, if evaluated at all, was not reported. They did not follow the true TT protocol described and discussed in this chapter because they were never asked to elicit their inner intention to heal. This omission raises questions about what technique was actually being assessed. Many of the sessions were videotaped in a brightly lit television studio, which could easily have generated performance anxiety in addition to electrical interference. More importantly, there was no control for experimenter bias and intention, a significant possibility given that the girl's parents, the article's coauthors, were members of Quackwatch Inc., a now discredited organization devoted to debunking alternative therapies.

It is a basic tenet of energy-based therapies that the frame of mind of the healer influences the degree of energy effect he or she creates (Brennan, 1992). If the girl had been a master healer emitting huge bursts of energy, it would be striking that the success rates were so low. However, if at some unconscious or conscious level she wanted negative results, she might have literally shut down her own energy field, making it even harder than normal to detect its presence. Perhaps this effect is the true significance of the low detection scores—the nurses may have been accurately responding to a negative intention and alteration in the test energy field. Contrast these apparently negative data with results from an earlier study (Schwartz, Russek, & Beltran, 1995) that reported a successful detection rate of more than 65% using a similar approach with a legitimate protocol. Interestingly, this study was not referenced in the otherwise exhaustive TT bibliography cited in the *JAMA* paper. *JAMA* authors summarily dismissed this research literature as being without significant scientific merit.

Also striking beyond the methodological problems is the authors' unwarranted conclusion that TT is clinically useless. No clinical outcomes were assessed in this study, so no conclusions could logically be made regarding clinical efficacy. One wonders what led the usually judicious editorial staff of *JAMA* to make a statement decrying the use of a therapeutic intervention, and then garner such strong publicity for a flawed middle school science project.

Another controversy concerns a body of research that was generally accepted within the energy medicine community as strongly validating the efficacy of TT in enhancing the normal physiologic process of wound healing. A study by Daniel Wirth, published in 1990, purported to show that even under double-blind conditions, TT could dramatically speed up the rate at which standardized punch biopsies of the skin could heal in normal healthy subjects (Wirth, 1990). Due to the tightly controlled conditions and strikingly positive statistics, this study and several other subsequent ones by the same author have been regarded as providing a foundation for energy medicine research.

However, in subsequent years, several researchers were troubled by their inability to obtain any information about the research protocol from Wirth directly and began to investigate his research methods more fully (Solfvin, Leskowitz, & Benor, 2005). They found that documentation could not be provided to show that the study was performed as described, and they came to believe that some, if not all, of Wirth's primary data was fabricated. However, they pointed out that sufficient subsequent research had established the validity of energy medicine, and of TT, to such an extent that even absent the entire body of Wirth's work, the field of energy medicine still has a strong research foundation.

REFERENCES

Achterberg, J. (1999). Clearing the air in the therapeutic touch controversy. *Alternative Therapies, 4*(4), 100–101.

Astin, J. A., Harkness, E., & Ernst, E. (2000). The efficacy of "distant healing": A systematic review of randomized trials. *Annals of Internal Medicine, 132*(11), 903.

Bennett, C. H. & DiVincenzo, D. P. (2000). Quantum information and computation. *Nature, 404*(6775), 247.

Benor, D. J. (2004). *Consciousness bioenergy and healing: Self-healing and energy medicine for the 21st century: (Vol. 2).* Medford, NJ: Wholistic Healing.

Bergson, H. (1911). *Creative evolution.* New York: Henry Holt (translated by Arthur Mitchell).

Birch, S. (2003). Trigger point-acupuncture point correlations revisited. *Journal of Alternative and Complementary Medicine, 9*(1), 91–103.

Blackwell, B., Bloomfield, S. S., & Buncher, C. R. (1972). Demonstration to medical students of placebo responses and non-drug factors. *Lancet, 1,* 1279–1282.

Brennan, B. (1992). *Hands of light*. New York: Bantam New Age.

Bruyere, R. (1994). *Wheels of light: Chakras, auras, and the healing energy of the body*. New York: Fireside/Harper Collins.

Cassidy, C. M. (1995). Social science theory and methods in the study of alternative and complementary medicine. *Journal of Alternative and Complementary Medicine, 1*(1), 19.

Colbert, A. P., Hammerschlag, R., Aickin, M., & McNames, J. (2004). Reliability of the Prognos electrodermal device for measurements of electrical skin resistance at acupuncture points. *Journal of Alternative and Complementary Medicine, 10*(4), 610–616.

de Craen, A. J., Moerman, D. E., Heisterkamp, S. H., Tytgat, G. N., Tijssen, J. G., & Kleijnen, J. (1999). Placebo effect in the treatment of duodenal ulcer. *British Journal of Clinical Pharmacology, 48*, 853–860.

de Craen, A. J., Tijssen, J. G., de Gans, J., & Kleijnen, J. (2000). Placebo effect in the acute treatment of migraine: Subcutaneous placebos are better than oral placebos. *Journal of Neurology, 247*, 183–188.

Dossey, L. (2003). Signal versus information in DMILS research protocols (response to Kevin Chen). *Journal of Non-Locality and Remote Mental Interactions, 2*(1).

Engebretson, J. & Wardell, D. W. (2007). Energy-based modalities. *Nursing Clinics of North America, 42*(2), 243.

Freinkel, A. (1999). An even closer look at therapeutic touch. *Journal of American Medical Association, 280*(22), 1905–1908.

Fries, E., Hesse, J., Hellhammer, J., & Hellhammer, D. H. (2005). A new view on hypocortisolism. *Psychoneuroendocrinology, 30*(10), 1010–1016.

Goldberg, R. T., Pachas, W. N., & Keith, D. (1999). Relationship between traumatic events in childhood and chronic pain. *Disability and Rehabilitation, 21*(1), 23–30.

Gracely, R. H. (1979). The effect of naloxone on multidimensional scales of postsurgical pain in nonsedated patients. *Society for Neuroscience Abstract, 5*, 609.

Hintz, K. J., Yount, G. L., Kadar, I., Schwartz, G., Hammerschlag, R., & Lin, S. (2003). Bioenergy definitions and research guidelines. *Alternative Therapies in Health and Medicine, 9*(3 suppl), A13.

Hyland, M. E. (2003). The meaning(s) of entanglement in entanglement theory. In H. Walach, R. Schneider, & R. A. Chez (Eds.), *Proceedings: generalized entanglement from a multidisciplinary perspective, Freiburg, Germany, October 9–11, 2003*. Alexandria, VA: Samueli Institute.

Jahn, R. G. & Dunne, B. J. (1986). On the quantum mechanics of consciousness, with applications to anomalous phenomena. *Foundation Physics, 16*, 721.

Jain, S., McMahon, G. F., Hasen, P., Kozub, M. P., Porter, V., King, R., et al. (2012). Healing Touch with Guided Imagery for PTSD in returning active duty military: A randomized controlled trial. *Military Medicine*, 1015–1021.

Jonas, W. B. & Crawford, C. C. (Eds.), (2003a). *Intention and energy medicine: Science, research methods and clinical implications*. London: Churchill Livingstone.

Jonas, W. B. & Crawford, C. C. (2003b). Science and spiritual healing: A critical review of spiritual healing, "energy" medicine, and intentionality. *Alternative Therapies in Health and Medicine, 9*(2), 56.

Julsgaard, B., Kozhekin, A., & Polzik, E. S. (2001). Experimental long-lived entanglement of two macroscopic objects. *Nature, 413*(6854), 400.

Kepner, J. (2002). *Energy and the nervous system in embodied experience*. Available from Pathways for Healing website, http://www.pathwaysforhealing.com/pdfs/Phenom%20of%20NS.pdf&gt.

Kirsch, I. (Ed.), (1999). *How expectancies shape experience*. Washington, DC: American Psychological Association.

Kreiger, D. (1993). *Accepting your power to heal*. Santa Fe, New Mexico: Bear.

Kwok, G., Cohen, M., & Cosic, I. (1998). Mapping acupuncture points using multi channel device. *Australasian Physical and Engineering Sciences in Medicine, 21*(2), 68–72.

Lazorthes, Y., Sol, J. C., Fowo, S., Roux, F. E., & Verdié, J. C. (2007). Motor cortex stimulation for neuropathic pain. *Acta Neurochirurgica, Suppl 97*(pt 2), 37.

Leskowitz, E. (1999). Phantom limb pain: Subtle energy perspectives. *Subtle Energy and Energy Medicine, 8*(2), 125–152.

Leskowitz, E. (2001a). Phantom limb pain: Subtle energy perspectives. *Subtle Energy and Energy Medicine, 8*(2), 125–152.

Leskowitz, E. (2001b). Nonlocal and subtle energetic aspects of chronic pain. *Alternative Therapies in Health and Medicine, 7*(5), 144–145.

Li, A., Lao, L., Wang, Y., Xin, J., Ren, K., & Berman, B. M., et al. (2008). Electroacupuncture activates corticotrophin-releasing hormone-containing neurons in the paraventricular nucleus of the hypothalamus to alleviate edema in a rat model of inflammation. *BMC Complementary and Alternative Medicine* 8:20.

Lopez-Ibor, J. J., Lopez-Ibor, M. I., & Pastrana, J. I. (2008). Transcranial magnetic stimulation. *Current Opinion in Psychiatry, 21*(6), 640.

Lu, Z. (1997). *Scientific qigong exploration: The wonders and mysteries of qi.* Malvern, PA: Amber Leaf Press.

Margo, C. E. (1999). The placebo effect. *Survey of Ophthalmology, 44*(1), 31.

May, E. (2003). Challenges for healing and intentionality research: Causation and information. In W. B. Jonas & C. C. Crawford (Eds.), *Healing, intention and energy medicine: Science, research methods and clinical implications.* London: Churchill Livingstone. p. 283.

Mayor, D. F. & Micozzi, M. S. (Eds.), (2011). *Energy medicine east and west.* Edinburgh: Churchill Livingstone.

McFadden, J. J. (February 11, 2016). It seems life really does have a vital spark: Quantum mechanics, Q3 Symposium. *Probing the Implications of Quantum Innovations.* Sydney, Australia: University of Sydney.

Meehan, T. (1993). Therapeutic touch and postoperative pain: A Rogerian research study. *Nursing Science Quarterly, 6*(12), 69–78.

Melzack, R., Stillwell, D. M., & Fox, E. J. (1977). Trigger points and acupuncture points for pain: Correlations and implications. *Pain, 3*(1), 3–23.

Mentgen, J. L. (2001). Healing touch. *Nursing Clinics of North America, 36*(1), 143.

Moldofsky, H. (1986). Sleep and musculoskeletal pain. *American Journal of Medicine, 81*(3A), 85–89.

Myss, C. & Shealy, C. N. (1998). *The Creation of Health: The emotional, psychological, and spiritual responses that promote health and healing.* New York: Three Rivers Press.

National Center for Complementary and Alternative Medicine (NCCAM): *Energy medicine: An overview,* 2007, http://nccam.nih.gov/health/whatiscam/energy/energymed.htm

North American Nursing Diagnosis Association (NANDA). (2008). *Nursing diagnoses: Definitions and classifications, 2007-2008.* Philadelphia: The Association.

Ochoa, J. L. & Verdugo, M. J. (1995). Reflex sympathetic dystrophy: A common clinical avenue for somatoform expression. *Neurology Clinics, 13*(2), 351–363.

Ohnishi, S. T. & Ohnishi, T. (2008). Philosophy, psychology, physics and practice of ki. *Evidence Based Complementary Alternative Medicine, 6*(2), 175.

O'Mathuna, D. P. & Ashford, R. L. (2003). Therapeutic touch for healing acute wounds. *Cochrane Database Systematic Reviews,* (4), CD002766.

O'Mathuna, D. P. & Ashford, R. L. (2012). Therapeutic touch for healing acute wounds. *Cochrane Database Systematic Reviews,* CD002766.

Peters, R. (1999). M. The effectiveness of therapeutic touch: A meta-analytic review. *Nursing Science Quarterly, 12*(1), 52.

Rein, G. (2004). Bioinformation within the biofield: Beyond bioelectromagnetics. *Journal of Alternative Complementary Medicine, 10*(1), 59.

Rosa, L., Rosa, E., Sarner, L., & Barrett, S. (1998). A close look at therapeutic touch. *JAMA, 279,* 1005–1010.

Rosenblum, B. & Kuttner, F. (2008). *Quantum enigma: Physics encounters consciousness.* New York: Oxford University Press.

Rubik, B. (2002). The biofield hypothesis: Its biophysical basis and role in medicine. *Journal of Alternative Complementary Medicine, 8*(6), 703.

Schlebusch, K. P., Maric-Oehler, W., & Popp, F. A. (2005). Biophotonics in the infrared spectral range reveal acupuncture meridian structure of the body. *Journal of Alternative and Complementary Medicine, 11*(1), 171–173.

Schwartz, G., Russek, L., & Beltran, J. (1995). Interpersonal hand-energy registration: Evidence for implicit performance and perception. *Subtle Energies, 6,* 183–200.

Smith, C. W. (1998). Is a living system a macroscopic quantum system? *Frontier Perspectives, 7*, 9.

Smith, C. W. (2003). Straws in the wind. *Journal Alternative Complementary Medicine, 9*(1), 1.

So, P. S., Jiang, Y., & Qin, Y. (2008). Touch therapies for pain relief in adults. *Cochrane Database Systematic Review,* (4), CD006535.

Solfvin, J., Leskowitz, E., & Benor, D., (letter). (2005). Questions concerning the work of Daniel P Wirth. *Journal of Alternative Complementary Medicine, 11*(6), 949–950. full report, http://www.wholisticheal-ingresearch.com/WirthQ.htm.

Sparber, A. G., Crawford, C. C., & Jonas, W. B. (2003). Laboratory research on bioenergy healing (p. 139). In W. B. Jonas & C. C. Crawford (Eds.), *Healing, intention and energy medicine: Science, research methods and clinical implications.* London: Churchill Livingstone.

Teitelbaum, J. E., Bird, B., Greenfield, R. M., Weiss, A., Muenz, L., & Gould, L. (2000). Effective treatment of chronic fatigue syndrome and fibromyalgia – a randomized, double-blind, placebo-controlled, intent-to-treat study. *Journal of Chronic Fatigue Syndrome, 8*(2), 3–15.

Tiller, W. A. (1997). *Science and human transformation: Subtle energies, intentionality and consciousness.* Walnut Creek, CA: Pavior.

Travell, J., & Simons, D. (1983). *Myofascial pain and dysfunction: The trigger point manual.* Baltimore, MD: Lippincott Williams & Wilkins.

Tsang, H. W., & Fung, K. M. (2008). A review on neurobiological and psychological mechanisms underlying the anti-depressive effect of qigong exercise. *Journal of Health Psychology, 13*(7), 857.

Turner, J., Clark, A. J., Gauthier, D. K., & Williams, M. (1998). The effect of therapeutic touch on pain and anxiety in burn patients. *Journal of Advanced Nursing, 28*(1), 10–20.

Ventura, C. (2005). CAM and cell fate targeting: Molecular and energetic insights into cell growth and differentiation. *Evidence-Based Complementary and Alternative Medicine, 2*(3), 277.

Walborn, S. P., Terra Cunha, M. O., Pádua, S., & Monken, C. H. (2002). Double-slit quantum erasure. *Physical Review A, 65*(033818), 1.

Walborn, S. P., Terra Cunha, M. O., Padua, S., & Monken, C. H. (2003). Quantum erasure. *American Science, 91*, 336.

Warber, S. L., Gordon, A., Gillespie, B. W., Olson, M., & Assefi, N. (2003). Standards for conducting clinical biofield energy healing research. *Alternative Therapies in Health and Medicine, 9*(3 suppl), A54.

Winstead-Fry, P. & Kijek, J. (1999). An integrative review and meta-analysis of therapeutic touch research. *Alternative Therapies in Health and Medicine, 5*(6), 58.

Wirth, D. (1990). The effect of noncontact therapeutic touch on the rate of healing of full thickness dermal wounds. *Subtle Energies, 1*(1), 1–21.

Yan, X., Shen, H., Jiang, H., Zhang, C., Hu, D., Wang, J., et al. (2008). External qi of yan xin qigong induces G2/M arrest and apoptosis of androgen-independent prostate cancer cells by inhibiting Akt and Nf-Kappa B pathways. *Molecular and Cellular Biochemistry, 310*(1-2), 227.

Yount, G., Solfvin, J., Moore, D., Schlitz, M., Reading, M., Aldape, K., et al. (2004). In vitro test of external qigong. *BMC Complementary and Alternative Medicine, 4*, 5.

Yu, T., Tsai, H. L., & Hwang, M. L. (2003). Suppressing tumor progression of in vitro prostate cancer cells by emitted psychosomatic power through Zen meditation. *American Journal of Chinese Medicine, 31*(3), 499.

Zha, L. (2001). *Review of history, findings and implications of research on exceptional functions of the human body in China.* In Proceedings: bridging worlds and filling gaps in the science of spiritual healing, Keauhou Beach Resort, Kona, Hawaii, November 29–December 4, 2001. Alexandria, VA: Samueli Institute.

Suggested Readings can be found on the companion website, http://www.micozzipainconditions.com.

Chapter 10

Electromagnetic Therapies

ELECTRICITY AND MAGNETISM

Human awareness of magnetism dates back in time, and extravagant claims of "magnetic" healing can be traced back to more than 4000 years ago. In historic periods, attempts were made to explain the efficacy of this invisible force by invoking arcane and unfounded quasi-scientific principles and properties. Coupled with commercial efforts to sell magnetic healing products, practices, and services, "magnetic healing" produced an interesting history of pseudoscience, sensationalism, and controversy, in addition to having substantial successes, during the 19th century. In the 21st century therapeutic use of magnets and electromagnetic treatments is receiving public enthusiasm. However, given the history of controversy and professional rivalries, the medical and scientific community remains somewhat skeptical of the current widespread claims. A major obstacle has been the usual inability to determine a mechanism of action within the accepted 20th-century biomedical paradigm. Fundamental questions regarding efficacy could potentially be resolved by rigorous, randomized, double-blind, placebo-controlled trials, if appropriately designed and funded. These kinds of controlled studies by the medical scientific community have only recently been done relative to the long history of magnetic healing. However, the French scientific commission convened to investigate "mesmerism," "animal magnetism," and "magnetic healing" in the 1780s actually did design controlled experiments to test the existence of this kind of healing—but the commission broke down over debates about "mechanism of action" before the experiments could be accomplished on the eve of the French Revolution (see the "Revolutionary Developments" section). The scientific community is now looking again at this revolutionary subject objectively and beginning to reverse their entrenched skepticism.

Historical perspectives on magnetism and healing have been provided by a number of sources (Armstrong & Armstrong, 1991; Geddes, 1991; Macklis, 1993; Markov, 2007; Mourino, 1991; Rosch, 2004; Weintraub, 2001, 2004a,b), which include several excellent reviews of this rich history. For example, in antiquity, according to

Acknowledgments to Marc Micozzi, Michael Weintraub, and Jennifer Gehl for prior contributions in Micozzi, M.S. (Ed.), (2016). *Fundamentals of commentary and alternative medicine* (5th ed.). St Louis: Elsevier Health Sciences/Saunders.

the Yellow Emperor's Canon of Internal Medicine (or the Yellow Emperor's "Inner Classic"), magnetic stones (lodestones) were applied to acupressure points as a means of pain reduction (see Section IV). Similarly the ancient Hindu Vedas ascribed therapeutic powers of ashmana and siktavati (instruments of stone).

ATTRACTIONS OF THE WORD AND WORLD OF MAGNETS

The term "magnet" was probably derived from the ancient Greek legend of Magnes, a shepherd who was walking on Mount Ida when suddenly the metallic tacks in his sandals were drawn toward specific rocks. Such magnetic rocks were apparently mineral lodestones that contain magnetite, a magnetic oxide of iron (Fe_3O_4). These natural magnetic stones were noted to influence other similar adjacent stones that were brought into close proximity, producing movements.

The ancients called them "alive stones" or "Herculean stones" because they were meant to lead the way. Various powers were attributed to these stones, as noted in the writings and artifacts of the ancient Greeks and Romans. For example, Plato, Euripides, and others indicated that these invisible powers of movement could be put to practical use, such as by building ships with iron nails and destroying opposing military ships and navies by maneuvering them close to magnetic mountains or magnetic rock.

Medicinal and healing properties were also attributed to these lodestones. Various magnetic rings and necklaces were sold in the marketplace in Samothrace around AD 200 to treat arthritis and pain. Similarly lodestones were ground up to make powders and salves to treat various pains and other health conditions. Numerous claims and anecdotal stories were accompanied by public embrace of these magical devices.

MEDIEVAL MAGNETISM

The Middle Ages in Europe witnessed the emergence of numerous myths that persist in certain segments of society. For example, it was believed that magnets could extract gold from wells and that application or ingestion of garlic could neutralize magnetic properties. In 1289, the first major treatise on magnetism was produced by Peter Peregrinus. He ascribed to lodestones curative properties for treating gout, baldness, and arthritis and spoke about its strong aphrodisiac powers. He also described drawing poison from wounds with close application of magnetic lodestones. His work contains the first drawing and description of a compass in the Western world. The idea that magnets could be used therapeutically resurfaced in the early 16th century when Paracelsus (Philippus Aureolus Theophrastus Bombast von Hohenheim), considered to be one of the most influential physicians and alchemists of his time, used lodestones (magnets) to treat conditions, such as epilepsy, diarrhea, and hemorrhage. He believed that every person is actually a living magnet, that they can attract good and evil, and that magnets are an important elixir of life, anticipating later ideas about a human bioenergy field.

Exploration and Enlightenment Ideas

Scientific enlightenment during the 17th century began on this topic with the work of Dr. William Gilbert, physician to Queen Elizabeth I of England. He wrote his classic text *De Magnete* in 1600, describing hundreds of detailed experiments concerning electricity and also terrestrial magnetism. He debunked many medicinal applications and was responsible for laying the groundwork for future research and study. Luigi Galvani and Alessandro Volta subsequently made significant contributions in studying electricity. However, for the next century there were no major documented advancements in the study of magnetism and healing. In the early 18th century there again developed significant interest in both magnetism and electricity. In 1705 Francis Hauksbee invented an electrostatic engine that, by rotating and spinning an attached globe, could transfer an electronic charge to various metallic objects brought close to it, such as chain, wire, and metal. This procedure induced electrical shocks. Refinements in this device led to more general usage, and by 1743 traveling circuses throughout Europe and the American colonies were providing individuals stimulating experiences with electric shocks for a small fee.

Benjamin Franklin (Again)

Legend suggests that Benjamin Franklin witnessed an "electrified boy" exhibition in a traveling circus in the mid-1700s and thus first became interested in his lifelong experiments on both electricity and magnetic phenomena. Franklin is also famed for his later experiments on electricity, by "capturing" lightning in a bottle, for which he attached a key to an airborne kite during a thunderstorm (as depicted in the heroic portrait by Benjamin West entitled "Franklin Taming Lightning") (Fig. 10.1). It was actually Franklin's young son who was sent out into the lightning storm with the kite. This action risked an exhibition of Franklin's personalized version of his own "electrified boy." (It appears Franklin did not like his son. Years later when the son was serving as British Colonial Governor of New Jersey, during the Revolutionary War, the father had him arrested.)

Much of the current terminology regarding electricity and magnetism actually originated with Franklin, such as charge, discharge, condenser, electric shock, electrician, positive, negative, plus, and minus. Franklin distinguished himself in studies primarily of electric "fluid" and charges. He concluded that all matter contained magnetic fields that are uniformly distributed throughout the body. He believed that when an object is magnetized, the fluid condenses in one of its extremities. That extremity becomes positively magnetized, whereas the donor region of the object becomes negatively magnetized. He felt that the degree to which an object can be magnetized depends upon the force necessary to start the fluid moving within it.

Revolutionary Developments

The scientific revolution brought to Europe the development of carbon-steel magnets (1743–1751). Father Maximilian Hell, and later his student Franz Anton Mesmer, applied these magnetic devices to patients, many of whom were

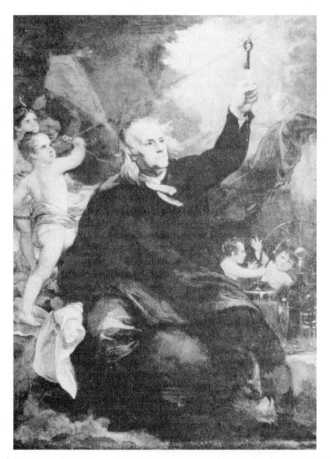

FIG. 10.1 | Poets, philosophers, and scientists of the late 18th and early 19th centuries were all interested in vitalism—finding the energy that animates life and the universe. Here Benjamin Franklin is shown in a heroic pose by Benjamin West figuratively "taming lightning." In fact, Franklin, like his contemporaries, was searching for insights into nature and human nature, not just exploring electricity in a contemporary utilitarian sense. Later, scientists thought that reductionist, materialist explanations substituted for the need for vitalist interpretations.

experiencing hysterical or psychosomatic symptoms (see Chapter 7). As discussed earlier in the book, Mesmer is known today as the founder of hypnotism (originally known as "mesmerism," or "animal magnetism"), but he was basically a student of magnetism, especially as applied to medicine. Specifically in his major treatise "On the Medicinal Uses of the Magnet," Mesmer described how he fed a patient iron filings and then applied specially designed magnets over the vital organs to generally stop uncontrolled seizures. His cures were astounding and provided good theater when they were performed in front of large groups (Fig. 10.2).

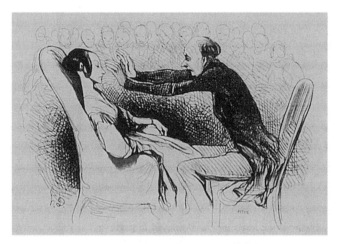

FIG. 10.2 | Mesmerism and hypnotism were the object of satire and a number of caricatures during the 19th century.

Relative to the later concept and term "hypnosis," the "power of suggestion" was clearly being displayed as it was ultimately transferred to nonferric objects, such as paper, wood, silk, and stone. Mesmer reasoned that he was not dealing with ordinary mineral magnetism but rather with a special vital force, or energy, called "animal magnetism." The term "mesmerization" was often applied to his displays of people overcoming illness and disease by mesmerizing their bodies' "innate magnetic poles" to induce a healing crisis, often in the form of convulsions. After such a crisis, health would be restored. Mesmer hailed this animal magnetism as a specific natural force of healing.

Mesmer's claims of success infuriated his conservative, "regular medicine" colleagues and motivated the French Academy of Sciences, under King Louis XVI, to convene a special study in 1784. The panel for this study included such distinguished figures Antoine-Laurent Lavoisier (who discovered the chemistry of combustion), Joseph-I. Guillotine, and Benjamin Franklin, then serving as ambassador to France from the newly independent United States of America. In a controlled set of experiments, blindfolded patients were to be exposed to a series of magnets or sham magnetic objects and asked to describe the induced sensation. Although there remains controversy as to whether and what experimental observations were actually made, the committee "lost their heads" in bickering about mechanisms of action (a process that was soon to be facilitated in reality by the invention of one of their members, Dr. Guillotine, as used on another, Lavoisier, among many others, in the coming French Revolution).

In the breach, the royal panel concluded that the efficacy of the magnetic healing resided entirely within the mind of the individual and that any healing was due to suggestion. Based on these conclusions, the medical establishment declared

Mesmer's theories "fraudulent," and mesmerism became equated for a time with medical "quackery." Mesmer left France in disgrace, and some members of the panel who remained in France, such as Lavoisier, literally lost their heads. However, "magnetic healing" had long and popular usage throughout the 19th and early 20th centuries in Europe and the United States. Two notable "magnetic healers" founded alternative schools of healing in the United States during the 1890s, as discussed later and in Chapter 12.

In Europe physicist Hans Christian Ørsted (1777–1851) continued electromagnetic studies and first noted that a compass needle was deflected when a current flowed through a nearby wire. He also discovered that a current-carrying wire coil exerts a force on a magnet. Also, a magnet exerts a force on the coil of wire, inducing an electrical current to pass through the wire. The coil also behaves like a magnet when electricity is conducted through the wire, as if it possessed magnetic north and south poles. Magnetism and electricity were thus observed to be somehow connected, giving rise to "electromagnetism."

AMPING UP RESEARCH

Ørsted was instrumental in creating a controlled scientific environment that led to further study. André-Marie Ampère deduced the quantitative relation between magnetic force and electric current. The term "amp" is used today to measure the amount of current. In the 1820s Michael Faraday and Joseph Henry (later founding secretary of the Smithsonian Institution in the 1850s) demonstrated more connections among magnetism and electricity, showing that a changing magnetic field could induce an electrical field perpendicularly. In 1896 Arsène D'Arsonval reported to the Société de Biologie back in Paris that when a subject's head (not decapitated) was placed in a strong time-varying magnetic field, phosphenes (sensations of light caused by retinal stimulation) were perceived. Some 15 years later, Thompson (1910) confirmed that visual phosphenes can be induced and also showed that exposure to a strong alternating magnetic field also produced taste sensation. Various coils were constructed by Dunlap and later by Magnusson and Stevens. They noted that magnetophosphenes were brightest at a low frequency of about 25 Hz and become fainter at higher frequencies.

MAGNETIC HEALING IN THE EARLY UNITED STATES

Meanwhile in the United States, magnetic therapy flourished. There were significant sales of magnets, magnetic salves, and liniments by traveling magnetic healers. Later in the 19th century Daniel David Palmer, the founder of chiropractic and self-described "magnetic healer," stated that putting down his hands for physical manipulation of the patient produced better results than the simple "laying on of hands" (see Chapter 12).

By 1886 the Sears catalogue advertised numerous magnetic products, such as magnetic rings, belts, caps, soles for boots, and girdles. In the 1920s Thacher created a mail-order catalogue advertising more than 700 specific magnetic garments and devices and products that he described as a "plain road to health without the use of medicine and was dependent on the magnetic energy of the sun." He believed that the iron content of red blood cells made blood the primary magnetic conductor of the body. Thus the most efficient way to recharge the body's magnetic field was by wearing his magnetic garments. The complete set was said to "furnish full and complete protection of all the vital organs of the body." Collier's Weekly Magazine dubbed Thacher the "king of the magnetic quacks." There was no government regulation of these devices or claims, and thus these types of promotions fueled skepticism. The US Food and Drug Administration (FDA), founded in 1906 for food and drug safety, had no jurisdiction yet over medical devices at that time, and there were no good scientific trials. (Problems with the purity and safety of drugs had led to the passage of the Pure Food and Drug Act of 1906 and the subsequent formation of the FDA.)

TWENTIETH-CENTURY RESEARCH WORLDWIDE

After WWII there was heightened interest and research in magnetotherapy in Japan and the former Soviet Union. Specifically in Japan magnetotherapeutic devices were accepted under the Drug Regulation Act of 1961. By 1976 various devices were commonly and commercially used to treat illnesses and promote health. Similar interests in Bulgaria, Romania, and Russia led to development of various therapeutic approaches, and physicians in those countries had available the use of magnetic fields to assist in treating pain and diseases. Germany, Japan, Russia, Israel, and at least 45 other countries currently consider magnetic therapy to be an official medical procedure for the treatment of pain and various neurological and inflammatory conditions (Whitaker & Adderly, 1998) (Box 10.1). By contrast, magnetotherapy has had limited acceptance in Western medicine. Unwarranted claims and promotion only led to further scientific skepticism.

BOX 10.1 *Innovative Treatment of Stroke Pain*

In a recent study, Japanese researchers found an innovative, effective, and noninvasive way to help stroke victims cope with pain. For the past century, fundamental sciences—such as physics and quantum mechanics, biology, and ecology—have begun to look at energetic interactions. These energetic interactions form the common basis for health and healing. So, in this view, all the other therapies just access the body's energy in ways that influence health and healing.

With this new understanding about energy, the medicine of the future will learn to bypass invasive drugs and surgeries. They will go straight to the source of energetic healing. Transcranial magnetic stimulation (TMS) is already available now. TMS is a noninvasive procedure that uses magnetic fields to stimulate nerve cells in the brain. Doctors use TMS to help treat depression, anxiety, migraines, and now—pain. For the procedure itself, doctors place an electromagnetic coil against the scalp near the forehead. The electromagnet used in TMS creates electric currents that stimulate nerve cells in the region of your brain involved in pain. The new study involved 18 patients

Continued

BOX 10.1 *Innovative Treatment of Stroke Pain—cont'd*

who had experienced a blood clot or bleeding in one side of the brain, called "unilateral ischemic" or "hemorrhagic strokes". Several weeks into recovery, patients began to experience severe hand or leg pain because of brain damage from the stroke. Indeed, stroke can cause severe pain sensations, such as uncomfortable numbness, prickling or tingling, as well as other pain.

All the patients in the study received repetitive TMS treatments—called rTMS—to the primary motor cortex for at least 12 weeks. After 12 weeks of rTMS, 11 patients achieved satisfactory-to-excellent pain relief. (Researchers defined "satisfactory" relief when a patient achieved a 40% to 69% reduction in pain scores [Kobayashi, Fujimaki, Mihara, & Ohira, 2015]. They defined "excellent" relief when a patient achieved a 70% or greater pain reduction.) The six study patients who continued treatment for 1 year achieved permanent pain relief.

The researchers for this study urge neurologists and pain management specialists to take an interest in this effective method, which has minimal side effects. In fact, none of the 18 patients reported any serious side effects from the weekly sessions.

MODERN MEDICAL MAGNETISM

The modern era of magnetic stimulation for medical applications can be said to have begun with the work of Bickford and colleagues (Bickford & Fremming, 1965). They considered the possibility of stimulation of the nervous system (experimental frog nerves and human peripheral nerves) in pain and healing. They also discussed generation of eddy currents in the brain that could reach a certain magnitude to stimulate cortical structures through an intact cranium (Bickford & Fremming, 1965). Barker and colleagues, at the University of Sheffield, developed the first commercial cranial magnetic stimulator in 1985 (Barker, 1991; Barker, Freeston, Jalinous, & Jarratt, 1987). They gave a practical demonstration at Queen's Square by stimulating "Dr. Merton's brain," which caused muscle twitches. As might be expected, the physiological and clinical possibilities became more apparent (Merton & Morton, 1980). Technical challenges were met with the development of devices capable of stimulating the brain focally at frequencies of up to 100 Hz using specific coil configurations (i.e., circular). Adaptations for focal therapy were created. Thus a new discipline developed using high and low repetitive stimulation frequencies directed to previously inaccessible areas of the brain and body (George et al., 2003; Kobayashi & Pascual-Leone, 2003; Pascual-Leone, Valls-Sole, Wasserman, & Hallett, 1994). By the end of the 20th century more than 6000 publications existed on basic neurophysiology, clinical syndromes, and therapeutic implications. Although most of the initial papers were results of open-label (nonplacebo) observations, many current publications report on randomized, double-blind, placebo-controlled trials. When all of this experimental and clinical information is pooled, the data strongly suggest that application of exogenous magnetic fields at low levels induces biological effects on a variety of systems, especially pain sensation and the musculoskeletal system.

Magnetism Terminology and Principles

Essential terms are defined to discuss and understand the role of magnetism in medicine. Biomagnetics refers to the field of science dealing with the application of magnetic fields to living organisms. Both basic research on cells in culture and clinical trials have provided a better understanding of mechanisms of action (Adey, 1992, 2004; Adey et al., 1999; Lednev, 1991; Markov, 2004; Markov & Colbert, 2001; Pilla, 2003; Pilla, Muehsam, & Markov, 1997; Timmel, Till, Brocklehurst, & Hore, 1998). Human tissues are dielectric and conductive and therefore can respond to electrical and magnetic fields that are oscillating or static. Cell membranes consist of paramagnetic and diamagnetic lipoprotein materials that respond to magnetic fields and serve as signaling (transduction) pathways by which external stimuli are sent and conveyed to the cell interior. Calcium ions are very important in transduction coupling at the cell membrane level. Electromagnetic fields can also alter the configuration of atoms and molecules in dielectric and paramagnetic-diamagnetic substances. Thus atoms in these substances polarize to a degree when placed in an electromagnetic field, act as a dipole, and align accordingly (Adey, 1988, 1992; Blumenthal et al., 1997; DeLoecker, Cheng, & Delport, 1990; Engstrom & Fitzsimmons, 1999; Farndale, Maroudas, & Marsland, 1987; Lednev, 1991; Maccabee et al., 1991; Pilla et al., 1997; Repacholi & Greenebaum, 1999; Rosen, 1992; Rossini et al., 1994; Timmel et al., 1998). Adey (1988, 1992, 2004) suggested that the presence of chemical free radicals is important for signal transduction.

The Chemistry of Magnetism

Chemical bonds are essentially electromagnetic bonds formed between adjacent atoms. The breaking of the chemical bonds of a singlet pair allows electrons to influence adjacent electrons with similar or opposite spins, which thereby become triplet pairs, and so on. Thus by imposing magnetic fields into this medium, one may influence the rate and amount of communication between cells. At the cell membrane level, free radicals of nitric oxide may play an essential role in this regulation of receptors specifically (Adey, 1988, 1992, 2004). Free radicals, and nitric oxide, are involved in the normal regulatory mechanisms in many tissues. Pain and certain diseases are associated with disordered free radical regulation producing oxidative stress. These diseases include Alzheimer's disease (dementia), Parkinson's disease, cancer, and coronary artery heart disease. This area remains incompletely understood and under intense research scrutiny.

Field Penetration

Magnetic field strength is indicated by magnetic flux density, which is the number of field lines (flux) that cross a unit of surface area. It is usually described in terms of the unit gauss (G) or tesla (T). There are 10,000 G in 1 T. There is an exponential decay of field strength with distance from a magnetic source according the inverse square law for electromagnetic (EM) radiation. The objective is to apply a static magnetic device as close to the skin as possible and to ensure that a magnet of sufficient size and surface field is used when the target is deep in tissue areas. Magnetotherapy is defined as the use of time-varying magnetic fields of low-frequency values (3 Hz to 3 kHz) to induce a sufficiently strong current to stimulate living tissue.

Faraday's law (1831) defines the fundamental relation between a changing magnetic field and a conductor (any medium that carries electrically charged particles). When a wire is used as an example of a conductor, Faraday's law basically states that any change in the magnetic environment of the coil of wire with time will cause a voltage to be induced in the wire. No matter how the change is produced, a voltage will be generated. Thus magnetic field amplitude may be varied by powering the electromagnet with sinusoidal or pulsing current; by moving a permanent magnet toward or away from the wire; moving the wire toward or away from the magnetic field; or rotating the wire relative to the magnet, and so on (DeLoecker et al., 1990; Goodman & Blank, 2002; Serway, 1998; Smith, 1996; Wittig & Engstrom, 2002).

Lenz's law states that the polarity of the voltage induced according to Faraday's law is such that it produces a current whose magnetic field opposes the applied magnetic field back (electromagnetic field [EMF]). Therefore when a current is passed through a coil that creates an expanding magnetic field around the coil, the induced voltage and associated electrical current flow produce a magnetic field in opposition to the directly induced magnetic field.

Eddy currents are induced by the voltage generated, according to Faraday's law, in any conducting medium. When the conducting medium does not contain defined current pathways, there is no induced current, only induced voltage. There is movement in a spiral, swirling fashion. This movement, in turn, may potentially penetrate the membranes of neurons associated with pain. If the induced current is of sufficient amplitude, an action potential, or an excitatory or inhibitory postsynaptic nerve potential may be produced.

The Hall effect and Lorentz force are related to the same physical phenomenon of electromagnetism. In the Hall effect, when charged particles in a conductor move along a path that is transverse to a magnetic field, the particles experience a force that pushes them toward the outer walls of the conductor. The positively charged particles move to one side, and the negatively charged particles move to the other side. This movement produces a voltage across the conductor known as the "Hall voltage." The human body is replete with charged ions, and the Hall effect would be expected to occur to varying degrees when a magnetic field is passed through the body. The strength of the Hall voltage produced depends on three factors: (1) the strength of the magnetic field; (2) the number of charged particles moving transverse to the magnetic field; and (3) the velocity of movement of the charged particles (ions). The pulsing and static magnetic fields in current therapeutic applications are much too weak and the endogenous currents much too small for the Hall effect to be considered of any significance in magnetic field biological effects (Pilla, Nasser, & Kaufman, 1992, 1993). However, this contention is somewhat controversial and not universally accepted. Clearly, cellular and neural components in the body normally provide conductive pathways for ions, so it is reasonable to assume that these components would be prime objects of attention in attempting to observe the Hall effect. It is presumed that this voltage might add to the nerve's resting potential of -70 mV and make it harder to depolarize. After the resting potential rises from its normal undisturbed voltage of approximately -70 mV to a voltage of approximately -55 mV (threshold potential), an action potential spike is initiated. When ions move under the influence of a voltage, they become an electric current the magnitude of which is determined by Ohm's law, which states that electric current equals voltage divided by resistance.

This phenomenon predicts the effects of ions exposed to a combination of exogenous alternating current/direct current (AC/DC) magnetic fields at approximately 0.1 G and the dynamics of ions in a binding site. A bound ion in a static magnetic field will precess at the Larmor frequency and will accelerate faster to preferred orientations in the binding site with increased magnetic field strength. (A Larmor precession, named after early 20th-century Irish scientist Sir Joseph Larmor, is the precession of the magnetic moment of any object with a magnetic moment about an external magnetic field). Thus an increased binding rate can occur with resulting acceleration in the downstream biochemical cascade.

PENETRATION OF TISSUES

Magnetic fields can penetrate all tissues, including epidermis, dermis, and subcutaneous tissue, as well as tendons, muscles, and even bone. The specific amount of magnetic energy and its effect at the target organ depends on the size, strength, and duration of contact of the device. Magnetic fields fall into two broad categories: (1) static (DC) and (2) time varying (AC). The strength of static magnetic devices varies from 1 to 4000 G. Static fields have zero frequency because the polarity and field strength do not change with time but rather remain constant. Permanent magnets produce only static fields unless they are rotated or otherwise moved, which causes the magnetic field amplitude to change with time at the tissue target. Static magnetic fields that are either permanent or electromagnetic are in the range of 1 to 4000 G and have been reported to have significant biological effects (Colbert, 2004; Markov & Colbert, 2001; Pilla, 2003; Pilla & Muehsam, 2003). The most common static magnets sold to the public are known as refrigerator or flat-button magnets. They are made of various materials and also have different designs. Configuration can be unidirectional so that only one magnetic pole is represented on one side of the surface (whereas the opposite pole is on the opposite side away from the applied surface), or the surface can have a bipolar north–south design that appears repetitively as concentric ring, multitriangular, or quadripolar configurations.

The term "bipolar magnet" refers to a repetitive north–south polarity created on the same side of a ceramic or plastic alloy or neodymium material. The term "unipolar" refers to only one magnetic pole at a given surface (i.e., north or south). Multipolar alterations of north and south have also been used. Each specific manufacturer makes claims as to the superiority of its product. However, the most important characteristic of the magnetic field is the field strength at the target site and also the duration of exposure that leads to biological effects. It is believed that tissues, cells, and other structures have a "biological window" within which they can interact with these invisible fields. Static magnetic fields of 5 to 20 G have been felt to be pertinent. Thus the gauss rating and field strength at the surface are irrelevant in predicting biological responses. Bipolar magnets, using a small arc, are capable of inducing biologically significant fields at a relatively short distance from the surface (1 to 1.5 cm), whereas the penetration of unipolar magnets is much deeper (4 to 8 cm) (Markov, 2007).

BIOLOGICAL AND CELLULAR EFFECTS

Static magnetic fields in a 1- to 4000-G range have significant biological effects. Basic science has demonstrated that static magnetic fields ranging from 23 to 3000 G can alter the electrical properties of aqueous solutions. In addition, weak static magnetic fields can modulate myosin (from muscle tissue) phosphorylation at the molecular level in a cell-free preparation (Markov & Pilla, 1997). At a cellular level, exposure to 300 G doubled alkaline phosphatase activity in osteoblast-like (bone) cells (McDonald, 1993). Neurite (nerve) outgrowth from embryonic chick ganglia was significantly increased by exposure to 225 to 900 G (Macias, Buttocletti, Sutton, Pintar, & Maiman, 2000; McLean, Holcomb, Wamil, Pickett, & Cavopol, 1995; Sisken, Walker, & Orgel, 1993). Several experiments using unidirectional and multipolar magnets demonstrated blockade of sensory nociceptive neuron action potentials (pain) by exposure to a static magnetic field in the 10-mT range. A minimum magnetic field gradient of 15 G/mm was required to cause approximately 80% action potential blockade in isolated nerve preparations (McLean et al., 1995). This blockade reversed when the magnetic exposure was removed. Protection against acid-induced neuronal swelling was also demonstrated with magnetic exposure (McLean et al., 2003). Others have demonstrated a biphasic response of the acute microcirculation in rabbits exposed to static magnetic fields (10 G) (Ohkubo & Xu, 1997; Okano, Gmitrov, & Ohkubo, 1999). Notwithstanding this provocative and promising data in both in vitro and in vivo studies, skepticism prevails because of design flaws (Holcomb, McLean, Engstrom, & McCullough, 2002; Ramey, 1998). Specifically, a rigorous, randomized, placebo-controlled, double-blind design has been lacking; basic mechanisms of action have not been identified; and optimum target dosage and optimum polarity have yet to be determined. The absence of non-magnetic placebos as controls has also been of concern.

Clinical Observations and Effects

Colbert (2004) reviewed 22 therapeutic trials reported in US literature from 1982 to 2002. Clinical improvement in subjects who wore permanent magnets on various parts of their bodies was demonstrated in 15 studies, whereas 7 reported limited or no benefit. Magnetic field strength varied from 68 to 2000 G, and time exposure varied from 45 minutes to constant wearing for 4 months. Thus the optimum treatment duration, as well as the optimal polarity (unidirectional, multipolar, etc.), had yet to be established. Complicating the issue even further is the observation by Blechman, Oz, Nair, and Ting (2001) that a significant number of the static magnets sold to the public had lower field flux density measurements than the manufacturers claimed. It is known that a large amount of cancellation occurs in multipolar arrays. Similarly Eccles (2005) conducted a critical review of the randomized controlled trials that used static magnets for pain relief. He found a 73% statistical reduction in pain. He also commented on the difficulty in performing double-blind studies using static magnets because of the obvious interaction with metallic objects.

Specific clinical trials using a double-blind, placebo-controlled design include that of Vallbona, Hazelwood, and Jurida (1997). They applied 300- to 500-G, concentric-circle, bipolar magnets over painful joints in patients with postpolio syndrome for 45 minutes and reduced pain by 76%. Carter, Aspy, and Mold (2002) applied unipolar 1000-G static magnets and placebos over the carpal tunnel for 45 minutes, and both groups experienced significant pain reduction, felt to represent a placebo effect. Unidirectional magnetic pads (150 to 400 G) were placed over liposuction sites immediately after the procedure and kept in place for 14 days; this treatment produced a 40% to 70% reduction of pain, edema, and discoloration (Man, Man, & Plosker, 1999). Brown, Ling, Wan, and Pilla (2002) demonstrated statistical reduction of pelvic pain with magnetic therapy. Patients with fibromyalgia who slept on a unidirectional magnetic mattress pad (800-G ceramic magnets) for 4 months experienced a 40% improvement (Colbert et al., 1999). Weintraub (1999) noted a 90% reduction in neuropathic pain in patients with diabetic peripheral neuropathy with constant wearing of multipolar 475-G insole devices. There was also a 30% reduction in neuropathic pain associated with nondiabetic peripheral neuropathy (Man et al., 1999; Weintraub, 1999). A nationwide study using placebo controls also confirmed these results in 275 patients with diabetic peripheral neuropathy (Weintraub et al., 2003).

Hinman, Ford, and Heyl (2002) found a 30% response to short-term application of unipolar static magnets positioned over painful knees. Greater movement was also noted. Holcomb et al. (2002), using a quadripolar array of static magnets with alternating polarity, demonstrated analgesic benefit in patients with low back pain and knee pain.

Saygili, Aydinlik, Ercan, Naldöken, and Ulutuncel (1992), in an investigation of the effect of magnetic retention systems in dental prostheses on buccal mucosal blood flow, failed to detect changes in capillary blood flow after continuous exposure to a magnetic field for 45 days. Hong et al. (1982) had 101 patients with chronic neck and shoulder pain wear magnetic necklaces or placebos for 3 consecutive weeks after baseline electrodiagnostic studies, but no significant improvement was seen in the magnetic therapy group. In a study using a randomized placebo crossover design, Martel, Andrews, and Roseboom (2002) could not identify any change in forearm blood flow after 30 minutes of exposure to bipolar magnets. Other randomized placebo-controlled trials producing negative results should be mentioned, including the use of bipolar devices in patients with chronic low back pain (Collacott, Zimmerman, White, & Rindone, 2000) and the use of magnetic insoles by patients with plantar fasciitis (Winemiller, Billow, Laskowski, & Harmsen, 2003). Weintraub and others commented on design flaws in both of these studies (Weintraub, 2000, 2004a,b). Simultaneous application of static magnets to the back and feet in patient with failed back syndrome was also ineffective (Weintraub, Steinberg, & Cole, 2005). Pilla independently assessed the strength of the magnetic devices and found them to be less than the manufacturer's claims, thereby confirming the observations of Blechman et al. (2001) regarding the discrepancy between claimed and measured field flux densities.

It is assumed that the biological benefits from static magnetic fields are similar to those from pulsed electromagnetic fields (PEMFs), but the correlation has been imperfect. The specific mechanism of biological benefit remains to be determined. At present the most generally accepted theory is that static magnetic fields on the order of 1 to 10 G can affect ion-ligand binding, producing modulation (Pilla, 2003; Pilla & Muehsam, 2003; Pilla et al., 1997). There may also be physical realignment and translational movement of diamagnetically anisotropic molecules. Despite these theoretical and scientific rationales for benefit, criticisms, and skepticism remain. Critics allege it is placebo effects, yet a more enlightened and open-minded appraisal would accept the positive in vitro and in vivo observations. Ramey (1998), a veterinarian, has been a noted critic of static magnetic therapy, yet these devices are used extensively in veterinary medicine (e.g., magnetic blankets for race horses), in which any placebo effects would not be expected to apply in the same way as in human medicine.

In terms of safety, the World Health Organization has stated that there are no adverse effects on human health from exposure to static magnetic fields, even up to 2 T, which equals 20,000 G (United Nations Environment Programme MF, 1987). Similarly in 2003 the FDA extended nonsignificant risk status to magnetic resonance imaging (MRI) using flux densities of up to 8 T (US Food and Drug Administration, Center for Devices and Radiological Health, 2003).

MAGNETIC THERAPY AS ENERGY MEDICINE FOR PAIN

The practical applications of magnetic therapy have been available for decades without getting into more innovative forms of energy medicine discussed elsewhere in the book, especially when it comes to the management of pain. This pragmatic area of research and practice has been nonetheless neglected relative to drug and surgical approaches to pain, and there remains the need to further evaluate the quality and type of information available on the relatively well-studied use of magnetic therapy for the treatment of pain.

Magnetic therapy is reportedly a safe, noninvasive method of applying magnetic fields to the body for therapeutic purposes. The use of magnets for relief of pain has become popular among consumers, with annual spending on such therapy having exceeded $500 million in the United States and Canada and $5 billion worldwide (Weintraub et al., 2003; Weintraub & Cole, 2008). There have been many clinical studies of magnetic therapy for pain. For example, Therion's Advanced Biomagnetics Database contains more than 300 clinical studies. Nonetheless, few of these were randomized controlled trials, and the quality of the research is uncertain.

TABLE 10.1 *Proportion of Subjects Reporting Improvement of Pain After 45 Minutes of Magnetic Therapy*

	Active Magnetic Device ($n = 29$)	Inactive Device ($n = 21$)
Pain improved	22 (76%)	4 (19%)
Pain not improved	7 (24%)	17 (81%)

Chi-squared (1 degrees of freedom) = 20.6; $p < 0.0001$.
From Vallbona, C., Hazlewood, C.F., & Jurida, G. (1997). Response of pain to static magnetic fields in postpolio patients: a double-blind pilot study. *Archives of Physical Medicine and Rehabilitation, 78*, 1200.

It has been known for some time that magnets reduce pain in subjects. Table 10.1 shows the data from a classic 1997 study by Vallbona et al. (1997) with highly significant analgesic effects demonstrated by these data. Overall, the evidence shows that patients with more severe pain appear to respond better to magnetic therapy than do patients with only milder symptoms. There appear to be no adverse effects from application of *static* or *dynamic pulsed magnetic therapy* (Harlow et al., 2004; Segal et al., 2001; Weintraub & Cole, 2008; Weintraub et al., 2003). In a randomized, double-blinded, placebo-controlled trial involving 36 symptomatic patients with refractory *carpal tunnel syndrome,* application of dynamic magnetic fields produced significantly greater pain relief than use of a placebo device as measured by short- and long-term pain scores, as well as better objective nerve conduction, without changing motor strength or sensitivity to electrical current (Weintraub & Cole, 2008;).

The Weintraub study on magnetic therapy (Weintraub et al., 2003) was the first multicenter, double-blind, placebo-controlled study to examine the role of static magnetic fields in treatment of *diabetic peripheral neuropathy* and *neuropathic pain.* The results confirmed those of two previous pilot studies showing that the antinociceptive (pain relief) effect was significantly enhanced with long-term exposure to magnetic therapy. Evidence continued to support magnetic therapy as an effective treatment for neuropathic pain (Segal et al., 2001)

Overall, 14 of 22 studies have reported a significant analgesic effect of static magnets. Of the 19 better-quality studies, 12 found positive results and 6 found negative results, and in 1 there was a nonsignificant trend toward a positive analgesic effect. The weight of evidence from published well-conducted controlled trials suggests that static magnetic fields are able to induce analgesia (Eccles, 2005).

Taken as a whole, the studies of magnetic therapy are of the type required by the evidence hierarchy for "energy healing" (discussed in Chapter 9) to qualify as good-to-best evidence and to demonstrate a causal link between magnetic therapy and analgesia. There are clear interactions of magnetic energy with the body. These interactions probably involve influences over electric potentials and action potentials across neuronal membranes with known and measurable forms of energy that are now being called "veritable" forms of energy medicine (see Chapter 9). Veritable energy medicine includes electromagnetic, sound, and light therapies.

PULSED ELECTROMAGNETIC FIELDS

The generation of PEMFs requires an electric current to produce a pulsating (time-varying) magnetic field in that the electric coil that produces the magnetic field is stationary. Regardless of how the waveforms are transmitted through the coil, the ensuing magnetic flux lines appear in space in exactly the same manner as do the flux lines from a permanent solid magnet. The magnetic field penetrates biological tissues without modification, and the induced electrical fields are produced at right angles to the flux lines. The ensuing current flow is determined by the tissue's electrical properties (impedance) and determines the final spatial dosimetry. Peak magnetic fields from PEMF devices are typically 5 to 30 G at the target tissue, with varying specific shapes and amplitudes of fields.

Cellular studies (in vitro, in vivo) have been most provocative. In reviewing this work, Markov summarized various cellular and structural changes in response to this PEMF exposure (Markov, 2004; Markov & Colbert, 2001). Specifically, changes in fibrinogen, fibroblasts, leukocytes, platelets, fibrin, cytokines, collagen, elastin, keratinocytes, osteoblasts, and free radicals are all noted. In addition, magnetic fields influence vasoconstriction, vasodilatation, phagocytosis, cell proliferation, epithelialization, and scar formation.

Similarly in a series of reviews, Pilla summarized the effects of these weak PEMFs on both signal transduction and growth factor synthesis as it relates to bone fractures (Pilla, 2003; Pilla & Muehsam, 2003; Pilla et al., 1992, Pilla, Nasser, & Kaufman, 1993). He noted that there is upregulation of growth factor production, calcium ion transport, self-proliferation, insulin-like growth factor II release, and insulin-like growth factor II receptor expression in osteoblasts as a mechanism for bone repair. He also cited increases both in transforming growth factor-β1 messenger RNA and in protein in osteoblast cultures, producing an effect on a calcium/calmodulin-dependent pathway. Other studies with chondrocytes (cartilage) confirm similar increases in transforming growth factor-β1 messenger RNA and protein synthesis with PEMF exposure, suggesting a therapeutic application for joint repair (Ciombor, Lester, Aaron, Neame, & Caterson, 2002; Pilla et al., 1996). PEMFs have also been successfully applied to stimulate *nerve regeneration*. Neurite outgrowth has been demonstrated in cell cultures exposed to electromagnetic fields. Eddy currents are generated that can depolarize, hyperpolarize, and repolarize nerve cells, which suggests that neuromodulation can result.

Back in 1979 the FDA first approved the use of PEMF as a means of stimulating and recruiting osteoblast cells at a bone fracture site. Application of coils around the fracture cast induces current flows through the fracture site, producing 80% success. It became apparent after early testing that intermittent exposure, rather than continuous exposure, was the optimal technique. Four FDA-approved devices were developed for treatment of nonunion fractures, and each has specific signal parameters, treatment time, and other features. It is not yet clear how long PEMF exposure must last to trigger a bioelectrical effect. Effective waveforms tend to be asymmetric, biphasic, and quasi-rectangular or quasi-triangular in shape. This property indicates that tissues have various windows of vulnerability and susceptibility to PEMF.

Based on the high success rate of PEMF therapy, it is currently considered part of the standard armamentarium of orthopedic spine surgeons and is recommended as an adjunct to standard fracture management. In addition, the results are equivalent to those of surgical repair with minimal risk, and the treatment is more cost-effective.

BONE, JOINT AND MUSCULOSKELETAL PAINS

PEMF therapy has also been used to treat orthopedic pain and other conditions, as well as painful musculoskeletal disorders. These include aseptic necrosis of the hips, osteoporosis, osteoarthritis, osteogenesis imperfecta, rotator cuff dysfunction, and low back pain (Aaron, Lennox, Bunce, & Ebert, 1989; Binder, Parr, Hazelman, & Fitton-Jackson, 1984; Fukada & Yasuda, 1957; Jacobson, Gorman, Yamanashi, Saxena, & Clayton, 2001; Linovitz et al., 2000; Mooney, 1990; Pipitone & Scott, 2001; Pujol et al., 1998; Wilson & Jagadeesh, 1974; Zdeblic, 1993). In their reviews Markov (2004, 2007) and Markov and Colbert (2001) stated (with the exception of periarthritis) reduced pain scores were noted in carpal tunnel pain (93%) (Battisti, Fortunato, Giananneshi, & Rigato, 1998) and rotator cuff tendinitis (83%) (Binder et al., 1984), and 70% of multiple sclerosis patients had reduced spasticity (Lappin, Lawrie, Richards, & Kramer, 2003). Pilla reports double-blind studies claiming benefit for chronic wound repair (Battisti et al., 1998; Kloth et al., 1999; Mayrovitz & Larsen, 1995; Todd, Heylings, Allen, & McMillin, 1991), acute ankle sprain (Ciombor et al., 2002; Pilla et al., 1996), and acute whiplash injuries (Foley-Nolan, Barry, Coughlan, O'Connor, & Roden, 1990; Foley-Nolan et al., 1992). Other research with a double-blind, placebo-controlled design, had demonstrated use of pulsed high-frequency (27-MHz) electromagnetic therapy to treat persistent neck pain produced significant improvement by the second week of therapy (Foley-Nolan et al., 1990, 1992). Pujol et al. (1998) targeted musculoskeletal pain using magnetic coils, which produced a benefit compared with placebo.

Neuropathy and Nerve Injury

Weintraub and Cole (2004) applied nine consecutive 1-hour treatments to patients with peripheral neuropathy, which induced a greater than 50% reduction in neuropathic pain in an open-label, nonplacebo trial. Pickering, Bayston, and Scammell (2003) demonstrated that the antibiotic effect of gentamicin against *Staphylococcus epidermidis* could be augmented by exposure to a PEMF. Raji and Bowden (1983) applied 27-MHz pulsed electromagnetic therapy to the transected common peroneal nerve of rats; 15 minutes of treatment daily produced accelerated healing with reduced scar tissue, increased growth of blood vessels, and increased maturation of myelin (Fukada & Yasuda, 1957).

Selecting a PEMF Device

There are a large number of different commercially available PEMF devices that generate low-frequency fields of different shapes and amplitudes. These features represent major variables in attempting to understand and analyze the biologic and clinical effects. It has been speculated that the target area receives 5 to 30 G and that each type of tissue has its own biophysical window and specific encoding susceptibility (Pilla & Muehsam, 2003). There is considerable uncertainty about the specific mechanisms involved, as well as the optimal approach in terms of frequency, amplitude, and duration of exposure. This issue may be moot based on available data because several different devices generating different frequencies and amplitudes and used for different durations have nonetheless been successful in producing similar nonunion fracture healing. In addition, there is an abundance of experimental and clinical data demonstrating that extremely low-frequency and static magnetic fields can have a profound effect on a large variety of biological systems, organisms, and tissues, as well as cellular and subcellular structures. There are many vastly different approaches to influencing pain and healing that appear to operate at many different physiologic, conscious, subconscious and unconscious levels. It appears likely the body is able to "tune" these vastly different kinds of influences to help stimulate a return to homeostasis with some proper encouragement.

For PEMF, it has been assumed that a target is the cell membrane with ion and ligand binding and that even small changes in transmembrane voltage can induce a significant modulation of cellular function. In a recent review, Pilla (2003) has attempted to provide a unifying approach for static and pulsating magnetic fields, as well as weak ultrasound, which also induces electrical fields comparable to those associated with PEMFs. Pilla has also used pulsed (nonthermal) radiofrequency fields at 27.12 Hz and has achieved soft-tissue healing, reduction of edema, and postoperative pain relief. Pulsed radiofrequency therapy was also approved by the FDA (Mayrovitz & Larsen, 1995). A novel device has been developed with time-varying, biaxial rotation that generates both simultaneous static (DC) and oscillating (AC) fields. The fields are constantly changing and thus produce variable exposure to tissues and varying amplitudes at the target tissue. Weintraub and coworkers have found this type of therapy to be effective in reducing *neuropathic pain* from diabetic *peripheral neuropathy* and *carpal tunnel syndrome* (Weintraub & Cole, 2007a,b).

Transcranial Magnetic Stimulation

Transcranial magnetic stimulation (TMS) is a specific adaptation of PEMF that creates a time-varying magnetic field over the surface of the head. TMS depolarizes underlying superficial neurons, which induce electrical currents in the brain. High-intensity current is rapidly turned on and off in the electromagnetic coil through the discharge of capacitors. Thus brief (microsecond), powerful magnetic fields are produced, which in turn induce current in the brain. Two magnetic stimuli are delivered, used in close sequence, to the same cortical region through a single stimulating coil. The first stimulus is a conditioning stimulus at below motor threshold intensity that influences the intracortical neurons and exerts a significant modulating effect on the amplitude of the motor-evoked potential induced by the second, above motor threshold stimulus. This modulating effect depends on the interval between the stimuli. Cortical inhibition consistently occurs at intervals between 1 and 5 ms, and facilitation is seen at intervals between 10 and 20 ms.

TMS is simple to perform, inexpensive, generally safe, and provides useful measures of neuronal excitability. It has also been used along the neuraxis and continues to provide important insights into basic neurological functions, neurophysiology, and neurobiology. Although TMS is generally used as a research tool, therapeutic use of TMS is being considered. The abnormalities revealed by TMS are not disease specific and require clinical correlation. TMS stimulation directed to the primary motor cortex in individuals with a number of movement disorders helped investigators to appreciate the role of the basal ganglia. Specific TMS studies looked at Parkinson's disease, dystonia, Huntington's chorea, essential tremor, Tourette's syndrome, myoclonus, restless legs syndrome, progressive supranuclear palsy, Wilson disease, stiff person syndrome, and Rett's syndrome, among others, with promising results.

TMS has also proved useful in investigating the mechanisms of epilepsy, and rTMS may prove to have a therapeutic role in the future (Osenbach, 2006).

TMS is used in preoperative assessment of specific brain areas to optimize the surgical procedure. Both inhibitory and facilitatory interactions in the cortex can be studied by combining a subthreshold conditioning stimulus with a suprathreshold test stimulus at different short (1 to 20 ms) intervals through the same coil. In addition, this paired-pulse TMS approach is used to investigate potential central nervous system–activating drugs, various neurological and psychological diseases, and so on. Left and right hemispheres often react differently (Cahn, Herzog, & Pascual-Leone, 2003). The clinical utility of this aspect has not yet been demonstrated. When TMS pulses are delivered repetitively and rhythmically, a process called "rTMS", it can be modified further to induce excitatory or inhibitory effects. In rare cases seizures may be provoked in epileptic patients, as well as in normal volunteers (Abbruzzese & Trompetto, 2002; Amassian, Cracco, & Maccabee, 1989; Cantello, 2002; Chae, Nahas, & Wasserman, in press; George, Lisanby, & Sackeim, 1999; Kobayashi & Pascual-Leone, 2003; Lisanby, Gutman, Luber, Schroeder, & Sackeim, 2001; Pascual-Leone, Wasserman, & Davey, 2002; Rollnik et al., 2002; Terao & Ugawa, 2002; Theodore, 2003; Wasserman, 1998; Walsh & Rushworth, 1999).

rTMS leads to modulation of cortical excitability. For example, high-frequency rTMS of the dominant hemisphere but not the nondominant hemisphere can induce speech arrest (Orpin, 1982). This effect also correlates with results of the Wada test. The higher the stimulation frequency, the greater the disruption of cortical function. Lower frequencies of rTMS in a 1-Hz range can suppress excitability of the motor cortex, whereas 20-Hz stimulation trains lead to a temporary increase in cortical excitability. Pascual-Leone et al. have been studying these effects in patients with neurologic disorders, such as Parkinson's disease, dystonia, epilepsy, and stroke.

Osenbach (2006) provides a comprehensive review of the use of motor cortex stimulation (MCS) to manage *intractable pain*, concluding "there is little doubt that MCS provides excellent relief in carefully selected patients with a variety of neuropathic pain but leaves many unanswered questions." Tinnitus has been recalcitrant to many therapies, but there has been increasing use of magnetic and electrical stimulation of the auditory cortex with benefit (DeRidder et al., 2004;

Whitaker & Adderly, 1998). Mood disorders and mental conditions, including *anxiety*, mania, *depression*, and schizophrenia, are also being treated with TMS (George et al., 1999, 2003, 2004). These early observations and data suggest potential therapeutic utility. Elucidation of the underlying neurobiology is a work in progress in various neuropsychiatric syndromes. Creating sham TMS is difficult, and there is some evidence to suggest that tilting of the coils produces some biological effect on the brain (George et al., 2004).

SAFETY

A controversial and legitimate concern relates to the possibility that exposure of living tissues to EMFs may play a causative role in malignancy and birth defects. Specifically, this concern has been raised due to foci of childhood leukemia cases reported adjacent to high power lines. During a 5-year period (1991–96), Congress appropriated $60 million for dedicated research to look for such a causal association. The result was that no significant risk from power line frequencies could be confirmed.

However, no funding was made available to explore and expand the beneficial effects of magnetics and EMFs. There is now a 37-year experience with the approved use of PEMF in promoting repair of recalcitrant fractures without any adverse effect reported. Similarly static magnetic fields have been used for therapeutic uses for centuries, and no adverse effects have been reported.

The FDA has received a number of reports and complaints through its Medical Device Reporting system concerning EMF interference with a variety of medical devices, such as pacemakers and defibrillators. In addition, the development of advanced magnetic resonance technology using ultra-high magnetic field systems of more than 3 T (although they were considered safe) led to a reassessment of biomedical implant devices, which were previously judged to be safe to use at 1.5 T. Of the 109 implants and devices tested, 4% were considered to have a magnetic field interaction at 3 T and were potentially unsafe to use with fields of this magnitude (Shellock, 2002). In light of potential concerns regarding radiofrequency-induced magnetic fields with thermal effects at the cellular and molecular levels, the FDA has limited switching rates for generation of these gradient fields to a factor of three below the mean threshold of peripheral nerve stimulation (Shellock & Crues, 2004). Weintraub, Khoury, and Cole (2007) looked at the biological effects of 3-T MRI machines compared with 1.5-T and 0.6-T machines and found that 14% of subjects experienced sensory symptoms (new or altered) with both the 3-T and 1.5-T systems.

RESEARCH DIRECTIONS

The study of magnetic fields (static and pulsed) has evolved from a medical curiosity into investigation of significant and specific medical applications. There are at least five major professional and scientific societies involved in the study of the biological and clinical effects of electromagnetic fields (Markov & Colbert, 2001):

(1) the Bioelectromagnetics Society (BEMS); (2) the European Bioelectromagnetics Association (EBEA); (3) the Bioelectrochemical Society (BES); (4) the Society for Physical Regulation in Biology and Medicine (SPRBM); and (5) Engineering in Medicine and Biology (IEMB).

PEMF and TMS can influence biological functions and serve as therapeutic interventions. However, judging the efficacy of static magnets for treatment of various clinical conditions remains challenging, particularly because the important dosimetry component has not been fully determined and documented. More attention should be focused on creating strong, randomized, placebo-controlled study designs and looking for biological markers.

A major obstacle to future progress has been the lack of research funding, especially National Institutes of Health (NIH) funding. The late Senator Arlen Specter (R/D-Pennsylvania) was a senior member of the Senate Appropriations Subcommittee on Health and Education, which had doubled the NIH budget. At the behest of one of us (Micozzi), he asked the leadership of NIH about funding research on bioenergy and was told that NIH "does not believe in bioenergy." Perhaps the US Department of Energy should sponsor research in this field. Its leaders cannot respond that they do not believe in energy. The medical device industry has been willing to support many innovative studies. However, if major scientific advancement of knowledge is to occur in the field of magnetotherapy, recent history shows that it will require a combination of government and industry support, as well as professional interest.

Appendix | *Brief catalogue of electromagnetic medical devices for diagnosis and treatment*

Practitioners of biophysical modalities use a number of noninvasive devices (i.e., devices that do not penetrate the skin) to measure electrical charges and magnetic fields of particular low frequencies. Such devices are also believed to promote healing by interacting with the body.

Biophysical properties of the body have long been observed and used in healing. For example, these properties have been known as "qi (chi)" in Traditional Chinese Medicine, "prana" in Ayurvedic medicine, and "vital force" in homeopathy. Acupuncturists, homeopathic doctors, chiropractors, and practitioners of biophysical medicine and magnetic field therapy (including medical doctors) are among the practitioners who use noninvasive devices to detect and influence biophysical properties of the body.

Although conventional medicine recognizes the presence of electrical charges and magnetic forces in the body, certain biophysical properties, also referenced as "subtle energy," have not generally been as studied or utilized by Western science and medicine.

Unlike other medical devices regulated by the FDA, many of the noninvasive devices used to detect and influence these biophysical properties fall into a gray area from a regulatory standpoint. In 1976 the FDA set standards for the regulation of acupuncture needles as an experimental device, and the needle was reclassified as a therapeutic device in 1996, based partly on clinical evidence published in a series of articles that Micozzi, as editor-in-chief, had published in the new *Journal of Alternative and Complementary Medicine: Research on Paradigm, Practice and Policy* during 1995. The FDA team working on reclassification specifically requested me, as founding editor of the journal at that time, to provide lists of references to accelerate the review process. That FDA action occurred before the NIH Consensus Conference on Acupuncture in 1997. However, the FDA did not adopt standards for electroacupuncture devices, a major category of biophysical devices. One of the challenges continues to be the inability of Western science to measure these biophysical properties. As a result, such devices, when cleared by the FDA, are generally approved for use for "investigational" or experimental, purposes, as in research studies, but not in the diagnosis or treatment of illness.

The following sections discuss four categories of devices: (1) electrical and magnetic devices used in conventional medicine for conventional purposes; (2) conventional devices used in innovative applications; (3) conventional devices used for both innovative and conventional applications; and (4) unconventional devices.

ELECTRICAL AND MAGNETIC DEVICES USED CONVENTIONALLY IN BIOMEDICINE

Devices that measure the electrical and magnetic properties of the physical body have been used conventionally in biomedicine for many years. These electrical devices include the electrocardiograph (ECG), electroencephalograph (EEG), and

> ## SIDEBAR
>
> ### Brain Tumor-Treating Fields
>
> Optune is a noninvasive therapy approved by the FDA that is intended for tumor and cancer treatment. Optune, as alternating electric field therapy, targets proliferating cancer cells in the brain. These new energy frequencies are also called "tumor-treating fields" or "TT Fields". It is similar to other brain-reading devices because it requires electrodes on the scalp to help to locate the tumor. The therapy includes low-intensity and intermediate-frequency electric impulses within the ranges of 1 to 3 V/cm and 100 to 300 kHz. These frequencies are directly at the site of the tumor. According to research very little or no harm is reported in the surrounding healthy tissues of the brain.
>
> In essence, these are electricity fields and are able to stop tumor cells from dividing and promote apoptosis. These frequencies promote healthier lifestyles, better quality of life, minute toxicity, and comparable effectiveness to chemotherapy (Davies, Weinberg, & Palti, 2013). The Optune device has reportedly decreased sizes of tumors related to glioblastoma, a deadly tumor that is highly aggressive and the most common brain tumor in adults (Ansstas & Tran, 2016; Domingo-Musibay & Galanis, 2015). Optune devices can cost over $20,000 per month unless a special payment plan is awarded.

electromyograph (EMG), used to measure heart, brain, and muscle activity, respectively, and skin galvanic response, for diagnostic purposes. The ECG reads the electrical rhythms of the heart, the EEG records electrical brain waves, and the EMG measures electrical properties of the muscles, which may be correlated to muscle performance. The EMG is often used in physical (rehabilitative) medicine to diagnose conditions that cause pain, weakness, and numbness.

In addition to devices that measure electrical charges, conventionally, biomedicine has made increasing use of MRI for diagnostic purposes. MRI measures the magnetic fields of the body to create images for the diagnosis of physical abnormalities. Another magnetic device, the superconducting quantum interference device (SQUID), combines magnetic flux quantization and Josephson tunneling to measure magnetic heart signals complementary to ECG signals.

Conventional Biomedical Devices for Alternative Applications

Some of the devices described previously have also been used in innovative ways (not as originally intended) for treatment purposes, such as the use of the ECG and EEG in biofeedback to monitor subconscious processes and "feedback" this information to support behavioral change. The ECG is also the basis of the Flexyx Neurotherapy System, an innovative approach to the modulation of central perception and the processing of afferent signals from the physical receptors in the body (pressure, pain, heat, cold).

MRI, used to diagnose a variety of medical abnormalities, is also being used in a number of innovative ways, as in neuroscience to show brain activity during performance of different tasks, such as reading or other language tasks, and during acupuncture. At NIH, basic science researchers have investigated innovative uses of MRI to measure physiologic changes, such as those involved in eye movement or brain activity.

Conventional Devices for Treatment in Both Conventional and Alternative Medicine

Some devices that use electrical charges and magnetic fields are being used by both conventional and biophysical medical practitioners.

Superconducting Quantum Interference Device

In addition to its use in conventional medicine, the SQUID has also been used to measure weak magnetic fields of the brain. In other studies, it has been used to measure large, frequency-pulsing biomagnetic fields that emanate from certain practitioners, such as polarity therapists. This biomagnetic field is thought to trigger biological processes at the cellular and molecular levels, helping the body repair itself.

Transcutaneous Electrical Nerve Stimulation Unit

Developed by Dr. C. Norman Shealy, the transcutaneous electrical nerve stimulation (TENS) unit is used by both conventional medical and biophysical practitioners for pain relief. The FDA approved the TENS unit as a device for pain management in the 1970s. The electronic unit sends pulsed currents to electrodes attached to the skin, displacing pain signals from the affected nerves and preventing the pain message from reaching the brain.

TENS has been suggested to stimulate the production of endorphins as one proposed mechanism of action. In 1990 TENS was the subject of a study published in the *New England Journal of Medicine*. Although it was found ineffective in that study, other studies have found TENS helpful for *mild-to-moderate pain*. TENS may have better results in relieving skin and connective tissue pain than muscle or bone pain.

Electro-Acuscope

Using a lower-amplitude electrical current than the TENS unit, the Electro-Acuscope device reduces pain by stimulating tissue rather than by stimulating the nerves or muscles. It is thought to relieve pain by running currents through damaged tissues. Medical doctors, chiropractors, and physical therapists use the Electro-Acuscope for treatment of muscle spasms, migraines, jaw pain, bursitis, arthritis, surgical incisions, sprains and strains, neuralgia, shingles, and bruises. As with the TENS unit the Electro-Acuscope has been approved by the FDA as a device for pain management.

Diapulse

The Diapulse device emits radio waves that produce short, intense electromagnetic pulses that penetrate the tissue. It is said to improve blood flow, *reduce pain*, and promote healing. The Diapulse is used in a variety of health care settings, especially in the treatment of postoperative swelling and pain.

Unconventional Devices Used in Alternative Medicine

The following devices are some of the more popular devices used in biophysical medicine. The FDA has not set standards for these devices, but some may be registered with the FDA as "biofeedback" devices.

Electroacupuncture Devices

Dermatron

Voll, a German physician, introduced the Dermatron in the 1940s. He believed that acupuncture points have electrical conductivity, and used this device to measure electrical changes in the body. This technique became known as "electroacupuncture according to Voll" (EAV) and is currently termed "electroacupuncture biofeedback". Used for diagnosis, the Dermatron became the basis for a number of devices manufactured in Germany, France, Russia, Japan, Korea, the United Kingdom, and the United States.

Vega

Another modified electroacupuncture device similar to the Voll device, the Vega, works much faster and is also used for diagnosis. Based on the belief that the first sign of abnormality in the body is a change in electrical charge, this device records the change in skin conductivity after the application of a small voltage. Computers have been added to recent models using different names, such as the Computron.

Mora

Franz Morel, MD, a colleague of Voll, developed the Mora, another variation of the Voll device. Morel believed that electromagnetic signals could be described by a complex waveform. The Mora reads "wave" information from the body. Proponents believe that the Mora can relieve headaches, migraines, muscular aches and pains, circulation disorders, and skin disease.

Other Devices

Modern variations of Voll's electroacupuncture devices include the Accupath 1000, Biotron, Computron, DiagnoMetre, Eclosion, Elast, Interro, LISTEN System, Omega AcuBase, Omega Vision, Prophyle, and Punctos III.

Devices Using Light and Sound Energy

See also Chapter 11, Emery Medicine Therapies: Light and Phototherapies.

Cymatic Instruments

In addition to the electroacupuncture, biofeedback, and other devices that measure electrical charges described earlier, there are also therapeutic *cymatic* devices, in which a sound transducer replaces the electrodes of the EAV devices. Each organ and tissue in the body emits sound at a particular harmonic frequency. The cymatic device recognizes and records the emitted sound patterns that are associated with each body part and bathes the affected area with sound to balance the disturbance. These devices are used for diagnosis and treatment.

Sound Probe

The sound probe emits a pulsed tone of three alternating frequencies. This device is thought to destroy bacteria, viruses, and fungi that are not in resonance with the body.

Light Beam Generator

The light beam generator is thought to work by emitting photons of light that help to restore a normal energy state at the cellular level, allowing the body to heal. The light beam generator is believed to promote healing throughout the body and to help to correct such problems as *depression*, insomnia, *headaches*, and menstrual disorders.

Infratonic Qui Gong Machine

The Infratonic Qui Gong Machine (QGM) uses electroacoustic technology to direct massage-like sound waves into the body. This device is used as a *pain management* tool in China, Japan, Taiwan, Singapore, France, Spain, Mexico, and Argentina. The FDA has approved this device for therapeutic massage in the United States.

Teslar Watch

Named after the researcher Nikola Tesla, the Teslar watch was developed to modulate the harmful effects of "electronic" pollution from modern sources, such as computers, cell phones, televisions, hair dryers, and electric blankets. It is believed that these products create magnetic energy that may destabilize the body's electromagnetic field. Although this energy is at extremely low frequencies, which range from 1 to 100 Hz, it is believed to affect humans adversely over time.

Kirlian Camera

The Kirlian camera records and measures high-frequency, high-voltage electrons using a gas visualization discharge (GVD) technique, also called the "corona discharge technique." The most experienced researchers in this technique are in Russia. Seymon and Valentina Kirlian pioneered this research in the 1970s. Other contributors included Nikola Tesla in the United States, J.J. Narkiewich-Jodko in Russia, and Pratt and Schlemmer in Prague. In 1995 Konstantin Korotkov and his team in St. Petersburg developed a new Kirlian camera using a Crown television set.

REFERENCES

Aaron, R. K., Lennox, D., Bunce, G. E., & Ebert, T. (1989). The conservative treatment of osteonecrosis of the femoral head. A comparison of core decompression and pulsing electromagnetic fields. *Clinical Orthopedics and Related Research, 249,* 209.

Abbruzzese, G. & Trompetto, C. (2002). Clinical and research methods for evaluating cortical excitability. *Journal of Clinical Neurophysiology, 19,* 307.

Adey, W. R. (1988). Physiological signaling across cell membranes and cooperative influences of extremely low frequency electromagnetic fields. In H. Frohlich (Ed.), *Biological coherence and response to external stimuli* (p. 148). Berlin, Heidelberg: Springer-Verlag.

Adey, W. R. (1992). *Resonance and other interactions of electromagnetic fields with living organisms.* Oxford, UK: Oxford University Press.

Adey, W. R. (2004). Potential therapeutic applications of non-thermal electromagnetic fields: Ensemble organization of cells in tissue as a factor in biological field sensing. In P. J. Rosch & M. S. Markov (Eds.), *Bioelectromagnetic medicine* (p. 1). New York: Marcel Dekker.

Adey, W. R., et al. (1999). Spontaneous and nitrosourea-induced primary tumors of the central nervous system in Fischer 344 rats chronically exposed to 836 MHz modulated microwaves. *Radiation Research, 152*(3), 293–302.

Amassian, V. E., Cracco, R. Q., & Maccabee, P. J. (1989). Focal stimulation of human cerebral cortex with the magnetic coil: A comparison with electrical stimulation. *Electroencephalography and Clinical Neurophysiology, 74,* 401.

Ansstas, G. & Tran, D. D. (2016). *Treatment with tumor-treating fields therapy and pulse dose bevacizumab in patients with bevacizumab-refractory recurrent glioblastoma: A case series.* http://www.ncbi.nlm.nih.gov/pmc/articles/PMC4748800/.

Armstrong, D. & Armstrong, E. M. (1991). *The great American medicine show.* New York: Prentice-Hall.

Barker, A. T. (1991). Introduction to the basic principles of magnetic nerve stimulation. *Journal of Clinical Neurophysiology, 8,* 26.

Barker, A. T., Freeston, I. L., Jalinous, R., & Jarratt, J. A. (1987). Magnetic stimulation of the human brain and peripheral nervous system: An introduction and the results of an initial clinical evaluation. *Neurosurgery, 20,* 100.

Battisti, E., Fortunato, M., Giananneshi, F., & Rigato, M. (1998). *Efficacy of the magnetotherapy in idiopathic carpal tunnel syndrome.* In D. Suminic (Ed.), *Proc IV EBEA: Proceedings of the fourth European Bioelectromagnetics Association Congress, Zagreb, Croatia, November 19–21.*(p. 34).

Bickford, R. G. & Fremming, B. D. (1965). Neuronal stimulation by pulsed magnetic fields in animals and man. In *Digest of sixth international conference on medical electronics and biological engineering* (p. 112).

Binder, A., Parr, G., Hazelman, B., & Fitton-Jackson, S. (1984). Pulsed electromagnetic field therapy of persistent rotator cuff tendinitis: A double-blind, controlled assessment. *Lancet, 1*(8379), 695.

Blechman, A. M., Oz, M. C., Nair, V., & Ting, W. (2001). Discrepancy between claimed field flux density of some commercially available magnets and actual gaussmeter measurements. *Alternative Therapies in Health and Medicine, 7,* 92.

Blumenthal, N. C., Ricci, J., Breger, L., Zychlinsky, A., Solomon, H., Chen, G. G., et al. (1997). Effects of low intensity AC and/or DC electromagnetic fields on cell attachment and induction of apoptosis. *Bioelectromagnetics, 18,* 264.

Brown, C. S., Ling, F. W., Wan, J. Y., & Pilla, A. A. (2002). Efficacy of static magnetic field therapy in chronic pelvic pain: A double-blind, pilot study. *American Journal of Obstetrics and Gynecology, 187,* 1581.

Cahn, S. D., Herzog, A. G., & Pascual-Leone, A. (2003). Paired-pulsed transcranial magnetic stimulation: Effects of hemispheric laterality, gender and handedness in normal controls. *Journal of Clinical Neurophysiology, 20,* 371–374.

Cantello, R. (2002). Applications of transcranial magnetic stimulation in movement disorders. *Journal of Clinical Neurophysiology, 19,* 272.

Carter, R., Aspy, C. B., & Mold, J. (2002). The effectiveness of magnet therapy for treatment of wrist pain attributed to carpal tunnel syndrome. *Journal of Family Practice, 51,* 38.

Chae, J. H., Nahas, Z., Wasserman, E. M., et al. (in press). A pilot study using rTMS to probe the functional neuroanatomy of tics in Tourette's syndrome. *Neuropsychiatry, Neuropsychology and Behavioral Neurology.*

Ciombor, D., Lester, G., Aaron, R., Neame, P., & Caterson, B. (2002). Low-frequency EMF regulates chondrocyte differentiation and expression of matrix proteins. *Journal of Orthopedic Research, 20,* 40.

Colbert, A. P. (2004). Clinical trials involving static magnetic field applications. In P. J. Rosch & M. S. Markov (Eds.), *Bioelectromagnetic medicine* (p. 781). New York: Marcel Dekker.

Colbert, A. P., Markov, M. S., Banerij, M., et al. (1999). Magnetic mattress pad use in patients with fibromyalgia: A randomized, double-blind pilot study. *Journal of Back and Musculoskeletal Rehabilitation, 13,* 19.

Collacott, E. A., Zimmerman, J. T., White, D. W., & Rindone, J. P. (2000). Bipolar permanent magnets for the treatment of low back pain: A pilot study. *Journal of American Medical Association, 283*, 1322.

Davies, A. M., Weinberg, U., & Palti, Y. (2013). *Tumor treating fields: A new frontier in cancer therapy.* http://www.ncbi.nlm.nih.gov/pubmed/23659608.

DeLoecker, W., Cheng, N., & Delport, P. H. (1990). Effects of pulsed electromagnetic fields on membrane transport. *Emerging Electromagnetic Medicine, Section I*, 45.

DeRidder, D., DeMulder, G., Walsh, W., Muggleton, N., Sunaert, S., & Møller, A. (2004). Magnetic and electrical stimulation of the auditory cortex for intractable tinnitus. *Journal of Neurosurgery, 100*, 560.

Domingo-Musibay, E., & Galanis, E. (2015). *What next for newly diagnosed glioblastoma?* http://www.ncbi.nlm.nih.gov/pubmed/26558493.

Eccles, N. J. (2005). A critical review of randomized controlled trials of static magnets for pain relief. *Journal of Alternative and Complementary Medicine, 11*, 495.

Engstrom, S. & Fitzsimmons, R. (1999). Five hypotheses to examine the nature of magnetic field transduction in biological systems. *Bioelectromagnetics, 20*, 423.

Farndale, R. W., Maroudas, A., & Marsland, T. P. (1987). Effects of low-amplitude pulsed magnetic fields on cellular ion transport. *Bioelectromagnetics, 8*, 119.

Foley-Nolan, D., Barry, C., Coughlan, R. J., O'Connor, P., & Roden, D. (1990). Pulsed high-frequency (27 MHz) electromagnetic therapy for persistent neck pain: A double-blind, placebo-controlled study of 20 patients. *Orthopaedics, 13*, 445.

Foley-Nolan, D., Moore, K., Codd, M., Barry, C., O'Connor, P., & Coughlan, R. J. (1992). Low-energy, high-frequency, pulsed electromagnetic therapy for acute whiplash injuries: A double-blind, randomized, controlled study. *Scandinavian Journal of Rehabilitation Medicine, 24*, 51.

Fukada, E. & Yasuda, I. (1957). On the piezoelectric effect of bone. *Journal of the Physical Society of Japan, 12*, 121.

Geddes, L. (1991). History of magnetic stimulation of the nervous system. *Journal of Clinical Neurophysiology, 8*, 3.

George, M. S., Lisanby, S. H., & Sackeim, H. A. (1999). Transcranial magnetic stimulation: Applications in neuropsychiatry. *Archives of General Psychiatry, 56*, 300.

George, M. S., Nahas, Z., Kozel, F. A., Li, X., Denslow, S., Yamanakka, K., et al. (2004). Repetitive transcranial magnetic stimulation (rTMS) for depression and other indications. In P. J. Rosch & M. S. Markov (Eds.), *Bioelectromagnetic medicine* (p. 293). New York: Marcel Dekker.

George, M. S., Nahas, Z., Kozol, F. A., Li, X., Yamanaka, K., Mishory, A., et al. (2003). Mechanisms and the current state of transcranial magnetic stimulation. *CNS Spectrums, 8*, 496.

Goodman, R. & Blank, M. (2002). Insights into electromagnetic interaction mechanisms. *Journal of Cell Physiology, 192*, 16.

Harlow, T., Greaves, C., White, A., Brown, L., Hart, A., & Ernst, E. (2004). Randomised controlled trial of magnetic bracelets for relieving pain in osteoarthritis of the hip and knee. *British Medical Journal (Clinical research ed.), 329*(7480), 1450–1454.

Hinman, M. R., Ford, J., & Heyl, H. (2002). Effects of static magnets on chronic knee pain and physical function: A double-blind study. *Alternative Therapies in Health and Medicine, 8*, 50.

Holcomb, R. R., McLean, M. J., Engstrom, S., & McCullough, B. A. (2002). Treatment of mechanical low back pain with static magnetic fields: Result of a clinical trial and implications for study design. *Magnetotherapy, 171*.

Hong, C. Z., Lin, J. C., Bender, L. F., Schaeffer, J. N., Meltzer, R. J., & Causin, P. (1982). Magnetic necklace: Its therapeutic effectiveness on neck and shoulder pain. *Archives of Physical Medicine and Rehabilitation, 63*, 462.

Jacobson, J. I., Gorman, R., Yamanashi, W. S., Saxena, B. B., & Clayton, L. (2001). Low-amplitude, extremely low frequency magnetic fields for the treatment of osteoarthritic knees: A double-blind clinical study. *Alternative Therapies in Health and Medicine, 7*, 54.

Kloth, L. C., Berman, J. E., Sutton, C. H., Jeutter, D. C., Pilla, A. A., & Epner, M. E. (1999). Effect of pulsed radiofrequency stimulation on wound healing: A double-blind, pilot clinical study. In F. Bersani (Ed.), *Electricity and magnetism in biology and medicine* (p. 875). New York: Plenum.

Kobayashi, M., Fujimaki, T., Mihara, B., & Ohira, T. (2015). Repetitive transcranial magnetic stimulation once a week induces sustainable long-term relief of central poststroke pain. *Neuromodulation, 18*(4), 249–254.

Kobayashi, M., & Pascual-Leone, A. (2003). Transcranial magnetic stimulation in neurology. *Lancet Neurology, 2,* 145.

Lappin, M. S., Lawrie, F. W., Richards, T. L., & Kramer, E. D. (2003). Effects of a pulsed electromagnetic therapy on multiple sclerosis, fatigue and quality of life: A double-blind, placebo-controlled trial. *Alternative Therapies in Health and Medicine, 9,* 38.

Lednev, L. L. (1991). Possible mechanism of weak magnetic fields on biological systems. *Bioelectromagnetics, 12,* 71.

Linovitz, R. J., Ryaby, J. T., Magee, F. P., Faden, J. S., Ponder, R., & Muenz, L. R. (2000). Combined magnetic fields accelerate primary spine fusion: A double-blind, randomized, placebo-controlled study. *Proceedings of the American Academy of Orthopedic Surgery, 67,* 376.

Lisanby, S. H., Gutman, D., Luber, B., Schroeder, C., & Sackeim, H. A. (2001). Sham TMS: Intracerebral measurement of the induced electrical field and the induction of motor-evoked potentials. *Biological Psychiatry, 49,* 460.

Maccabee, P. J., Amassian, V. E., Cracco, R. Q., Cracco, J. B., Eberle, L., & Rudell, A. (1991). Stimulation of the human nervous system using the magnetic coil. *Journal of Clinical Neurophysiology, 8,* 38.

Macias, M. Y., Buttocletti, J. H., Sutton, C. H., Pintar, F. A., & Maiman, D.J. (2000). Directed and enhanced neurite growth with pulsed magnetic field stimulation. *Bioelectromagnetics, 21,* 272.

Macklis, R. M. (1993). Magnetic healing, quackery and the debate about the health effects of electromagnetic fields. *Annals of Internal Medicine, 118,* 376.

Man, D., Man, B., & Plosker, H. (1999). The influence of permanent magnetic field therapy on wound healing in suction lipectomy patients: A double-blind study. *Plastic and Reconstructive Surgery, 104,* 2261.

Markov, M. S. (2004). Magnetic and electromagnetic field therapy: Basic principles of application for pain relief. In P. J. Rosch & M. S. Markov (Eds.), *Bioelectromagnetic medicine* (p. 251). New York: Marcel Dekker.

Markov, M. S. (2007). Magnetic field therapy: A review. *Electromagnetic Biology and Medicine, 26,* 1.

Markov, M. S. & Colbert, A. P. (2001). Magnetic and electromagnetic field therapy. *Journal of Back and Musculoskeletal Rehabilitation, 15,* 17.

Markov, M. S. & Pilla, A. A. (1997). Weak static magnetic field modulation of myosin phosphorylation in a cell-free preparation: Calcium dependence. *Bioelectrochemistry and Bioenergetics, 43,* 233.

Martel, G. F., Andrews, S. C., & Roseboom, C. G. (2002). Comparison of static and placebo magnets on resting forearm blood flow in young, healthy men. *Journal of Orthopedics and Sports Physical Therapy, 32,* 518.

Mayrovitz, H. N. & Larsen, P. B. (1995). A preliminary study to evaluate the effect of pulsed radiofrequency field treatment on lower extremity peri-ulcer skin microvasculature of diabetic patients. *Wounds, 7,* 90.

McDonald, F. (1993). Effect of static magnetic fields on osteoblasts and fibroblasts in-vitro. *Bioelectromagnetics, 14,* 187.

McLean, M., Holcomb, R. R., Engstrom, S., et al. (2003). A static magnetic field blocks action potential firing and kainic acid-induced neuronal injury in vitro. In M. J. McLean, S. Engstrom, & R. R. Holcomb (Eds.), *Magnetotherapy: Potential therapeutic benefits and adverse effects* (p. 29). New York: TFG Press.

McLean, M. J., Holcomb, R. R., Wamil, A. W., Pickett, J. D., & Cavopol, A. V. (1995). Blockade of sensory neuron action potentials by a static magnetic field in the mT range. *Bioelectromagnetics, 16,* 20.

Merton, P. A. & Morton, H. B. (1980). Stimulation of the cerebral cortex in the intact human subject. *Nature, 285,* 227.

Mooney, V. (1990). A randomized, double-blind, prospective study of the efficacy of pulsed electromagnetic fields for interbody lumbar fusions. *Spine, 15,* 708.

Mourino, M. R. (1991). From Thales to Lauterbur, or from the lodestone to MR imaging: magnetism and medicine. *Radiology, 180,* 593.

Ohkubo, C. & Xu, S. (1997). Acute effects of static magnetic fields on cutaneous microcirculation in rabbits. *In Vivo, 11,* 221.

Okano, H., Gmitrov, J., & Ohkubo, C. (1999). Biphasic effects of static magnetic fields on cutaneous microcirculation in rabbits. *Bioelectromagnetics, 20*, 161.

Orpin, J. A. (1982). False claims for magnetotherapy. *Canadian Medical Association Journal, 15*, 1375.

Osenbach, R. K. (2006). Motor cortex stimulation for intractable pain. *Neurosurgical Focus, 21*, 1.

Pascual-Leone, A., Valls-Sole, J., Wasserman, E. M., & Hallett, M. (1994). Responses to rapid-rate transcranial magnetic stimulation of the human motor cortex. *Brain, 117*, 847.

Pascual-Leone, A., Wasserman, E. M., & Davey, N. J. (Eds.), (2002). *Handbook of transcranial magnetic stimulation.* London: Oxford University Press.

Pickering, S. A. W., Bayston, R., & Scammell, B. E. (2003). Electromagnetic augmentation of antibiotic efficacy in infection of orthopaedic implants. *Journal of Bone and Joint Surgery, 85*, 588.

Pilla, A. A. (2003). Weak time-varying and static magnetic fields: From mechanisms to therapeutic applications. In P. Stavroulakis (Ed.), *Biological effects of electromagnetic fields* (p. 34). New York: Springer-Verlag.

Pilla, A. A., Martin, D. E., Schuett, A. M., et al. (1996). Effect of pulsed radiofrequency therapy on edema from grades I and II ankle sprains: A placebo-controlled, randomized, multi-site, double-blind, clinical study. *Journal of Athletic Training, S31*, 53.

Pilla, A. A. & Muehsam, D. J. (2003). Pulsing and static magnetic field therapeutics: From mechanisms to clinical application. *Magnetotherapy, 30*, 119.

Pilla, A. A., Muehsam, D. J., & Markov, M. S. (1997). A dynamical systems/Larmor precession model for weak magnetic field bioeffects: Ion binding and orientation of bound water molecules. *Bioelectrochemistry, 43*, 241.

Pilla, A. A., Nasser, P. R., & Kaufman, J. J. (1992). The sensitivity of cells and tissues to weak electromagnetic fields. In M. J. Allen, S. F. Cleary, & A. E. Sowers (Eds.), *Charge and field effects in biosystems—3* (p. 231). Boston: Birkhäuser.

Pilla, A. A., Nasser, P. R., & Kaufman, J. J. (1993). The sensitivity of cells and tissues to therapeutic and environmental EMF. *Bioelectrochemistry and Bioenergetics, 30*, 161.

Pipitone, N. & Scott, D. L. (2001). Magnetic pulsed treatment for knee osteoarthritis: A randomized, double-blind, placebo-controlled study. *Current Medical Research and Opinion, 17*, 190.

Pujol, J., Pascual-Leone, A., Dolz, C., Delgado, E., Dolz, J. L., & Aldomà, J. (1998). The effect of repetitive magnetic stimulation on localized musculoskeletal pain. *Neuroreport, 9*, 1745.

Raji, A. R. M. & Bowden, R. E. M. (1983). Effects of high pulsed power electromagnetic field on the degeneration and regeneration of the common peroneal nerve in rats. *Journal of Bone and Joint Surgery, 65*, 478.

Ramey, D. W. (1998). Magnetic and electromagnetic therapy. *The Scientific Review of Alternative Medicine, 2*, 13.

Repacholi, M. H. & Greenebaum, B. (1999). Interaction of static and extremely low frequency electric and magnetic fields with living systems: Health effects and research needs. *Bioelectromagnetics, 20*, 133.

Rollnik, J. D., Wusterfeld, S., Dauper, J., Karst, M., Fink, M., Kossev, A., et al. (2002). Repetitive transcranial magnetic stimulation for the treatment of chronic pain: A pilot study. *European Neurology, 48*, 6.

Rosch, P. (2004). Preface. In P. J. Rosch (Ed.), *A brief historical perspective in bioelectromagnetic medicine* (p. III). New York: Marcel Dekker.

Rosen, A. D. (1992). Magnetic field influence on acetylcholine release at the neuromuscular junction. *American Journal of Physiology, 262*, 1418.

Rossini, P. M., Barker, A. T., Berardelli, A., Caramia, M. D., Caruso, G., Cracco, R. Q., et al. (1994). Noninvasive electrical and magnetic stimulation of the brain, spinal cord and roots: basic principles and procedure for routine clinical application: Report of an IFCN committee. *Electroencephalography and Clinical Neurophysiology, 91*, 79.

Saygili, G., Aydinlik, E., Ercan, M. I., Naldöken, S., & Ulutuncel, N. (1992). Investigation of the effect of magnetic retention systems used in prostheses on buccal mucosal blood flow. *International Journal of Prosthodontics, 5*, 326.

Segal, N. A., Toda, Y., Huston, J., Saeki, Y., Shimizu, M., Fuchs, H., et al. (2001). Two configurations of static magnetic fields for testing rheumatoid arthritis of the knee: A double-blind clinical trial. *Archives of Physical Medicine and Rehabilitation, 82*, 1453.

Serway, R. A. (1998). *Principles of physics* (2nd ed., p. 636). Fort Worth, Tex: Saunders College Publishing.

Shellock, F. G. (2002). Biomedical implants and devices: Assessment of magnetic field interactions with a 3.0 T MR system. *Journal of Magnetic Resonance Imaging, 16*, 721.

Shellock, F. G. & Crues, J. V. (2004). MR procedures: Biological effects, safety and patient care. *Radiology, 232*, 635.

Sisken, B. F., Walker, J., & Orgel, M. (1993). Prospects on clinical applications of electrical stimulation for nerve regeneration. *Journal of Cell Biochemistry, 52*, 404.

Smith, W. F. (1996). *Principles of materials science and engineering* (3rd ed., p. 659). New York: McGraw-Hill.

Terao, Y. & Ugawa, Y. (2002). Basic mechanisms of TMS. *Journal of Clinical Neurophysiology, 19*, 322.

Theodore, W. H. (2003). Transcranial magnetic stimulation in epilepsy. *Epilepsy Currents, 3*, 191.

Thompson, S. P. (1910). A physiological effect of an alternating magnetic field. *Proceedings of the Royal Society B, 82*, 396–399.

Timmel, C. R., Till, U., Brocklehurst, B., & Hore, P. J. (1998). Effects of weak magnetic fields on free radical recombination reactions. *Molecular Physics, 95*, 71.

Todd, D. J., Heylings, D. J., Allen, G. E., & McMillin, W. P. (1991). Treatment of chronic varicose ulcers with pulsed electromagnetic fields: A controlled pilot study. *Irish Medical Journal, 84*, 54.

United Nations Environment Programme MF. (1987). *The International Labour Organization.* Geneva: World Health Organization.

US Food and Drug Administration, Center for Devices and Radiological Health. (April 1, 2003). *Medical Device Reporting data files.* http://www.FDA.gov/CDRH/MDRFILE/html.

Vallbona, C., Hazelwood, C. F., & Jurida, G. (1997). Response of pain to static magnetic fields in postpolio patients: A double-blind pilot study. *Archives of Physical Medicine and Rehabilitation, 78*, 1200.

Walsh, V., & Rushworth, M. (1999). A primer of magnetic stimulation as a tool for neuropsychology. *Neuropsychologia, 37*, 125.

Wasserman, E. M. (1998). Risk and safety of repetitive transcranial magnetic stimulation: Report and suggested guidelines from the International Workshop in the Safety of Repetitive Transcranial Magnetic Stimulation: June 5-7, 1996. *Electroencephalography and Clinical Neurophysiology, 108*(1).

Weintraub, M. I. (1999). Magnetic bio-stimulation in painful diabetic peripheral neuropathy: A novel intervention. A randomized, double-blind, placebo, cross-over study. *American Journal of Pain Management, 9*, 8.

Weintraub, M. I. (2000). Are magnets effective for pain control? *Journal of American Medical Association, 284*, 565.

Weintraub, M. I. (2001). Magnetic biostimulation in neurologic illness. In M. I. Weintraub (Ed.), *Alternative and complementary treatment in neurologic illness* (p. 278). New York: Churchill Livingstone.

Weintraub, M. I. (2004a). Magnetotherapy: Historical background with a stimulating future. *Critical Reviews in Physical and Rehabilitation Medicine, 16*, 95.

Weintraub, M. I. (2004b). Magnets for patients with heel pain. *Journal of American Medical Association, 291*, 43.

Weintraub, M. I. & Cole, S. P. (2004). Pulsed magnetic field therapy in refractory neuropathic pain secondary to peripheral neuropathy: Electrodiagnostic parameters—Pilot study. *Neurorehabilitation and Neural Repair, 18*, 42.

Weintraub, M. I. & Cole, S. P. (2007a). Novel device generating static and time-varying magnetic fields in refractory diabetic peripheral neuropathy: subset analysis of cohort with long-term exposure in nationwide, double-blind, placebo-controlled trial. *Diabetes, 56*(Suppl. 1), A-610.

Weintraub, M. I. & Cole, S. P. (2007b). A randomized, controlled trial of the effects of a combination of static and dynamic magnetic fields on carpal tunnel syndrome. *Neurology, 68*(Supp. 1), A180.

Weintraub, M. I. & Cole, S. P. (2008). A randomized controlled trial of the effects of a combination of static and dynamic magnetic fields on carpal tunnel syndrome. *Pain Medicine, 9*(5), 493.

Weintraub, M. I., Khoury, A., & Cole, S. P. (2007). Biologic effects of 3 Tesla (T) MR imaging comparing traditional 1.5 T and 0.6 T in 1023 consecutive outpatients. *Journal of Neuroimaging, 17*, 241.

Weintraub, M. I., Steinberg, R. B., & Cole, S. P. (2005). The role of cutaneous magnetic stimulation in failed back syndrome. *Seminars in Integrative Medicine, 3*, 101.

Weintraub, M. I., Wolfe, G. I., Barohn, R. A., Cole, S. P., Parry, G. J., Hayat, G., et al. (2003). Static magnetic field therapy for symptomatic diabetic neuropathy: A randomized, double-blind, placebo-controlled trial. *Archives of Physical Medicine and Rehabilitation*, *84*, 736.

Whitaker, J. & Adderly, B. (1998). *The pain relief breakthrough* (pp. 24–38). Boston: Little, Brown.

Wilson, D. H. & Jagadeesh, O. (1974). The effect of pulsed electromagnetic energy on peripheral nerve regeneration. *Annals of the New York Academy of Sciences*, *238*, 575.

Winemiller, M. H., Billow, R. G., Laskowski, E. R., & Harmsen, W. S. (2003). Effect of magnetic vs. sham-magnetic insoles on plantar heel pain: A randomized controlled trial. *Journal of American Medical Association*, *290*, 1474.

Wittig, J. E. & Engstrom, S. (2002). Magnetism and magnetic materials. In M. J. McLean, S. Engstrom, & R. R. Holcomb (Eds.), *Magnetotherapy: Potential therapeutic benefits and adverse effects* (p. 3). New York: TFG Press.

Zdeblic, T. D. (1993). A prospective randomized study of lumbar fusion: Preliminary results. *Spine*, *18*, 983.

Suggested Readings can be found on the companion website, http://www.micozzipainconditions.com.

Chapter 11

Electromagnetic Therapies

LIGHT AND PHOTOTHERAPIES

BIOENERGETICS AND ELECTROMAGNETIC THERAPIES

There is a bioenergetic or biophysical aspect to many healing modalities that has long been observed clinically. Contemporary fundamental physics is now in the process of providing explanatory models, mechanisms, and paradigms for the biophysical basis of many healing phenomena (see Chapter 10). Contemporary biophysics remains useful for understanding the basis of many contemporary diagnostic and therapeutic approaches. These biophysical characteristics extend beyond the current paradigm of biomedical science, which is expressed in reductionist biochemical and molecular biological terms. Biophysical models may be more consistent with many scientific observations in whole-organism biology, physiology, and homeostasis. Biophysics, rather than biochemistry or molecular biology, may better provide explanatory mechanisms for the observed effectiveness of such clinical practices as acupuncture, herbalism (including vibrational energies of plants), homeopathy, healing touch, meditation, and mind-body modalities, as discussed throughout this textbook.

However, it is not necessary to travel into the nonconventional realms of "energy medicine" (see Chapter 9) to observe the effects of energy on healing. For example, in conventional energy terms, nonthermal, nonionizing electromagnetic fields in low frequencies have long been observed to have the following effects on the physical body:
- stimulation of bone repair,
- nerve stimulation,
- promotion of soft-tissue wound healing,
- treatment of osteoarthritis and pain,
- tissue regeneration,
- immune system stimulation, and
- neuroendocrine modulation.

Contemporary biophysically based diagnostic/therapeutic modalities include electrodermal screening, applied kinesiology, bio-resonance, and radionics.

Acknowledgments to Marc Micozzi and Michael I. Weintraub for prior contributions in Micozzi, M.S. (Ed.), (2016). *Fundamentals of commentary and alternative medicine* (5th ed.). St Louis: Elsevier Health Sciences/Saunders.

Utilization of these approaches requires the availability of suitable medical devices and clinical practitioners.

Many well-established historical healing traditions have drawn on diagnostic and therapeutic approaches that may now be interpreted in the light of contemporary biophysics. The ancient and complex healing traditions of China and India make reference to and use practices that are currently thought to be based on biophysical modalities (see Section IV). Acupuncture, acupressure, jin shin do, t'ai chi, reiki, qigong, tui na, and yoga may be seen today to operate on a biophysical basis. In addition, Asian medical systems have also used sound, light, and color for their healing properties, which may now be viewed in biophysical perspective. However, these methods developed over three millennia in widespread clinical practice and observation around the world without the benefit of 19th- and 20th-century discoveries and theories about electromagnetic radiation. Contemporary outcomes-based clinical trials have been demonstrating the efficacy of these modalities in management of many medical conditions (Lanzl, Rozenfeld, & Wootton, 2003). It is not only traditional Asian medical modalities and practices that may be seen in the light of bioenergy. Several schools of health theory and practice have emerged in the West around the idea of bioenergy.

WESTERN SCHOOLS OF BIOENERGY

Bioenergetic and biophysical medical modalities have been prominent in the more recent history of American and European medicine. Several schools of thought were organized in the United States, or brought from Europe, that center around healing approaches, which we may now associate in whole or in part with emerging biophysical explanations. Such schools and their founders have often influenced each other through time (Box 11.1). In addition,

BOX 11.1 *Western Schools and Their Founders*

Influences on the Development of Bioenergetics
- Homeopathy (Samuel Hahnemann, 1830–60)
- Faith healing (Phineas Quimby, 1830–60)
- Christian Science (Mary Baker Eddy, 1861–80)
- Theosophy (Helena Blavatksy/Henry Steel Olcott, 1861–80)
- Movement therapy (Matthias Alexander, 1861–80)
- Iridology (Nils Liljequist, Ignaz von Peczely, 1861–1900)
- Zone therapy/reflexology (William Fitzgerald, 1901–20)
- Anthroposophical medicine (Rudolf Steiner, 1901–20)
- Polarity therapy (Randolph Stone, 1921–40)
- Bach flower remedies (Edward Bach, 1921–40)
- Electromagnetism (Semyon and Valentine Kirlian, 1921–40)
- Movement therapy (Moshé Feldenkrais, 1941–60)
- Shiatsu (Tokujiro Namikoshi, 1941–60)
- Jin shin jyutsu (Jiro Murai, 1941–60)
- Orgone therapy (Wilhelm Reich, 1941–60)
- Structural integration (Ida Rolf, 1960–80)

interpretations of herbal, nutritional, and even pharmacological therapies have been extended to include "vibrational energy" or "biological information" as a mechanism of action.

There have been many adherents, clients, practitioners, and clinical observations of these bioenergetic schools of medical thought and practice over time. They have been held outside the realm of regular medical practice, partially because the mechanisms of action of these approaches have not been explained within the prevailing biomedical paradigm. Hypnosis is an example of an effective therapeutic modality with widespread effectiveness and acceptance within medicine. However, there remains no explanation for its mechanism of action. An alternative approach to explaining hypnosis has been developed on a statistical basis, describing the profiles of clients and conditions likely to benefit by developing "hypnotic susceptibility scales" (see Chapter 7). This same approach is potentially available for the clinical study of any therapeutic modality with observable outcomes even in the absence of an identified "mechanism of action." Application of the science of psychometrics provides an approach similar to that taken toward hypnosis, and has been successfully applied to a spectrum of "mind-body" approaches, as well as acupuncture (see Appendix I, pp. 572–579).

Concepts of mechanism of action are always bounded by the prevailing scientific paradigm and may not provide the most clinically useful questions. With the development of new scientific observations, a new paradigm may emerge that is more inclusive in its explanation of observed phenomena.

INDIVIDUAL PRACTITIONERS

In addition to the fairly widespread, organized schools of thought and practice, there are many intuitive healers whose practices are highly individualized and highly eclectic. These practitioners represent approaches used by many clients. The knowledge and practices of such gifted healers must be passed on or they will be lost. This situation in the contemporary United States may be seen as analogous to that of herbal remedies in the rainforest and regions of great biodiversity. Environmentalists are rightly concerned about the loss of biodiversity when unique plants disappear; ethno-botanists are concerned about the loss of the peoples whose cultural knowledge alone can convert the rain forest plants to cures. Much of this kind of knowledge is essentially intuitive as typically applies to individual practitioners of bioenergetic approaches.

EMPIRICAL ASSUMPTIONS OF BIOENERGETICS

1. The human body has a biophysical component.
2. What has been scientifically defined as the "mind" is biophysically linked to the human body.
3. Every part of the human body is biophysically linked to every other part of the body.

4. Mental states (thoughts, emotions) generate physiological responses in the human body through neurological, hormonal, and immunological mechanisms (psychoneuroimmunology).
5. Biophysically based modalities are noninvasive by currently measurable and clinically observable criteria.

ELECTROMAGNETIC RADIATION: LIGHT

IDENTITY OF LIGHT

Light has one identity as electromagnetic waves characterized by wavelengths of electromagnetic in the visual spectrum. Light also exists as tiny energy bundles, or photons. As discussed in previous chapters, light is paradoxically both a particle and a wave. Visible light, called the "visual spectrum" is electromagnetic radiation at wavelengths of 400 to 700 nanometers (nm) detected by the retina of the human eye. The retina is sensitive to approximately 90% of the spectrum of electromagnetic radiation that propagates through the atmosphere and reaches the Earth's surface. As a sensory organ, the eye developed to detect that portion of the electromagnetic spectrum that is there to be seen in the terrestrial environment. Because of the elevation of the path of the sun through the sky at different times of year (seasons) at different latitudes, beneficial and/or harmful wavelengths of radiation, such as ultraviolet light, may or may not penetrate the atmosphere. In the temperate zones of the planet (between the Arctic and Tropic Circles), the months and weeks around the equinoxes generally provide a good balance of healthful wavelengths without excessive harmful wavelengths of light passing through the atmosphere.

MEASURING LIGHT AND ITS ENERGY

The size of the waves of light (wavelengths) are typically measured in nanometers. One nanometer equals 1 billionth of a meter. According to Planck's law, the energy level is the inverse of the wavelength multiplied by the Planck constant. The shorter the wavelength and higher the energy, the greater the ability of light to penetrate tissues. For example, a blue-violet light (toward the ultraviolet side of the spectrum) has a shorter wavelength, and a red light (toward the infrared side of the spectrum) has a longer wavelength. Infrared light is even longer in wavelength (lower energy), and ultraviolet light is even shorter in wavelength (higher energy), than the visible spectrum. The high energy of ultraviolet light is the reason dermatologists are concerned that DNA-damaging ultraviolet light with a shorter wavelength and higher "ionizing" energy is dangerous. By contrast, we have the notion that using infrared light with a longer wavelength and lower energy for tanning is a "safer" form of exposure. (See "Human Photosynthesis: Light and Vitamin D.")

X-rays, gamma rays, ultraviolet rays, cosmic rays, and other EM radiation fall below visible light on the electromagnetic spectrum. Longer wavelengths such as infrared rays, microwaves, television signals, and FM/AM radio waves have different characteristics. Laser beams are a particular kind of amplified light. The atomic models that led to the discovery of lasers were conceptualized and developed in 1917 by Albert Einstein. His discovery became known as "LASER" for *l*ight *a*mplification by *s*timulated *e*mission of *r*adiation. When an atom is in an excited state and an incoming light particle reaches it, it may eject an additional photon instead of absorbing the particle. This theory was a revolutionary concept that proved to be true, and Einstein received the Nobel Prize for explaining the photoelectric effect. By 1960, the first practical ruby red laser was developed by Maiman, who used crystals and mirrors to produce a monochromatic, nondivergent light beam in which all waves were parallel and in phase (Maiman, 1960). These characteristics were subsequently referred to as "mono-chromaticity", "collimation", and "coherence", respectively. The original ruby red beam was a visible red light with a wavelength of 694 nm. Since then, various crystals and gases have been used to develop lasers in other regions of the electromagnetic spectrum, including infrared and visible-light lasers.

HEALING LIGHT

The application of light for medicinal purposes (healing) has been understood for thousands of years. The ancient Greeks observed that exposure to sunlight induced strength and health. During the Middle Ages, the disinfectant properties of sunlight were used to combat plague and other illnesses. During the 19th century, cutaneous tuberculosis (scrofula) was treated with ultraviolet light exposure and, more generally, exposure to light and sunshine as part of the popular nature cure for a wide range of ailments (see later). Currently, conventional light therapy is used to treat psoriasis, hyperbilirubinemia, seasonal affective disorder, and vitamin D deficiency.

HUMAN PHOTOSYNTHESIS: LIGHT AND VITAMIN D

One of the most salient aspects of the effects of light energy for human health is the photosynthesis of vitamin D in the skin. Although labeled as a vitamin, vitamin D behaves more like a hormone (with typical hormonal biochemical structure) throughout the body.

Although the biochemistry of vitamin D has been understood only relatively recently, it has been a part of biology for a very long time. A microorganism that is estimated to have lived in the oceans for 750 million years is able to synthesize vitamin D, which possibly makes vitamin D the oldest hormone on the planet.

It was recognized over 150 years ago that people, especially children, who lived and worked in dark urban areas where there was little light were susceptible to bone diseases such as rickets. In Boston in 1889, it was estimated that 80% of infants had rickets. This pattern marked a shift away from a US population that had been primarily engaged in agriculture (Thomas Jefferson's idea of an agrarian democracy) during the 1800s and exposed to plenty of light on the farms and in the fields. The lack of light in dank, dark urban environments was compounded by the lack of fresh foods and unavailability of food distribution.

At that time, it was noted that an extended visit to the country with clean air, clean water, abundant sunlight, and the benefits of nature would often cure medical disorders. Thus the idea of the nature cure was born. One of the many famous beneficiaries of the nature cure in the late 1800s was future president Theodore Roosevelt, who was well known for saying that he was literally "Dee-lighted" with any number of things, including the results of his cure for his lung disease. One of the most common lung diseases in the late 1800s was tuberculosis (TB). Sanitariums and solariums were created in wilderness areas away from the cities so that TB patients could benefit from the nature cure. Although no antibiotic treatments were available at that time, many patients with TB benefitted from exposure to nature, including sunlight.

As early as 1849, cod liver oil was also used in the treatment of TB, according to the Brompton Hospital Records, Volume 38 (Table 11.1).

We now know cod liver oil to be one of the few rich dietary sources of vitamin D. We also now know that vitamin D activates the immune system cells that can fight TB. So the nature cure of sun and fish oil, which delivered increased vitamin D, was the right treatment for the times.

The direct connection between sunlight and bone metabolism was also established in 1919 when Huldschinsky treated rickets with exposure to a mercury arc lamp. In 1921, Hess and Unger observed that sun exposure cured rickets.

In the 1930s medicine began to directly appreciate the connection between sunlight and the metabolic activities we now associate with vitamin D.

TABLE 11.1 *Historic Milestones in Recognition of the Relations Among Sunlight, Vitamin D Activity, and Health*

Year	Observation/Milestone	Vitamin D Pioneers
1849	Cod liver oil (vitamin D) treats tuberculosis	Brompton Hospital
1889	Nature cure treats rickets	Weir Mitchell, et al.
1919	Mercury arc lamp (ultraviolet B light) treats rickets	Huldschinsky
1921	Sun exposure cures rickets	Hess and Unger
1920s	Vitamin D discovered	Windaus
1920s	Vitamin D photosynthesized in laboratory	Windaus (Nobel Prize, 1928)
1940s	Sunlight protects against cancer	Apperly
1970	25-Hydroxyvitamin D3 isolated	Holick
1971	1,25-Dihydroxyvitamin D3 isolated	Holick
1979	Vitamin D receptors found	De Luca, et al.
1980	Vitamin D treats psoriasis	Holick, et al.
2002	Vitamin D regulates blood pressure	Li, et al.

This decade also saw the actual identification and labeling of the many metabolically active constituents we now call vitamins. Vitamin D was discovered in the early 1920s by Windaus, who was later awarded the Nobel Prize for synthesizing vitamin D in the laboratory by replicating the photo-activation process that occurs in the skin.

In the 1930s the federal government set up an agency to recommend to parents, especially those living in the Northeast, that they send their children outside to play and get some exposure to the sun.

The fortification of milk with vitamin D also began at that time. Unfortunately, the last 40 years have actually seen a reversal of some of the sensible public health recommendations regarding adequate vitamin D and sun exposure.

There Goes the Sun

Many physicians and public health organizations, including the biomedically oriented World Health Organization, have been trying to go one better on Moby Dick's Captain Ahab, who "would strike the sun if it insulted" him. For 40 years, there has been a concerted campaign to make people avoid sun exposure. Because ultraviolet B (UVB) light from the sun is responsible for the photo-activation of vitamin D in the skin, sunblockers that "protect" the skin also virtually eliminate photo-activation of vitamin D. A sunscreen with a sun protection factor (SPF) of 8 is supposed to absorb 92.5% of UVB light, whereas doubling the SPF to 16 absorbs 99%. This sun block essentially shuts down vitamin D production. (It also demonstrates that SPF formulations above 16 have little marginal utility and calls into question the appropriateness of the ever-increasing SPF numbers found on the pharmacy shelves.) People have become photophobic, and dermatologists have been on a campaign to "strike the sun."

A study in Australia, which has high levels of sunlight and high rates of skin cancer, found 100% of dermatologists to be deficient in vitamin D. In fact, most people should go outside in the sun for reasonable periods of time to get the many benefits of sunlight. It is always wise to protect the face and head with a hat and sunglasses, because less than 10% of UVB light absorption happens above the neck and the face is the most cosmetically sensitive. It is best to expose the entire body in a bathing suit for 10 to 15 minutes at least three times per week. African Americans require more sun exposure because their natural skin pigmentation provides an SPF equivalent of 8 to 15.

Health benefits of sunlight:
- Improves bone health
- Improves mental health
- Improves heart health
- Prevents many common cancers
- Alleviates skin disorders
- Decreases risk of autoimmune disorders
- Decreases risk of multiple sclerosis
- Decreases risk of diabetes

Global Dimensions of Deficiency

Essentially little or no active vitamin D is available from regular dietary sources. It is principally found in fish oils, sun-dried mushrooms, and fortified foods like milk and orange juice. However, many countries worldwide forbid the fortification of foods. There is potentially plenty of vitamin D in the food chain, because both phytoplankton and zooplankton exposed to sunlight make vitamin D. Wild-caught salmon, which feeds on natural food sources, for example, has available vitamin D. However, farmed salmon fed food pellets with little nutritional value have only 10% of the vitamin D of wild fish. The "perfect storm" of photophobia, lack of exposure to sunlight, and insufficiency of available dietary vitamin D has led to a national and worldwide epidemic of vitamin D deficiency.

Estimates are that at least 30% and as much as 80% of the US population is vitamin D deficient. In the United States, at latitudes north of Atlanta, the skin cannot make (photo-convert) any vitamin D from November through March (i.e., essentially outside of daylight saving time). During this season the angle of the sun in the sky is too low to allow UVB light to penetrate through the atmosphere, where it is absorbed by the ozone layer. Even in the late spring, summer, and early fall, most vitamin D is made between 10 a.m. and 3 p.m., when UVB from the sun penetrates the atmosphere and reaches the earth's surface.

It might be expected that vitamin D deficiency would be a problem limited to northern latitudes. In Bangor, Maine, among young girls 9 to 11 years old, nearly 50% were deficient at the end of winter and nearly 20% remained deficient at the end of summer. At Boston Children's Hospital, over 50% of adolescent girls and African American and Hispanic boys were found to be vitamin D deficient year round. In another study in Boston 34% of whites, 40% of Hispanics, and 84% of African American adults over age 50 were found to be deficient.

Vitamin D deficiency is also a national problem. The US Centers for Disease Control and Prevention completed a national survey at the end of winter and found that nearly 50% of African American women aged 15 to 49 years were deficient. These are women in the critical childbearing years. A growing fetus must receive adequate vitamin D from the mother, especially because breast milk does not provide adequate vitamin D. A study of pregnant women in Boston found that in 40 mother-infant pairs at the time of labor and delivery, over 75% of mothers and 80% of newborns were deficient. This observation was made despite the fact that pregnant women were instructed to take a prenatal vitamin that included 400 IU of vitamin D and to drink two glasses of milk per day.

Further, vitamin D deficiency is a global problem. Even in India, home to 1 billion of the earth's people, where there is plenty of sun, 30% to 50% of children, 50% to 80% of adults, and 90% of physicians are deficient. In South Africa, vitamin D deficiency is also a problem even though Cape Town is situated at 34 degrees latitude.

Although there are many new bilateral and multilateral governmental and private efforts to export Western medical technology and pharmaceuticals to the Third

World to combat infectious diseases such as AIDS, there is no comparable effort to acknowledge and address the global dimensions of the vitamin D deficiency epidemic. The US Congress and President deemed it as a great achievement to give $40 billion in tax dollars to US pharmaceutical companies to send expensive drug treatments for AIDS (a preventable disease) overseas. By contrast, addressing the vitamin D deficiency epidemic could be accomplished with much safer and less expensive nutritional supplements together with sunlight, the only source of energy that is still free.

EFFECTS OF LIGHT ON TISSUES

Every object has optical properties that determine the effectiveness of light and the interaction of light with that object. For example, the light from mid-infrared and far-infrared lasers, such as carbon dioxide, holmium, and yttrium-aluminum-garnet (yag) lasers, is primarily absorbed by water in the tissues. This absorption of the infrared light energy produces heat, which leads to local vaporization that does not spread to adjacent tissues.

The light from near-infrared and visible-light lasers such as neodymium and argon lasers is poorly absorbed by water, but is rapidly absorbed by pigments such as hemoglobin and melanin. This optical property makes these lasers effective in the heat ablation of tissues that are rich in pigment, such as retina, gastric mucosa, and pigmented cutaneous lesions. These so-called "high-powered" surgical lasers, using heat and energy, lead to highly specific and targeted tissue changes.

Over the past 30 years, numerous animal and laboratory experiments have been carried out using these high-energy lasers. These experiments produced results that ultimately led to human testing and approval by the US Food and Drug Administration (FDA) for the use of lasers in humans. Despite more than 30 years of similar experiments using weak or low-level nonthermal lasers, there remains controversy concerning the effectiveness of low-level laser therapy (LLLT) as a treatment modality because of a lack of randomized, double-blind, placebo-controlled trials and publication of findings in peer-reviewed journals. Various articles have made claims, but the studies reported by many have flawed methodology, use different time and dosage schedules, and do not have a strict placebo-controlled design. Despite all these shortcomings, several investigations were brought to the attention of the FDA. In 2002 the FDA approved an application for the use of laser light as a therapeutic device for pain relief.

Tissue Optical Properties and Pain

Musculoskeletal tissues appear to have optical properties that respond to light between 500 and 1000 nm. Sufficient specific laser dosages and the numbers of treatments needed are still the subject of investigation. It is hypothesized that light-sensitive organelles, or chromatophores, absorb light (Walsh, 1997) and that ultimately the energy produces a biological reaction. It has been suggested that chromatophores are present on the myelin sheath or nerves and in mitochondria of cells. It is proposed that monochromatic wavelength properties, rather than the coherency and collimation of laser light, induce biological changes. It is presumed that the collimation and coherency lead to rapid degradation by scatter. Others have theorized that the primary tissue photoreceptors are flavins and porphyrins. Thus, therapeutic benefits for pain reduction that are produced by a combination of red and near-infrared light is caused by an increase in β-endorphins, blocking depolarization of C-fiber afferents, reduction in bradykinin levels, and ionic channel stabilization.

Biostimulation

Cold laser therapy, or LLLT, is based on the idea that monochromatic light energy, which depends on its wavelength for tissue penetration, can alter cellular functions. The original European studies on wound healing in animals yielded positive results, and the technique was described as "biostimulation." Mester, Toth, and Mester (1982) and Lyons et al. (1987) found that light could be stimulatory at low power and could elicit an opposite inhibitory effect at higher power. In addition, the cumulative dosages of the radiation could sometimes be inhibitory. Today, a variety of lasers are available. The two most popular are helium-neon (HeNe) (632 nm) and gallium-aluminum-arsenide (GaAlAs) (830 nm). In practice, these visible and infrared lasers have powers of 30 to 90 mW and deliver from 1 to 9 J/cm^2 to tissue treatment sites. To date, they have been shown to be safe within this range. They have also been used at higher doses.

Since tissue penetration depends on the wavelength (energy), the shorter wavelength (higher energy) HeNe laser beam (632 nm) penetrates several millimeters into tissue. The GaAlAs (830 nm) at 30 mW allows photons to penetrate more than 3 cm. Several authors have stated that an infrared laser beam travels about 2 mm into tissue and that this represents one penetration depth with a loss of 1/e (37%) of beam intensity (Basford, 1998). However, the shorter visible HeNe red beam is attenuated the same amount in 0.5 to 1 mm (Anderson & Parrish, 1981; Basford, 1995; Kolari, 1985).

Therefore, in addition to the energy of the light beam corresponding to the wavelength, the energy intensity drops off as the beam passes deeper into tissue. How does one measure the decay in the amount of energy with distance? At the surface of the skin, the laser delivers from 1 to 9 J/cm^2. Karu (1987) demonstrated that light of 0.01 J/cm^2 can alter cellular processes. As a result, approximately six penetration depths (3 to 6 mm for HeNe red light and about 24 mm for GaAlAs infrared light) are possible before the strength of the beam stream drops from 9 J/cm^2 to 0.01 J/cm^2. Thus, the threshold and specific therapeutic amount needed for stimulation differs for the superficial nerves and tissues and for the deeper structures. There is also a scattering of energy that influences non-neural adjacent tissues (i.e., flexor tendons in the forearm and wrist with stimulation at the level of the carpal tunnel).

Tissue Penetration, Pain, and Thresholds

Tissue penetration and tissue saturation with pulsed frequency settings of 1 to 100 Hz are key elements that influence pain and neuralgia. A setting of 1000 Hz was observed to influence edema and swelling, and 5000 Hz influenced inflammation.

Light from a super-pulsed laser using a gallium arsenide (GaAs) infrared diode provides the deepest penetration in body tissues. It operates at a wavelength of 904 nm. Super-pulsing is defined as the generation of continuous bursts of very-high-power pulses of light energy (10–100 watts) of extremely short duration (100–200 nanoseconds). This approach allows GaAs penetration to tissue depths of 3 to 5 cm and deeper. Some versions of GaAs therapeutic lasers actually penetrate to tissue depths of 10 to 14 cm (Kneebone, 2007). There have been many claims and studies regarding laser therapy, and the varied quality of trials has led to controversy. Basford (1986, 1995, 1998) was a major critic of the deficiencies of many studies, and noted that research on cold laser, LLLT, has developed along the following three separate lines:

1. Cellular functions.
2. Animal models.
3. Human trials.

Effects on Cellular Functions

Perhaps the strongest and most well-established research has been on changes in cellular functions. There is a strong body of direct evidence indicating that LLLT can significantly alter cellular processes. The following are specific areas of treatment in which benefits have been claimed:

- Stimulation of collagen formation leading to stronger scars (Mester, Mester, & Mester, 1985), increased recruitment of fibroblasts and formation of granulation tissue (Mester & Jaszsagi-Nagy, 1973), increased neovascularization (Mester et al., 1982), and faster wound healing (Lam et al., 1986; Lyons et al., 1987; Rochkind, Barrnea, Razon, Bartal, & Schwartz, 1987).
- Pain relief and reduced firing frequency of nociceptors (Mezawa, Iwata, Naito, & Kamogawa, 1988).
- Enhanced remodeling and repair of bone (Rochkind et al., 1987; Walsh, 1997)
- Stimulation of endorphin release (Yamada, 1991).
- Modulation of the immune system via prostaglandin synthesis (Kubasova, Kovacs, & Somosy, 1984; Mester et al., 1982).

Basic animal and cellular research with red-beam, low-level lasers has produced both positive and negative results. Passarella (1989) believed that the optical properties of cellular mitochondria are influenced by HeNe laser irradiation, with new mitochondrial conformations produced that ultimately lead to increased oxygen consumption. Walker (1983) suggested that HeNe laser light affects serotonin metabolism. Yu, Naim, McGowan, Ippolito, and Lanzafame (1997) demonstrated an increased phosphate potential and energy charge with light exposure. Further research continues at the cellular level. Fibroblast, lymphocyte, monocyte, and macrophage cells have been studied, and bacterial cell lines of *Escherichia coli* have served as models for investigation (Karu, 1988). The most popular laser in such cellular research has been the HeNe laser with a wavelength of 632.8 nm. However, some major discrepancies have been found in the results reported in existing literature related to the wide variation in the laser parameters employed, particularly dosages and treatment times. Imprecise dosimetry has clouded the issues. The optimal dose for achieving biological benefits has yet to be definitively determined.

ANIMAL MODELS

Notwithstanding a lack of standardization, controls, and imprecise dose and treatment schedules for in vivo experimental work, results from cellular research have been extrapolated to research on animals. Subsequently, a wide variety of animal models have been employed to assess the biostimulatory effects of laser irradiation on wound healing. Small, loose-skinned rodents such as mice, rats, and guinea pigs have been used most often, but studies using pig models have led to different results. It has been argued that pigskin represents a more suitable model for extrapolation to humans, because it is similar in character to human skin, which has led to its use in human skin grafts, for example (Basford, 1986; Hunter, Leonard, Wilson, Snider, & Dixon, 1984).

Baxter (1997) provides an excellent review of the animal models used in the wound-healing literature. The details of experimental and irradiation procedures are numerous and variable. Reproduction of results and intertrial comparisons are usually not practical. Research groups have reported either acceleration in healing or no effect on the healing process. Two criteria frequently used to assess wound healing are collagen content and tensile strength. Rochkind et al. (1989) conducted one of the largest series of controlled animal trials, comparing the recovery of LLLT-treated crushed sciatic nerves with that of nonirradiated nerves in rats. Constant low-intensity laser irradiation ($7.6-10 \, \text{J/cm}^2$ daily for up to 20 days) demonstrated highly beneficial effects as judged from recordings of compound action potentials. Wound-healing rates in both irradiated and nonirradiated wounds were accelerated. However, the amplitude of nerve action potentials in crushed sciatic nerves was raised substantially only in the irradiated groups. The laser treatment also greatly reduced the degeneration of motor neurons, which suggested that these results might be extrapolated for application in human research trials.

The information gained from trials of in vivo animal exposure to laser photo-biostimulation indicated that wound healing could be achieved. However, variations existed in methodology, techniques, dosimetry, exposure time, and frequency of treatments.

HUMAN TRIALS

Many clinicians have been persuaded by the cellular and animal data to conduct human trials. A number of pain disorders, including neurological, rheumatological, and musculoskeletal conditions, have been treated with LLLT with various results. The FDA had previously been a major obstacle because of the absence of randomized, placebo-controlled trials and the varying methodology, dosages and techniques, and the absence of objective parameters. However, as mentioned earlier, in February 2002 it approved the application for the use of LLLT for pain relief. Research studies on various specific pain conditions are described subsequently.

Laser acupuncture using a HeNe diode was reported to be successful in the treatment of experimentally induced arthritis in rats. Vocalization and limb withdrawal in response to noxious stimulation were the parameters measured (Zhu, Li, Ji, & Li, 1990). As noted earlier, Naeser, Hahn, and Lieberman (1996) and Branco and Naeser (1999) were successful in applying this procedure to treatment of carpal tunnel syndrome. Similarly, Weintraub (1997) saw additional improvement when he combined Naeser's acupressure points with his protocol in treating this syndrome.

One of the major economic burdens in the United States has been caused by the high incidence of soft-tissue injuries and low back pain and subsequent work disability. Numerous studies using HeNe and infrared laser diodes (830-nm range) have reported varying results (Basford, 1986, 1995; Gam, Thorsen, & Lonnberg, 1993; Klein & Eek, 1990), but randomized, controlled, and blinded studies have been difficult to carry out.

ARTHRITIS PAIN

Rheumatologists in the United States have had encouraging results in laser treatment of rheumatoid arthritis (Goldman et al., 1980). Similar results have been reported in the Soviet Union/Russia, Eastern Europe, and Japan. Walker, Akhanjee, and Cooney (1986) reported success after a 10-week course of treatment with HeNe lasers. Using a GaAlAs 830-nm laser, Asada, Yutani, and Shimazu (1989) found 90% improvement in an uncontrolled trial in 170 patients with rheumatoid arthritis. Despite these generally positive results, Bliddal, Hellesen, Ditlevsen, Asselberghs, and Lyager (1987) did not see any significant change in symptoms of morning stiffness or joint function in such patients. Improvement was noted in pain scale ratings. Similar positive results for laser therapy have been reported for osteoarthritis pain and other conditions. Critics have argued, however, that because rheumatoid arthritis is inherently a disease of exacerbation and remission, it is difficult to assess the efficacy of the therapy over the short term.

CARPAL TUNNEL SYNDROME

Carpal tunnel syndrome is a common clinical disorder, seen in 5% to 10% of the population, caused by compression of the median nerve at the wrist. Acroparesthesia (numbness, tingling, and burning) in the first three fingers often arises and may interfere with sleep. When resistant to conservative treatment, the disorder often progresses, with weakness and atrophy. There are nine flexor tendons adjacent to the median nerve, and they often intersect the nerve fascicles in the carpal tunnel. Thus, nerve compression or tendinitis may serve as a cause.

Basford et al. (1993), using laser light of only 1 J of energy, found that both sensory and motor distal latencies could be significantly decreased in normal volunteers. Basford et al.'s study was a double-blind controlled trial using a GaAlAs percutaneous laser. Weintraub (1997) used a similar laser at higher energy levels of 9 J and measured compound motor nerve action potential/sensory nerve action potential electrophysiological parameters. He reported a nearly 80% success rate in resolving the symptoms of carpal tunnel syndrome with laser therapy. There were no control subjects in the study, but almost 1000 sensory and motor nerve latencies were analyzed before and after each treatment in a cross-over design. Distal latency was prolonged in 40% of subjects, yet they remained asymptomatic. This prolonged latency suggests that non-neural tissues were stimulated and could be responsible for symptoms of tendonitis. At the dose used, a significant number of individuals showed immediate prolongation of distal latency (nerve conduction). They remained asymptomatic, however, and by the next visit, the distal latency was back to baseline or improved. A similar observation has also been made by others (Snyder-Mackler & Bork, 1988). In addition, several reports of studies using higher doses of 10 to 12 J of infrared laser light (40 to 50 mW) revealed alterations in conduction in both the median and superficial radial nerves (Baxter, Walsh, Allen, Lowe, & Bell, 1994; Bork & Snyder-Mackler, 1988; Walsh, Baxter, & Allen, 1991).

Naeser et al. (1996) and Branco and Naeser (1999) used a combination of two noninvasive, painless treatment modalities—red-beam laser and microampere-level transcutaneous electrical nerve stimulation (TENS)—to stimulate acupuncture points on the hand of patients with carpal tunnel syndrome or wrist pain. Sham treatments were used as a control. A significant reduction in median nerve sensory latencies in the treated hand and a 92% reduction in pain were observed. Postoperative failures also decreased with this protocol. A laser treatment protocol ($9 J/cm^2$) also stimulated various acupressure points (Naeser et al., 1996; Branco & Naeser, 1999), as well as the flexor tendons in the upper wrist. Up to 85% improvement in wrist pain was achieved in patients with carpal tunnel syndrome.

NERVE PAIN

Superficial nerves also respond to laser biostimulation. Disorders such as meralgia paresthetica, cubital tunnel syndrome, tarsal tunnel syndrome, radial nerve palsy, and traumatic digital neuralgias have responded to this treatment (Weintraub, 1997; Padua, Padua, & Aprile, 1998). Because of the small number of individuals treated, these observations are considered anecdotal. However, Weintraub believes that his observations that non-neural structures play an important yet unappreciated role in symptomatic carpal tunnel syndrome, and probably other nerve entrapments, are indeed significant. For example, the distal latency of the median nerve could be longer than 5 ms in patients who have become asymptomatic with laser treatment. Either a threshold exists for the median nerve or the tendons and blood vessels surrounding the median nerve exert some influence. Franzblau and Werner (1999) raised similar issues in a provocative editorial titled, "What Is Carpal Tunnel Syndrome?"

LOW BACK PAIN

Low back pain syndrome is the most common cause of pain and disability in the United States, affecting 75% to 85% of Americans at some point in their lifetimes. Low back pain provides an example where a host of noninvasive, nonsurgical therapies have been shown to be more effective and cost-effective, such as spinal manual therapy, acupuncture, bodywork and massage, physical therapy, active herbal ingredients for joints, such as Ashwaganda, Bosewellia, and Curcumin (see Chapter 23) as well as biophysical modalities. Common causes include herniated disks, spinal stenosis, spondylosis, facet joint dysfunction, and failed back syndrome secondary to surgery. As with chronic neck pain, the small C-nociceptive afferents and A delta fibers are involved, with localized chemical dysfunction producing altered signal transduction. Use of a high-output GaAlAs infrared laser at 9 J/cm, and/or a GaAs super-pulsed infrared laser, may be effective in treating the deeper tissues. Usually the nerve irritation occurs deep, around 60 mm, secondary to a herniated disk. Acupressure point stimulation may also be used concurrently.

LOWER LIMB PAIN

Meralgia paresthetica is an often disabling symptom caused by compression of the lateral anterior femoral cutaneous nerve at the level of the inguinal ligament. Weintraub treated 10 patients with this condition by applying laser stimulation from the level of the inguinal ligament to the level of the knee anterolaterally. Significant pain reduction was noted in 8 of the 10 patients by the fourth treatment, but there have been recurrences. The soles of the feet and various acupressure points were stimulated by laser without providing relief in 10 cases of nondiabetic peripheral neuropathy. The use of monochromatic infrared and visible light phototherapy to treat diabetic peripheral neuropathy has been reported to be successful in inducing temporary or permanent relief from pain and inflammation (Leonard, Farooqi, & Myers, 2004).

MIGRAINE HEADACHE
Cerebral Circulation, Auditory and Vestibular Function

Application of laser light to the hegu point on the side of the head contralateral to the pain may be effective for treating migraine headaches. Treatment with an intraoral HeNe laser directed along the zone of maxillary alveolar tenderness also achieves success in the range of 78%. Stimulation is repeated three times at intervals of 1 minute to 90 seconds.

Weintraub has achieved benefit by stimulating naguien acupressure points with an 830-nm laser. Naeser (1999), in a review of the highlights of the Second Congress of the World Association for Laser Therapy, reported that Wilden treated inner ear disorders, including vertigo, tinnitus, and hearing loss, with a combination of 630- to 700-nm and 830-nm lasers. The total dose was at least 4000 J. Daily 1-hour laser treatments to both ears were performed for at least 3 weeks. The lasers were applied to the auditory canal and the mastoid and petrosal bones. Wilden said that he used this approach for more than 9 years in 800 patients, and except in very severe cases, most patients reported improvement in hearing.

Naeser et al. (1995) improved blood flow in stroke patients using laser acupuncture treatment and noted improvement in symptoms.

NECK PAIN

Chronic neck pain is common and is often associated specifically with a herniated disc, degenerative disc disease, degenerative spine disease, spinal stenosis, or facet joint dysfunction. The small C-nociceptive afferents and the larger myelinated A delta fibers usually innervate these areas. Local chemical dysfunction with release of substance P, phospholipase A, cytokines, nitric oxide, and so on is probably also involved. It is theorized that direct photoreception by cytochromes produces elevated production of adenosine triphosphate and changes in cell membrane permeability. Anti-edema affects and anti-inflammatory responses have been alleged to occur in response to laser therapy through reduction in bradykinin levels and increase in β-endorphin levels. Both the depth of penetration and the total dose influence the success of the laser treatment at the target tissue level. Thus, combinations of high-output (centiwatt) GaAlAs and GaAs (super-pulsing) lasers can achieve penetration of 3 to 5 cm and even deeper (10 to 14 cm). In addition, acupressure point stimulation (2 to 4 J of energy) to the ear, hand, or body should be used.

NEURALGIA AND PAIN SYNDROMES

The efficacy of laser therapy in treating various pain syndromes has been investigated by several groups. Preliminary double-blind studies by Walker (1983) demonstrated improvement in seven out of nine patients with trigeminal neuralgia. Two out of five patients with post-herpetic neuralgia showed improvement, and five out of six patients with radiculopathy improved. Baxter, Bell, Allen, and Ravey (1991) also believed that laser therapy was effective for post-herpetic neuralgia. Moore, Hira, Kumar, Jaykumar, and Oshiro (1988) investigated the efficacy of GaAlAs laser therapy in the treatment of post-herpetic neuralgia in a double-blind, crossover trial involving 20 patients. The result was an apparently significant reduction in pain. Hong, Kim, and Lim (1990) validated these results in their study, in which 60% of patients with post-herpetic neuralgia felt improvement within 10 minutes. Trigeminal neuralgia was successfully treated with HeNe laser by Walker et al. (1986). In the 35 patients studied in this double-blind, placebo-controlled trial, a significant difference was found in visual analogue scale pain ratings between patients receiving active laser treatment and placebo-treated patients.

Friedman, Weintraub, and Forman (1994) used an intraoral HeNe laser directed at a specific maxillary alveolar tender point to significantly abort atypical facial pain. Using an intraoral HeNe laser directed at a specific maxillary alveolar tender point, Weintraub (1996) was able to abort acute migraine headaches in 85% of cases in a study that included a sham-treatment control condition. These findings support the trigeminovascular theory of migraine with a maxillary (V2) provocative site. The results achieved rival those of pharmacotherapy. Interestingly, Friedman

(1998) used cryotherapy (cold water) applied to the same maxillary alveolar tender point to treat atypical facial pain and migraine headache. The treatment produced a striking reduction in discomfort.

Several groups have investigated the efficacy of laser therapy in the treatment of radicular and pseudoradicular pain syndromes. Bieglio and Bisschop (1986) and Mizekami et al. (1990) reported positive effects in treating these conditions. Low-power laser therapy has also been used successfully to induce preoperative anesthesia in both veterinary practice and dental surgery (Christensen, 1989). In contrast to the numerous clinical human studies of laser-mediated analgesia, there have been relatively few laboratory studies. Most of the experiments have been completed in China in a variety of animals, including rats, goats, rabbits, sheep, and horses. There are no English abstracts or translations of most of these works. Other studies in animals that were published in English and used tail-flick methodology to assess pain have reported variable findings.

SPORTS INJURIES

A number of reports document the apparent efficacy of laser therapy in reducing pain associated with sports injuries. These reports initially came from Russia and Eastern Europe. The results were subsequently confirmed by Morselli et al. (1985) and Emmanoulidis and Diamantopoulos (1986). It is notable that in the latter study, improvement was accompanied by a decrease in thermographic readings.

The use of laser therapy to treat tendinopathies, especially lateral humeral epicondylitis (tennis elbow), has been studied by numerous groups. There has usually been a relatively rapid response to therapy; however, Haker and Lundberg (1990) failed to show any effect of laser acupuncture treatment on tennis elbow.

SAFETY

No detrimental effects are produced by low-output, nonthermal lasers, although direct retinal exposure is to be avoided. Pregnancy does not appear to be a contraindication with LLLT, but investigators have been advised to avoid treating pregnant women and individuals with local tumors in the area of treatment. Individuals who are taking photosensitizing drugs such as tetracycline or who have photosensitive skin should probably avoid this treatment. It has also been suggested that the use of phototherapy after steroid injections is contraindicated, because anti-inflammatory medication is well documented to reduce the effectiveness of photo-biostimulation (Lopes et al., 2006).

Medicine is faced with many pain conditions that respond poorly or marginally to pharmacological therapy in addition to the side effects inherent. Thus, there is appeal of noninvasive therapeutic laser and other phototherapy devices that are both effective and safe. They are an addition to the physician's armamentarium. Therapeutic laser treatment has been used successfully in a number of fields and is a popular modality worldwide. Critical analysis of the literature indicates that the majority of studies suffer from methodological flaws such as the absence of controls, and variable duration and intensity of laser treatment. Consequently, many observations are to be considered anecdotal pending more appropriate randomized control trials. In the interim, laser therapy appears to be safe and worthy of further investigation for the management of pain and other medical conditions.

REFERENCES

Anderson, R. R. & Parrish, J. A. (1981). The optics of human skin. *Journal of Investigative Dermatology,* 77, 13–19.

Asada, K., Yutani, Y., & Shimazu, A. (1989). Diode laser therapy for rheumatoid arthritis: A clinical evaluation of 102 joints treated with low reactive laser therapy (LLLT). *Laser Therapy, 1,* 147–151.

Basford, J. (1986). Low-energy laser treatment of pain and wounds: Hype, hokum? *Mayo Clinic Proceedings, 61,* 671–675.

Basford, J. R. (1995). Low intensity laser therapy: Still not an established tool. *Lasers in Surgery and Medicine, 16,* 331–342.

Basford, J. (April 27, 1998). Laser therapy. Minneapolis: Paper presented at the 50th annual meeting of the American Academy of Neurology.

Basford, J. R., Hallman, H. O., Matsumoto, J. Y., Moyer, S. K., Buss, J. M., & Baxter, J. D. (1993). Effects of 830 nm continuous wave laser diode irradiation on median nerve function in normal subjects. *Lasers in Surgery and Medicine, 13,* 597–604.

Baxter, G. D. (1997). *Therapeutic lasers: Theory and practice.* New York: Churchill Livingstone.

Baxter, G. D., Bell, A. J., Allen, J. M., & Ravey, J. (1991). Low level laser therapy: Current clinical practice in Northern Ireland. *Physiotherapy, 77,* 171–178.

Baxter, G. D., Walsh, D. M., Allen, J. M., Lowe, A. S., & Bell, A. J. (1994). Effects of low intensity infrared laser irradiation upon conduction in the human median nerve in vivo. *Experimental Physiology, 79,* 227–234.

Bieglio, C. & Bisschop, C. (1986). Physical treatment for radicular pain with low-power laser stimulation. *Lasers in Surgery and Medicine, 6,* 173.

Bliddal, H., Hellesen, C., Ditlevsen, P., Asselberghs, J., & Lyager, L. (1987). Soft laser therapy of rheumatoid arthritis. *Scandinavian Journal of Rheumatology, 16,* 225–228.

Bork, C. E. & Snyder-Mackler, L. (1988). Effect of helium-neon laser irradiation on peripheral sensory nerve latency. *American Physical Therapy Association, 68,* 223.

Branco, K. & Naeser, M. A. (1999). Carpal tunnel syndrome: Clinical outcome after low-level laser acupuncture, microamps transcutaneous electrical nerve stimulation and other alternative therapies: an open protocol study. *Journal of Alternative and Complementary Medicine, 5,* 5–26.

Christensen, P. (1989). Clinical laser treatment of odontological conditions. In J. Kert & L. Rose (Eds.), *Clinical laser therapy: low level laser therapy.* Copenhagen: Scandinavian Medical Laser Technology.

Emmanoulidis, O. & Diamantopoulos, C. (1986). CW IR Low-power laser applications significantly accelerates chronic pain relief rehabilitation of professional athletes: A double-blind study. *Lasers in Surgery and Medicine, 6,* 173.

Franzblau, A. & Werner, R. A. (1999). What is carpal tunnel syndrome? *Journal of American Medical Association, 282,* 186–187.

Friedman, M. H. (1998). Intra-oral maxillary chilling: A non-invasive treatment in acute migraine and tension-type headache treatment. *Headache Quarterly, Current Treatment and Research, 9,* 274.

Friedman, M. H., Weintraub, M. I., & Forman, S. (1994). Atypical facial pain: A localized maxillary nerve disorder? *American Journal of Pain Management, 4,* 149–152.

Gam, A. N., Thorsen, H., & Lonnberg, F. (1993). The effect of low-level laser therapy on musculoskeletal pain: A meta-analysis. *Pain, 52,* 63–66.

Goldman, J. A., Chiapella, J., Casey, H., Bass, N., Graham, J., McClatchey, W., et al. (1980). Laser therapy of rheumatoid arthritis. *Lasers in Surgery and Medicine, 1,* 93–101.

Haker, E. & Lundberg, T. (1990). Laser treatment applied to acupuncture point in lateral humeral epicondylalgia: A double-blind study. *Pain, 43,* 243–248.

Hong, J. N., Kim, T. H., & Lim, S. D. (1990). Clinical trial of low reactive level laser therapy in 20 patients with post-herpetic neuralgia. *Laser Therapy, 2,* 167–170.

Hunter, J., Leonard, L., Wilson, R., Snider, G., & Dixon, J. (1984). Effects of low energy laser on wound healing in a porcine model. *Lasers in Surgery and Medicine, 3,* 285–290.

Karu, T. I. (1987). Photobiological fundamentals of low power laser therapy. *IEEE Journal of Quantum Electronics, QE-23,* 1703–1717.

Karu, T. I. (1988). Molecular mechanisms of the therapeutic effect of low intensity laser irradiation. *Lasers in the Life Sciences, 2,* 53–74.

Klein, R. G. & Eek, B. C. (1990). Low-energy laser treatment and exercise for chronic low back pain: Double-blind control trial. *Archives of Physical Medicine and Rehabilitation, 71,* 34–37.

Kneebone, W. J. (2007). Treatment of chronic neck pain utilizing low-level laser therapy. *Practical Pain Management,* 64–66.

Kolari, P. J. (1985). Penetration of unfocused laser light into the skin. *Archives of Dermatological Research, 277,* 342–344.

Kubasova, T., Kovacs, L., & Somosy, Z. (1984). Biological effect of He-Ne laser investigations on functional and micromorphological alterations of cell membranes, in vitro. *Lasers in Surgery and Medicine, 4,* 381–388.

Lam, T. S., Abergel, R. P., Meeker, C. A., Castel, J. C., Dwyer, R. M., & Uitto, J. (1986). Laser stimulation of collagen synthesis in human skin fibroblast cultures. *Lasers in the Life Sciences, 1,* 61–77.

Lanzl, L. H., Rozenfeld, M., & Wootton, P. (2003). The radiation therapy dosimetry network in the United States. *Medical Physics, 30*(10), 2762–2792.

Leonard, D. R., Farooqi, M. H., & Myers, S. (2004). Restoration of sensation, reduced pain and improved balance in subjects with diabetic peripheral neuropathy: A double-blind, randomized, placebo-controlled study with monochromatic near-infra-red treatment. *Diabetes Care, 27,* 168–172.

Lopes, A., Albertini, R., Lopes-Martins, P. S. L., Aimbire, F., Neto, H.C.C.F., & Iversen, V. (2006). Steroid receptor antagonist mifepristone inhibits the anti-inflammatory effect of photoradiation. *Photomedicine and Laser Surgery, 24,* 197–201.

Lyons, R. F., Abergel, R. P., White, R. A., Dwyer, R. M., Caste, J. C., & Uitto, J. (1987). Biostimulation of wound healing in vivo by a helium-neon laser. *Annals of Plastic Surgery, 18,* 47–50.

Maiman, T. H. (1960). Stimulated optical radiation in ruby. *Nature, 187,* 493–494 (letter).

Mester, E. & Jaszsagi-Nagy, E. (1973). The effect of laser radiation on wound healing and collagen synthesis. *Studia Biophysica, 35,* 227–230.

Mester, E., Mester, A. F., & Mester, A. (1985). The biomedical effects of laser applications. *Lasers in Surgery and Medicine, 5,* 31–39.

Mester, E., Toth, N., & Mester, A. (1982). The biostimulative effect of laser beam. *Laser Basic Biomededical Research, 22,* 4–7.

Mezawa, S., Iwata, K., Naito, K., & Kamogawa, H. (1988). The possible analgesic effect of soft-laser irradiation on heat nociceptors in the cat tongue. *Archives of Oral Biology, 33,* 693–694.

Micozzi, M. S. (Ed.). (2015). *Fundamentals of complementary and alternative medicine,* (5th ed.). (pp. 213–239). St Louis: Elsevier Health Sciences/Saunders.

Mizekami, T., Yoshii, N., Uhikubo, Y., Sato, T., Iwabuchi, S., Aoki, K., et al. (1990). Effect of diode laser for pain: A clinical study on different pain types. *Laser Therapy, 2,* 171–174.

Moore, K. C., Hira, N., Kumar, P. S., Jaykumar, C. S., & Oshiro, T. (July, 1988). A double-blind crossover trial of low level laser therapy in the treatment of post-herpetic neuralgia. *Lasers in Medical Science, 301* (abstract).

Morselli. (1985). Very low energy-density treatment by CO_2 laser in sports medicine. *Lasers in Surgery and Medicine, 5,* 150.

Naeser, M. A. (1999). Review of second congress: World Association for Laser Therapy (WALT) meeting. *Journal of Alternative and Complementary Medicine, 5,* 177–180.

Naeser, M. A., Alexander, M. P., Stiassny-Eder, D., Galler, V., Hobbs, J., Bachman, D., et al. (1995). Laser acupuncture in the treatment of paralysis in stroke patients: A CT scan lesion site study. *American Journal of Acupuncture, 23,* 13–28.

Naeser, M. A., Hahn, K. K., & Lieberman, B. (1996). Real vs. sham laser acupuncture and microamps TENS to treat carpal tunnel syndrome and worksite wrist pain: pilot study. *Lasers in Surgery and Medicine*, (Suppl. 8), 7.

Padua, L., Padua, R., & Aprile, I. (1998). Noninvasive laser neurolysis in carpal tunnel syndrome. *Muscle & Nerve, 21,* 1232–1233.

Passarella, S. (1989). HeNe laser irradiation of isolated mitochondria. *Journal of Photochemistry and Photobiology, 31,* 642–643.

Rochkind, S., Barrnea, L., Razon, N., Bartal, A., & Schwartz, M. (1987). Stimulating effect of HeNe low dose laser on injured sciatic nerves of rats. *Neurosurgery, 20,* 843–847.

Rochkind, S., Rousso, M., Nissan, M., Villarreal, M., Barr-Nea, L., & Rees, D. G. (1989). Systemic effects of low-power laser irradiation on the peripheral and central nervous system, cutaneous wounds and burns. *Lasers in Surgery and Medicine, 9,* 174–182.

Snyder-Mackler, L. & Bork, C. E. (1988). Effect of helium-neon laser irradiation on peripheral sensory nerve latency. *Physical Therapy, 68,* 223–225.

Walker, J. B. (1983). Relief from chronic pain by low-power laser irradiation. *Neuroscience Letters, 43,* 339–344.

Walker, J. B., Akhanjee, L. K., & Cooney, M. M. (1986). Laser therapy for pain of rheumatoid arthritis. *Lasers in Surgery and Medicine, 6,* 171.

Walsh, J. (1997). The current status of low level laser therapy in dentistry: Part I—Soft tissue applications. *Australian Dental Journal, 42,* 247–254.

Walsh, D. M., Baxter, G. K., & Allen, J. M. (1991). *The effect of 820 nm laser upon nerve conduction in the superficial radial nerve.* London: Abstract presented at fifth International Biotherapy Laser Association Meeting.

Weintraub, M. I. (1996). Migraine: A maxillary nerve disorder? A novel therapy: Preliminary results. *American Journal of Pain Management, 6,* 77–82.

Weintraub, M. I. (1997). Non-invasive laser neurolysis in carpal tunnel syndrome. *Muscle & Nerve, 20,* 1029–1031.

Yamada, K. (1991). Biological effects of low-power laser irradiation on clonal osteoblastic cells (MC3T-E1). *Nippon Siekeigeka Gakkai Zasshi, 65,* 787–799.

Yu, W., Naim, J. O., McGowan, M., Ippolito, K., & Lanzafame, R. J. (1997). Photomodulation of oxidative metabolism and electron chain enzymes in rat liver mitochondria. *Photochemistry and Photobiology, 66,* 866–871.

Zhu, L., Li, C., Ji, C., & Li, W. (1990). The effect of laser irradiation on arthritis in rats. *Pain, 5*(1), 385.

Chapter 12

Spinal Manual Therapy and Chiropractic

Spinal manipulation has been practiced for centuries among cultures throughout the world and has included prominent figures in the history of medicine. In the United States, its formal practice was established by a 19th-century "magnetic healer" originating from the historical traditions described in Chapter 10.

Hippocrates was an early practitioner of spinal manipulation (Withington, 1959), and according to some scholars, he used manipulation "not only to reposition vertebrae, but also thereby to cure a wide variety of dysfunctions" (Leach, 1994). Galen was a Greek-born Roman physician who lived in the 2nd century AD. His approach to healing set a recognized standard in Western medicine for 1500 years after his death. He also used spinal manipulation and reported the successful resolution of a patient's hand weakness and numbness through manipulation of the seventh cervical vertebra (Lomax, 1975).

When Europe entered the Middle Ages, these healing traditions were preserved in the learning centers of the Middle East by the ascendant Arabic civilization. This body of knowledge returned to Europe, and the preserved works of Hippocrates and Galen, together with new insights from Avicenna (Ib'n Sina) and Unani Medicine (Abu-Asab, Amri, & Micozzi, 2013) helped form the foundations of Renaissance medicine. Ambroise Paré, sometimes called the "father of surgery," used manipulation to treat French vineyard workers in the 16th century (Lomax, 1975; Paré, 1968).

In the centuries that followed, to the beginning of the modern era, manipulative techniques were passed down from generation to generation within families. These "bone setting" methods, transmitted from father to son and often from mother to daughter, played an important role in the history of nonmedical healing in Great Britain, and similar methods are common in the folk medicine of many nations (Bennett, 1981).

During the 19th century, the new United States became a vibrant center of "magnetic" and natural healing theory and practice. Two organized manipulation-based healing practices, osteopathy and chiropractic, had their origins during that era.

Acknowledgment to Dan Redwood for prior contributions in Micozzi, M.S. (Ed.), (2016). *Fundamentals of complementary and alternative medicine* (5th ed.). St Louis: Elsevier Health Sciences/Saunders.

They arose in close proximity in time and place in the American Midwest, which was still on the edge of the American frontier.

ORIGINS FROM MAGNETIC HEALING

Daniel David Palmer, a self-educated "magnetic" or "mesmeric" healer in the Mississippi River town of Davenport, Iowa, founded the chiropractic profession in 1895 with two fundamental premises: (1) vertebral subluxation (which he defined as spinal misalignment causing abnormal nerve transmission) is the primary cause of virtually all disease; and (2) chiropractic adjustment (manual manipulation of the subluxated vertebra) is its cure (Palmer, 1910). This "one cause–one cure" philosophy played a central role in chiropractic history, first as a guiding principle, then later as a historical remnant, while providing a target for the slings and arrows of organized medicine (Fig. 12.1).

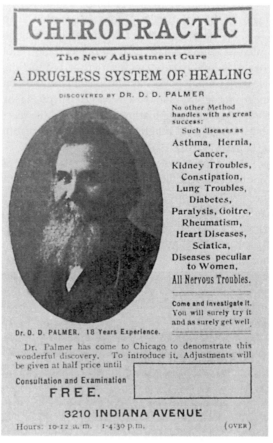

FIG. 12.1 | In this 1904 advertisement, Dr. Palmer touted chiropractic as a cure for virtually all human ailments. Such claims engendered great controversy.

Contemporary chiropractors do not follow a simplistic and all-encompassing formulation. However, subluxations (now commonly defined as spinal joint dysfunctions or segmental dysfunctions [SDFs]; see later discussion) and their adjustment by spinal manual therapy (SMT) are still central to chiropractic practice. Chiropractors may do more, but their ability to evaluate and adjust the spine with great expertise has allowed this healing art and practice to survive for more than a century despite a barrage of medical opposition, some justified, and some not.

The one cause–one cure proponents among early chiropractors had two major effects on the development of the professional practice. First, their deep faith in the truth of their message, combined with the positive results of chiropractic adjustments, created a strong and steadily growing activist constituency of patients and supporters. They generated a grassroots movement that enabled the survival of the profession through difficult years during the first half of the 20th century. Civil disobedience was an important part of the early development of the

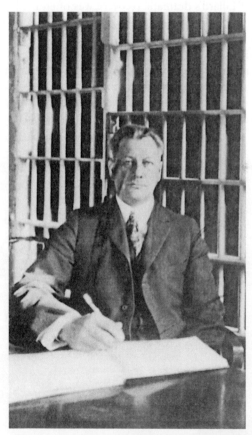

FIG. 12.2 | Dr. D.S. Tracy behind bars in Los Angeles. Hundreds of chiropractors served time in jail to secure the right to practice their healing art freely.

chiropractic profession. Hundreds, including Palmer, the founder, went to jail, charged with practicing medicine without a license (Fig. 12.2). They persisted and ultimately prevailed, winning licensure throughout the United States, North America, and in many other nations worldwide.

PUTTING DOWN OF HANDS

Chiropractic was controversial from its inception. In the first chiropractic adjustment, the patient sought treatment for deafness and attained results that greatly exceeded expectations. Harvey Lillard was a deaf janitor in the building where Palmer had an office, and came to him for help. Noting an apparent misalignment in the patient's spine, Palmer administered the first chiropractic adjustment, after which Lillard is reported to have been able to hear for the first time in nearly two decades (Fig. 12.3).

Similar results were not forthcoming when other deaf people sought his assistance. There have been other rare reports through the years of hearing restored through spinal manipulation, including one by a Canadian orthopedist (Bourdillion, 1982). The story of Lillard's dramatic recovery was often used to disparage chiropractic, with charges that such an event is impossible, because no spinal nerves supply the ear, which is supplied by a cranial nerve.

Current knowledge of neurophysiology provides a credible theoretical basis for this observation and other apparent visceral organ responses to spinal adjustments. The physiological mechanism lies in the somato-autonomic (or somatovisceral) reflex. Chiropractors and osteopaths assert that signals initiated by spinal manipulation are transmitted through autonomic pathways to internal organs.

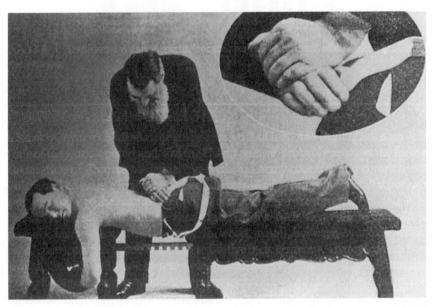

FIG. 12.3 | Daniel David Palmer, the founder of chiropractic, adjusting a patient (c.1906).

Such autonomic pathways exist, but whether spinal manipulation can elicit such healing responses via these pathways remains in dispute. In the case of Palmer's first adjustment, the relevant nerve pathway begins in the thoracic region, coursing up through the neck and into the cranium along sympathetic nerves that eventually lead to the blood vessels of the inner ear. (The sensory nerve for auditory sensation originates higher in the central nervous system [CNS] as a cranial nerve, but normal function of the hearing apparatus also depends on an adequate blood supply, which in turn depends on a properly functioning sympathetic nerve supply; see Fig. 4.1).

There are sometimes dramatic positive somatovisceral responses to chiropractic spinal adjustments, while most such cases appear to be nonresponsive. Marked individual variations in response to virtually all complementary and alternative medicine (CAM) therapies remains a hallmark of these practices—an issue that has yet to be seriously addressed by the profession (although guidance is offered in Appendix I, pp. 572–579). There have been some recent advancements in the application of psychometric assessments to match personality boundary types, or "emotional types," to the most effective treatment(s) for pain.

All healing arts face the need to maintain the enthusiasm generated by positive therapeutic results while clearly and consistently distinguishing among proven, probable, and speculative findings. Some of the harshest criticism of chiropractic has been in reaction to the tendency of some chiropractors to "globalize" (Gellert, 1994), making broad, overarching claims on the basis of limited, albeit powerful, anecdotal evidence.

Whatever the validity of medical critiques, the American medical establishment's policy on chiropractic was not that of a disinterested group seeking to serve the public health and well-being. A century-long campaign against chiropractic impeded medical advancement and at times posed a severe threat. Until relatively recently, allopathic medical students were taught that chiropractic is harmful, or at best worthless, and they in turn passed along these prejudices to their own patients.

A staunchly antichiropractic policy was pursued by the American Medical Association (AMA). In 1990, the US Supreme Court affirmed a lower court ruling in which the AMA was found liable for federal antitrust violations for having engaged in a conspiracy to "contain and eliminate" (the AMA's own words) the chiropractic profession (Wilk v AMA, 1990). The process that culminated in this landmark decision began in 1974 when a large packet of confidential AMA documents was provided anonymously to leaders of the American Chiropractic Association and the International Chiropractors Association. As a result of the ensuing Wilk v AMA litigation, the AMA reversed its long-standing ban on interprofessional cooperation between medical doctors and chiropractors, agreed to publish the full findings of the court in the *Journal of the American Medical Association,* and paid an undisclosed sum, most of which was earmarked for chiropractic research.

This ruling has not completely reversed the effects of organized medicine's boycott, especially when it comes to application of the most effective and cost-effective treatments for common pain conditions. Nonetheless, progress has accelerated substantially in the years since the Wilk decision, as men and women of goodwill in both professions strive to inaugurate a new era in which their patients are the beneficiaries of their mutual cooperation in the management of pain (e.g., in multidisciplinary spine centers that have appeared across the United States). Outside the United States, historically, relations between the medical and chiropractic professions were also less than cordial. However, international collaborations developed among chiropractors and allopathic physicians earlier than it happened in the United States. This cooperation has had particularly beneficial effects in the research area. Many of the key clinical trials that first established chiropractic's scientific credibility were conducted in Europe and Canada. Nearly all of the major universities in Canada now have endowed research chairs held by dual-degreed chiropractors (primarily DC-PhDs).

Gradually, the tide has turned in the United States as well. Research projects funded by the federal government (through the National Center for Complementary and Alternative Medicine, the Health Resources and Services Administration, the Agency for Health Care Policy and Research [AHCPR], the Agency for Healthcare Quality, and the Department of Defense) have encouraged an atmosphere of growing medical-chiropractic cooperation. Multidisciplinary organizations such as the American Back Society, as well as "integrative" spine centers, back centers, and related clinical practices and facilities, also reflect a new common ground in the battle against chronic pain. The American Public Health Association, which previously had an explicitly antichiropractic policy, reversed course in the 1980s and now has a thriving Chiropractic Health Care section which, during the 2000s, presented landmark studies on the effectiveness of SMT for low back pain (LBP) (e.g., Lawrence et al., 2008). The incorporation of chiropractic into the health care systems serving active duty members of the US military, and military veterans through the Veterans Health Administration (VHA), provides opportunity for interprofessional cooperation as well as models for multidisciplinary team-based care. In 2013, the VHA initiated postdoctoral residency training programs for doctors of chiropractic.

BREAKTHROUGHS FOR TREATING PAIN

One of the breakthrough moments in the history of pain control was the 1994 publication of the Guidelines for Acute Lower Back Pain, developed for the AHCPR of the US Department of Health and Human Services. The panel that developed the guidelines included primarily medical physicians and was chaired by an orthopedic surgeon (2 of the 23 members were chiropractors), and the guidelines included a powerful endorsement of spinal manipulation for the treatment of pain (Bigos, Bowyer, & Braen, 1994).

Based on an extensive literature review and consensus process, the AHCPR Guidelines concluded that spinal manipulation "hastens recovery" from acute LBP and recommended it either in combination with, or as a replacement for, nonsteroidal anti-inflammatory drugs (NSAIDs). At the same time, the panel rejected as unsubstantiated numerous methods (including bed rest, traction, and various other physical therapy and pharmaceutical modalities) that for years had constituted the foundation of conventional medicine's approach to acute LBP. The panel further endorsed the use of such self-care measures as exercise, ergonomic seating, and wearing low-heeled shoes. The panel also cautioned against back surgery except in the most severe cases.

The AHCPR Guidelines stated that spinal manipulation offers both "symptomatic relief" and "functional improvement," and that none of the other recommended medical interventions offers both. Spinal manipulation should be the treatment of choice for patients with acute LBP who show none of the guideline's diagnostic "red flags," such as fractures, tumors, infections, or cauda equina syndrome (Micozzi, 1998). Standards for the treatment of LBP, the most prevalent musculoskeletal ailment in the United States and the most frequent cause of disability for persons under age 45, establish a pivotal role for spinal manipulation (Shekelle & Adams, 1991). This outcome provides an important contemporary example of an "alternative" health care method achieving entry into the health care mainstream, especially for the treatment of pain.

Assessments by government agencies in Canada (Manga, Angus, Papadopoulos, & Swan, 1993), Great Britain (Rosen, 1994), Sweden (Commission on Alternative Medicine, 1987), Denmark (Danish Institute for Health Technology Assessment, 1999), Australia (Thompson, 1986), and New Zealand (Hasselberg, 1979) have brought about similar approvals of spinal manipulation for LBP.

Following investigations by the American College of Physicians (ACP) in Philadelphia (e.g., Micozzi, 1998), guidelines jointly issued in 2007 by the ACP and the American Pain Society (APS) similarly recommend spinal manipulation based on its "proven benefits" for acute, subacute, and chronic LBP (Chou et al., 2007). The ACP-APS guidelines state that spinal manipulation is the only nonpharmacologic method with proven benefits for acute LBP. They also recognize benefits of both manipulation and other methods within the chiropractic scope of practice for subacute and chronic LBP—intensive interdisciplinary rehabilitation, exercise therapy, acupuncture, massage therapy, and yoga. The ACP-APS LBP guidelines have essentially replaced the AHCPR Guidelines, and are currently the most influential LBP guidelines worldwide.

With special funding through the US Health Resources and Services Administration, provided in the Congressional budget by former Sen. Tom Harkin (D-Iowa) for the Policy Institute for Integrative Medicine (Bethesda, MD) and the Palmer College Chiropractic Research Consortium (Davenport, IA) consisting of over a dozen chiropractic and medical schools also convened an expert consensus development panel to review nearly 1000 studies worldwide on the treatment of back pain and confirmed these findings, as reported to the American Public Health Association and others (Lawrence et al., 2008).

THEORETICAL PRINCIPLES

Chiropractic uses concepts with other "magnetic," energetic, and natural healing arts such as acupuncture and naturopathy. The following core constructs form the basis of chiropractic theory:
1. Structure and function exist in intimate relation with one another.
2. Structural distortions can cause functional abnormalities.

3. Vertebral subluxation (spinal joint dysfunction with neurologic effects) is a significant form of structural distortion and leads to a variety of functional abnormalities.
4. The nervous system occupies a central role in the restoration and maintenance of proper bodily function.
5. Subluxation influences bodily function primarily through neurologic means.
6. Chiropractic spinal adjustment is a specific and definitive method for reduction or correction of vertebral subluxation.

Chiropractic is best known for its success in the relief of musculoskeletal pain, but its basic axioms do not directly address the treatment of pain. Instead, they focus on the correction of structural and functional imbalances, which in many cases cause pain. This profession is renowned for the relief of musculoskeletal pain but does not define its basic purpose in those terms.

BONE-OUT-OF-PLACE THEORY

Early chiropractors, following Palmer's lead, assumed that their adjustments worked by moving misaligned vertebrae back into line, thereby relieving pressure caused by direct bony impingement on spinal nerves. The standard explanation given to patients was the analogy of stepping on a garden hose: if you step on the hose, the water cannot get through; then when you lift your foot off the hose, the free flow of water is restored. Similarly, it was claimed that adjustment removes the pressure of bone on nerve, thus allowing free flow of nerve impulses.

Based on the information available at the time, such 19th-century concepts were considered plausible. Chiropractors were able to feel interruptions in the symmetry of the spinal column with their experienced hands, as many times verified on x-ray examination. (The x-ray technique was developed by Roentgen in Germany at about the same time chiropractic arose in the United States during the late 1890s.) More often than not, when they adjusted the subluxated vertebra with manual pressure, patients reported significant functional improvements in pain and healing effects.

Problems exist with this theory. After an adjustment results in dramatic relief from headaches or sciatica pain, an x-ray study rarely shows any discernible change in spinal alignment. (The American Chiropractic Association Council on Diagnostic Imaging now considers such comparative x-ray films inappropriate because of the unnecessary radiation exposure.) Positive health changes have not consistently correlated with vertebral alignment and the issue has not been fully resolved. A 2007 randomized clinical trial, the first to demonstrate significant benefit from chiropractic in cases of hypertension, used a technique that places great reliance on x-ray analysis of upper cervical vertebral alignment (Bakris et al., 2007).

SEGMENTAL DYSFUNCTION

Alternative hypotheses have been proposed to replace the bone-out-of-place concept. The theory of intervertebral motion and SDF was the dominant chiropractic model of the contemporary era, as advocated by a minority of chiropractors for many decades. This model first achieved profession-wide attention among chiropractors in the 1980s and now has broad acceptance in chiropractic college curricula throughout the world. This theory also offers a coherent explanation of chiropractic and the vertebral subluxation complex (VSC), which can also be communicated in familiar terms to medical practitioners and researchers.

Motion theory contends that loss of proper spinal joint mobility, rather than positional misalignment, is the key factor in joint dysfunction. It posits that the subluxation always involves more than a single vertebra and that subluxation mechanics involve SDF, an interruption in the normal dynamic relations between two articulating joint surfaces (Schafer & Faye, 1989).

Anatomically, the vertebral motor unit (or motion segment) consists of an anterior segment, with two vertebral bodies separated by an intervertebral disc, and a posterior segment, consisting of two adjacent articular facets, along with muscles, ligaments, blood vessels, and nerves, interfacing with one another. Restriction of joint motion, a common feature of a manipulatable lesion or subluxation, is termed a fixation. Fixation-subluxations are the clinical entity most amenable to spinal manipulation.

L. John Faye, DC, a pioneer in moving the dynamic or motion model into the chiropractic mainstream, identified a five-component model for the VSC. In Faye's original formulation (Schafer & Faye, 1989), these are the neurologic, kinesiologic, myologic, biochemical, and histologic components. Faye later amended his model to replace the final two components with inflammatory and stress components (as presented at Cleveland Chiropractic College, Kansas City, Kansas in 2009).

Former college president and national spokesperson for the American Chiropractic Association, J.F. McAndrews, DC, an early advocate of motion theory and practice, described a visual model of spinal motion principles (Fig. 12.4) as follows:

The reader may view a mobile hanging from the ceiling, with many strings on which ornaments are suspended. As the mobile hangs there, it is in a state of dynamic equilibrium. Then, if you cut one of the strings, the whole mobile starts moving, because its balance has been upset. Eventually, it slows down and reaches a new state of dynamic equilibrium. But things have changed. It does not look the same. All those ornaments have shifted, in relation to the central axis and also in relation to each other.

The body's musculoskeletal system works in much the same way. When normal balance is disrupted, it must compensate. Structural patterns become altered to a greater or lesser degree, depending on the nature and intensity of the forces that threw off the old pattern of balance.

Leach (1994) cites three signs accepted as evidence of the existence of SDF: (1) point tenderness or altered pain threshold to pressure in the adjacent para-spinal musculature or over the spinous process; (2) abnormal contraction or tension within the adjacent para-spinal musculature; and (3) loss of normal motion in one or more planes. Chiropractic education includes extensive training in the

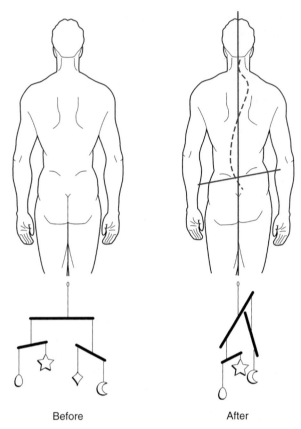

Before   After

FIG. 12.4 | Visual model of spinal motion principles comparing a mobile hanging from ceiling to the body's musculoskeletal system before and after imbalance is introduced.

development of the psychomotor skills necessary to diagnose the VSC or SDF and to perform the manipulative maneuvers best suited to its correction.

More problematic than fixations are subluxations involving joint hypermobility, characterized by ligamentous laxity, frequently of traumatic etiology. Hypermobility can be clinically diagnosed by eliciting a repeated click when a joint is moved through its normal range of motion (ROM). Hypermobile joints should not be forcibly manipulated because this action can further increase the degree of hypermobility. However, nearby articulations that have become fixated to compensate for the hypermobile joint, may require manipulation. Muscles in the area should be strengthened and toned to minimize the workload of the overstressed hypermobile joint. The motion segment is the initial focus of chiropractic therapeutic intervention and is the site where the most direct and immediate effects of manipulation are likely to be noted. More far-reaching effects are possible, however, through neural facilitation.

Neural Segmental Facilitation and Chronic Inflammation

Segmental facilitation has been defined as a lowered threshold for firing in a spinal cord segment, caused by afferent bombardment of the dorsal horn of the spinal cord associated with spinal lesions (Korr, 1976). Once a segment is facilitated, effects may include local somatic pain or visceral organ dysfunction. Segmental facilitation is the dominant hypothesis proposed as the neurophysiological basis by which the VSC or SDF influences autonomic function. Some models for the specific mechanisms postulate that inflammation is a key factor (Dvorak, 1985; Gatterman & Goe, 1990; Mense, 1991). Others have proposed neurological models through which such facilitation could occur even in the absence of inflammation (Korr, 1975; Patterson & Steinmetz, 1986). When present, chronic inflammation alters the local environment of the nerve, causing chemical, thermal, and mechanical changes. Inflammation surrounding a nerve is likely to compromise its function. Aberrant nerve activity may disrupt the homeostatic mechanisms essential to normal somatic or visceral organ function. A facilitated segment may result in either parasympathetic vagal dominance or excessive sympathetic output. Leach (1994) concludes:

"It appears that SDF is capable of initiating segmental facilitation and that certainly this is the most logical explanation for the use of [chiropractic] adjustment … for other than pain syndromes; certainly the segmental facilitation hypothesis is gaining greater acceptance and is based upon a large body of acceptable scientific research" (Leach, 1994).

EVALUATION AND ADJUSTMENT

In the clinical setting, the chiropractic model demonstrates both similarities and differences compared with the standard medical approach. Foremost, chiropractors seek to evaluate individual symptoms in a broad context of health and body balance, not as isolated symptoms to be suppressed. This holistic viewpoint shares much with both ancient and emerging models elsewhere in the complementary and alternative healing arts. Chiropractors nonetheless recognize the need for thorough evaluation of symptoms. They are trained to take medical histories and perform physical examinations in a manner similar to a typical medical office physical exam (or what used to be done at the typical medical office). However, the chiropractic paradigm does not hold the elimination of symptoms to be the sole or ultimate goal of treatment. Health is more than the absence of disease symptoms. The true goal is sustainable balance, as recognized by chiropractors and other holistically oriented health practitioners.

Chiropractors are trained in state-of-the-art diagnostic techniques, and examination procedures overlap significantly with those used by orthodox medical physicians. Chiropractors evaluate the information obtained from these methods through a perspective that places greater emphasis on the intricate structural and functional interplay among different parts of the body. The central focus of chiropractic practice is the analytical process for determining (1) when and where spinal manual therapy (SMT) is appropriate, and (2) the type of adjustment most appropriate in a given situation.

PROPOSED ALGORITHMS

Proposed algorithms for this process detail procedures whereby the chiropractor arrives at an overall clinical impression (not limited to the spine, and methodically ruling out pathologies that contraindicate SMT), and proceeds to evaluate SDF to arrive at a specific chiropractic diagnosis (Leach, 1994). This diagnostic process takes into account subluxations that are present, along with other clinical entities (e.g., degeneration, disc involvement, carpal tunnel syndrome). In certain cases, conditions may require treatment in addition to SMT, or may affect the style of SMT that is appropriate. For example, the presence of advanced degenerative joint disease would not render SMT inappropriate, but would rule out forms of SMT that introduce substantial amounts of force on the arthritic joint. According to the Guidelines for Chiropractic Quality Assurance and Practice Parameters (Haldeman, Chapman-Smith, & Peterson, 1993), the high-velocity low-amplitude (HVLA) thrust adjustment, the most common form of chiropractic SMT, is "absolutely contraindicated" in anatomical areas where the following occur:

- Malignancies
- Bone and joint infections
- Acute myelopathy or acute cauda equina syndrome
- Acute fractures and dislocations, or healed fractures and dislocations with signs of ligamentous rupture or instability
- Acute rheumatoid, rheumatoid-like, or nonspecific arthropathies, including ankylosing spondylitis characterized by episodes of acute inflammation, demineralization, and ligamentous laxity with anatomical subluxation or dislocation
- Active juvenile avascular necrosis
- Unstable os odontoideum

These guidelines rate in descending order of severity conditions in the following categories: "relative to absolute contraindication," "relative contraindication," and "not a contraindication." Listing all conditions in each category is beyond the scope of this chapter. The key point is that chiropractic diagnosis is geared toward evaluating where each case falls along this spectrum, and then proceeding with appropriate medical referral, chiropractic treatment, or concurrent care. Chiropractic practice standards mandate timely referral to a medical physician for diagnosis and treatment for conditions beyond the chiropractor's domain, or when a reasonable trial of chiropractic care (current standards in most cases limit this approach to about one month) fails to bring satisfactory results (Baker, Farabaugh, Augat, & Hawk, 2012; Haldeman et al., 1993). In addition, chiropractors frequently seek second opinions in less dramatic cases when chiropractic treatment, although helpful, fails to bring full resolution. Referrals from chiropractors to neurologists, neurosurgeons, orthopedic surgeons, internists, and other medical specialists are common. Referrals to complementary practitioners such as acupuncturists, massage therapists, and naturopaths also occur when appropriate, in areas where such practitioners are available. An increasing number of practicing chiropractors are also dually trained and licensed to provide acupuncture, Ayurvedic medicine, and other areas of CAM.

APPROACHES TO PAIN

In widespread experience, conventional medical physicians engage in symptom suppression more than chiropractors do. Medical physicians also more frequently assume that the site of a pain is also the site of its cause; knee pain is generally assumed to be a knee problem, shoulder pain is assumed to be a shoulder problem, and so forth. This pain-centered diagnostic logic frequently leads to increasingly sophisticated and invasive, albeit misdirected, diagnostic and therapeutic procedures. For example, if physical examination of the knee fails to define the problem clearly, the knee is radiographed. If the x-ray film fails to offer adequate clarification, magnetic resonance imaging (MRI) of the knee is performed, and in many cases an invasive surgical procedure follows, which may or may not alleviate the problem.

As with their allopathic colleagues, chiropractors use diagnostic tools such as radiography and MRI. The point is not to criticize these useful technologies when appropriately used, but to present an alternative diagnostic model. Chiropractors are familiar with many patients to whom this entire high-tech diagnostic and therapeutic scenario (as in the previous knee example) is played out. After the failures of this scenario the knee problem discovered to be a compensation for a mechanical disorder in the lower back, a common condition that too often remains outside the medical diagnostic loop. When the lower back is mechanically dysfunctional and in need of spinal adjustment, it typically places unusual stress on one or both knees, causing pain. In these patients, medical physicians can and often spend months or years medicating the knee symptoms or performing surgery, while never addressing the actual source of the problem.

NEUROLOGY AND BIOMECHANICS

The chiropractic approach to musculoskeletal pain involves evaluating the site of pain in a regional and whole-body context. Shoulder, elbow, and wrist problems can be caused by injuries or pathologies in these areas. Pain in and around each of the shoulder, elbow, and wrist joints can also have its origin in SDF in the cervical spine. Similarly, symptoms in the hip, knee, and ankle can originate at the site of the pain, but in many cases, the source lies in the lumbar spine or sacroiliac joints. Besides pain, other neurologically mediated symptoms (e.g., paresthesia) can have a similar etiology. Consideration of this chain of causation is built into the core of chiropractic training, evaluation, and practice.

Chiropractors intentionally avoid the simple assumption that the site of a symptom is the site of its cause. Instead, they seek the source of the pain along the path of the nerves leading to and from the site of the symptoms. Pain in the knee might come from the knee itself, but tracing the nerve pathways between the knee and the spine can reveal possible areas of causation in and around the hip, in the deep muscles of the buttocks or pelvis, in the sacroiliac joints, or in the lumbar spine.

When segmental joint dysfunction does exist, for example, at the fourth and fifth lumbar levels, it might have its primary source at L4-L5, or it might represent compensation for another subluxation elsewhere in the spine, perhaps in the lower or middle thoracic vertebrae or in a mechanical dysfunction of the muscles and joints of the feet. Such an integrative, whole-body approach to structure and function is of great value. For patients whose presentation includes visceral organ symptoms, chiropractic diagnostic logic includes (once medical contraindications to manipulation have been ruled out) evaluation of the spine. Particular attention is paid to spinal levels providing autonomic nerve supply to the involved areas and consideration of possible nutritional, environmental, and psychological factors.

RESEARCH STUDIES

For years, chiropractors were criticized for offering only anecdotal evidence in support of their methods. For more nearly three decades, since the early 1990s, only those ignorant of the scientific literature can still make such criticisms. As summarized by Bronfort, Haas, Evans, Leiniger, and Triano (2010) in their comprehensive UK Evidence Report, there are now over 100 randomized clinical trials of manual manipulation, virtually all of which were conducted after the mid-1970s. A substantial majority are LBP studies, most of which found manipulation to be more effective than all methods to which it was compared. The current literature also contains a substantial number of studies on neck pain and headaches, along with a smaller number on musculoskeletal conditions of the extremities and nonmusculoskeletal or visceral conditions.

RESEARCH METHODOLOGY

Two challenging methodological questions in chiropractic research are as follows:
1. What constitutes a genuine control or placebo intervention?
2. How can practitioners properly interpret data collected in trials that compare active and control treatments?

These questions also apply to a broad range of procedures, particularly nonpharmaceutical modalities such as massage, acupuncture, physical therapy, and surgery. Depending on how one defines the placebo effect, the same set of research data can be interpreted as supporting or refuting the value of the therapeutic method under study (Redwood, 1999).

Appropriate Placebo Control

Two widely publicized studies illustrate the potential difficulties of defining the placebo or control too broadly. In their research on children with mild to moderate asthma, Balon et al. (1998) randomly assigned individuals to either active manipulation or simulated manipulation groups. Both groups experienced substantial improvement in symptoms and quality of life, reduction in the use of beta-agonist medication, and statistically insignificant increases in peak expiratory flow. These two groups did not differ significantly in regard to these improvements, however, and the researchers concluded "chiropractic spinal manipulation provided no benefit." If the simulated manipulation had no therapeutic effect, this conclusion is reasonable. However, closer reading of the article's text reveals the following:

"For simulated treatment, the subject lay prone while soft tissue massage and gentle palpation were applied to the spine, paraspinal muscles, and shoulders. A distraction maneuver was performed by turning the patient's head from one side to the other, while alternately palpating the ankles and feet. The subject was positioned on one side, a nondirectional push, or impulse, was applied to the gluteal region, and the procedure was repeated with the patient positioned on the other side; then the subject was placed in the prone position, and a similar procedure was applied bilaterally to the scapulae. The subject was then placed supine, with the head rotated slightly to each side, and an impulse was applied to the external occipital protuberance. Low-amplitude, low-velocity impulses were applied in all these nontherapeutic contacts, with adequate joint slack so that no joint opening or cavitation occurred. Hence, the comparison of treatments was between active spinal manipulation as routinely applied by chiropractors and hands-on procedures without adjustments or manipulation."

(Balon et al., 1998)

The validity of this study's conclusion hinges entirely on the assumption that these "placebo" procedures are therapeutically inert. The following questions must be answered to evaluate this conclusion:

1. Would massage therapists view all these hands-on procedures as "nontherapeutic"?
2. Would acupuncturists or practitioners of Shiatsu concur that direct manual pressure on multiple areas rich in acupuncture points is inconsequential, and allow its use as a "placebo"?
3. Would the average chiropractor agree that these pressures, impulses, and stretches are an appropriate placebo, particularly in light of the fact that they overlap with typical "low-force" chiropractic adjustments and mobilization procedures?

The authors of the study addressed these concerns as follows:

"We are unaware of published evidence that suggests that positioning, palpation, gentle soft tissue therapy, or impulses to the musculature adjacent to the spine influence the course of asthma."

(Balon et al., 1998)

A reasonable alternative interpretation of this study's results, however, is that various forms of hands-on therapy, including joint manipulation and various forms of movement, mobilization, and soft tissue massage, appear to have a mildly beneficial effect for asthmatic patients (Redwood, 1999). There are also powerful as yet unexplained benefits for acupuncture in asthma, which were used as part of the basis for the reclassification of acupuncture needles from an experimental to a therapeutic device 20 years ago in light of its superior safety profile compared to drug treatments, including in the treatment of asthma (see Chapter 15).

Active Pain Controls

Another study that raises similar questions involves manipulation for episodic tension-type headache (ETTH) (Bove & Nilsson, 1998). Patients were randomized into two groups. One received soft tissue therapy (deep friction massage) plus spinal manipulation, and the other (the "active control" group) received soft tissue therapy plus application of a low-power laser to the neck. All treatments were applied by the same chiropractor. Both groups had significantly fewer headaches and decreased their use of analgesic medications. As in the asthma study, differences between the two groups did not reach statistical significance. Thus the authors concluded that "as an isolated intervention, spinal manipulation does not seem to have a positive effect on tension-type headache."

Unlike the asthma study (Balon et al., 1998), Bove and Nilsson's carefully worded conclusion is justified by their data, but it would have been more informative to include the equally accurate conclusion that hands-on therapy, whether massage or manipulation, plus massage demonstrated significant benefits. Shortly after his paper's publication, Bove noted the following in a message to an Internet discussion group:

"Our study asked one question [whether manipulation as an isolated intervention is effective for ETTH] and delivered one answer, a hallmark of good science.…
We stressed that chiropractors do more than manipulation, and that chiropractic treatment has been shown to be somewhat beneficial for ETTH and very beneficial for cervicogenic headache. The message was that people should go to chiropractors with their headaches, for diagnosis and management."

(Bove & Nilsson, 1998)

The mass media's reporting on Bove and Nilsson's headache study provided a telling illustration of why defining the placebo or control correctly is more than an academic exercise. Media reports on this study put forth a message quite different from Bove's nuanced analysis, with headlines concluding that chiropractic does not help headaches. Reports on the asthma study were similar. Moreover, future Medline searches will include the authors' tersely stated negative conclusions, with no mention of any controversy surrounding their interpretation.

The best way to avoid such confusion in the future is to emphasize increased usage of other valid methodologies, particularly direct comparisons of CAM procedures with standard medical care. Comparative studies have shown that manipulation is equal or superior to conventional medical procedures, with fewer side effects (Boline, Kassak, Bronfort, Nelson, & Anderson, 1995; Meade, Dyer, Browne, & Frank, 1995; Meade, Dyer, Browne, Townsend, & Frank, 1990; Nelson et al., 1998; Wiberg, Nordsteen, & Nilsson, 1999; Winters, Sobel, Groenier, Arendzen, & Meyboom-de Jong, 1997). When fairly constructed (and "deconstructed"), such studies yield data that allow health practitioners and the general public to place CAM procedures into proper context. Comparing chiropractic and other nonpharmaceutical procedures to highly questionable active placebos confuses the issues and delays the advent of a "level playing field."

UNIVERSITY OF COLORADO PROJECT

Contemporary chiropractic research can be seen as beginning at the University of Colorado in the 1970s, initially with grants from the International Chiropractors

Association and later with added financial support from the American Chiropractic Association and the US government. Chung Ha Suh and colleagues at the Biomechanics Department undertook a series of studies that provided an extensive body of chiropractic-related, basic science research.

Suh was the first US university professor willing to defy the AMA boycott and pursue chiropractic research. He was a native of Korea, where he had not been subjected to the same antichiropractic bias as were the US health care academics of his era. Launching this research, he withstood intense pressure from powerful political forces within the American medical and academic establishments. They condemned chiropractic for lack of scientific underpinning, while concurrently striving to prevent chiropractors from obtaining the funding and university affiliations necessary for the development of any such research base (Wilk v AMA, 1990).

The University of Colorado team pursued research in two major areas. First, Suh (1974) developed a computer model of the cervical spine that allowed a deeper understanding of spinal joint mechanics and their relations to spinal chiropractic adjustment. The second area involved a range of studies on nerve compression and various aspects of neuron function (Kelly & Luttges, 1975; Luttges, Kelly, & Gerren, 1976; MacGregor & Oliver, 1973; MacGregor, Sharpless, & Luttges, 1975; Sharpless, 1975; Simske & Schmeister, 1994; Triano & Luttges, 1982). Sharpless (1975) and demonstrated that minuscule amounts of pressure (10 mm Hg) on a nerve root resulted in up to a 50% decrease in electrical transmission down the course of the nerve supplied by that root.

Low Back Pain

A substantial body of research addressed the effectiveness of SMT in the treatment of LBP. As referenced earlier, consensus panels evaluating the data have consistently placed spinal manipulation on the list of most recommended procedures for LBP.

The use of spinal manipulation as a treatment for acute, subacute, and chronic LBP received the rating "A: Supported by good evidence from relevant studies" from the Council on Chiropractic Guidelines and Practice Parameters" (Globe, Morris, Whalen, Farabaugh, & Hawk, 2008; Lawrence et al., 2008). Current joint guidelines from the ACP and the APS, as noted earlier, endorse manipulation for both chronic and acute LBP (Chou et al., 2007).

Research on Criteria for Referral

A primary care physician's decision about whether and where to refer LBP patients hinges on which treatments are expected to yield the most satisfactory outcomes. A summary of studies on spinal manipulation for LBP is provided to aid this decision-making process.

In an influential trial with more than 700 patients, British orthopedic surgeon T.W. Meade compared chiropractic manipulation with standard hospital outpatient treatment for LBP, which consisted of physical therapy and wearing a corset (Meade et al., 1990, 1995). He concluded, "For patients with low back pain in whom manipulation is not contraindicated, chiropractic almost certainly confers worthwhile, long-term benefit in comparison to hospital outpatient management." He described the applicability of these findings for primary care physicians as follows:

"Our trial showed that chiropractic is a very effective treatment, more effective than conventional hospital outpatient treatment for LBP, particularly in patients who had back pain in the past and who [developed] severe problems. So, in other words, it is most effective in precisely the group of patients that you would like to be able to treat. One of the unexpected findings was that the treatment difference—the benefit of chiropractic over hospital treatment—actually persists for the whole of that three-year period [of the study] the treatment that the chiropractors gives does something that results in a very long-term benefit."

(Meade, 1992)

Meade's study was the first large randomized clinical trial to demonstrate substantial short-term and long-term benefits from chiropractic care. It dealt with both acute LBP patients and chronic LBP patients, and Meade's data support the use of SMT for both populations.

Besides Meade et al. (1990, 1995), a major prospective study of LBP was performed at the University of Saskatchewan hospital orthopedics department by Kirkaldy-Willis, a world-renowned orthopedic surgeon, and Cassidy, the chiropractor who later became the department's research director (Kirkaldy-Willis & Cassidy, 1985). The approximately 300 subjects in this study were "totally disabled" by LBP, with pain present for an average of 7 years. All had gone through extensive, unsuccessful medical treatment before participating as research subjects. After 2 to 3 weeks of daily chiropractic adjustments, more than 80% of the patients without spinal stenosis had good to excellent results, reporting substantially decreased pain and increased mobility. After chiropractic treatment, more than 70% were improved to the point of having no work restrictions. Follow-up a year later demonstrated that improvements were long-lasting. Even those with a narrowed spinal canal, a particularly difficult subset, showed a notable response. More than half the patients improved, and about one in five was pain free and on the job 7 months after treatment.

In a randomized trial of 209 patients, Triano, McGregor, Hondras, and Brennan (1995) compared SMT to education programs for chronic LBP, which was defined as pain lasting 7 weeks or longer, or more than six episodes in 12 months. These investigators found greater improvement in pain and activity tolerance in the SMT group, noting that "immediate benefit from pain relief continued to accrue after manipulation, even for the last encounter at the end of the 2-week treatment interval. There appears to be clinical value to treatment according to a defined plan using manipulation even in low back pain exceeding 7 weeks duration."

The UK Back Pain Exercise and Manipulation study (UK BEAM Trial Team, 2004a,b) was a large randomized trial with over 1300 patients. As noted earlier, a previous study by orthopedic surgeon Thomas Meade and colleagues, also published in the *British Medical Journal* (Meade et al., 1990, 1995), had a dramatic impact in the United Kingdom and beyond. It showed that chiropractic care brought better outcomes for LBP patients than did standard medical care. One key criticism of Meade's landmark study was that the medical care group was treated in National Health Service facilities, while the chiropractic group was treated in private practice settings. Concern was quite vocal from certain conventional medicine advocates that this factor may have compromised Meade's findings by creating higher expectations of success among the patients randomized to chiropractic care. The UK BEAM study was partly aimed at answering the questions raised by those skeptical of Meade's positive evaluation of chiropractic care. UK BEAM brought a remarkable and unprecedented collaboration among chiropractors, physical therapists, and osteopaths (the scope of osteopathic practice in the United Kingdom is closer to that of chiropractors in the United States than to osteopaths in the United States). In the United Kingdom, spinal manipulation is within the scope of practice of these three disciplines.

The investigators set out to replicate some of the other essentials of Meade's research approach by pragmatically comparing manual therapy and other treatment approaches. To address the concern raised by Meade's critics, they arranged for some spinal manipulation patients to receive care in private practices while others were treated in National Health Service settings, and divided the medical care group similarly. The UK BEAM treatment package (Brealey et al., 2003) was agreed to among representatives of the professional associations representing chiropractors, osteopaths, and physiotherapists. The treatment package foundation was evidence-based recommendations that patients should have early access to physical treatments and should return to normal activities as soon as possible. The interdisciplinary planning group also strongly recommended that the spinal manipulation arm of the trial not involve the use of manipulation in isolation, but should include "care that reflected the holistic nature of their approaches." Moreover, they urged that practitioners be permitted to exclude patients from manipulative treatment who were found to be unsuitable candidates according to the practitioner's assessment.

The patients were randomized into one of the following groups: (1) exercise classes, (2) spinal manipulation, or (3) spinal manipulation followed by exercises. The manipulation group was divided in two, with care delivered at a private practice or a National Health Service (NHS) facility. Members of all groups also received "usual care" from a medical physician, based on UK national guidelines; such care consisted of advice to continue normal activities and avoid bed rest, and included a copy of *The Back Book*. Both manipulation (delivered by chiropractors, osteopaths, and physiotherapists) and manipulation plus exercise produced statistically significant gains at 3 months and at 12 months. The exercise-only group had statistically significant improvements at 3 months but not 12. Also, for those who had already received manipulation for 6 weeks, the addition of exercise starting at that point appeared to be less helpful than for those who had not previously had manipulation. In terms of addressing the objections to Meade's earlier study, there were no significant differences between manipulation delivered in NHS facilities or private locations.

As a follow-up to UK BEAM, a smaller study by Wilkey, Gregory, Byfield, and McCarthy (2008) featured a head-to-head comparison of chiropractic care (pragmatically defined to allow all procedures the participating chiropractors would normally employ) versus medical care in the British National Health Service hospital's pain clinic (defined in similarly pragmatic terms). The chiropractic and pain clinic groups started at baseline with similar levels of pain, although the chiropractic group was on average a decade older than the pain clinic group and chiropractic subjects had endured their pain for a mean of 3 years longer (7.3 vs. 4.0 years) than the pain clinic group.

Nevertheless, improvement in pain intensity at week 8 was 1.8 points greater (on a 0–10 scale) for the chiropractic group than for the pain clinic group, a dramatic difference. Disability scores (which measure the impact of pain on daily activities) measured with the Roland Morris Disability Questionnaire also demonstrated a far larger benefit from chiropractic care, with a greater than fivefold difference in the degree of improvement. These data measured effects through the end of the 8-week treatment period. Shortly after publication of Wilkey et al.'s study, the British National Health Service began to cover spinal manipulation for LBP.

In the first randomized controlled trial of chiropractic care for older adults, and one of the first to compare different methods of chiropractic adjustment to each other and to conservative medical care, Hondras, Long, Cao, Rowell, and Meeker (2009) evaluated the effects of these three approaches for 240 people with subacute or chronic LBP. High-velocity and low-velocity chiropractic techniques (combined with standardized exercise recommendations) resulted in similar levels of improvement, with both chiropractic methods substantially outperforming the medical care group, who received the same exercise instructions along with pain medication.

A multidisciplinary team at the National Spine Center in Canada (Bishop, Quon, Fisher, & Dvorak, 2010) compared chiropractic guidelines-based care (including spinal manipulation) versus usual care by family practice medical physicians for acute LBP, defined as 16 weeks or less in duration. They found that guidelines-based care was far more effective and that typical medical care was poorly adherent to guidelines, with 78% of medical patients receiving prescriptions for narcotics (e.g., Tylenol 3 with codeine), which are not guideline endorsed. This result alarmed the editors of *Spine Journal* and they included a "grey box" on "Evidence and Methods" commentary with Bishop et al.'s article. They implored medical physicians to adhere more closely to evidence-based guidelines, with regard to their excessive prescription of opioids (which has emerged as a major public health hazard) and passive modalities, as well as their reluctance to recommend spinal manipulation and exercise.

Preventing Acute From Becoming Chronic Pain

The prognosis for patients with acute LBP is better than for those with chronic pain. Thus high priority should be given to preventing acute cases from becoming chronic. However, there is a key factor leading physicians to minimize this concern. Conventional medical wisdom is that 90% of LBP resolves on its own within a short time. Findings published in a landmark *British Medical Journal* study (Croft, Macfarlane, Papageorgiou, Thomas, & Silman, 1998) call for urgent reassessment of the assumption that most LBP patients seen by primary care physicians attain res-olution of their complaints. Contrary to prevailing assumptions, Croft et al. (1998) found that at 3-month and 12-month follow-up, only 21% and 25%, respectively, had completely recovered in terms of pain and disability. However, only 8% con-tinued to consult their physician for longer than 3 months. In other words, the oft-quoted 90% figure actually applied to the number of patients who simply stopped seeing and seeking help from their physicians, and just gave up. It is not the number who actually recovered from back pain. The dissatisfaction with conventional med-ical care was also reminiscent of Cherkin's earlier work (Cherkin & MacCornack, 1989; Cherkin, Deyo, & Berg, 1991). Croft et al. (1998) stated the following:

"We should stop characterizing low back pain in terms of a multiplicity of acute problems, most of which get better, and a small number of chronic long-term problems. Low back pain should be viewed as a chronic problem with an untidy pattern of grumbling symptoms and periods of relative freedom from pain and disability interspersed with acute episodes, exacerbations, and recurrences. This takes account of two consistent observations about low back pain: firstly, a previous episode of low back pain is the strongest risk factor for a new episode, and, secondly, by the age of 30 years almost half the population will have experienced a substantial episode of low back pain. These figures simply do not fit with claims that 90 percent of episodes of low back pain end in complete recovery."

The patients in Croft's study were not referred for manual manipulation, and most developed chronic LBP. Based on the AHCPR Guidelines, which emphasize the functionally restorative qualities of SMT, it is reasonable to expect that early chiropractic adjustments would have prevented this progression in many patients. Recall that follow-up in both the Meade (1 year and 3 years) and the Kirkaldy-Willis (1 year) studies showed that the beneficial effect of manipulation was sustained for extended periods (Kirkaldy-Willis & Cassidy, 1985; Meade et al., 1990, 1995). The decision not to refer patients to chiropractors probably means that many LBP patients will develop long-standing problems that could have been avoided.

Low Back Pain With Leg Pain

Differential diagnosis is crucial for cases in which LBP radiates into the leg. Specifically, motor, sensory, and reflex testing should be used to screen for signs of radiculopathy and cauda equina syndrome. Such factors play a central role in de-termining which patients should be referred directly for surgical consultation and which should be referred for manual manipulation. A growing body of research ev-idence indicates that, even in cases where radicular signs such as muscle weakness or decreased reflex response are present, chiropractic can yield beneficial results. In a series of 424 consecutive cases, Cox and Feller (1994) reported that 83% of 331 lumbar disc syndrome patients completing care (13% of whom had previous un-successful low back surgeries) had good to excellent results. "Excellent" was defined as greater than 90% relief of pain and return to work with no further care required, and "good" as 75% relief of pain and return to work with periodic manipulation or analgesia required. There was a median of 11 treatments and 27 days to attain maximal improvement. BenEliyahu (1996) followed 27 patients receiving chiropractic care for cervical and lumbar disc herniation (LDH), the majority being lumbar cases. Pretreatment and posttreatment MRI studies were performed; 80% of patients had a good clinical outcome, while 63% of the post-MRI studies showed the herniation was either reduced in size or completely resorbed. In a study of 14 patients with lumbar disc herniation, Cassidy, Thiel, and Kirkaldy-Willis (1993) reported that all but one obtained significant clinical improvement and relief of pain after a 2- to 3-week regimen of daily side-posture manipulation of the lumbar spine, directed toward improving spinal mobility. All patients received computed tomography (CT) scans before and 3 months after treatment. In most patients the CT appearance of the disc herniation remained unchanged after successful treatment, although five showed a small decrease in the size of the herniation, and one patient showed a large decrease.

Subsequently, Santilli, Beghi, and Finucci (2006) assessed the short- and long-term effects of spinal manipulation and simulated manipulation on acute back pain and sciatica with disc protrusion. They performed a randomized trial on 102 ambulatory patients with acute lumbar disc syndrome verified with clinical findings and MRI. Treatments were given 5 days per week by experienced chiropractors using a rapid thrust technique. The number of treatment sessions depended on the level of pain relief achieved, up to a maximum of 20 sessions. Manipulations appeared more effective on the basis of the percentage of pain-free cases (local pain, 28% vs. 6%; radiating pain, 55% vs. 20%). McMorland, Suter, Casha, du Plessis, and Hurlbert (2010) compared spinal manipulation versus micro-diskectomy for sciatica secondary to LDH in 40 patients who met participating neurosurgeons' inclusion criteria for surgery (having failed at least 3 months of nonoperative management including treatment with analgesics, lifestyle modification, physiotherapy, massage therapy, and/or acupuncture). Patients were randomized to either surgical micro-diskectomy or standardized chiropractic spinal manipulation. Crossover (where each patient acts as his or her own control) to the alternate treatment was allowed after 3 months. Sixty percent of patients with sciatica who failed other medical management benefited from spinal manipulation to the same degree as those who underwent surgical intervention. Of the other 40%, subsequent surgical intervention conferred an excellent outcome, countering the hypothesis that a course of manipulation may be harmful by causing a delay in surgery. The authors (a chiropractor and three neurosurgeons) concluded that patients with symptomatic LDH failing medical management should consider spinal manipulation, then followed by surgery if warranted. Evidence of this kind, combined with its own cost-benefit analyses, led the University of Pittsburgh Medical Center to institute a policy under which patients with chronic LBP must be treated with a 3-month course of care including both chiropractic and physical therapy, before any spine surgery is approved (Redwood, 2013).

Chronic Pain Management

Senna and Machaly (2011) performed a prospective, single-blind, randomized, controlled clinical trial to assess the effectiveness of SMT for the management of chronic nonspecific LBP and to determine the effectiveness of maintenance SMT in long-term reduction of pain and disability levels associated with chronic low back conditions after an initial phase of treatments. Sixty patients with chronic, nonspecific LBP lasting at least 6 months were randomized to receive: (1) 12 treatments of sham SMT over a 1-month period; (2) 12 treatments, consisting of SMT over a 1-month period, but no treatments for the subsequent 9 months; or (3) 12 treatments over a 1-month period, along with "maintenance spinal manipulation" every 2 weeks for the following 9 months. Patients in the second and third groups experienced significantly lower pain and disability scores compared to the first group at the end of one month. Only the third group, who received maintenance manipulation during the follow-up period, showed more improvement in pain and disability scores at the 10-month evaluation. In the nonmaintenance SMT group, the mean pain and disability scores returned to levels close to their pretreatment level.

Cifuentes, Willetts, and Wasiak (2011) at the Center for Disability Research at the Liberty Mutual Research Institute for Safety explored the effectiveness of various approaches from medicine, physical therapy and chiropractic for the prevention of injury recurrence when "health maintenance care" is provided to workers who have returned to their jobs after a work-related low back injury (Cifuentes et al., 2011). The authors define health maintenance care as:

"a clinical intervention approach thought to prevent recurrent episodes of LBP … it blends the public health concepts of secondary prevention (treatment and prevention of recurrences) with tertiary prevention (obtaining the best health condition while having an incurable disease). Health maintenance care can include providing advice, information, counseling and specific physical procedures. Health maintenance care is predominantly and explicitly recommended by DCs, although some physical therapists also advocate health maintenance procedures to prevent recurrences."

After controlling for demographics and severity, patients treated by chiropractors were significantly less likely to have a disabling recurrence compared to those treated by medical doctors or physical therapists. Chiropractic care fared best, and its hazard ratio (HR) was used as the reference point (1.0). In comparison, the HR was 1.6 for medical physicians and 2.0 for physiotherapists. However, the HR for those not receiving any health maintenance care at all after they returned to work was 1.2, which was described as similar to the HR for chiropractic in terms of statistical significance, and might suggest that patients were better off not seeking any medical or physical therapy.

Cost Effectiveness for Low Back Pain
A retrospective claims analysis of 85,000 LBP patients insured by Tennessee Blue Cross/Blue Shield found that those initiating care with chiropractors had 40% lower treatment costs for LBP episodes than those initiating care with medical physicians. When severity was factored in, those who initiated care with chiropractors still had 20% lower costs (Liliedahl, Finch, Axene, & Goertz, 2010).

A systematic review of guideline-endorsed treatments for LBP found that spinal manipulation was cost effective for patients with subacute or chronic LBP, but that there was insufficient evidence for the cost effectiveness of spinal manipulation for acute LBP (Lin, Haas, Maher, Machado, & van Tulder, 2011). In contrast, the epidemiologist authors of this study reported that they could find "no evidence" of cost effectiveness of medications for LBP.

A systematic review found spinal manipulation was cost effective for neck and back pain, used alone or combined with other therapies (Michaleff, Lin, Maher, & van Tulder, 2012). A prospective cohort study of Washington State workers found that 1.5% of workers who saw a chiropractor first for work-related back pain review, later had surgery, compared to 42.7% of those who first saw a surgeon. This dramatic difference was for cases equivalent in severity (Keeney et al., 2013), suggesting on its face that nearly half of back surgeries may be inappropriate.

Neck Pain

Neck pain is the second most common reason that patients seek chiropractic care. Chiropractic care can be clinically observed as helpful to individuals with acute or chronic neck pain. Currently, the research from randomized trials on spinal manipulation is equivocal, which is actually true for all other neck pain treatments as well. In contrast to the strong evidence on LBP, neck pain is a disorder for which no single method can be said to have sufficiently strong research support at this time.

World Health Organization Bone and Joint Decade

By far the most comprehensive recent evaluation of all neck pain therapies was that performed by the Bone and Joint Decade 2000 to 2010 Task Force on Neck Pain and Its Associated Disorders of the World Health Organization (Haldeman, Carroll, Cassidy, Schubert, & Nygren, 2008; Hurwitz et al., 2008). The panel concluded:

"Our best evidence synthesis suggests that therapies involving manual therapy and exercise are more effective than alternative strategies for patients with neck pain; this was also true of therapies which include educational interventions addressing self-efficacy."

Chiropractors consistently include exercise advice and share relevant self-care educational materials with patients as part of overall care (Jamison, 2002). Management of neck pain substantially embodies the full range of noninvasive therapeutic approaches recommended by the Bone and Joint Decade Task Force.

A team of Dutch researchers led by Koes et al. (1993) studied patients with persistent back and neck complaints. In a randomized trial, they were treated with manual therapy (spinal manipulation and mobilization), physiotherapy (exercises, massage, electrotherapy, ultrasound, shortwave diathermy), treatment by a general practitioner (analgesics, posture advice, home exercise, and bed rest), or a placebo treatment consisting of detuned shortwave diathermy and detuned ultrasound. For neck and back complaints together, improvements in severity of the main complaint were larger with manipulative therapy than with physiotherapy; for neck complaints only, the mean improvement in the main complaint as shown by the visual analog scale was slightly better for manipulative rather than physical therapy. Both manual therapy and physiotherapy (both of which are part of the chiropractor's scope of practice) were superior to medical care and placebo. In this study, the placebo actually yielded results superior to medical care, suggesting that patients are better off doing nothing than seeking regular medical care.

In a randomized clinical trial, Palmgren, Sandstrom, Lundqvist, and Heikkila (2006) found that a group of chronic neck pain patients who received 15 to 25 chiropractic treatments over a 5-week period had significantly lower pain scores and greater head repositioning accuracy than another group with the same condition given a similar examination but no treatment. Chiropractic care included high- and low-velocity techniques, myofascial release (see Chapter 13), and spine-stabilizing exercises. The researchers concluded that chiropractic care could be effective in reducing pain originating in the cervical spine and enhancing proprioceptive sensibility (movement and position sense).

Bronfort et al. (2012), at Northwestern University of Health Sciences (NWUHS), hypothesized that: "SMT is more effective than medication or home exercise with advice (HEA) for acute and subacute neck pain."

In a randomized trial, they found that neck pain patients receiving spinal manipulation achieved significantly more pain relief than those receiving medication. They also found that a group receiving a few instructional sessions of home exercise advice achieved results that were, for all practical purposes, equal to the manipulation group. Regarding adverse side effects, Bronfort's group reported that while

"the frequency of reported side effects was similar among the 3 groups (41% to 58%), the nature of the side effects differed, with participants in the SMT and HEA groups reporting predominantly musculoskeletal events and those in the medication group reporting side effects that were more systemic in nature. Of note, participants in the medication group reported higher levels of medication use after the intervention".

Also worth noting is that the medication group, which had to use more medications, reported the most side effects and the manipulation group reported the least.

A second neck pain study from a team at NWUHS (Evans et al., 2012) looked at chronic neck pain, in contrast to the Bronfort et al. study, which focused on acute and subacute neck pain. The chronic neck pain project compared two different exercise regimes: "high-dose" supervised exercise and "low-dose" home exercise. In addition, they divided the high-dose exercise group in half, with one subgroup also receiving chiropractic spinal manipulation while the other was treated solely with intensive exercise. Unlike the Bronfort et al. trial, there was no additional group randomized to receive medication as a primary treatment. In the Evans et al. trial, all groups showed improvement, with the two supervised strengthening groups improving significantly more than the home exercise group. However, "no significant differences were found between supervised exercise with or without spinal manipulation, suggesting that spinal manipulation confers little additional benefit."

The authors appropriately note that this finding "differs from the conclusion of the Task Force on Neck Pain and Its Associated Disorders and systematic reviews (Gross et al., 2007; Kay et al., 2005), which found an advantage for exercise combined with manual therapy for chronic neck pain," adding, "importantly, our study was not designed to assess the effect of spinal manipulation alone." A recent Cochrane systematic review has found limited evidence to support spinal manipulation alone for the short-term relief of chronic neck pain.

HEADACHE

In a practice guideline for chiropractic care of adults with headaches, Bryans et al. (2011) provide a systematic review of the relevant literature. Based on the 21 articles that met their inclusion criteria, spinal manipulation and multimodal multidisciplinary interventions including massage are recommended for management of patients with episodic or chronic migraine. They reported that the literature does not support spinal manipulation for the management of ETTH, and that no recommendation can be made for or against the use of spinal manipulation for patients with chronic tension-type headache. Instead, they found that low-load craniocervical mobilization may be beneficial for longer term management of patients with episodic or chronic tension-type headaches. For cervicogenic headache, spinal manipulation is recommended, and joint mobilization or deep neck flexor exercises may improve symptoms.

Overall, Bryans et al. (2011) concluded that "evidence suggests that chiropractic care, including spinal manipulation, improves migraine and cervicogenic headaches. The type, frequency, dosage, and duration of treatment(s) should be based on guideline recommendations, clinical experience, and findings. Evidence for the use of spinal manipulation as an isolated intervention for patients with tension-type headache remains equivocal." Probably the most noteworthy chiropractic research on headaches to have emerged from the United States is the work on headaches conducted by Boline et al. (1995). Chiropractic was shown to be more effective than the tricyclic antidepressant (TCA) amitriptyline used for long-term relief of headache pain. During the treatment phase of this trial, pain relief among those treated with medication was comparable to the SMT group. However, the chiropractic patients maintained their levels of improvement after treatment was discontinued, whereas those taking medication returned to pretreatment status in an average of 4 weeks after its discontinuation. This finding strongly implies that although medication suppressed the symptoms, chiropractic addressed the problem at a more causal level. A subsequent trial by this group of investigators employing a similar protocol for patients with migraine headaches demonstrated that migraines were similarly responsive to chiropractic, and that adding amitriptyline to chiropractic treatment conferred no additional benefit (Nelson et al., 1998).

ARM AND LEG PAINS

Chiropractic focus on the spine is enhanced through attention to the roles of the limbs and extremities (arms and legs). Since the earliest days of the profession, chiropractors have adjusted extremity joints. In some cases, adjustment is done to address local problems at the ankle, knee, or shoulder. In other cases it is done to influence the overall balance of the body, including the spine. Causation runs in both directions—spinal adjustments can influence the extremities, and extremity manipulation can influence the spine.

Two comprehensive reviews have evaluated the status of extremity manipulation research, which is currently much less extensive than research on manipulation of the spine. Brantingham et al. (2009), in an expert panel appointed by the Scientific Commission of the Council on Chiropractic Guidelines and Practice Parameters, reviewed all available research on lower extremity conditions. They found fair evidence for manipulative therapy of the knee and/or full kinetic chain, and of the ankle and/or foot, combined with multimodal or exercise therapy for knee osteo-arthritis, patella-femoral pain syndrome, and ankle inversion sprain. They found limited evidence for manipulative therapy of the ankle and/or foot combined with multimodal or exercise therapy for foot conditions such as plantar fasciitis, meta-tarsalgia, and hallux limitus and hallux rigidus.

Bronfort et al. (2010) included, in their comprehensive UK Evidence Report, review of research on manual therapies for upper and lower extremity problems. For lower extremity conditions, they reached conclusions similar to the Brantingham review. For upper extremity conditions (which were not included in the Brantingham review), Bronfort's group found moderate evidence supporting the addition of manipulation or joint mobilization to usual medical care for shoulder girdle pain. Evidence was inconclusive but tended in a favorable direction on manipulation and mobilization for rotator cuff pain. There was moderate evidence that long-term benefits from elbow mobilization with exercise exceed those from corticosteroid injections. Evidence was inconclusive but tended in a favorable direction, for manipulation and mobilization in the treatment of carpal tunnel syndrome. Specific trials on manual methods for extremity (arm and leg) conditions are as follows.

SHOULDER

In a study from the Netherlands, published in the *British Medical Journal,* Winters et al. (1997) found that for "shoulder girdle" pain, manipulation was superior to physical therapy. For "synovial" pain at the shoulder's ball-and-socket joint, corticosteroid injections were the most effective approach. Another Dutch study by Bergman et al. (2004) found that adding manipulative therapy to usual medical care yielded superior outcomes in patients with shoulder dysfunction and pain. In a study from the United States published in the *Journal of the American Chiropractic Association,* Munday et al. (2007) conducted a randomized, single-blinded, placebo-controlled, clinical trial on shoulder impingement syndrome in which one group received shoulder adjustments and the other a placebo (detuned ultrasound). Participants were treated 8 times over 3 weeks, resulting in a significant pain reduction for the group receiving chiropractic care (Munday et al., 2007).

Hip

One major study on hip manipulation was conducted by Hoeksma et al. (2004) who compared hip manipulation and mobilization to an exercise program. Patients were treated once a week for 9 weeks. Success rates (perceived improvement) after 5 weeks were 81% in the manual therapy group and 50% in the exercise group. Patients in the manual therapy group had significantly better outcomes in pain, stiffness, hip function, and ROM. Effects of manual therapy on improvement of pain, hip function, and ROM endured after 29 weeks (Hoeksma et al., 2004).

Knee

At a military medical center in Texas, Deyle et al. (2000) analyzed a program of manual therapy applied to the knee and to the lumbar spine, hip, and ankle as required, plus standardized knee exercises. They compared this program to a placebo involving subtherapeutic ultrasound applied to the knee. Both clinical and statistically significant improvements were observed in the 6-minute walking distance and Western Ontario and McMaster Universities Arthritis Index (WOMAC) score (for osteoarthritis symptoms) at 4 weeks and 8 weeks in the treatment group, but not the placebo group. By 8 weeks, average 6-minute walking distances had improved by 13% and the WOMAC scores had improved by 56%. At 1 year, patients in the treatment group had clinically and statistically significant gains over baseline WOMAC scores and walking distance. Meanwhile, 20% of patients in the placebo group and 5% of patients in the treatment group had undergone knee surgery. The researchers concluded that "a combination of manual physical therapy and supervised exercise yields functional benefits for patients with osteoarthritis of the knee and may delay or prevent the need for surgical intervention" (Deyle et al., 2000).

Deyle et al. also performed a large study on knee osteoarthritis compared a home-based physical therapy regime with a clinic-based program that included both supervised exercise and manual therapy (Deyle et al., 2005). These investigators concluded that a home exercise program was effective for patients with osteoarthritis of the knee and that clinical visits with manual therapy and supervised exercise increased the benefit.

Ankle

Pellow and Brantingham (2001) performed the first chiropractic trial on ankle inversion sprains. They compared results of an ankle mortise separation adjustment to a placebo intervention of detuned ultrasound. Patients received 8 treatment sessions over 4 weeks. The researchers found that "although both groups showed improvement, statistically significant differences in favor of the adjustment group were noted with respect to reduction in pain, increased ankle ROM, and ankle function."

Standard treatment for ankle sprains is based on the rest, ice, compression, and elevation (RICE) protocol. Green, Refshauge, Crosbie, and Adams (2001) found that adding mobilization to RICE was more effective than RICE alone for decreasing pain and increasing ankle mobility. Patients were treated every second day for

2 weeks or until discharge criteria were met. The experimental group had greater improvement in range of movement before and after each of the first three treatment sessions. The experimental group also had greater increases in stride speed during the first and third treatment sessions.

SOMATOVISCERAL DISORDERS

Although the bulk of chiropractic research focuses on musculoskeletal disorders, some investigators have studied the effects of SMT for somatovisceral disorders. There is currently no visceral disorder for which more than one randomized trial has shown a benefit from spinal manipulation. A systematic review by Hawk, Khorsan, Lisi, Ferrance, and Evans (2007) summarized the literature on chiropractic treatment of nonmusculoskeletal disorders, applying both conventional methods of analysis and a whole-systems perspective. Research on visceral disorders involving pain is summarized subsequently.

Infantile Colic

A randomized trial by chiropractic and medical investigators at the University of Southern Denmark showed chiropractic spinal manipulation to be more effective for treating infantile colic than water-soluble dimethicone, an antifoaming agent for the gastrointestinal (GI) tract (Wiberg et al., 1999). An estimated 23% of newborns suffer from colic, a painful condition marked by prolonged, intense, high-pitched crying. Numerous studies have explored a possible GI etiology, but the cause of colic has long remained a mystery.

The mean daily hours of colic in the chiropractic group were reduced by 66% on day 12, which is virtually identical to the 67% reduction in a previous prospective trial. In contrast, the dimethicone group showed a 38% reduction. The Danish study on infantile colic was the first randomized controlled trial to demonstrate effectiveness of chiropractic manipulation for a disorder generally considered to be nonmusculoskeletal in nature. Addressing this issue, the authors concluded that their data led to two possible interpretations: "Either spinal manipulation is effective in the treatment of the visceral disorder infantile colic or infantile colic is, in fact, a musculoskeletal disorder" (Wiberg et al., 1999).

A contrasting view is provided by a study performed under the auspices of a university pediatrics department in Norway (Olafsdottir, Forshei, Fluge, & Markestad, 2001). In this study, 86 infants were randomly assigned to chiropractic care or placebo (held for 10 minutes by a nurse, rather than given a 10-minute visit with a chiropractor). In the chiropractic group, adjustments were administered by light fingertip pressure. Both groups experienced substantial decreases in crying, the primary outcome measure; 70% of the chiropractic group improved versus 60% of those held by nurses. However, no statistically significant differences were found between the two groups in terms of the number of hours of crying, or as measured on a five-point improvement scale (from "getting worse" to "completely well"). The researchers concluded that "chiropractic spinal manipulation is no more effective than placebo in the treatment of infantile colic." This conclusion raises a significant methodological issue regarding the role of control or placebo interventions in chiropractic and other nonpharmacological research, as discussed in this chapter.

Otitis Media

A pilot study by Fallon, a New York pediatric chiropractor, evaluating chiropractic treatment for children with otitis media demonstrated improved outcomes compared to the natural course of the illness. Using both parental reports and tympanography with a cohort of more than 400 patients, data suggest a positive role for spinal and cranial manipulation in the management of this challenging condition (Fallon, 1997; Fallon & Edelman, 1998).

Menstrual Pain

Two small controlled clinical trials evaluating the effects of chiropractic manipulation for primary dysmenorrhea showed encouraging results. Both pain relief and changes in certain prostaglandin levels were noted (Kokjohn, Schmid, Triano, & Brennan, 1992; Thomasen, Fisher, Carpenter, & Fike, 1979). However, a much larger randomized trial concluded no significant benefit from manipulation (Hondras, Long, & Brennan, 1999). The validity of this larger trial's comparison group intervention has been criticized (Hawk et al., 2007) on methodological grounds.

SAFETY

All health care interventions entail some risk, which is best evaluated in relation to other common treatments for similar conditions (i.e., adjustment/manipulation vs. anti-inflammatory medications for neck pain). Medications with a safety profile comparable to that of spinal manipulation are considered quite safe. Although minor, temporary soreness after a chiropractic treatment is not unusual, major adverse events resulting from chiropractic treatment are few and infrequent. As one reliable metric, chiropractic malpractice insurance premiums are substantially lower than those for medical and osteopathic physicians and surgeons.

Stroke

A rare, potential reaction to chiropractic treatment that has raised the greatest concern is that of vertebrobasilar accident (VBA), or stroke, following cervical spine manipulation. Stroke following manipulation occurs so rarely that it is virtually impossible to study other than on a retrospective basis. The cohort necessary for a prospective study would have to be so large as to involve hundreds of thousands or millions of patients in order to observe a minimum number of cases for study. Statistical correlation does not equal causation. Such correlations have been based on events involving numbers of stroke patients (in single digits) interspersed among millions of chiropractic visits. Conclusions about direct causation are not possible.

Lauretti (2003) provided a summary of chiropractic safety issues based on the information available several years ago, putting forth the following key points: All reliable published studies estimating the incidence of stroke from cervical adjustment or manipulation agree that the risk is less than 1 to 3 incidents per 1 million treatments and approximately 1 incident per 100,000 patients. Haldeman, Carey, Townsend, and Papadopoulos (2001) found the rate of stroke to be 1 in 8.0 million office visits, 1 in 5.9 million cervical adjustments/manipulations, 1 in 1430 chiropractic practice years, and 1 in 48 chiropractic practice careers. NSAIDs, which are also widely used for neck pain and headaches, have a much less desirable safety record than manipulation.

Since then, relevant analysis of an unusually large database in Canada has been completed. The two most important and revealing studies exploring the possible relation between chiropractic and stroke were based on a retrospective review of hospital records in the province of Ontario, Canada.

Rothwell, Bondy, and Williams (2001) reviewed all records from 1993 to 1998 and found a total of 582 VBA cases. Each was age and sex matched to four controls from the Ontario population with no history of stroke at the event date. Public health insurance billing records were used to document utilization of chiropractic services during the year prior to VBA onset. Health care in Canada is publicly funded and this data is presumed to be comprehensive. Slightly more than 90% of the entire cohort (525 of 582 cases) had no chiropractic visits in the year preceding their VBA. Of the 57 individuals with VBAs who did visit a chiropractor in the 365 days preceding the VBA (out of 50 million chiropractic visits during the 5-year period studied), 27 are believed to have had cervical manipulation. Of these, 4 individuals visited a chiropractor on the day immediately preceding the VBA, 5 in the previous 2 to 7 days, 3 in the previous 8 to 30 days, and 15 in the previous 31 to 365 days. Compared to the controls, there was an increased association of VBA among patients who saw a chiropractor 1 to 8 days prior to the VBA event, but a decreased association of CVA among patients who saw a chiropractor 8 to 30 days before the event. Parsing their data for age-related differences, Rothwell et al. (2001) found no positive association between recent chiropractic visits and VBAs in patients over 45 years of age. However, patients under age 45 were 5 times more likely to have visited a chiropractor within the week prior to the VBA and five times more likely to have had three or more visits with a cervical diagnosis in the month preceding the VBA. "Despite the popularity of chiropractic therapy," the authors wrote in their conclusion;

"the association with stroke is exceedingly difficult to study. Even in this population-based study, the small number of events was problematic. Of the 582 VBA cases, only 9 had a cervical manipulation within one week of their VBA. Focusing on only those aged 45 years or younger reduced our cases by 81%; of these, only 6 had cervical manipulation within 1 week of their VBA. "

Regarding incidence, they add, "Our analysis indicates that, for every 100,000 persons aged 45 years or younger receiving chiropractic, approximately 1.3 cases of VBA attributable to chiropractic would be observed within 1 week of their manipulation." Recognizing that such a temporal association does not imply causation, Rothwell et al. (2001) "caution that such rate estimates can easily be overemphasized … this study design does not permit us to estimate the number of cases that are truly the result of trauma sustained during manipulation."

Several years later, Cassidy et al. (2008) completed a review of the same records evaluated by Rothwell's group and extended the time period covered in the review by three years. They performed additional analyses to determine whether patients who had seen a chiropractor were more likely to have had a stroke than patients who had seen a medical physician. This question, which had not been part of the earlier Rothwell et al. (2001) review, was crucial because patients in the early stages of stroke commonly experience symptoms (headache, neck pain) that may well lead them to consult a chiropractor or a medical doctor. Cassidy et al. (2008) found that it was no more likely for a stroke patient to have seen a chiropractor than to have seen a primary care medical physician. The authors concluded,

"The increased risks of VBA stroke associated with chiropractic and PCP visits is likely due to patients with headache and neck pain from VBA dissection seeking care before their stroke. We found no evidence of excess risk of VBA stroke associated chiropractic care compared to primary care."

Any claims or criticisms that the benefits of spinal manual therapy are not supported by research evidence must at this point be considered the result of scientific ignorance or bias. Scientific studies have not been able to substantiate claims of any dangerous side effects of SMT or provide any evidence that adjustments of the neck cause any increased risk of cerebral strokes. Rather, research evidence indicates that spinal manual therapy, especially for acute, subacute, and chronic LBP is safe, effective, and cost-effective, and that standard medical care and back surgery may well be ineffective, useless, and dangerous. SMT is provided by some physical therapists and all chiropractors. There are approximately 60,000 chiropractors in the United States, licensed in all 50 states and Washington, DC. Spinal manual therapy is also available worldwide. Scientific evidence supports SMT as the treatment of choice for LBP, the most common cause of pain and disability in working-age Americans today.

REFERENCES

Abu-Asab, M., Amri, H., & Micozzi, M. S. (2013). *Avicenna's medicine: A new translation of the 11th-century canon with practical applications for integrative health care.* Rochester VT: Healing Arts Press. 462 p.

Baker, G. A., Farabaugh, R. J., Augat, T. J., & Hawk, C. (2012). Algorithms for the chiropractic management of acute and chronic spine-related pain. *Topics in Integrative Healthcare, 3*(4). http://www.tihcij.com/Articles/Algorithms-for-the-Chiropractic-Management-of-Acute-and-Chronic-Spine-Related-Pain.aspx?id=0000381.

Bakris, G., Dickholtz, M., Sr., Meyer, P. M., Kravitz, G., Avery, E., Miller, M., et al. (2007). Atlas vertebra realignment and achievement of arterial pressure goal in hypertensive patients: A pilot study. *Journal of Human Hypertension, 21,* 347–352.

Balon, J., Aker, P. D., Crowther, E. R., Danielson, C., Cox, P. G., O'Shaughnessy, et al. (1998). A comparison of active and simulated chiropractic manipulation as adjunctive treatment for childhood asthma. *New England Journal of Medicine, 339*(15), 1013–1020.

BenEliyahu, D. J. (1996). Magnetic resonance imaging and clinical follow-up: Study of 27 patients receiving chiropractic care for cervical and lumbar disc herniations. *Journal of Manipulative and Physiological Therapeutics, 19*(9), 597–606.

Bennett, G. M. (1981). *The art of the bonesetter*. Isleworth: Tamor Pierston.

Bergman, G. J., Winters, J. C., Groenier, K. H., Pool, J. J., Meyboom-de Jong, B., Postema, K., et al. (2004). Manipulative therapy in addition to usual medical care for patients with shoulder dysfunction and pain: A randomized, controlled trial. *Annals of Internal Medicine, 141*(6), 432–439.

Bigos, S., Bowyer, O., & Braen, G. (1994). *Acute lower back pain in adults. Clinical practice guideline, Quick reference guide No 14, AHCPR Pub No 95-0643*. Rockville, Md: US Department of Health and Human Services, Public Health Service, Agency for Health Care Policy and Research.

Bishop, P. B., Quon, J. A., Fisher, C. G., & Dvorak, M. F. S. (2010). The Chiropractic Hospital-based Interventions Research Outcomes (CHIRO) study: A randomized controlled trial on the effectiveness of clinical practice guidelines in the medical and chiropractic management of patients with acute mechanical low back pain. *The Spine Journal, 10*(12), 1055–1064.

Boline, P. D., Kassak, K., Bronfort, G., Nelson, C., & Anderson, A. V. (1995). Spinal manipulation vs. amitriptyline for the treatment of chronic tension-type headaches: A randomized clinical trial. *Journal of Manipulative and Physiological Therapeutics, 18*(3), 148–154.

Bourdillion, J. F. (1982). *Spinal manipulation* (3rd ed.). East Norwalk, Conn: Appleton-Century-Crofts.

Bove, G., & Nilsson, N. (1998). Spinal manipulation in the treatment of episodic tension-type headache: A randomized controlled trial. *Journal of American Medical Association, 280*(18), 1576–1579.

Brantingham, J. W., Globe, G., Pollard, H., et al. (2009). Manipulative therapy for lower extremity conditions: Expansion of literature review. *Journal of Manipulative and Physiological Therapeutics, 32*(1), 53–71.

Brealey, S., Burton, K., Coulton, S., Farrin, A., Garratt, A., Harvey, E., et al. (Aug 1 2003). UK back pain exercise and manipulation (UK BEAM) trial–national randomised trial of physical treatments for back pain in primary care: Objectives, design and interventions [ISRCTN32683578]. *BMC Health Services Research, 3*(1), 16.

Bronfort, G., Evans, R., Anderson, A. V., Svendsen, K. H., Bracha, Y., & Grimm, R. H. (2012). Spinal manipulation, medication, or home exercise with advice for acute and subacute neck pain. *Annals of Internal Medicine, 156*(1 Part 1), 1–10.

Bronfort, G., Haas, M., Evans, R., Leiniger, B., & Triano, J. (2010). Effectiveness of manual therapies: The UK evidence report. *Chiropractic and Osteopathy, 18*(1), 3.

Bryans, R., Descarreaux, M., Duranleau, M., Marcoux, H., Potter, B., Ruegg, R., et al. (2011). Evidence-based guidelines for the chiropractic treatment of adults with headache. *Journal of Manipulative and Physiological Therapeutics, 34*(5), 274–289.

Cassidy, J. D., Boyle, E., Cote, P., et al. (2008). Risk of vertebral-basilar stroke and chiropractic care: Results of a population-based case-control and case-crossover study. *Spine, 33*(4 Suppl.), S176–S183.

Cassidy, J. D., Thiel, H. W., & Kirkaldy-Willis, W. H. (1993). Side posture manipulation for lumbar intervertebral disk herniation. *Journal of Manipulative Physiological Therapeutics, 16*(2), 96–103.

Cherkin, D., Deyo, R. A., & Berg, A. O. (1991). Evaluation of a physician education intervention to improve primary care for low back pain. I. Impact on physicians. *Spine, 16*(10), 1168–1172.

Cherkin, D. C., & MacCornack, F. A. (1989). Patient evaluations of low back pain care from family physicians and chiropractors. *Western Journal of Medicine, 150*(3), 351–355.

Chou, R., Qaseem, A., Snow, V., Casey, D., Cross, J. T., Jr., Shekelle, P., et al. (2007). Diagnosis and treatment of low back pain: A joint clinical practice guideline from the American College of Physicians and the American Pain Society. *Annals of Internal Medicine, 147*(7), 478–491.

Cifuentes, M., Willetts, J., & Wasiak, R. (2011). Health maintenance care in work-related low back pain and its association with disability recurrence. *Journal of Occupational and Environmental Medicine/ American College of Occupational and Environmental Medicine, 53*(4), 396–404.

Commission on Alternative Medicine. (1987). Social Departementete: Legitimization for vissa kiropraktorer. *Stockholm, 12*, 13–16.

Cox, J. M., & Feller, J. A. (1994). Chiropractic treatment of low back pain: A multicenter descriptive analysis of presentation and outcome in 424 consecutive cases. *Journal of the Neuromusculoskeletal System, 2*, 178–190.

Croft, P. R., Macfarlane, G. J., Papageorgiou, A. C., Thomas, E., & Silman, A. J. (1998). Outcome of low back pain in general practice: A prospective study. *British Medical Journal, 316*(7141), 1356–1359.

Danish Institute for Health Technology Assessment. (1999). Low-back pain: Frequency, management, and prevention from an HTA perspective. *Danish Health Technology Assessment, 1*(1), 1–106.

Deyle, G. D., Allison, S. C., Matekel, R. L., Ryder, M. G., Stang, J. M., Gohdes, D. D., et al. (2005). Physical therapy treatment effectiveness for osteoarthritis of the knee: A randomized comparison of supervised clinical exercise and manual therapy procedures versus a home exercise program. *Physical Therapy, 85*(12), 1301–1317.

Deyle, G. D., Henderson, N. E., Matekel, R. L., Ryder, M. G., Garber, M. B., & Allison, S. C. (2000). Effectiveness of manual physical therapy and exercise in osteoarthritis of the knee. A randomized, controlled trial. *Annals of Internal Medicine, 132*(3), 173–181.

Dvorak, J. (1985). Neurological and biomechanical aspects of pain. In A. A. Buerger & P. E. Greenman (Eds.), *Approaches to the validation of spinal manipulation* (pp. 241–266). Springfield, IL: Charles C Thomas.

Evans, R., Bronfort, G., Schulz, C., Maiers, M., Bracha, Y., Svendsen, K., et al. (2012). Supervised exercise with and without spinal manipulation performs similarly and better than home exercise for chronic neck pain: A randomized controlled trial. *Spine, 37*(11), 903–914.

Fallon, J. (1997). The role of the chiropractic adjustment in the care and treatment of 332 children with otitis media. *Journal of Clinical Chiropractic Pediatrics, 2*(2), 167–183.

Fallon, J., & Edelman, M. J. (1998). Chiropractic care of 401 children with otitis media: A pilot study. *Alternative Therapies in Health and Medicine, 4*(2), 93.

Gatterman, M. I., & Goe, D. R. (1990). Muscle and myofascial pain syndromes. In M. I. Gatterman (Ed.), *Chiropractic management of spine related disorders* (pp. 285–329). Baltimore: Lippincott Williams & Wilkins.

Gellert, G. (1994). Global explanations and the credibility problem of alternative medicine. *Advances in Mind Body Medicine, 10*(4), 60–67.

Globe, G. A., Morris, C. E., Whalen, W. M., Farabaugh, R. J., & Hawk, C. (2008). Council on chiropractic guidelines and practice parameter. Chiropractic management of low back disorders: Report from a consensus process. *Journal of Manipulative and Physiological Therapeutics, 31*(9), 651–658.

Green, T., Refshauge, K., Crosbie, J., & Adams, R. (2001). A randomized controlled trial of a passive accessory joint mobilization on acute ankle inversion sprains. *Physical Therapy, 81*(4), 984–994.

Gross, A. R., Goldsmith, C., Hoving, J. L., Haines, T., Peloso, P., Aker, P., et al. (2007). Conservative management of mechanical neck disorders: A systematic review. *Journal of Rheumatology, 34*(5), 1083–1102.

Haldeman, S., Carey, P., Townsend, M., & Papadopoulos, C. (2001). Arterial dissections following cervical manipulation: The chiropractic experience. *Canadian Medical Association Journal, 165*, 905.

Haldeman, S., Carroll, L., Cassidy, J. D., Schubert, J., & Nygren, A. (2008). The bone and joint decade 2000-2010 task force on neck pain and its associated disorders: Executive summary. *Spine, 33*(4 Suppl.), S5–S7.

Haldeman, S., Chapman-Smith, D., & Peterson, D. M. (Eds.), (1993). Guidelines for chiropractic quality assurance and practice parameters. In *Proceedings of the mercy center consensus conference.* Gaithersburg, Md: Aspen.

Hasselberg, P. D. (1979). *Chiropractic in New Zealand: Report of a commission of inquiry.* Wellington, NZ: Government Printer.

Hawk, C., Khorsan, R., Lisi, A. J., Ferrance, R. J., & Evans, M. W. (2007). Chiropractic care for nonmusculoskeletal conditions: A systematic review with implications for whole systems research. *Journal of Alternative and Complementary Medicine, 13*(5), 491–512.

Hoeksma, H. L., Dekker, J., Ronday, H. K., Heering, A., van der Lubbe, N., Vel, C., et al. (2004). Comparison of manual therapy and exercise therapy in osteoarthritis of the hip: A randomized clinical trial. *Arthritis and Rheumatism, 51*(5), 722–729.

Hondras, M. A., Long, C. R., & Brennan, P. C. (1999). Spinal manipulative therapy versus a low force mimic maneuver for women with primary dysmenorrhea: A randomized, observer-blinded, clinical trial. *Pain, 81*(1–2), 105–114.

Hondras, M. A., Long, C. R., Cao, Y., Rowell, R. M., & Meeker, W. C. (2009). A randomized controlled trial comparing 2 types of spinal manipulation and minimal conservative medical care for adults 55 years and older with subacute or chronic low back pain. *Journal of Manipulative and Physiological Therapeutics*, *32*(5), 330–343.

Hurwitz, E. L., Carragee, E. J., van der Velde, G., Carroll, L. J., Nordin, M., Guzman, J., et al. (2008). Treatment of neck pain: Noninvasive interventions: Results of the bone and joint decade 2000-2010 task force on neck pain and its associated disorders. *Spine*, *33*(4 Suppl.), S123–S152.

Jamison, J. R. (2002). Health information and promotion in chiropractic clinics. *Journal of Manipulative and Physiological Therapeutics*, *25*, 240–245.

Kay, T. M., Gross, A., Goldsmith, C., Santaguida, P. L., Hoving, J., & Bronfort, G. (2005). Exercises for mechanical neck disorders. *Cochrane Database of Systematic Reviews*, *3*. CD004250.

Keeney, B. J., Fulton-Kehoe, D., Turner, J. A., Wickizer, T. M., Chan, K. C., & Franklin, G. M. (2013). Early predictors of lumbar spine surgery after occupational back injury: Results from a prospective study of workers in Washington State. *Spine*, *38*(11), 953–964.

Kelly, P. T., & Luttges, M. W. (1975). Electrophoretic separation of nervous system proteins on exponential gradient polyacrylamide gels. *Journal of Neurochemistry*, *24*, 1077–1079.

Kirkaldy-Willis, W., & Cassidy, J. (1985). Spinal manipulation in the treatment of low back pain. *Canadian Family Physician*, *31*, 535–540.

Koes, B. W., Bouter, L. M., van Mameren, H., Essers, A. H., Verstegen, G. J., Hofhuizen, D. M., et al. (1993). A randomized clinical trial of manual therapy and physiotherapy for persistent back and neck complaints: Subgroup analysis and relationship between outcome measures. *Journal of Manipulative and Physiological Therapeutics*, *16*(4), 211–219.

Kokjohn, K., Schmid, D. M., Triano, J. J., & Brennan, P. C. (1992). The effect of spinal manipulation on pain and prostaglandin levels in women with primary dysmenorrhea. *Journal of Manipulative and Physiological Therapeutics*, *15*(5), 279–285.

Korr, I. M. (1975). Proprioceptors and the behavior of lesioned segments. In E. H. Stark (Ed.), *Osteopathic medicine* (pp. 183–199). Acton, Mass: Publication Sciences Group.

Korr, I. M. (1976). The spinal cord as organizer of disease processes: Some preliminary perspectives. *Journal of American Osteopathic Association*, *76*, 89–99.

Lauretti, W. J. (2003). Comparative safety of chiropractic. In D. Redwood, Cleveland, C. S.III (Eds.), *Fundamentals of chiropractic* (pp. 561). St Louis: Mosby.

Lawrence, D. J., Meeker, W., Branson, R., Haas, M., Haneline, M., Micozzi, M. S., et al. (2008). Chiropractic management of low back pain and low back-related leg complaints: A literature synthesis. *Journal of Manipulative and Physiological Therapeutics*, *31*(9), 659–674.

Leach, R. A. (1994). *The chiropractic theories: Principles and clinical applications* (3rd ed.). Baltimore: Lippincott Williams & Wilkins.

Liliedahl, R. L., Finch, M. D., Axene, D. V., & Goertz, C. M. (2010). Cost of care for common back pain conditions initiated with chiropractic doctor vs medical doctor/doctor of osteopathy as first physician: Experience of one Tennessee-based general health insurer. *Journal of Manipulative and Physiological Therapeutics*, *33*(9), 640–643.

Lin, C. W., Haas, M., Maher, C. G., Machado, L. A., & van Tulder, M. W. (2011). Cost-effectiveness of guideline-endorsed treatments for low back pain: A systematic review. *European Spine Journal*, *20*(7), 1024–1038.

Lomax, E. (1975). Manipulative therapy: A historical perspective from ancient times to the modern era. In M. Goldstein (Ed.), *The research status of spinal manipulation: 1975* (pp. 11–17). Washington, DC: US Government Printing Office.

Luttges, M. W., Kelly, P. T., & Gerren, R. A. (1976). Degenerative changes in mouse sciatic nerves: Electrophoretic and electrophysiological characterizations. *Experimental Neurology*, *50*, 706–733.

MacGregor, R. J., & Oliver, R. M. (1973). A general-purpose electronic model for arbitrary configurations of neurons. *Journal of Theoretical Biology*, *38*, 527–538.

MacGregor, R. J., Sharpless, S. K., & Luttges, M. W. (1975). A pressure vessel model for nerve compression. *Journal of Neurolological Sciences*, *24*, 299–304.

Manga, P., Angus, E. D., Papadopoulos, C., & Swan, W. R. (1993). *The effectiveness and cost-effectiveness of chiropractic management of low-back pain.* Richmond Hill, VA: Kenilworth.

McMorland, G., Suter, E., Casha, S., du Plessis, S. J., & Hurlbert, R. J. (2010). Manipulation or microdiskectomy for sciatica? A prospective randomized clinical study. *Journal of Manipulative and Physiological Therapeutics, 33*(8), 576–584.

Meade, T. W. (1992). Interview on Canadian Broadcast Corporation. In *Chiropractic: A review of current research.* Arlington, VA: Foundation for Chiropractic Education and Research.

Meade, T. W., Dyer, S., Browne, W., & Frank, A. O. (1995). Randomised comparison of chiropractic and hospital outpatient management for low back pain: Results from extended follow up. *British Medical Journal, 311*(7001), 349–351.

Meade, T. W., Dyer, S., Browne, W., Townsend, J., & Frank, A. O. (1990). Low back pain of mechanical origin: Randomised comparison of chiropractic and hospital outpatient treatment. *British Medical Journal, 300*(6737), 1431–1437.

Mense, S. (1991). Considerations concerning the neurobiological basis of muscle pain. *Canadian Journal of Physiology Pharmacology, 69,* 610–616.

Michaleff, Z. A., Lin, C. W., Maher, C. G., & van Tulder, M. W. (2012). Spinal manipulation epidemiology: Systematic review of cost effectiveness studies. *Journal of Electromyography and Kinesiology, 22*(5), 655–662.

Micozzi, M. S. (1998). Complementary medicine: What is appropriate? Who will provide it? *Annals of Internal Medicine, 129,* 65–66.

Munday, S., Jones, A., Brantingham, J., Globe, G., Jensen, M., & Price, J. (2007). A randomized, single-blinded, placebo-controlled clinical trial to evaluate the efficacy of chiropractic shoulder girdle adjustment in the treatment of shoulder impingement syndrome. *Journal of American Chiropractic Association, 44*(6), 6–15.

Nelson, C. F., Bronfort, G., Evans, R., Boline, P., Goldsmith, C., & Anderson, A. V. (1998). The efficacy of spinal manipulation, amitriptyline and the combination of both therapies for the prophylaxis of migraine headache. *Journal of Manipulative and Physiological Therapeutics, 21*(8), 511–519.

Olafsdottir, E., Forshei, S., Fluge, G., & Markestad, T. (2001). Randomised controlled trial of infantile colic treated with chiropractic spinal manipulation. *Archives of Disease in Childhood, 84,* 138–141.

Palmer, D. D. (1910). *Textbook of the science, art, and philosophy of chiropractic.* Portland, OR: Portland Printing House.

Palmgren, P. J., Sandstrom, P. J., Lundqvist, F. J., & Heikkila, H. (2006). Improvement after chiropractic care in cervicocephalic kinesthetic sensibility and subjective pain intensity in patients with nontraumatic chronic neck pain. *Journal of Manipulative and Physiological Therapeutics, 29*(2), 100–106.

Paré, A. (1968). *The collected works of Ambroise Paré.* New York: Milford House.

Patterson, M. M., & Steinmetz, J. E. (1986). Long-lasting alterations of spinal reflexes: A potential basis for somatic dysfunction. *Manual Medicine, 2,* 38–42.

Pellow, J. E., & Brantingham, J. W. (2001). The efficacy of adjusting the ankle in the treatment of subacute and chronic grade I and grade II ankle inversion sprains. *Journal of Manipulative and Physiological Therapeutics, 24*(1), 17–24.

Redwood, D. (1999). Same data, different interpretation. *Journal of Alternative and Complementary Medicine, 5*(1), 89–91.

Redwood, D. (2013). DC receives federal grant to study nonsurgical alternatives to surgery for spinal stenosis: Interview with Michael Schneider, DC, PhD. *Health Insights Today, 6*(2). http://www.cleveland. edu/media/cms_page_media/811/MichaelSchneiderInterview.pdf.

Rosen, M. (1994). *Back pain: Report of a clinical standards advisory group committee on back pain.* London: HMSO.

Rothwell, D. M., Bondy, S. J., & Williams, I. (2001). Chiropractic manipulation and stroke: A population-based case-control study. *Stroke, 32,* 1054–1060.

Santilli, V., Beghi, E., & Finucci, S. (2006). Chiropractic manipulation in the treatment of acute back pain and sciatica with disc protrusion: A randomized double-blind clinical trial of active and simulated spinal manipulations. *The Spine Journal: Official Journal of the North American Spine Society*, 6(2), 131–137.

Schafer, R. C., & Faye, L. J. (1989). *Motion palpation and chiropractic technique*. Huntington Beach, CA: Motion Palpation Institute.

Senna, M. K., & Machaly, S. A. (2011). Does maintained spinal manipulation therapy for chronic nonspecific low back pain result in better long-term outcome? *Spine*, 36(18), 1427–1437.

Sharpless, S. (1975). Susceptibility of spinal roots to compression block. In M. Goldstein (Ed.), *The research status of spinal manipulation: 1975* (pp. 155–161). Washington, DC: US Government Printing Office.

Shekelle, P. G. & Adams, A. H. (1991). *The appropriateness of spinal manipulation for low-back pain: Project overview and literature review*. Report No R-4025/1-CCR/FCER Santa Monica, CA: RAND.

Simske, S. J. & Schmeister, T. A. (1994). An experimental model for combined neural, muscular, and skeletal degeneration. *Journal of Neuromusculoskeletal System*, 2, 116–123.

Suh, C. H. (1974). The fundamentals of computer aided x-ray analysis of the spine. *Journal of Biomechanics*, 7, 161–169.

Thomasen, P. R., Fisher, B. L., Carpenter, P. A., & Fike, G. L. (1979). Effectiveness of spinal manipulative therapy in treatment of primary dysmenorrhea: A pilot study. *Journal of Manipulative and Physiological Therapeutics*, 2, 140–145.

Thompson, C. J. (1986). *Second report: Medicare Benefits Review Committee*. Canberra, Canada: Commonwealth Government Printer.

Triano, J. J. & Luttges, M. W. (1982). Nerve irritation: A possible model of sciatic neuritis. *Spine*, 7, 129–136.

Triano, J. J., McGregor, M., Hondras, M. A., & Brennan, P. C. (1995). Manipulative therapy versus education programs in chronic low back pain. *Spine*, 20, 948–955.

UK BEAM Trial Team. (2004a). United Kingdom back pain exercise and manipulation (UK BEAM) randomised trial: Effectiveness of physical treatments for back pain in primary care. *British Medical Journal*, 329(7479), 1377.

UK BEAM Trial Team. (2004b). United Kingdom back pain exercise and manipulation (UK BEAM) randomised trial: Cost effectiveness of physical treatments for back pain in primary care. *British Medical Journal*, 329(7479), 1381.

Wiberg, J. M., Nordsteen, J., & Nilsson, N. (1999). The short-term effect of spinal manipulation in the treatment of infantile colic: A randomized controlled clinical trial with a blinded observer. *Journal of Manipulative and Physiological Therapeutics*, 22(8), 517–522.

Wilk v AMA (1990). 895 F2D 352 Cert den, 112.2 ED 2D 524.

Wilkey, A., Gregory, M., Byfield, D., & McCarthy, P. W. (2008). A comparison between chiropractic management and pain clinic management for chronic low-back pain in a National Health Service outpatient clinic. *Journal of Alternative and Complementary Medicine*, 14(5), 465–473.

Winters, J. C., Sobel, J. S., Groenier, K. H., Arendzen, H. J., & Meyboom-de Jong, B. (1997). Comparison of physiotherapy, manipulation, and corticosteroid injection for treating shoulder complaints in general practice: Randomised, single blind study. *British Medical Journal*, 314(7090), 1320–1325.

Withington, E. T. (1959). *Hippocrates*. (Vol. 3). Cambridge, MA: Harvard University Press.

Suggested Readings can be found on the companion website, http://www.micozzipainconditions.com.

Chapter 13

Massage, Manual Therapies, and Bodywork

Essentially all massage, manual therapy, and bodywork approaches are directed toward tissue and musculoskeletal pain and inflammation, soreness, stiffness, and related physical conditions. The inclusion in this chapter and integration of some Asian manual therapies in continuity with other approaches also serves as transition to Section IV, "Asian Medical Systems."

Massage and related treatments include a variety of approaches that come under a definition of "manual therapies." These manual modalities use the practitioner's hands, and may potentially include the use of elbows, forearms, and even feet, to directly apply techniques (sometimes called "manual manipulation") to the patient's body for the purpose of enhancing health and wellness. Spinal manual therapy, chiropractic techniques, as well as aspects of physical, occupational therapy, and athletic training can all be broadly be included in this category. Those modalities are often combined with massage and other therapies to synergistically enhance health and healing.

Massage has a wide spectrum of therapeutic applications. Different theoretical concepts can be used to understand the body, including structure, function, movement, neural communications, and bioenergetic models. The practitioner's perspective influences which applications and techniques are best used to achieve the goals. The rate or speed of movements of the hands on the skin, the depth of pressure used, whether lubrication is employed, or whether the hands even contact the body at all can be combined to achieve the outcomes intended for a given session.

Manual manipulation has existed for thousands of years as a therapeutic practice. Origins of the earliest forms of manual therapy are not precisely known. More than 2000 years ago in ancient Greece, it was recorded that Hippocrates was skilled in the use of therapeutic manipulation and taught it in his school of medicine. There are ancient illustrations that suggest the use of manual therapies prior to written historical records. In ancient China, the use of manual therapy *(tui na)*, possibility to influence "acupuncture" points and energy channels on the body ("acupressure"), predates the development of the technology necessary to produce the fine filiform needles used for acupuncture, over 2000 years ago (Fig. 13.1).

Acknowledgment to Judith Walker DeLany for prior contributions in Micozzi, M.S. (Ed.), (2016). *Fundamentals of complementary and alternative medicine* (5th ed.). St Louis: Elsevier Health Sciences/ Saunders.

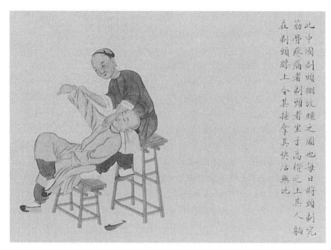

FIG. 13.1 | A patient receiving manipulation of the shoulder. Joint manipulation has always been an important feature of Chinese medical treatment.

Almost all world cultures apply some use of manual and manipulative therapy. Some of these practices have been passed along only in oral tradition, and documentation is difficult or impossible to find. The types of manual and manipulative therapy in this book are those for which historically documented information is available. Today manual therapies and bodywork incorporate diverse applications from around the world, with numerous methods to learn and practice them. In addition to conducting traditional live class or apprentice forms of teaching and learning, techniques are also taught on DVD, online, in webinars, and through live broadcasts.

The development of new science-based theories and models, and research investigations and data reflect the continuing inquiry and evolving understanding of the body and the way that manual therapies affect it. This investigation is now taking into account bioenergy and the consciousness approach to health and healing, especially involving pain perception and processing, as discussed in the previous chapters. This chapter describes the basic principles and theories of well-known manual modalities and their applications to pain. Understanding the body's connective tissues and fascia as a matrix is important to these approaches.

THE MATRIX OF THE BODY

Whether the manual modality addresses the osseous, muscular, visceral, bioenergetic, or "acupuncture" channel structures, it always affects the common integral component of fascia. Fascia is the contiguous colloidal matrix and connective tissue of the whole body. A colloid exists in a kind of "in-between" state of matter, having physical-chemical properties between a liquid (like body fluids) and a solid (like bone, muscle, and body tissues). Fascia, from a fluid standpoint, comprises a single, continual, integrated, and totally connected network, from the soles of the feet (plantar fascia) to the attachments on the inner aspects of the skull. From a solid standpoint, it "divides" the body by diaphragms, septa, and sheaths. However, fascia is more than just a background substance with an obvious supporting role. It is a ubiquitous, tenacious, living tissue deeply invested and involved in the bodies most fundamental processes, including structure, function, and metabolism. Patients often experience a feeling of "release" during manual manipulations of this matrix, from the head or thorax all the way to the tips of the toes. One way to consider it, from a craniosacral perspective (discussed later), is by the subtle manual pressures on fluid dynamics of the cerebrospinal fluid (CSF) of the central nervous system (CNS) enveloping the brain and nervous system down through the spinal canal, to the cauda equina (Latin for "tail of the horse," to describe the spinal nerves of the lower body as they exit the spinal canal at the sacrum), down through the peripheral nerves, and out to the body. Another way to consider it is through the subtle pressures and influences on the interconnected matrix of the connective tissues themselves all through the body.

The therapeutic approach does not consider muscles as being separate structures from fascia since they are so intimately related. Chaitow and DeLany (2008) state:

- Fascia attaches extensively to and invests into muscles, by providing individual muscle fibers with an envelope of endomysium that blends with the stronger perimysium surrounding the fasciculi, which, in turn, merges into an even stronger epimysium that surrounds the muscle as a whole and attaches to adjacent fascial tissues. The fascial planes provide pathways for nerves, blood and lymphatic vessels and a supporting matrix for more highly organized structures, such as the viscera.
- Fascia comprises the intermuscular septa and interosseous membranes, which provide surfaces for muscular attachments. Restraining mechanisms, such as retention bands, fibrous pulleys, and check ligaments, are invested with fascia that assists in the creation and control of movement. Where the texture is loose, it allows movement between adjacent structures and can also mitigate the effects of pressure, forming fluid-filled sacs, called bursae, which reduce friction of tendons against underlying bones.
  - Fibroblastic activity in fascia aids in the repair of injuries by the deposition of collagenous fibers (scar tissue). Superficial fascia allows for the storage of fat (panniculus adiposis), which aids in the conservation of body heat (and appears as the "marbling" of meaty tissue).
  - Connective tissue contains nearly a quarter of all body fluids, providing an essential medium through which the cellular elements of other tissues are brought into functional relation with blood and lymph. Fluids, as well as infectious processes, often travel along fascial planes. Phagocytic activity of the white blood cell histiocytes in fascia provides an important defense mechanism against bacterial invasion and plays a role as scavengers in removing cell debris and foreign material.
  - Removing connective tissue from the complex would leave any muscle as a jelly-like structure without form and no longer capable of performing its function.

When any part of the fascial network becomes distorted, resulting and compensating adaptive stresses can be imposed on structures that it divides, envelopes, enmeshes, and supports, and with which it connects. The consequences of a stress cascade are not limited just to the structural elements of muscle, tendon, ligament, bone, and disk. Pressure can also be imposed on the neural, blood, and lymphatic components, which course alongside and through fascia, as well as the visceral organs and glands invested by fascia. Fascial entrapment of neural structures can, in turn, produce pain and a wide range of symptoms and dysfunctions by triggering neural receptors within the fascia that connect to the CNS. Sources of pain signaling may include the pacinian corpuscles, which inform the CNS about the rate of acceleration of movement taking place in the area. There are also highly specialized, sensitive mechanoreceptors and proprioceptive reporting sites contained in the tendons and ligaments as well as peptides released by cells and hormones excreted by the glands, which serve as the chemical messengers of metabolism and can influence pain and inflammation.

Massage and other manual techniques are used primarily to alleviate pain and restore function. Manipulation of connective tissues affects the fascia by altering its ground substance, elongating for shortened tissues, and rebalancing the biochemical environment surrounding individual cells. A range of massage techniques and systems offer a variety of effects on isolated tissues, overall structural integrity, and general well-being of the individual that help eliminate, reduce, and manage pain.

CLASSICAL MASSAGE

Uses of massage as therapy may predate written history (Fig. 13.2). The ancient Greeks are credited in the West as inventors of the art of gymnastics, which may have included therapeutic massage to restore the free movement of body fluids and return the patient to a state of health. During the European Renaissance, physician Ambroise Paré authored a widely used surgery text in which he espoused the application of massage and manipulation and was reportedly the first to use the term "subluxation." In 1813, Pehr Henrik Ling, a gymnastics instructor, founded the Royal Gymnastic Central Institute, where he developed a systematic routine of formal movements and passive gymnastics known as "Swedish Movement Cure." His work actually contained minimal massage techniques but is identified as the forerunner of Swedish massage. Ling's student Johann Georg Metzger (Casanelia & Stelfox, 2009; Pettman, 2007) was a Dutch physician who developed a basic classification of massage techniques. Metzger's own work was never published, but his students von Mosengeil and Helleday in turn wrote and published descriptions of the techniques and the classifications, using the French terms still used today (effleurage, petrissage, tapotement, etc.) (Orstrom, 1918). In the late 19th century the prominent French physician Marie Marcellin Lucas-Championnière (perhaps being the only one who could read and understand these terms) advocated consideration of soft-tissue union in the healing process of traumatic injury. His students, in turn, the English physicians William Bennett and Robert Jones, effectively brought massage to England. Bennett incorporated the use of massage at St. George's Hospital in

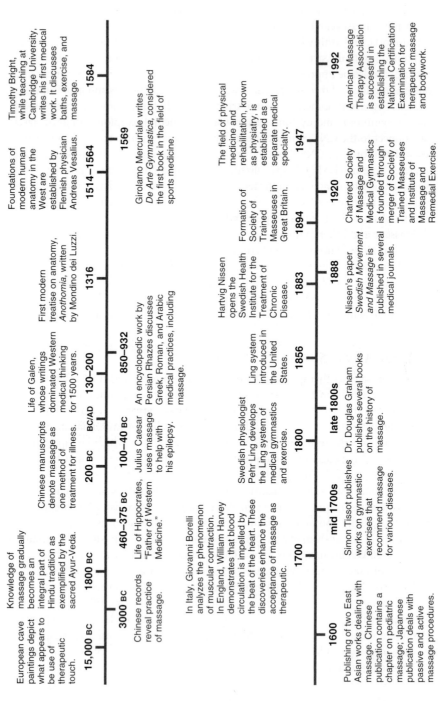

FIG. 13.2 | Massage timeline.

London at the turn of the 20th century. Jones used massage therapy at the Southern Hospital in Liverpool. Jones taught James Mennell, who authored the text *Physical Treatment by Movement, Manipulation, and Massage* (1917) and became a tireless advocate of massage in England. Jones also taught Mary McMillan, who was very influential in the introduction and promotion of massage in the United States. Around the turn of the 20th century, the German scientist Zabludowski, a professor of massage at the University of Berlin, brought science and credibility to the application of massage. Dr. John Harvey Kellogg compiled extensive documentation regarding the effects of massage at his "nature cure" institute in Battle Creek, Michigan at the turn of the 20th century.

During the first half of the 20th century, several others continued to make significant contributions:

- Albert Hoffa's techniques, described in his German text *Technik der Massage* (1900), are still in use today. Hoffa advocated limiting massage to only 15-minute treatments and ensuring that no pain was experienced by the client. Like Ling before him, Hoffa stated massage should be applied from distal to proximal, outward to inward, with the heart as the point of reference. His manual adaptations included knuckling and circular effleurage, two-finger pétrissage, and other forms.
- Mary McMillan, aforementioned, is credited with categorization of massage into five basic techniques and introduced innovative variations in each of those categories. She advocated the use of olive oil as a lubricant for its nutrient value when absorbed through the skin. Her techniques have been widely adopted by massage therapists in the United States and elsewhere.
- Elisabeth Dicke was a proponent of *Bindegewebsmassage* ("binding webs" massage) as a student of Hoffa who had described massage based on the connective tissue system of the body. She described areas of referred pain on the back that indicate internal pathology but do not necessarily correspond to nerve segmental distributions. Areas of tenderness correspond to certain acupuncture points as well. This treatment is given with the middle finger in a series of sequenced strokes without lubricant.
- James Cyriax was an advocate of friction as the most effective technique in massage. He developed the "transverse friction massage" technique, which is widely used by manual therapists. Deep friction massage is used to stimulate increased circulation to affected areas applied to muscles, tendons, ligaments, and bones. Cyriax (1984 a,b) described these methods in detail in his book *Textbook of Orthopaedic Medicine*, volume 2.
- Janet Travell (one of US President John F. Kennedy's physicians in the 1950s and early 1960s) and David Simons were medical doctors who researched myofascial "trigger points" for decades, documenting their locations and patterns of referral. Their efforts produced two textbooks: *Myofascial Pain and Dysfunction* and *The Trigger Point Manual*, volume 1 on the upper body and volume 2 on the lower body (Simons, Travell, & Simons, 1999; Travell & Simons, 1992). Their work provided foundations for a new branch of pain medicine and topics for researchers worldwide who continue to uncover new elements of understanding of myofascial and trigger points in pain.

ESSENTIAL THEORY IN PRACTICE

The science of physiology became entwined with the study of pain and the structures of the body in the growth of the Western model of biomedicine. Some attribute the development of the physical therapy profession as an outgrowth of massage. Many other forms of so-called bodywork, an assortment of which are discussed later in next chapter, are also ultimately outgrowths of massage and its various techniques and styles.

One essential theory of massage therapy is based on the principle that the tissues of the body function at optimal levels when arterial supply and venous and lymphatic drainage are unimpeded ("rule of the artery"). When the flow of body fluids becomes unbalanced, muscle tightness and changes in the nearby skin and fascia ensue, resulting in pain. The basic techniques of massage are designed to re-establish proper fluid dynamics as can be directed primarily through the skin, muscles, and fascia. Nerve pathways are also occasionally addressed. Aside from passive or active range of motion (ROM), joint articulations are generally not directly addressed in this form of therapy, although they may be affected by the applied techniques.

Areas to avoid during the application of massage include skin infections or melanoma skin tumors, sites of bleeding and bruising (especially within 48 hours of a traumatic event), acute inflammation (e.g., rheumatoid arthritis, appendicitis), thrombophlebitis, atherosclerosis, varicose veins, and immunocompromised states (to avoid transmission of infection from patient to massage practitioner or vice versa). Certain medical procedures (e.g., radiation therapy), medications (e.g., blood thinners), or conditions (e.g., osteoporosis, recent fractures) may limit or contraindicate the use of deep pressure, friction, or ROM work. A number of locations require extra caution, such as the region of the carotid artery, suboccipital triangle, supraclavicular fossa, posterior knee, femoral triangle, and abdominal cavity. Specific training may also be required for intraoral applications or for work with lymphedema and cancer patients.

In accordance with the body fluid dynamic theory, techniques of massage are generally applied in the direction of the heart to stimulate increased venous and lymphatic drainage from involved tissues. Muscle groups are addressed together, with one group usually being treated before advancing to the next. Different combinations of techniques are used depending on the objectives of treatment. Treatment typically begins with more gentle, superficial techniques before progressing to deeper or more aggressive applications. Traditional massage is often performed with powder, oil, or another type of lubricant applied to the skin of the client, who lies prone, supine, or laterally on a table, or who may be seated in a massage chair. A variety of techniques also exist that use no lubricant or only a thin film (e.g., Rolfing, structural bodywork), and entire approaches may be performed without lubrication (e.g., lymphatic drainage, craniosacral therapy, discussed later). Verbal communication between the practitioner and patient is important because the practitioner relies on cues given by the patient to help guide the treatment. The visceral effects of massage include general vasoactivity in somatic tissues as regulated by the autonomic nervous system. Also, effects on blood pressure and/or heart rate (usually decreases in both) can be observed as the person relaxes during the treatment.

FIVE BASIC TECHNIQUES

There are five basic techniques of massage. They are all passive techniques, meaning the practitioner does the work while the client sits or lays back and relaxes. The five basic techniques are effleurage, pétrissage, friction, tapotement, and vibration. There are variations of these basic techniques, which may create different outcomes within the tissue for pain relief. Effleurage applied at a moderate pace with lubrication increases blood flow and lymphatic drainage. However, effleurage applied with almost no lubrication at a very slow pace produces a shearing force on the tissue that focuses on the ground substance of the fascia. These variations provide a wide array of styles, methods, and versions of massage, each with its own foundation and applications, drawing their common roots in the basic techniques.

Effleurage is the most frequently applied massage technique typically used to begin a treatment session and introduce the patient to the process of touching (Fig. 13.3). Effleurage uses a gliding stroke applied with light to moderate pressure (superficial or deep), serving to modulate the arterial supply and venous and lymphatic drainage

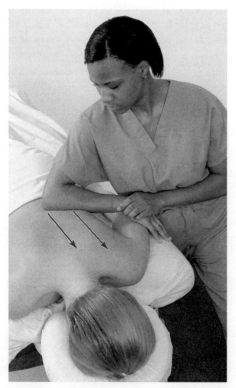

FIG. 13.3 | Effleurage can be applied with thumbs, fingers, palms, or forearm (as shown).

of the tissues contacted. The amount of pressure applied determines the layer(s) of the body contacted; very light pressure affects primarily the skin, deeper pressure the superficial fascia, and even deeper pressure the deep fascia. The thumbs, fingers, or entire palmar surface of the hand is used. A "knuckling" technique may also be used or the proximal half of the ulnar surface of the arm can be used to provide a very broad surface of application. During the initial stages of treatment, effleurage is also used as a palpation diagnostic tool, as the practitioner searches for areas of altered texture or density, asymmetry, or tenderness. Specific long strokes are often used at the conclusion of treatment, especially if sleep induction is desired.

Pétrissage is somewhat more aggressive than effleurage, with the thumb and fingers working together to lift and "milk" the underlying fascia and muscles in a kneading motion. Care is taken not to pinch or produce bruising. Pétrissage also increases venous and lymphatic drainage of the muscles and breaks up adhesions (small areas of local fibrosis) that may be present in the fascia. Depending on the direction of application and any motion restriction, this technique can be considered direct or indirect.

Frottage (friction) can be considered the most deeply applied massage technique (Fig. 13.4). The tips of the fingers or thumb are used in circular, longitudinal, or transverse movements. If deeper pressure is desired, or if the practitioner becomes fatigued, the heel of the hand, or sometimes even the elbow, can be used. Friction can be employed when production of heat is desired, when adhesions are present, or when the target tissue is too deep for pétrissage. Cyriax developed the technique of transverse friction massage, which is widely used by physical therapists. As with pétrissage, the direction of the applied technique, relative to any motion restriction, determines whether the application is direct or indirect.

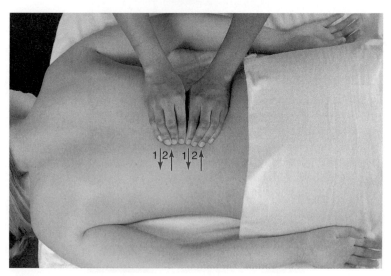

FIG. 13.4 | Friction applied to paraspinal muscles.

Tapotement, often depicted in classic boxing films, involves rapid, repeated blows of varying strength delivered with the tips of the fingers, with the sides or palms of the hands, with the hands cupped, or with the fists. Occasionally, rapid pinching of the skin is done. The purpose of tapotement is to stimulate arterial circulation to the area. It has considerable ability to inhibit reflexive spasms or to restore tone to hypotonic muscles. The technique should not produce bruising and should not be applied over the area of the kidneys, on the chest, or over any recent incisions or areas of inflammation or contusion.

Vibration that is manually applied is usually considered one of the more difficult of the massage techniques to perform without rapidly becoming fatigued. The modern application of vibration typically employs a mechanical vibrator or oscillator of some type. When the hands are used, a light, rhythmic, quivering effect is achieved. Brisk snapping or strumming across certain tissues, such as erector spinae muscles, can also be considered a form of vibration, an effect that can be likened to the vibration of a guitar string when strummed.

Manual pressures and forces may be applied to the tissue that alters its length, mobility, and density. For instance, a shear force can be applied to a superficial muscle layer to slide it laterally across the underlying muscle and disengage it from a deeper layer, which results in more mobility between the two (Fig. 13.5). Stretching a muscle's fibers can elongate the muscle and result in decompression of the associated joint(s). Elongation of a fascial plane can alter postural alignment and result in improved biomechanics of the region or the structure body as a whole.

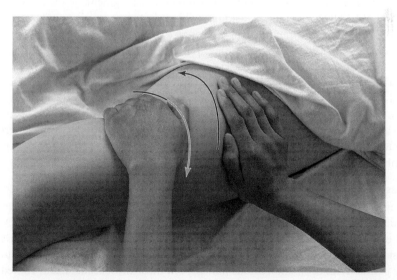

FIG. 13.5 | Shearing forces applied to the fascia of the anterior thigh.

CLINICAL APPLICATIONS

Variations of these basic techniques produce different outcomes within the tissues. A multitude of methods, versions, and styles of massage have emerged, with many having broad applications.

Burman and Friedland (2006) suggest basic techniques that form a central, unifying skill set for all massage applications that crosses global, cultural, philosophical, and theoretical foundations. While the depth of pressure, tension applied, sequence, and order may vary among the applications, or even within an application, the techniques themselves contribute to this fundamental set of skills. This skill set can be distilled to eight components engaging with the body, starting with attention to breathing, consciousness, and bioenergy, as well as the manual manipulations, all of which are important for pain. DeLany (2012) offers the following succinct list from Burman and Friedland's work:

BREATHING (tracking, directing, pacing) engages the mechanism of respiration, which creates waves that impact every system of the body.

COGNITIVE (visualizing, inquiring, intending, focusing transmitting) are tools for assessment, enhancement, modification, and change.

ENERGY (sensing, intuiting, balancing) is effective in detecting distortions and assisting the body to establish balance.

COMPRESSION (pressing/pushing, squeezing/pinching, twisting/wringing) applies a force to the body, reducing the space within and between structures and pressing fluid out.

EXPANSION (pulling, lifting, rolling) opens up space within and between the structures, bringing fluid into them.

KINETICS (holding/supporting, mobilizing, letting go/dropping, stabilizing) focuses on the movement relationship between segments of the body.

OSCILLATION (vibrating, shaking, striking) initiates waves by applying intermittent or continuous vibratory contact.

GLIDING (sliding/planing, rubbing) follows the contours of skin, muscle, tendon, ligament, bone, and fascial layers.

The practitioner combines and blends these basic elements to achieve the desired changes within the myofascial tissues. Whether viewing massage as simply five basic manual techniques, or all tangible and intangible components as mentioned previously, the goals remain constant. The practitioner can move seamlessly from one technique or skill to another as needed, with decisions being driven in the moment by what is discovered within the body and tissues.

Massaging Channels: Energy Anatomy and Physiology of Pain

Many applications are centuries old, far exceeding experience in the practice of modern biomedicine. In particular, Asian theoretical foundations (see Section IV) contain concepts that may not appear to relate to 20th-century Western understanding, especially those involving energy, channels, meridians, and acupuncture points. With open and curious minds, even those most academically rooted in the 20th-century Western biomedical paradigm can find evidence to support the

Eastern principles. The following discussion (Chaitow & DeLany, 2008) provides one example of how Asian medical concepts fit easily into a Western model where physiological research provides support.

Many Western experts believe that trigger points (see the "Neuromuscular Therapy" section later in this chapter) and acupuncture points represent the same phenomenon (Kawakita, Itoh, & Okada, 2002; Melzack, Stillwell, & Fox, 1977; Plummer, 1980). When both traditional and "ah shi" acupuncture points (see Chapter 15) are included, approximately 80% of common trigger point sites have been claimed to lie precisely where traditional acupuncture points have been situated on meridian maps (Wall & Melzack, 1990). Some researchers (Birch, 2003; Hong, 2000) find this percentage to be flawed, particularly when the trigger points are correlated with acupuncture points that are seen to be "fixed" anatomically, as on myofascial meridian maps. When examining the validity of the findings reported by Birch (2003), Dorsher (2008) reviewed references and literature to conclude that the overlap is significant, perhaps as high as 95%. While this debate over percentage of overlap may never be settled, some authors agree that so-called acupuncture points may well represent some of the same phenomena as reflected in trigger points—and others do not.

"Ah shi" points do not appear on the classical acupuncture meridian maps but refer to "spontaneously tender" points that, when pressed, create a response in the patient of "Oh yes!" (ah shi) or "Ouch, that's it." In Chinese medicine, ah shi points are treated as "honorary acupuncture points" and, when tender or painful, are generally addressed in the same manner as regular acupuncture points (see Chapter 15). Could they be, in all but name, identical to trigger points?

In attempting to understand trigger points more fully, it is useful to consider current research into acupuncture points and connective tissue in general. Ongoing research at the University of Vermont, led by Dr. Helene Langevin, has produced remarkable new information regarding the function of fascia/connective tissue as well as its relation to the locations of acupuncture points and energy meridians or channels (Ahn et al., 2010; Langevin, Bouffard, Badger, Iatridis, & Howe, 2005; Langevin, Churchill, & Cipolla, 2001; Langevin, Cornbrooks, & Taatjes, 2004; Langevin & Yandow, 2002).

Langevin and colleagues present evidence that links the network of acupuncture points and meridians to a network formed by interstitial connective tissue. Using a unique dissection and charting method for location of connective tissue (fascial) planes, acupuncture points, and acupuncture meridians of the arm, they note that more than 80% of acupuncture points and 50% of meridian intersections of the arm appear to coincide with intermuscular or intramuscular connective tissue planes (Langevin & Yandow, 2002).

Langevin's research further shows microscopic evidence that when an acupuncture needle is inserted and rotated (as classically performed in acupuncture treatment), a "whorl" of connective tissue strands forms around the needle, thereby creating a tight mechanical coupling between the tissue and the needle. The tension placed on the connective tissue as a result of further movements of the needle delivers mechanical stimuli at the cellular level. Changes in the extracellular matrix may, in turn, influence various cell populations sharing the connective tissue matrix (e.g., fibroblasts, sensory afferent cells, immune cells, and vascular cells).

Chaitow and DeLany (2008) summarized key elements of Langevin's research as follows:

- Acupuncture points, and many of the effects of acupuncture, appear to relate to the locations of "points" directly over areas where there is fascial cleavage, where sheets of fascia diverge to separate, surround, and support different muscle bundles (Langevin et al., 2001).
- Connective tissue comprises a communication system of as yet unknown potential. Ingber and Folkman (1989), Ingber (1993), and Chen and Ingber (1999) demonstrated integrins (tiny projections emerging from each cell) to comprise a cellular signaling system. Integrins can modify their functions depending on the relative normality of the shapes of cells. The structural integrity (shape) of individuals' cells depends on the overall state of normality (e.g., deformed, stretched) of the fascia as a whole.
- Langevin et al. (2004) reported "loose" connective tissue forms a network extending throughout the body including subcutaneous and interstitial connective tissues. The existence of a cellular network of fibroblast cells within loose connective tissue may have considerable significance, as it may support yet unknown body-wide cellular signaling systems. Our findings indicate that soft-tissue fibroblasts form an extensively interconnected cellular network, suggesting they may have important, and so far unsuspected integrative functions, at the level of the whole body.
- Cells change their shapes and behaviors following stretching (and crowding or deformation). The observation of these researchers is that "the dynamic, cytoskeleton-dependent responses of fibroblasts to changes in tissue length demonstrated in this study have important implications for our understanding of normal movement and posture, as well as therapies using mechanical stimulation of connective tissue, including physical therapy, massage and acupuncture" (Langevin et al., 2005).

To understand the role that fascia plays in chronic pain, structural deterioration, and illness, researchers are finding evidence of cellular, structural, and systemic components of this complex matrix. The International Fascia Research Congress is composed of scientists, researchers, and clinicians worldwide sharing an interest in human fascial tissues. More information can be found at http://www.fasciacongress.org.

The following manual methods offer significant relief to pain and suffering with virtually no risk for potential injury. In an environment in which the costs of health care, as well as the widespread use of opioid pain drugs, are out of control and harm from medical error is seriously increasing, use of these therapeutic interventions for pain is practical, prudent, economical, and effective. The massage styles and methods included are arranged alphabetically. The order is not an indication of which are most useful or more popular and does not imply success, value, or appropriate use. Appropriate manual therapies have intrinsic value, the degree of which is likely to be dependent on the practitioner's mastery and the patient's receptivity.

MANUAL ACUPRESSURE AND JIN SHIN DO

Acupressure is the application of the fingers to acupuncture points on the body, or "acupuncture without needles." It is based on the meridian or channel system, which is an integral component East Asian medical arts and philosophy. According to this system, there are 12 major channels through which flows the body's energy, or qi (chi). Although most of the channels are named for specific organs, they do not necessarily correspond to the anatomical body part but rather are more functional in nature. Interruptions in the flow of qi (prana, ki, vital energy, as described in other cultures) cause functional aberrations associated with that particular channel. These interruptions can be released and flow rebalanced by specific application of needles or fingers.

Jin shin do, or the "way of the compassionate spirit," was developed by psychotherapist Teeguarden (1978) as a form of acupressure in which the fingers are used to apply deep pressure to hypersensitive acupuncture points. Jin shin do represents a synthesis of Taoist philosophy, psychology, breathing, and acupressure techniques. In accordance with this philosophy, the body is linked to the mind and spirit, and tender points found in the body can represent expressions of emotional trauma or locked memories (i.e., somatoemotional component) (Fig. 13.6).

The theory of jin shin do states that various stimuli cause energy to accumulate at acupuncture points. Repeated stress in turn causes a layering of tension at the point, known as "armoring." The most painful point is termed the local point as a frame of reference. Other related tender points are referred to as distal points. Deep pressure applied to the point ultimately causes a release, and the tension dissipates. The overall effect is to re-establish flow in the channel and balance body energy. The context of the jin shin do treatment is as much psychological as physical and reiterates the importance of the body-mind-spirit connection for this treatment.

During the treatment session, the practitioner identifies a local point and nonverbally "asks permission" to treat it. A finger is placed on the local point while another finger is applied to a distal point. Gradually increasing pressure is applied to the local point. After 1 or 2 minutes, the practitioner feels the muscle relaxing, followed by a pulsation (practitioners of craniosacral therapy refer to this phenomenon as the "therapeutic pulse"). When the pulsing stops, the patient usually reports a decreased sensitivity at the point, indicating a successful treatment. Myofascial releases are sometimes accompanied by emotional releases as painful or emotional memories are brought to consciousness.

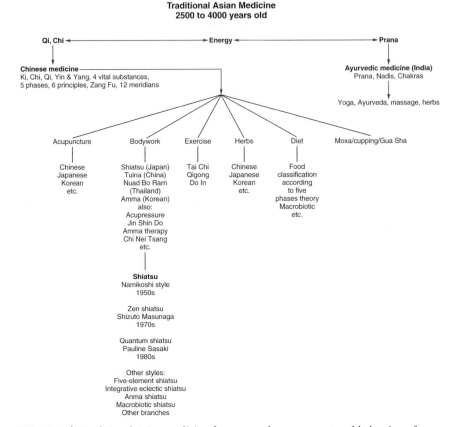

FIG. 13.6 | Traditional Asian medicine focuses on the assessment and balancing of energetic systems.

AYURVEDIC MANIPULATION

In Sanskrit, Ayurveda means "the study or science of life." As a healing art, Ayurveda is one of the world's oldest and, like the Hindu culture, probably predates the formal organization of Chinese Medicine. Ayurveda has many concepts and components, as discussed elsewhere in this book (see Chapter 18). Several principles that pervade Ayurveda apply to the manual components of Ayurvedic treatment.

Both Ayurvedic and Chinese theory present five basic elements. In contrast to those of Chinese theory (fire, water, earth, wood, metal), however, Ayurveda defines space (ether), air, fire, water, and earth as the five basic elements. These elements flow through the body with one or more predominating in certain areas, corresponding to specific organs, emotions, and other categories. Prana, or the life force (cf, qi, ki), also flows through the body, permeating the organs and tissues, and is especially concentrated at various points along the midline of the body, known as "chakras."

The unity and balance of body, mind, and spirit have deep cultural roots in Ayurveda. Body structure and a person's actions, feelings, and beliefs all reflect, and are reflected in, body constitution. The human constitution is based on the relative proportions and strengths of these three constituents (mind, body, spirit) and the five elements. Three basic types of constitutions (doshas) are recognized, which are based on different combinations of the five elements. The first, *vata*, is a combination of air and space and is reflected in kinetic energy. The second, *pitta*, combines fire and water and reflects a balance between kinetic and potential (stored) energy, which is expressed in the third constitution, *kapha*, a combination of earth and water.

The manipulative treatment developed within the Ayurvedic tradition offers three types of touch. *Tamasic* is strong and solid, firmly rooted in the earth (and might be well suited for a kapha constitution). The application is fast, and time is needed for the mind and spirit to "catch up." Tamasic might correspond to a high-velocity, low-amplitude technique (in osteopathy or chiropractic), tapotement (massage), or rubbing and thumb rocking (in Chinese medicine). The second type of touch, *rajasic*, is slower and is used to expand and integrate initial manual explorations and findings. It is considered to be more in resonance with the mind and spirit. As mentioned earlier, greater depth can be achieved with less tissue resistance due to the makeup of the body fascia. Effleurage (massage) and myofascial release (osteopathy, massage) might correspond to this type of touch, which in turn might be more suited to a pitta constitution. The vata constitution might benefit from the third type of touch, *satvic*, in which the application is very slow and gentle and can follow the intention of the mind and spirit. This might correspond to cranial osteopathy, sacro-occipital technique (chiropractic), counterstrain (osteopathy), the Trager approach, the Feldenkrais method, or healing or therapeutic touch (massage).

In a massage-oriented treatment, different essential oils (see also Chapter 24) are used as lubricants according to the constitution of the individual and the problem to be treated. The patient is prone or supine, lying on either side or sitting up, with the positions arranged in a specific sequence. Strokes are applied either toward or away from the heart, also in a specific sequence. Another technique, rarely encountered, uses the feet to perform the manipulation. The practitioner stands above the patient, who is lying prone on a reed mat, and applies the technique with the feet. Oils again are used as lubricants, and to maintain balance, the practitioner holds onto a cord strung lengthwise above the patient. The strokes go from the sacrum up the spine and out to the fingers, then back down to the feet. One side is done, then the other. The patient then lies supine, and the process is repeated.

Techniques can be direct or indirect relative to motion barriers. They can also be active or passive. Both the patient and the practitioner act as partners during treatment, exploring tissue and motion in an attempt to unlock the body and restore the unimpeded flow of prana and constitutional balance. Visualization, nonverbal communication, and mind intent are elements of treatment, regardless of the technique employed.

CRANIOSACRAL THERAPY

Craniosacral therapy originated from cranial osteopathy (osteopathic techniques applied to the cranium), as developed by W. G. Sutherland in the mid-1900s (see also "Osseous Techniques" later). Sutherland's work was based on observations that the joints between the skull bones (cranial sutures) are meant to permit some motion, just as joints in other areas of the body. While palpating the cranial bones and joints, he discovered the existence of a very subtle rhythm in the body unrelated to cardiovascular or breathing rhythms. Sutherland named this rhythm the cranial rhythmic impulse (CRI). This impulse, he learned, was capable of moving the cranial bones through a ROM that, although very small, was palpable to well-trained hands (Fig. 13.7). Cranial theory posits that there is inherent motility of the CNS, resulting in fluctuations of the cerebrospinal fluid, which bathes the brain and spinal cord. This fluctuation, in turn, moves the cranial bones through their small yet palpable ROM.

These concepts were expanded further in the 1970s by the findings of a research team at Michigan State University supervised by Dr. John Upledger. They confirmed that the motion associated with this rhythm is not restricted to the cranial bones. The cranium is linked to the spine and sacrum by the dural membranes, which cover the CNS, and the motion is palpable in the sacrum as well. In addition, through the fascial-fluid system, this motion affects the whole body. Motion restrictions in this system can be palpated and corrected (either directly or indirectly) through very gentle cranial manipulations that also have global effects on the body. Craniosacral therapy has emerged as a separate and distinct modality.

When "releases" are produced in this fascial system, and throughout the body, memories (sometimes emotionally painful) can be reawakened and produce "somatoemotional release," through mind-body connections. Clinical experience suggests that these experiences occur frequently. It is not understood whether this effect is related to the proximity of the membranes to the brain, stimulation of associated neural circuitry in peripheral tissues, or some other mechanism.

Craniosacral therapy has been controversial from its inception. Research studies that could conclusively evaluate the effectiveness of cranial therapies have not been performed. Evidence of effectiveness comes primarily in the form of clinical case reports and testimonials. Improvements in a variety of conditions have been reported, including chronic headache, cerebral palsy, autism, and behavioral disturbances. Data gathered through feasibility studies (Mann et al., 2012) and outcome-based studies lend credence to the effectiveness of craniosacral therapy (Mehl-Madrona, Kligler, Silverman, Lynton, & Merrell, 2007; Raviv, Shefi, Nizani, & Achiron, 2009).

Considerable time and effort are necessary to develop this skill. There are some osteopaths in the United States practicing cranial osteopathy. The practice of craniosacral therapy has also expanded to other manual therapy fields, including chiropractic, physical and massage therapies, and dentistry. Training has been offered by the Upledger Institute (Palm Beach Gardens, FL) and others.

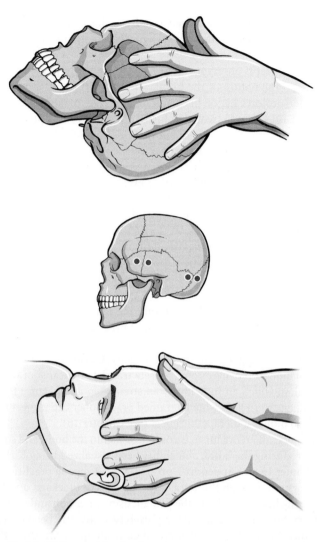

FIG. 13.7 | Vault hold for cranial palpation.

MANUAL ENERGY WORK

Energy work can be used to refer to either the techniques that have developed as part of ancient traditions (e.g., qigong) or recently developed methods in which the practitioner manipulates the bioenergy of the patient. The theory of bioenergy basically states that a life force, or vital energy, permeates the entire universe (see Chapters 2 and 3). This energy flows through all living things in coherent, distinct patterns. These patterns of flow are reflected in the meridian system (where qi, or chi, is the Chinese name given for the life force) and in the chakra system of Hindu tradition (where the word prana is used to indicate this force). Various forms of exercise have been developed for the cultivation of bioenergy, including yoga, internal qigong, and tai chi (see Section IV).

Three basic concepts are important in understanding energy work: intention, cooperation, and the nature of the human being. Intention is important in that the practitioner projects his or her consciousness, or mental intention, to heal into the patient. Intention to treat goes further than the proscriptive "do no harm" doctrine of Western therapeutics to embrace an affirmative attitude of love and concern. Intent also assumes a high level of mental visualization. Cooperation implies the partnership between the practitioner and patient as participants in the healing process, with neither being exclusively active or passive. The tripartite concept refers to recognition of three parts of the human being: body, mind, and spirit. This concept is envisioned in the much older Asian cultures as going beyond religion, whereas Western cultures have often relied on belief systems driven by organized faiths. In addition, the "scientific," reductionist approach of conventional Western medicine has been rather dismissive of spiritual aspects and has only recently begun acknowledging the mind-body connection (see Chapter 7). There are many systems of energy work, as discussed elsewhere in this book; four are included here among the massage and manual therapies. Two are rooted in Asian medical teaching and practice, and two are developed in Western application.

The Chinese term "qigong" (or qi gong, Qigong, Qi Gong) may be taken to refer to the manipulation of bioenergy and, loosely translated, means "qi work." Qigong can be internal, in which an individual can strengthen and balance the flow of qi within the self, or external, in which a trained practitioner can project his or her qi into a patient to induce a therapeutic effect (see Chapter 16).

The vital energy of an organism is contained within the body, and some radiates off the skin, producing the "aura," which has been visualized using Kirlian photography (see Chapter 11 and Appendix I, pp. 572-579). A qigong practitioner palpates the meridian system through this aura, locates points of blockage, and frees blockages by projecting his or her qi into the patient, using intention and visualization, or mental imagery. Specific "external qigong" exercises have also been developed that, when performed by the individual, serve to cultivate qi within the self (as in the Trager approach, the Feldenkrais method, and other bodywork techniques; see later in this chapter) Qigong can also arise naturally from long-term "internal" martial arts training, in which practitioners are capable of seemingly superhuman feats of strength and balance by channeling and projecting this energy.

HYDROTHERAPY AND THERMAL THERAPY

Hydrotherapy and thermal therapy are often considered to be an adjunct treatment to massage and other manual techniques, as well as part of traditional nature cure, naturopathy, and naturopathic medicine. They may be applied prior to, during, or after manual therapies, or may be stand-alone treatments in some cases. Some, such as aquatic massage, include techniques that may achieve significant results similar to that of massage.

Hydrotherapy is the use of water, in its many forms, either internally or externally, as a medical treatment. This modality is broadly defined and includes diverse approaches, such as application of or submersion in hot, cold, or neutral temperature water; application of vapocoolant spray or ice; or floating in a saltwater tank, or in or on the surface of a pool of water. The determination of which application(s) to use depends on the case presentation, type of trauma, consistency, and fluid levels in the tissues, as well as desired outcome goals. A few general guidelines help prevent injury and may improve desired results.

Generally speaking, muscles relax and blood vessels dilate when anything warm or hot is applied to tissues, resulting in increased blood flow and oxygen levels, and decreased pain nociceptive metabolites, segmental reflexes, and sympathetic tone. Unless there is a contraindication, such as recent trauma or tissue bruising, vasodilation is beneficial in many ways, reducing muscle spasms and joint stiffness, as well as softening muscles, connective tissues, and adhesions. After the application of heat, the tissues may become congested unless light exercise or gliding strokes of effleurage massage are applied. Alternatively, cold application of some sort can follow application of heat to decongest the area.

When a cold pack treatment is applied to tissues, it causes vasoconstriction of the local blood vessels and will increase small-fiber activity, flooding afferent pathways and causing brain stem inhibition of pain nociceptive information. After the removal of the cold treatment, blood vessels dilate slowly and tissues are again flushed with fresh, oxygen-rich blood. Additional benefits may include a reduction of pain, inflammation, and swelling of tissue often associated with trauma.

Accordingly, effective thermotherapy treatments are highly effective using alternately applied hot and cold, or contrast hydrotherapy, where heating and cooling the tissues is (usually rapidly) alternated to stimulate profound flushing of blood and lymph in muscles, skin, or organs.

The general principles of hot and cold applications are as follows:
- Cold is defined as 55 °F to 65 °F or 12.7 °C to 18.3 °C; anything colder is considered to be very cold and may damage the skin if inappropriately applied.
- Short cold applications (<1 minute) stimulate circulation; long cold applications (>1 minute) depress circulation and metabolism.
- Hot is defined as 98 °F to 104 °F or 36.7 °C to 40 °C; anything hotter than that is undesirable and dangerous.
- Short hot applications (<5 minutes) stimulate circulation; long hot applications (>5 minutes) vasodilate so well that they can result in congestion and require a cold application or massage to drain the area.
- Short hot followed by short cold applications cause alternation of circulation and may produce a profound flushing of the tissues.
- Cool is defined as 66 °F to 80 °F or 18.5 °C to 26.5 °C, and tepid is defined as 81 °F to 92 °F or 26.5 °C to 33.3 °C.

- Neutral/warm (93 °F to 97 °F or 33.8 °C to 36.1 °C) applications or baths at body heat are very soothing and relaxing.

Hot/cold packs, hot tubs, steam rooms, saunas, and cold plunges are the most commonly used applications of thermal therapy. Ancient in origin, massage applied with hot and/or cold stones enjoys popularity in modern times. Stones (usually smooth river rocks) of varying sizes allow for precise placement over small portions of a muscle. The stones are heated or cooled and then placed in strategic locations to alter the temperature of the skin and influence the underlying muscles (Wuttke, 2012).

Cryotherapy agents, such as vapocoolant sprays, are also used as surface anesthetics in the treatment of trigger points. Spray and stretch technique (S&S) can be seamlessly integrated with trigger point pressure release and other techniques, to release stubborn trigger points, spasms, or ischemic regions that are not readily responding to manual techniques. The goal of S&S is to inhibit pain signals of short, painful muscles or from trigger points, which then allows the tissues to be manually lengthened. Among other effects, it is thought to provoke a continual barrage of alarming impulses perceived and transmitted by A-delta fibers (cutaneous thermal receptors), which has an inhibitory effect on C-fibers (which transmit pain) and on facilitated neural pathways. It is suggested that counterirritants, such as Biofreeze, work under similar principles.

Sensory deprivation tanks, or flotation tanks, have been used to suspend the body in a solution of heavily salted water, which causes the body to float (as can be seen in the Great Salt Lake or the Dead Sea). Coupled with darkness and lack of sound, this weightless suspension from gravitational forces induces deep relaxation and pain-relieving affects.

Similarly, aquatic bodywork, such as Watsu, is conducted in a fluid matrix usually in a swimming pool or lake and may include specialized features and equipment, such as jets or waterfalls. The patient is usually supported by specially designed, strategically placed flotation devices and moved in the water by one or more trained practitioners.

Friedland (2012) describes this water therapy:

"Specific movements, rhythms, patterns, and waveforms are created by the therapist's own kinetic actions and transmitted to the patient. These movements, rhythms, patterns, and waveforms rebound onto, across, through, around, and out from the patient and are countered by the practitioner, who responds by transmitting more movements, rhythms, waves, and patterns. One of the greatest advantages of using the water is that it allows individuals with many types of injuries to receive treatment."

LYMPHATIC DRAINAGE TECHNIQUES

Manually applied lymph drainage techniques incorporate application of light pressure to the skin and superficial fascia in a particular pattern that encourages an increase in the movement of lymph. In addition, lymphatic pumps are rhythmic techniques applied over organs, such as the liver and spleen, to increase drainage.

The thoracic diaphragm is also sometimes used as a lymphatic pump because movement of this large muscular structure creates increased intra-abdominal pressure, which "pumps" the nearby cisterna chyli, a distended portion of the thoracic lymph duct that serves as a temporary reservoir for lymph from the lower half of the body (Fig. 13.8).

The hand stroke used in lymph drainage is distinctly different from effleurage. Effleurage applied in the direction of the heart can also increase the venous and lymphatic drainage of the involved structure(s). However, deeply applied effleurage can inhibit lymph movement and even result in damage to the lymphatic vessels, particularly if the region is already distended with excess lymph fluid. Using very light pressure, lymph drainage applies a rhythmic short stroke that creates a short pulling action on the skin and superficial fascia, which is then abruptly released. A turgor effect (local accumulation of fluid) encourages the movement of lymph into the lymph capillary. The lymph then moves along the vessels, which empty into

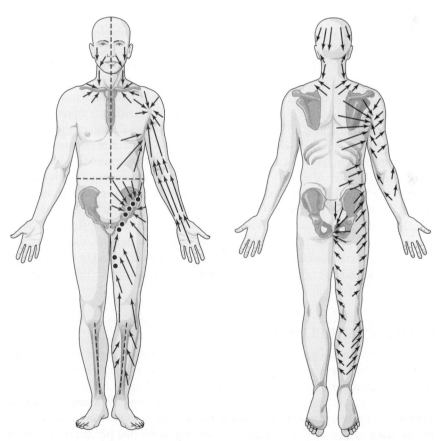

FIG. 13.8 | Lymphatic flow can be enhanced with manual lymph drainage techniques.

progressively larger lymph vessels, until the lymph eventually rejoins the vascular system at the subclavian vein for return into the blood circulation back to the heart.

Lymph drainage therapy (LDT) is useful in a variety of clinical settings to encourage overall health and is profoundly useful in postsurgical and posttrauma care. The edema associated with sprains, strains, and a variety of sport injuries can often be quickly reduced with these techniques. The Vodder method (manual lymph drainage, MLD) and the Chikly method (LDT) are the two most common methods for this effective and broadly applicable modality. Although the aims of the two methods are similar, the styles of application and of teaching are moderately different. Developers of both methods have published textbooks and journal articles to support their concepts and approaches.

MUSCLE ENERGY TECHNIQUE

Muscle energy technique (MET) can be applied directly or indirectly to individual muscles as well as to muscle groups (Chaitow, 2013). MET may be applied directly toward the motion barrier, or in an attempt to lengthen a shortened or spastic muscle. The technique is based on the principle of reciprocal inhibition, which states that a muscle (e.g., flexor) reflexively relaxes as its antagonist (e.g., the associated extensor) contracts. Conversely, if a muscle in spasm is contracted against resistance and then relaxed, the effect often results in increased ROM or reduction of the motion barrier. This indirect application is based on the principle of postisometric relaxation (also known as "postcontraction relaxation") (Lewit & Simons, 1984).

The MET technique is one of the few "active" techniques in manual therapy. The patient does the work and a distinction of MET is the amount of effort exerted by the patient. Usually, less than 20% of the total strength of the muscle is brought to bear during the interval of contraction. Another way of demonstrating this effect is through the "one-finger rule," in which the amount of force necessary is the force needed to move a single finger of the practitioner when the practitioner lightly resists the contraction. This effect is in contradistinction to the proprioceptive neuromuscular facilitation (PNF) technique often used in physical therapy, which employs a maximal muscle contraction and may expose the patient to risk of injury. A thorough knowledge of muscle attachments and their motion vectors is necessary to apply MET effectively and efficiently.

MYOFASCIAL RELEASE

Myofascial release is a gentle technique that uses knowledge of the physical properties of the fascia as it relates to muscles (Fig. 13.9). Although skill is necessary to apply this technique effectively, it is simple to learn and easily applied. The practitioner uses light and deep pressure, depending on the target structures, to palpate motion restriction within the fascia and moves toward or away from the restriction. The position is held until a "release," or softening, is felt, the perception of which is the most difficult aspect of application. The tissues are then slowly returned to

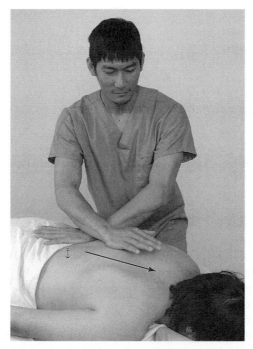

FIG. 13.9 | A crossed-arm myofascial release (MFR) can be applied broadly to the tissues to alter the ground substance of the fascia.

their original position. The release can involve relaxation of muscles, changes in the viscosity of the ground substance of the fascia, slow disengagement of fascial adhesions, or realignment of the fascia to a more appropriate orientation.

Myofascial–Soft-Tissue Technique

The myofascial–soft-tissue technique is a combination direct-indirect massage technique for reducing muscle spasm and fascial tension. It is similar to pétrissage, except that more parts of the hand are typically employed. This technique can be used as a prelude to the high-velocity, low-amplitude technique.

NEURAL MOBILIZATION AND MANIPULATION

Nerves, blood vessels, and lymphatic structures course throughout the body ensheathed in fascia. During movement, structures (e.g., bones, spinal discs, muscles) and fascia not only move but also must allow for the movement of the nerves within the sheath. The relationship of the surrounding structures to the nerves is known as the "mechanical interface."

When tissues are strained, overused, or incur trauma, or when patterns of use result in distorted movement patterns, painful mechanical deformation of the nerves (compression, stretching, angulation, torsion) can occur. In addition to motor and sensory impulses that are transmitted along neural pathways, a host of important trophic substances also flow along the nerves. Any abnormality in the mechanical interface can impede neuronal axoplasmic transport, as well as interfere with normal neural firing.

A number of techniques have emerged that focus on identifying fascial and muscular restriction of the nerves. Additionally, neurodynamic testing, an assessment tool, is often used with these techniques. David Butler, a physical therapist from Australia, contributed significantly through his work with neural mobilization techniques that slide, glide, or "floss" the nerves through their sheaths (Butler, 1991, 2000). This technique is accomplished by the use of specific repetitious body movements performed passively or actively, which gently free the nerves from fascial restrictions.

Neural manipulation, developed by French osteopath/physical therapist Jean-Pierre Barral and fellow osteopath Alain Croibier (Barral & Croibier, 1997), focuses more directly on the neural connective tissues to create more space around the neural and vascular structures (Barral, 2012).

Mechanical neural lesion is often the cause of a broad range of symptoms. However, other serious conditions can mimic neuropathy, some of which are contraindicated for direct techniques. For those interested in incorporating neural assessment and treatment as discussed here, instructor-supervised training is suggested. Precise positioning as well as fundamental training will help avoid further irritation to peripheral neuropathy and related problems.

NEUROMUSCULAR THERAPY TECHNIQUES

Neuromuscular therapy (NMT) involves precise, thorough examination and treatment of the soft tissues of a joint or region that is experiencing pain or dysfunction. As a medically oriented technique, it is primarily used for the treatment of chronic pain or as a treatment for recent (but not acute) trauma; however, it can also be applied to prevent injury or to enhance performance.

NMT emerged on two continents almost simultaneously, but the methods had little connection to each other until recent years. In the mid-20th century, European "neuromuscular technique" emerged, primarily through the work of Stanley Lief and Boris Chaitow. For the last several decades, it has been carried forward through the writing and teaching of Leon Chaitow, DO. The protocols of North American "neuromuscular therapy" also derived from a variety of sources, including chiropractic (Raymond Nimmo), myofascial trigger point therapy (Janet Travell, David Simons), and massage therapy (Judith DeLany, Paul St. John). Over the last decade, Chaitow and DeLany (2008, 2011) have combined presentation of the two methods in a two-volume text that comprehensively integrates the European and American versions. NMT continues to evolve, with many individuals teaching the techniques worldwide.

One of the main features of NMT involves step-by-step protocols that address all muscles of a region while also considering factors that may play a role in the presenting pain condition. Like osteopaths, neuromuscular therapists use the term "somatic dysfunction" when describing what is found during the examination. Somatic dysfunction is usually characterized by tender tissues and limited and/ or painful ROM. Causes of these lesions include but are not limited to connective tissue changes, ischemia, nerve compression, and postural disturbances, all of which can result from trauma, stress, and repetitive microtrauma (stress due to habitual occupational and recreationally related activities). A distinct focus of treatment is the identification and treatment of trigger points, noxious hyperirritable nodules within the myofascial that, when provoked by applied pressure, needling, and so on, radiate sensations (usually pain) to a defined target zone (Fig. 13.10). Consideration is also given to nutrition, hydration, hormonal balance, breathing patterns, and numerous other factors that impact neuromusculoskeletal health. When indicated, professional referral for treatment of these "perpetuating factors" is required.

Although the European and American versions have unifying philosophical threads, there are subtle yet distinct differences in the palpation methods. Both methods examine for taut bands that are often associated with trigger points, and both use applied pressure to treat the pain-producing nodules. However, European NMT uses a slow-paced, thumb-drag method, whereas the American version uses a medium-paced gliding stroke of the thumb or fingers. There is also a slightly different emphasis on the manner of application of trigger point pressure release (specific compression applied to the tissues) for deactivation of trigger points. In addition, American NMT offers a more systematic method of examination and treatment, whereas European methods use less detail in palpation of deeper structures,

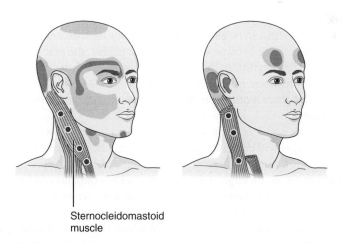

Sternocleidomastoid
muscle

FIG. 13.10 | Neuromuscular therapy focuses attention on locating and treating trigger points (TrPs). TrP referrals from sternocleidomastoid muscle can produce a variety of symptoms, including facial neuralgia, headache, sore throat, voice problems, hearing loss, vertigo, ear pain, and blurred vision.

preferring to incorporate positional release and other methods for deeper treatment. European methods also focus significantly more on superficial tissue texture changes than do their American counterparts.

Both European and American NMT support the use of hydrotherapies (hot and cold applications), movement, and self-applied (home care) therapies. Both suggest homework to encourage the patient's participation in the recovery process, which might include stretching, changes in habits of use, and alterations in lifestyle that help to eliminate perpetuating factors. Patient education may also be offered to increase awareness of static and dynamic posture in work and recreational settings and to teach the value of healthy nutritional choices. Referral to another health care practitioner may also be considered, especially when visceral pathology is suspected.

A successful foundation includes taking a thorough case history, including the patient's account of the precipitating factors, and performing a complete examination of the soft tissues. Although many decisions are individualized to each patient, the NMT protocols are performed while keeping a few basic rules in mind. Superficial tissues are treated before deeper layers, and proximal areas in an extremity are treated before distal regions. Every palpable muscle in the region is assessed—not just those whose referral patterns are consistent with the person's pain or which are thought by the practitioner to be the cause of the problem. This comprehensive approach helps to reveal muscles that may be substituting for the use of those which are dysfunctional or weak.

The first aim is to increase blood flow and soften fascia. Although gliding strokes are often the best choice, sometimes tissue manipulation (sliding the tissues between the thumb and finger to create shear) works better. Depending on the stiffness of the tissues, hot packs may be used to further encourage softening. Then gliding strokes and manipulation can be repeated, alternating with application of heat, or a few moments can be allowed in between for fluid exchange.

Once the tissues have become softer and more pliable, the practitioner palpates for taut bands. These bands, in which select fibers are locked in a foreshortened position, vary in diameter from that of a toothpick to larger than a finger. At the center of the band, there is often a thicker, denser area associated with central trigger point formation.

Once the fiber center is located, the region is evaluated for a trigger point, to which pressure is applied until a degree of resistance (like an "elastic barrier") is felt. Sufficient pressure is applied to match the tension, which provokes or intensifies the referral pattern to the target zone. The applied pressure should be monitored so that what is felt by the patient is no more than a moderate level of discomfort (7 on a scale of 10). Although the patient may feel some tenderness in the area being pressed, usually the focus is on pain, tingling, numbness, burning, or other sensations in the associated target zone of the trigger point. The well-documented, common target zones are usually distant from the location of the trigger point, and predictable. They have been well illustrated in numerous books and charts.

As the applied pressure is sustained, within 8 to 12 seconds, the sensations being reported should begin to fade as the practitioner feels a softening of the compressed nodule or (more rarely) a profound release. The pressure can be sustained for up to approximately 20 seconds, but longer than this is not recommended because this "ischemic compression" is further reducing blood flow in tissues that are already blood deprived.

Trigger point treatment (by pressure, needling, S&S, or other methods) can be repeated several times within the therapy session, with a few moments between each application to allow fluid exchange to occur. Each time treatment is reapplied, the practitioner should note the need to increase the level of applied pressure to stimulate the same level of sensation. In some cases, tenderness and referred sensations will be completely eliminated within one session.

As the final step, the fibers associated with the taut band should be lengthened. This might include passive or active stretching if the associated attachment sites are not too sensitive. If the attachments are moderately tender, inflammation is possible and elongation should be performed manually to avoid putting stress on the attachments. This elongation can be achieved by using a precisely applied myofascial release or a double-thumb gliding stroke, in which each thumb simultaneously slides from the central nodule to a respective attachment, applying tension to the band as the thumbs slide away from each other.

Specific training in the use of NMT protocols is necessary because many contraindications and precautions are associated with NMT techniques. The protocols can be incorporated into any manual practice setting and are particularly useful when interfaced with medical procedures. Many complex conditions can benefit from the thorough protocols and treatment strategies used in NMT.

ORTHOPEDIC MASSAGE

Orthopedic massage (OM) is a comprehensive assessment and treatment system that, like NMT, uses a methodological approach that may incorporate several techniques. Since it has a broad application based on patient presentation, it can be incorporated into relaxation massage, sports injury care, a diverse range of medical settings, and advanced rehabilitative therapy. Although there are different styles of orthopedic massage, they all fundamentally require skills in orthopedic assessment, variability of treatment, advanced knowledge of pain and injuries, and, in some cases, protocols for rehabilitation (Lowe, 2012).

OM drew its roots from sports massage, which emerged in the United States in the 1970s and 1980s. In particular, the standard orthopedic assessment protocols developed by Cyriax (1984 a,b) and the OM protocols written by Lowe (1997) provide the fundamental components that are known as "orthopedic massage." Many schools have adopted Lowe's textbooks as the basis for training, resulting in a move toward standardization of orthopedic massage. Practice settings are as diverse as the application itself and include private practices, physical therapy clinics, medical settings, chiropractic offices, spas, and sport facilities.

Lowe (2012) defines the core of orthopedic massage:

Assessment is at the very foundation of orthopedic massage. It is paramount to identify the tissues most likely at the root of a problem for effective management of soft tissue pain and injuries. Without an accurate assessment, there cannot be a sound or physiological rationale for the treatment and, thus, the treatment will be far less effective.... Skilled OM therapists have good knowledge of what tissues are involved and which therapeutic techniques would best treat those tissues. Thus, they are not limited by their "technique toolbag" and can employ established, as well as newly developed, techniques and methods, and hence are adaptable to the patient's condition. Their advanced education and knowledge leads to outcome-based therapeutic treatments and effective solutions.

OM and NMT (discussed previously) have long been established as successful medically oriented interventions that require comprehensive training and deliver highly effective results. These should not be confused with "medical massage," a term that has become popular in the last 15 years as a result of the aim of national massage organizations to standardize protocols being integrated into the medical communities. There is no one style of massage that makes up "medical massage." Clearly, OM and NMT practitioners are performing outcome-based massage targeted to specific conditions, the broad definition of medical massage. However, it is best to refer to them as OM and NMT practitioners, as this better defines the degree of training that they have received and the protocols that they use.

REFLEXOLOGY

In the Asian meridian system of the body, major meridians or channels are represented in the hands and feet. Acupuncture is usually not done on the soles of the feet in light of their sensitivity; thus, a system of foot massage was developed in China. William H. Fitzgerald, who called it "zone therapy," introduced this approach to the United States in 1913. Subsequently referred to by Byers (2001) and others as reflexology, the technique involves the application of deep pressure to various points on the hands and feet by the thumbs and fingers of the practitioner.

The feet receive the preponderance of attention in this method, with various identified points noted to correspond not only to the energy channels of the body but also to specific organs and systems. When treatment is given, areas of tenderness or texture change are identified and pressure is applied. It is suggested that this treatment opens the associated channel and allows body energy to flow unimpeded. When all points are successfully treated, the energy system is flowing and balanced (see also Chapter 16).

SPORTS MASSAGE

Sports massage has emerged throughout the world as a valuable tool in prevention of and recovery from injury and for enhancing performance and increasing skills in sports. Professional sports teams have long recognized the value of sports massage applications, employing athletic trainers, physical therapists, and massage therapists who often travel with the teams to administer care during the season and also work on team members during the off-season. The practitioners are responsible for assessing the tissues using manual techniques but also must consider the habits of use during the associated sport, determine which dysfunctional mechanics are actually useful adaptations by the body in response to stresses imposed by the sport, and incorporate particular strategies and methods of treatment and prevention of injury, depending on what is discovered.

It is important that the practitioner understand the biomechanics of the sport and the way in which the body might adapt to the imposed stresses. What might seem like a dysfunctional mechanic to be released in a nonsporting body might be a necessary or normal occurrence for that athlete. For instance, the external and internal ROM is often displaced posteriorly in a baseball pitcher's shoulder. This displacement potentially occurs in the humeral shaft as a result of the torsional forces imposed on it through years of windup movements, particularly when these forces are placed on the youthful bone. If normal ROM tests are used, the external rotation would appear to be excessive and the internal ROM would appear to be reduced, although overall the degree of ROM is the same as in a nonpitching shoulder. The uninformed practitioner might attempt to increase internal ROM, believing it to be reduced, and thereby destabilize the joint and overstretch the joint capsule, making the shoulder more vulnerable to injury.

Sports massage therapists often appear at neighborhood sports events to provide pre- and postevent massage. The techniques used warm up the tissues close to the time of event participation are significantly different from those used after the event to enhance recovery. Likewise, those used in the off-season to alter mechanics or those used in injured players differ from those used to prepare participants for play. It is important that the practitioner understand when to use which techniques, when ice and heat are appropriate, and just how much therapy is enough without overtreating the tissues. Professional sports massage training is suggested for all practitioners who work with athletes, whether in the field or in the clinic.

A number of stretching protocols can be incorporated to increase length in shortened tissues or restore balance between hypotonic and hypertonic tissues. Active isolated stretching (AIS), PNF, and MET are just a few of the many stretching protocols used by manual therapists and athletic trainers to achieve greater balance within the musculoskeletal system.

In the past few decades, athletes (including Olympians) have appeared with brightly colored tape placed in unusual patterns on the skin. Kenso Kase developed the application of kinesio tape to the skin for treatment purposes, and the Kinesio

Taping Method has emerged globally as a treatment method not only during sports activity and in recovery but also in the general population.

McGillicuddy (2012) explains, "Kase and others found that the Kinesio Taping applications not only reduced muscle tension, but also improved blood and lymphatic circulation and were effective in reducing neurological symptoms through skin stimulation. As Kase had studied kinesiology, he knew that muscles not only contribute to movement of the body but also help with circulation of the blood, lymphatic flow, and body temperature. By using the elastic tape, it was proposed that the muscles, fascia, and other tissues could be helped by outside assistance creating a gentle lifting of the skin, allowing for better lymphatic and vascular movement."

Kase, Wallis, and Kase (2003) suggested that the application of the Kinesio Tex Tape to the skin may affect mechanical receptors, fascia, subcutaneous space, ligaments, tendons, sensory perception, and lymphatic flow.

STRAIN-COUNTERSTRAIN OR POSITIONAL RELEASE TECHNIQUE

The strain-counterstrain (SCS) technique, originally called the "positional release technique (PRT)," is a very gentle, passive technique developed by Lawrence Jones, DO. The practitioner usually palpates a muscle in spasm (often associated with strain) while the patient reports on his or her sense of discomfort. The patient is next brought into a position that shortens the muscle or eases the dysfunctional joint (counterstrain), which exaggerates the motion restriction. The patient then reports on the level of ease. This position is held usually for 90 to 120 seconds, and the patient is then slowly returned to the original position. The technique is designed to interrupt the reflex spasm loop by altering proprioceptive input into the CNS and can be followed by gentle stretching of the involved muscle. Tender points are also treated in this manner: the patient is brought to a position of ease, held in the position until a "softening" or change in tissue texture is felt or the tenderness subsides, and then slowly returned to the original position.

Similar to SCS/PRT is a functional technique (functional positional release), which relies a little more on the practitioner's palpation skills than on the patient's reporting. The practitioner places a hand or finger on a tender area and searches for the most distressed tissue. The patient is then positioned until a "position of ease" is produced or until the discomfort is significantly reduced, and the patient holds this position for a certain period, usually at least 90 to 120 seconds and sometimes considerably longer. The patient is then brought slowly back to the original position. It is possible that as the position of ease reduces nociceptive and aberrant proprioceptive input to the CNS, an interruption of facilitation associated with pain and spasm is achieved. Realignment of fascia is also a result of the functional technique, and it is possible that the actin and myosin filaments are able to "unlatch" due to approximation of the two ends of the fibers.

RESORT-SPA THERAPIES

"Spa" is not actually a type of massage; it is a setting in which massage and many other therapies are practiced. Since it is profoundly popular throughout the world, incorporates a unique atmosphere that promotes deep relaxation, and involves a number of adjunct therapies, it is appropriately included alongside many of the massage styles that are used within its walls. The large and growing resort-spa facilities represent potential housing capacity for overnight and residential care that provides more natural approaches to pain and chronic diseases compared to the costly and toxic environments of hospitals.

Deep relaxation massage is the primary massage protocol used in most US-based spas. One form, Swedish massage, was discussed earlier in this chapter, together with the five main massage techniques that it uses: effleurage, pétrissage, friction, tapotement, and vibration. Heat, essential oils, dim lights, soft music, and other elements are often combined with the long, slow strokes and rhythmic kneading hand movements that are characteristic of relaxation massage. For many decades, this was the style of massage provided at spas and was mainly reserved for the "rich and famous." In the last 30 years, resort-spa stays and massage have become more openly available to a broad population, accessible in almost all regions and communities and marketed openly for its healing properties and as stress reduction.

Any of the styles of massage discussed in this chapter can be found in spa settings. Independent as well as predominant spas, such as Canyon Ranch and Massage Envy, may offer broad menus that include a very wide variety of massage styles. Many also offer a diverse range of classes involving exercise, healthy cooking, stress management, and self-care. Additionally, spas often incorporate skin treatments (e.g., facials, scrubs, wraps, waxing), water treatments (e.g., steam, sauna, cold plunge), and the application of an array of products that serve to exfoliate, polish, and hydrate the skin. Whether lying on a massage table, seated in a massage chair, or floating in water, the varied forms of spa-based treatment serve to relax the mind and body and to enhance a greater sense of well-being.

VISCERAL MANIPULATION

Visceral manipulation generally involves specific placement of gentle manual forces to encourage tone, mobility, and motion of the abdominopelvic viscera and their supporting connective tissues. Although not indicated in patients with tumors or inflammatory disease, visceral manipulation can be useful in stabilizing and balancing blood flow and autonomic innervation and can even dislodge certain obstructions of the gastrointestinal system.

Methods that address manual manipulation of the viscera have been a component of some therapeutic systems in Asian medicine for centuries and are now practiced extensively by European osteopaths, physical therapists, and other manual practitioners throughout the world. Osteopath and physical therapist Jean-Pierre

Barral of the Barral Institute in West Palm Beach, Florida, developed a system of training and practice of this technique that is available to all manual practitioners.

OSSEOUS TECHNIQUES

In addition to methods applied to the soft tissues, a variety of techniques can be used to normalize the position of the osseous structure. Although some are discussed elsewhere in this book, the following are often used in conjunction with the aforementioned myofascial methods. Their inclusion as a supporting modality here is meant to encourage the synergistic integration of manual modalities.

ARTICULATORY TECHNIQUE

In the articulatory technique, the practitioner moves the affected joint through its ROM in all planes, gently encountering motion barriers and gradually moving through them to establish normal motion. This low-velocity, moderate- to high-amplitude method would be considered a passive, direct/indirect, oscillatory technique used to restore as much motion as possible to a dysfunctional joint.

CRANIAL OSTEOPATHY

Cranial osteopathy (see also "Craniosacral Therapy") is the study of the anatomy and physiology of the cranium, as well as its relationship with the body as a whole. William Garner Sutherland developed and taught cranial osteopathy in the early to mid-1900s. He considered his cranial concepts to be an extension of Andrew Taylor Still's science of osteopathy and not separate from it. Where textbooks taught that cranial bones were fused and immovable, Dr. Sutherland perceived a subtle palpable movement and suggested that there was a continuity of this rhythmic fluid movement not only throughout the cranium but also throughout all body tissues.

The Osteopathic Cranial Academy website (http://www.cranialacademy.com) describes Sutherland's dilemma:

"While a student at the American School of Osteopathy in 1899, Dr. Sutherland pondered the fine details of a separated or 'disarticulated' skull. He wondered about the function of this complex architecture. Dr. Still taught that every structure exists because it performs a particular function. While looking at a temporal bone, a flash of inspiration struck Dr. Sutherland: 'Beveled like the gills of a fish, indicating respiratory motion for an articular mechanism.'"

Consumed by this idea, Sutherland was inspired and motivated toward a singular, detailed, and prolonged study of the cranium and often experimented on his own head. Over many years of intense study, he developed the concepts of "The Primary Respiratory Mechanism" with its five components: (1) the rhythmic movement of the brain and spinal cord, (2) fluctuations of cerebrospinal fluid, (3) the reciprocal tension membrane, (4) the osteo-articular mechanism, and (5) the involuntary motion of the sacrum. Dr. Sutherland described these activities of the CNS as having a motion with "inhalation" and "exhalation" phases and that a practitioner connecting directly (through specific palpation) with the primary respiratory mechanism could bring about a therapeutic response.

Northup (1949) recognized Sutherland's work in the 1949 yearbook of the Academy of Applied Osteopathy:

"Without doubt Dr. William G. Sutherland has made the greatest single contribution to the advancement of manipulative osteopathy since Dr. Andrew Taylor Still established it three quarters of a century ago, and in recognition of his great contribution to the osteopathic profession, we affectionately dedicate this 1949 Year Book to him."

High-Velocity, Low-Amplitude Technique

The high-velocity, low-amplitude (HVLA) technique is probably the most publicly recognized techniques of the osteopath or chiropractor (see Chapter 12). This is a thrust-oriented technique designed to aggressively break through a motion barrier. More often than not, an audible pop is heard, the result of a brief sonic cavitation of the involved joint. The HVLA technique can be applied directly (toward the barrier) or indirectly (away from the barrier), using short or long levers. Although often associated with manipulation of the spine, the HVLA technique can also be performed on the extremities.

Use of the HVLA technique is contraindicated in patients with osteoporosis, bone tumors, or severe atherosclerosis, and in those who are taking certain medications that make bones more brittle, such as many forms of chemotherapy. Recently, much discussion has focused on the safety of the HVLA technique when performed in the high cervical (neck) region due to potential risk to the vertebral artery. Controversy has expanded to include questions regarding the safety and accuracy of manual screening tests for vertebral artery insufficiencies (such as George's Test and the DeKlynes Test). In March 2004, all US chiropractic schools agreed to abandon the teaching and use of provocation tests such as these due to the inherent risks and high level of false data.

SPECIAL POPULATIONS

Age-related and condition-specific care has been a growing part of manual therapy professions for decades. While these special patients may require techniques from the many styles given in the chapter, they also have unique characteristics that require approaches based on age-related factors or medical conditions. These cases require special training and ongoing requirements so the practitioners can stay current regarding information, techniques, medications, and other pertinent data for these special circumstances.

Prenatal and Infant

Prenatal massage is therapeutic massage and bodywork given during pregnancy to promote both maternal and fetal well-being. Although cultures around the world show various forms of the use of prenatal and perinatal touch, pregnancy massage was considered as contraindicated until as recent as the 1970s.

Osborne (2012) describes how this circumstance has changed:

"In the last few decades, women and some maternity professions have increasingly demanded a more holistic and woman-centered approach to childbearing. As a result, in many circumstances, partners and other family members are now in close physical contact with the birthing mother. Labor assistants, or doulas, provide continuous physical and emotional support to laboring women, with impressive positive results for mothers, babies, hospitals, and other birth settings."

Beginning in the 1980s, several massage therapists and instructors began in-depth exploration of massage therapy for childbearing concerns. Most notably, Carole Osborne, Kate Jordan, Suzanne Yates, Elaine Stillerman, and Claire Marie Miller each developed their own guidelines for safe prenatal applications of massage therapy.

As massage therapy resumes its place in integrated health care and at multidisciplinary clinics, prenatal massage therapy has surfaced as an optimal specialization. It is strongly suggested that those working with pregnant clients study with an experienced instructor and stay current with developing research and continuing education in regards to this field.

Infant massage is a unique style whose main purpose is to create and support the emotional bond between parent and child (McClure, 2012). Additionally, gastrointestinal, respiratory, and circulatory functions may be enhanced. Although massage therapists may offer infant massage, a long-lasting standard is for a parent to be trained to apply the techniques. This step is usually accomplished while sitting on the floor with the adult's legs crossed and baby lying on the floor in front of him/her. McClure describes, if the baby becomes fussy, they are comforted, and then the massage is continued. If the baby indicates they have "had enough," the parent ends the massage with a positive, soothing movement that is familiar to the baby, and often the baby will drift off to sleep. If the baby is enjoying the massage, after massaging the face and arms, the baby is turned over and strokes are completed on the back and buttocks. During the massage, the parent often gently stops stroking and lays their hands on the baby's body, a movement called "resting hands."

Considerable research has been conducted in the field of infant massage, particularly in the area of weight gain in premature infants and in prenatal substance abuse. A considerable amount of favorable research has been published regarding research conducted by Dr. Tiffany Field and others at the Touch Research Institute, Miami, Florida. A complete list can be found at http://www6.miami.edu/touch-research.

AGING

As the body ages into elderly years, conditions such as thinning skin, changes in muscle tone, joint deterioration, osteoporosis, and sensorineural deficits may warrant specific approaches and precautions. Elderly care training helps ensure appropriate strategies are used for those who face the issues of aging, such as being frail and less mobile. In the United States, there are three main organizations that conduct training specific to elderly care: Day-Break Geriatric Massage Institute, Comfort Touch, and Compassionate Touch.

Discussing elderly care, Salvo (2012) states,

"The elderly may present the therapist with unique challenges. There are obvious physical changes, such as thinning skin, reduced muscle mass, and impairments of vision and hearing. Sensorineural deficits may also predispose the elderly to accidental injury, such as slips and falls. This population faces lifestyle and emotional changes, such as retirement, reduced income, and loss of loved ones. To better serve the elderly, the therapist needs to cultivate attitudes of patience, tolerance, loving kindness, and attentiveness."

ONCOLOGY

Oncology massage designates a special set of skills used in the care of a person affected by cancer and its related treatments and complications. Patients may be in active treatment, recovery, survivorship, or at the end of life. Practitioners pursuing this field should develop a broad understanding of the pathophysiology of cancer; side effects of treatment (medications, radiation, chemotherapy, surgery); and an ability to modify protocols to adapt for each unique case, such as for the presence of lymphedema or with scar mobilization. Treatments may take place in private practice, a patient's home, oncology clinics, hospitals, and in hospice care.

Du Rand (2012) addresses the myth that massage is contraindicated for cancer patients:

"Earlier massage training did not take into consideration the pathophysiology of the disease, and mistakenly hypothesized that pressure could stimulate the spread of cancer. Cancer starts and spreads because of a highly complicated accumulation of mutations on a genetic level in a cell's DNA and/or RNA. There is currently no evidence that massage will influence the development or proliferation of this mutation."

While that debate continues in some arenas, the effectiveness of massage therapy at reducing symptoms such as pain and anxiety has been demonstrated in ongoing research and clinical studies, with strong implications that massage will also reduce the fatigue, stress, nausea, and depression associated with cancer treatments.

For those joining the field of oncology massage, qualified training with supervised instruction is a must. Although textbooks, articles, and webinars offer a strong support for comprehensive understanding, there is no substitute for a qualified, experienced oncology massage instructor and ongoing continuing education to stay abreast of the latest information in this ever-changing field.

HOSPICE

Death is an integral part of life, and at the end stage for terminally ill people and their families, intensive palliative care that provides a loving touch, comfort, pain relief, and peaceful rest is priceless. With a history of more than 50 years in the United States, hospice care has provided physical, emotional, psychological, and spiritual support for those approaching the end of their lives. Hospice-based massage therapy is a natural and integral part of this care.

Puszko (2012) shares her insights:

The hospice patient receiving massage therapy may experience more immediately noticeable psychosocial benefits than physical benefits. The reason why touch is so powerful is based on the recognition that tactile experiences are the first sensations that greet us at the time of birth, and are the last perception to leave us at the end of life. Touch can penetrate the semi-comatose state produced by a painkiller, giving the treatment a modicum of human contact and reminding the patient that they are not alone. In fact, patients sometimes reduce their demand for drugs when massage is an integral part of the treatment protocol.

Puszko suggests that gentle massage reduces feelings of isolation and loneliness and supports self-acceptance and self-esteem when the body has been invaded by a debilitating disease: "The benefit of massage therapy for the hospice patient is to experience peace, joy, and love, and general feelings of comfort while actively dying."

Massage touches lives at all ages, from birth to death, and offers specific and effective techniques to those who suffer from chronic illness, express themselves through athletics or the arts, or just live a normal life with the distortions, bumps, and bruises that come with modern life. Whatever the individual's lifestyle or life circumstances, massage can be an integral part of living it comfortably and to the fullest.

MASSAGE PRACTICE SETTINGS AND AVAILABILITY

Massage therapy is used in a variety of clinical settings, spas, private practices, and sport arenas. The expertise of the massage therapist or practitioner is essential in determining which techniques may or may not be appropriate and how the massage may be delivered. Application choices will also be based on the case presentation and may be influenced by the environment, such as a hospital or spa, as well as the allocation of time, prescribed therapy, other associated modalities (e.g., stretching, exercise, biofeedback) that may be needed or desired and scope of practitioner's license. Massage is routinely applied to pediatric, adolescent, and geriatric patients. Frequently, massage therapists expand their therapeutic horizons by taking postgraduate study in other forms of bodywork or specific methods for application to certain pathologies. It is not uncommon to find a therapist who not only does Swedish massage but also employs the Trager approach, the Feldenkrais method, and craniosacral therapy, moving seamlessly from one to the other, as indicated by the response of the tissues and recipient.

The application of massage therapy in medical settings has recently expanded at a dramatic rate, perhaps because of the growing use of "multidisciplinary approaches" to patient care, and coverage under Medicare for specified conditions up to twice per week. Massage therapists and other manual practitioners now render their skills in hospitals, physical therapy clinics, rehabilitation centers, and the offices of physicians, osteopaths, chiropractors, dentists, and multidisciplinary clinics.

In professional sport arenas; Olympic competitions; and college, high school, and little league teams, massage and manual techniques have emerged as valued tools for rehabilitation, enhancement of performance, and prevention of injury. These professions are no longer considered to be on the outskirts of medicine but are now incorporated as an integral part of treatment options. All manual medicine modalities are areas that are ripe for research, with much being done worldwide to validate them and explore their breadth of application in patient care.

BODYWORK

FELDENKRAIS METHOD

Awareness Through Movement and Functional Integration

Moshé Feldenkrais (1904–84) was an Israeli physicist who developed a system of movement and manipulation over several decades (Feldenkrais, 1991; Rywerant & Feldenkrais, 2011). The Feldenkrais method is divided into two "educational" processes. The first, *awareness through movement*, is a sensorimotor balancing technique that is taught to "students" who are active participants in this process. The students are verbally guided through a series of very slow movements designed to create a heightened awareness of motion patterns and to re-educate the CNS to new patterns, approaches, and possibilities (e.g., learning t'ai chi).

The second process is referred to as *functional integration*. This process employs a passive technique using a didactic approach, not unlike Trager table work (see discussion later in this chapter). The practitioner acts as "teacher" and the patient as "student." The teacher brings the student through a series of manipulons to re-establish proper neuromotor patterning and balance. Manipulons are a manipulative sequence of information, action (as initiated by the practitioner), and response. They are gentle and are treated as exploratory, with the therapist introducing new motion patterns to the patient. Manipulons are referred to as "positioning," "confining," "single," or "repetitive." They can also be "oscillating." In all cases, the teacher plays a supportive and guiding role while creating a nonthreatening environment for change. Functional integration can be considered a combination of passive, articulatory, and functional techniques.

ROLFING

Structural Integration Methods

Rolfing is a form of structural integration that was developed by Ida Rolf in the middle of the 20th century. Rolf, who had a PhD in biochemistry, sought help from an osteopath after being dissatisfied with conventional medical treatment of her pneumonia. After this experience, Dr. Rolf embarked on a lengthy period of study, including yoga study, which resulted in the manual system that now bears her name (Rolf 1975, 1997; Rolf & Thompson, 1989). In 1971, she founded the Rolf Institute of Structural Integration in Boulder, Colorado, which now trains and certifies practitioners of this style.

The theory of Rolfing is based primarily on physical consideration of the inter-action of the human body with the gravitational field of the earth (see Chapters 2 and 3). As a dynamic entity, the human body moves around and through this field in a state of equilibrium, storing potential energy and releasing kinetic energy. In this system, form (potential energy) is in direct proportion to function (kinetic energy), and the balance between the two is equivalent to the amount of energy available to the body. In simple terms, the worse the posture, the more energy consumed at a baseline level, and thus the less there is available for normal activity. Furthermore, the physical energy of the body is in direct proportion to the "vital energy" of the person. Ideally, the body is always in a position of "equipoise," but this is seldom, if ever, the case.

Rolfing traditionally involves a 10-session treatment protocol designed to inte-grate the entire myofascial system of the body. Photographs are taken of the patient before and after each session or at the beginning and end of a series of treatments to evaluate progress. The body is treated as a system of integrated segments con-solidated by the myofascial system. Attempts are made through "processing," as the treatment is called, to lengthen and center through the connective tissue system by a series of direct myofascial release techniques. As distortions in the system are released, the patient may experience pain. The pain experienced is not merely struc-tural, however. It is thought that emotions are expressed in behavior of the mus-culoskeletal system, which is reflected in various postures and movement patterns (e.g., the widely accepted psychological concepts of Pavlovian conditioning and body language).

In other words, the musculoskeletal system is viewed as a link between the body and mind. Emotional or physical traumas are stored in the body as postures, which mirror a withdrawal response from the offending or painful agent. Over time, com-pensatory reactions occur, but the body ultimately decompensates (fails in adap-tation to the imposed stresses), which results in somatic or visceral dysfunction. The direct technique seeks to put the energy of the practitioner into the system of the patient in an attempt to overcome the resistance to change embodied in the withdrawal response. As releases are affected through the treatment, the emotional component may also be expressed (somato-emotional release).

The result of the treatment is a feeling of balance and "lightness" experienced by the patient. In addition, the patient should experience a heightened sense of well-being because the treatment releases the effects of emotional trauma. Thus, the feeling of lightness is more than simply an increase in the basal physical energy in the body but an increase in the body's vital energy as well.

Following Rolf's work, a number of other systems of structural integration developed. Among those who developed their own styles, several stand out with innovative thinking. Tom Myers, a distinguished teacher of structural integration, suggests that we consider the body to be a tensegrity structure. "Tensegrity," a term coined by architect-engineer Buckminster Fuller, describes a system characterized by a discontinuous set of compressional elements (struts) that are held together and/or moved by a continuous tensional network. Art student Kenneth Snelson attended Fuller's lectures and applied his concepts to build a three-dimensional tensegrity structure. His new-style sculpture was the first to exemplify the concepts of discontinuous-compression, continuous-tension structures, although Fuller usually receives the credit. The muscular system similarly supplies the tensile forces that erect the human frame by using contractile mechanisms embedded within the fascia to place tension on the compressional elements of the skeletal system, thereby providing a tensegrity structure capable of maintaining varying vertical postures, as well as carrying out significant and complex movements.

Myers (1997 a,b) described a number of clinically useful sets of myofascial chains. He sees the fascia as continuous through the muscle and its tendinous attachments, blending with adjacent and contiguous soft tissues, and with the bones, providing supportive tensional elements between the different compressional structures (bones) and thereby creating a tensegrity structure. These fascial chains are of particular importance in helping draw attention to (for example) dysfunctional patterns in the lower limbs that may impact structures in the upper body via these "long functional continuities."

Chaitow and DeLany (2008) note, "The truth, of course, is that no tissue exists in isolation but acts on, is bound to and interwoven with other structures. The body is inter- and intra-related, from top to bottom, side-to-side and front to back, by the inter-connectedness of this pervasive fascial system. When we work on a local area, we need to maintain a constant awareness of the fact that we are potentially influencing the whole body."

TRAGER APPROACH

Psychophysical Integration and Mentastics

Milton Trager, MD, was originally a boxer and gymnast and developed (almost by accident) his technique of psychophysical integration more than 50 years ago (Trager & Hammond, 1995). To obtain the credentials he believed were necessary to bring his technique to the medical community, he obtained a medical degree from the University of Guadalajara in 1955. While at medical school, he was able to demonstrate his technique and treat polio patients with a relatively high degree of success. After developing the technique over many years in his medical practice, he began to teach the method in 1975. The Trager Institute (Mill Valley, CA) was founded shortly thereafter and is responsible for dissemination of information and certification programs.

The Trager approach is a two-tiered approach, along the lines of the Feldenkrais method (see previous discussion). The psychophysical integration phase, also known as "table work," consists of a single treatment or a series of treatments. Mentastics, as described later, is an exercise taught to patients so that they may continue the work on their own.

Psychophysical integration is essentially an indirect, functional technique. The patient lies on a table, and the practitioner applies a very gentle rocking motion to explore the body for areas of tissue tension and motion restriction. No force, stroking, or thrust is used in this technique, merely a light, rhythmic contact. The purpose is to produce a specific sensory experience for the patient, one that is positive and pleasurable. Any discomfort serves to break the continuum of "teaching" and "learning."

The focus of the treatment, however, is not on any specific anatomical structure or physiological process, but rather on the psyche of the patient. An attempt is made to bring the patient into a position (or motion) of ease, in which a sensation of lightness or freedom is experienced. This sensation is "learned" by the patient during the process of sensorimotor repatterning. In the words of Dr. Trager, the patient learns "how the tissue should feel when everything is right." This mind-body interaction is the core of the treatment and plays an exceptional role to induce a change. The result is deep relaxation and increased ROM (i.e., a sense of lightness).

Patterns of behavior and posture are learned during a person's lifetime in part as reactions to trauma or withdrawal from pain, either physical or emotional (see the "Structural Integration Methods" section). Initially, the body may be able to compensate for such reactions, but it will eventually decompensate, which results in various somatic or visceral symptoms. The Trager treatment "allows" the patient to re-experience what is normal through this exploratory process.

The practitioner seeks to integrate with the patient by entering a quasi-meditative state of awareness referred to as the "hookup." This allows the practitioner to attend acutely to the work at hand and feel very subtle changes in tissue texture and movement, not unlike the level of attention necessary to practice cranial osteopathy (see earlier). Without any specific anatomical protocol, the work is very intuitive, and "letting go" is necessary by both parties. The practitioner maintains a position of "neutrality" and makes no attempt to "make anything happen," because it is actually the patient who is sensing and learning. The practitioner's role is one of a facilitator, in which he or she seeks to provide a safe and nurturing environment for the patient to explore new and pain-free patterns of motion.

Mentastics, the continuing phase of the Trager approach, is short for "mental gymnastics" and follows table work. A basic exercise set is taught, and patients are instructed to practice on their own. These exercises consist of repetitive and sequential movements of all the joints, designed to relieve tension in the body. They are to be performed in an effortless, relaxed state of awareness, in which the individual "hooks up" with the self. The basic principles of hatha-yoga and t'ai chi are used in these exercises. Once the set is learned, individuals can then continue to explore independently, creating their own custom-designed series.

Practitioners of the Trager approach have reported success (not necessarily cures) in patients with multiple sclerosis, muscular dystrophy, and other debilitating diseases. Athletes have also reported significant improvements in performance as a result of applying Trager techniques.

It is important to note the value of the preventive aspect of manipulation as a holistic practice. Manipulative treatment can be used for proactive general maintenance as well as for reactive treatment of dysfunction. To use an automobile analogy, most consumers think nothing of periodically getting a car tuned up and paying considerable sums for the privilege. Why not do the same for their own bodies? In addition, the value of manual treatment for young persons cannot be overstated. Structural corrections can be made before fascial distortions become relatively locked in or before continuous aberrant sensory input results in facilitated sensorimotor patterning. Corrections can be made before compensatory reactions in muscles, fascia, and behavior can create unbalanced anatomy and physiology that function poorly and eventually lead to structural remodeling or a decreased resistance to disease (pathology). As Alexander Pope once proclaimed, "Just as the twig is bent, the tree's inclined."

The importance given to this information should be tied to awareness that, as the body ages, adaptive forces cause changes in the structures of the body, with the occurrence of shortening, crowding, and distortion. With this change, we can see—in real terms within our own bodies and those of our patients—the environment in which cells change shape. As they do so, they change their potential for normal genetic expression, as well as their abilities to communicate and to handle nutrients efficiently.

Reversing or slowing undesirable processes is the potential of appropriate bodywork and movement approaches. It is yet to be precisely established to what degree functional health can be modified by soft-tissue techniques, such as those discussed in this chapter. However, the normalizing of structural and functional features of connective tissue by addressing myofascial trigger points, chronic muscle shortening and fibrosis, as well as perpetuating factors such as habits of use, has clear applications for pain treatment. Well-designed research to assess cellular, structural, and functional changes that follow the application of manual techniques is clinically relevant and sorely needed.

REFERENCES

Ahn, A. C., Park, M., Shaw, J. R., McManus, C. A., Kaptchuk, T. J., & Langevin, H. (2010). Electrical impedance of acupuncture meridians: The relevance of subcutaneous collagenous bands. *PLoS ONE*, 5(7). http://dx.doi.org/10.1371/journal.pone.0011907.

Barral, J. P. (2012). Neural manipulation. In J. DeLany, et al. (Eds.), *3D Anatomy for massage and manual therapies*. London: Primal Pictures.

Barral, J. P. & Croibier, A. (1997). *Approche osteopathique du traumatisme*. St. Etienne, France: Editions ATSA, CIDO & Actes Graphiques.

Birch, S. (2003). Trigger point–acupuncture point correlations revisited. *Journal of Alternative and Complementary Medicine*, 9(1), 91–103.

Burman, I. & Friedland, S. (2006). *TouchAbilities essential connections*. Clifton Park, NY: Thomson Delmar Learning.

Butler, D. S. (1991). *Mobilisation of the nervous system*. Melbourne, Australia: Churchill Livingstone.

Butler, D. S. (2000). *The sensitive nervous system*. Unley, South Australia: Noigroup Publications.

Byers, D. (2001). *Better health with foot reflexology* (revised ed.). St. Petersburg FL: Ingham Publishing, Inc.

Casanelia, L. & Stelfox, D. (2009). *Foundations of massage* (3rd ed.). Australia: Churchill Livingston, Elsevier.

Chaitow, L. (2013). *Muscle energy techniques* (4th ed.). Edinburgh: Elsevier/Churchill Livingstone.

Chaitow, L. & DeLany, J. (2008). *Clinical application of neuromuscular techniques, vol. 1. The upper body* (2nd ed.). Edinburgh: Elsevier Health Sciences.

Chaitow, L. & DeLany, J. (2011). *Clinical application of neuromuscular techniques, vol. 2. The lower body* (2nd ed.). Edinburgh: Elsevier Health Sciences.

Chen, C. & Ingber, D. (1999). Tensegrity and mechanoregulation: From skeleton to cytoskeleton. *Osteoarthritis and Cartilage, 7*(1), 81–94.

Cyriax, J. (1984a). *Textbook of orthopaedic medicine, vol. 2. Treatment by manipulation, massage and injection* (11th ed.). London: Bailliere Tindall.

Cyriax, J. (1984b). *Textbook of orthopaedic medicine, vol. 2. treatment by manipulation, massage and injection* (2nd ed.). London: Saunders.

DeLany, J. (2012). Intro to manual therapy. In J. DeLany, et al. (Eds.), *3D Anatomy for massage and manual therapies*. London: Primal Pictures.

Dorsher, P. T. (2008). Can classical acupuncture points and trigger points be compared in the treatment of pain disorders? Birch's analysis revisited. *The Journal of Alternative and Complementary Medicine, 14*(4), 353–359.

du Rand, J. (2012). Oncology massage. In J. DeLany, et al. (Eds.), *3D Anatomy for massage and manual therapies*. London: Primal Pictures.

Feldenkrais, M. (1991). *Awareness through movement: Easy-to-do health exercises to improve your posture, vision, imagination, and personal growth*. San Francisco: Harper Collins.

Friedland, S. (2012). Aquatic bodywork. In J. DeLany (Ed.), *3D Anatomy for massage and manual therapies*. London: Primal Pictures.

Hong, C. Z. (2000). Myofascial trigger points: pathophysiology and correlation with acupuncture points. *Acupuncture in Medicine, 18*(1), 41–47.

Ingber, D. E. (1993). The riddle of morphogenesis: A question of solution chemistry or molecular cell engineering. *Cell, 75*, 1249.

Ingber, D. E. & Folkman, J. (1989). Tension and compression as basic determinants of cell form and function: Utilization of a cellular tensegrity mechanism. In W. Stein & F. Bronner (Eds.), *Cell shape: determinants, regulation and regulatory role* (p. 1). San Diego, CA: Academic Press.

Kase, K., Wallis, J., & Kase, T. (2003). *Clinical therapeutic applications of the Kinesio taping method* (2nd ed.). Tokyo, Japan: Ken Ikai.

Kawakita, K., Itoh, K., & Okada, K. (2002). The polymodal receptor hypothesis of acupuncture and moxibustion, and its rational explanation of acupuncture points. In A. Sato, L. Peng, & J. L. Campbell (Eds.), *Exerpta medica, international congress series: Vol. 1238. Acupuncture—Is there a physiological basis?* (p. 63).

Langevin, H., Bouffard, N., Badger, G., Iatridis, J. C., & Howe, A. K. (2005). Dynamic fibroblast cytoskeletal response to subcutaneous tissue stretch ex vivo and in vivo. *American Journal of Physiology-Cell Physiology, 288*, C747–C756.

Langevin, H., Churchill, D., & Cipolla, M. (2001). Mechanical signaling through connective tissue: A mechanism for the therapeutic effect of acupuncture. *The FASEB Journal, 15*, 2275.

Langevin, H., Cornbrooks, C., & Taatjes, D. (2004). Fibroblasts form a body-wide cellular network. *Histochemistry and Cell Biology, 122*(1), 7.

Langevin, H. M. & Yandow, J. A. (2002). Relationship of acupuncture points and meridians to connective tissue planes. *The Anatomical Record, 269*(6), 257–265.

Lewit, K. & Simons, D. G. (1984). Myofascial pain: Relief by post-isometric relaxation. *Archives of Physical Medicine and Rehabilitation, 65*(8), 452.

Lippincott, H. A. (1949). *The Osteopathic Technic of Wm. G. Sutherland D.O.*, Academy of Applied Osteopathy Yearbook. p. 1-24.

Lowe, W. (1997). *Functional assessment in massage therapy* (3rd ed.). Bend, OR: OMERI.

Lowe, W. (2012). Orthopedic massage. In J. DeLany, et al. (Eds.), *3D Anatomy for massage and manual therapies*. London: Primal Pictures.

Mann, J., Gaylord, S., Fourot, K., Suchindran, C., Coeytaux, R., Wilkinson, L., et al. (2012). Craniosacral therapy for migraine: A feasibility study. *BMC Complementary and Alternative Medicine, 12*(Suppl 1), 111.

McClure, V. (2012). Infant massage. In J. DeLany, et al. (Eds.), *3D Anatomy for massage and manual therapies*. London: Primal Pictures.

McGillicuddy, M. (2012). Kinesiotaping. In J. DeLany, et al. (Eds.), *3D Anatomy for massage and manual therapies*. London: Primal Pictures.

Mehl-Madrona, L., Kligler, B., Silverman, S., Lynton, H., & Merrell, W. (2007). The impact of acupuncture and craniosacral therapy interventions on clinical outcomes in adults with asthma. *The Journal of Science & Healing, 3*(1), 28.

Melzack, R., Stillwell, D. M., & Fox, E. J. (1977). Trigger points and acupuncture points for pain: Correlations and implications. *Pain, 3*, 3.

Myers, T. (1997a). The 'Anatomy trains'. *Journal of Bodywork and Movement Therapies, 1*(2), 91–101.

Myers, T. (1997b). The 'Anatomy trains': Part 2. *Journal of Bodywork and Movement Therapies, 1*(3), 135–145.

Northup, T. (1949). *Forward*. In *Academy of applied osteopathy yearbook* (p. ix).

Orstrom, K. (1918). *Massage and the original Swedish movements* (8th ed.). Philadelphia, PA: P. Blakinston's Son & Co.

Osborne, C. (2012). Prenatal massage. In J. DeLany, et al. (Eds.), *3D Anatomy for massage and manual therapies*. London: Primal Pictures.

Pettman, E. (2007). A history of manipulative therapy. *Journal of Manual and Manipulative Therapy, 15*(3), 165–174.

Plummer, J. (1980). Anatomical findings at acupuncture loci. *The American Journal of Chinese Medicine, 8*, 170.

Puszko, S. (2012). Hospice-based massage therapy. In J. DeLany, et al. (Eds.), *3D Anatomy for massage and manual therapies*. London: Primal Pictures.

Raviv, G., Shefi, S., Nizani, D., & Achiron, A. (2009). Effect of craniosacral therapy on lower urinary tract signs and symptoms in multiple sclerosis. *Complementary Therapies in Clinical Practice, 15*(2), 72.

Rolf, I. P. (1997). *The integration of human structures*. Santa Monica, CA: Dennis-Landman.

Rolf, I. P. (1975). *What in the world is rolfing?*. Santa Monica, CA: Dennis-Landman.

Rolf, I. P. & Thompson, R. R. (1989). *Reestablishing the natural alignment and structural integration of the human body for vitality and well-being*. Rochester, VT: Inner Traditions International.

Salvo, S. (2012). Massage of the elderly. In J. DeLany, et al. (Eds.), *3D Anatomy for massage and manual therapies*. London: Primal Pictures.

Simons, D., Travell, J., & Simons, L. (1999). *Myofascial pain and dysfunction: The trigger point manual, vol. 1: upper half of body* (2nd ed.). Baltimore: Lippincott Williams & Wilkins.

Teeguarden, I. (1978). *Acupressure way of health: Jin Shin Do*. Tokyo: Japan Publications.

Trager, M. & Hammond, C. (1995). *Movement as a way to agelessness: A guide to Trager mentastics*. Barryton, NY: Station Hill Press.

Travell, J. & Simons, D. (1992). *Myofascial pain and dysfunction: The trigger point manual, vol. 2: lower half of body*. Baltimore, MD: Williams and Wilkins.

Wall, P. & Melzack, R. (1990). *Textbook of pain* (2nd ed.). Edinburgh: Churchill Livingstone.

Wuttke, R. (2012). Hot/cold stone therapy. In J. DeLany, et al. (Eds.), *3D Anatomy for massage and manual therapies*. London: Primal Pictures.

Suggested Readings can be found on the companion website, http://www.micozzipainconditions.com.

Section IV

ASIAN MEDICAL SYSTEMS

Traditional Asian medical systems offer highly potent nondrug treatments for pain, based on the manipulation of the body's energy, or qi, as in Chinese medicine. As explained in Chapter 14, the therapeutic manipulation and balancing of qi has both a material/physical aspect and an immaterial/spiritual aspect. In ancient texts it is called the "spiritual pivot". Like Chinese medicine itself, balancing of qi to address pain conditions is essentially a "mind-body" approach, addressing both—albeit unified—aspects. A classic safe and effective approach for treating pain is acupuncture, which is addressed in Chapter 15. Although we have found psychometric evaluation of personality boundary types to be useful in assessing the susceptibility of different patients to different mind-body therapies (as had been done previously with hypnosis; see Chapter 7 and Appendix I, pp. 572–579), the potency of acupuncture for pain relief appears to cross all boundaries.

Chapter 14

Foundations of Chinese and East Asian Medicine

ORIGINS

More than 5000 years ago the people of the Yellow River Valley, in what is currently China, became organized as a cohesive society that would come to permanently characterize the southeast quadrant of the Asian continent, and eventually extend its influence thousands of miles to the east and south over successive centuries. In the ethnomedical history of East and Southeast Asia, it is useful to consider the concept of "Greater China" radiating outward from the Yellow River Valley and encompassing the contiguous areas of Manchuria, Korea, Japan, Indochina (Cambodia, Laos, Vietnam), the Malay Peninsula, and the Indonesian Archipelago. This vast area came under Chinese influence through mercantile and military expansion in the long period between the earlier phase of Vedic and Hindu influences from ancient India and the later waves of Islamic influence in much of this part of the globe. The peoples of this Chinese civilization also would eventually travel to every corner of the earth, taking their traditional culture, including traditional medicine, and spreading it around the globe. Together with modern Western biomedicine, it is currently the only other form of medicine that can be said to be available in virtually every urban setting in the world.

Conversely, when foreign cultures encountered the dominant Chinese civilization, they would usually be brought under the fold. A famous example is when the Mongol invader from the northwest, Genghis Khan, conquered China. Within two generations, his grandson Kublai Khan had become thoroughly "sinified"—that is, he proverbially became more Chinese than the Chinese. He eventually came to symbolize the prototypical Chinese Emperor in the eyes of 18th- and 19th-century Western literary figures, such as Samuel Taylor Coleridge, who used Kublai Khan in his poem of the same name as the symbol of oriental despotism, eroticism, exoticism, and splendor, all at once. This type of depiction of China came to be understood as actually a Western image of China and Asia, labeled *Orientalism* by Edward Said (in his book of the same name) in the 20th century.

CONSISTENCY IN DIVERSITY

The ability of China to incorporate valuable new discoveries and ideas was at the same time central to maintaining the core of their culture and cosmology. An important example of China encountering and incorporating new ideas was the influence of Gautama the Buddha from India, who traveled into China and profoundly influenced its cosmology, culture and medicine. The spiritual tradition of Buddhism came to exist side by side with Confucianism and Daoism, again illustrating the ability of Chinese civilization to accommodate and incorporate diverse traditions, existing side by side. An emperor of the Ming Dynasty (1368 to 1644) wrote these lines in a poem:

"In my garden
Side-by-side
Native plants
Foreign plants"

Beyond the limits of accommodation and assimilation, the Chinese also made efforts to protect the identity of their culture and civilization and to keep out foreign "barbarians." Such efforts are dramatically illustrated by the huge project for the construction of the Great Wall (the only manmade artifact that can be seen from outer space). At places it is as close as only 50 miles from Beijing (*Bei*: northern; *jing*: capital), for example, at Ba Da Ling. While keeping out the Islamic religious influence of the "Moslem hordes" of the Middle Ages, the Chinese nonetheless picked up a few new ideas from the animal kingdom, just outside the Great Wall for the menu of classic Northern Chinese cuisine, such as duck and lamb, as well as transportation, such as the camel, for the important trade route, *the Silk Road*. Later when 16th- to 19th-century Europeans were the potential colonizers, the Chinese created "cantonments" for each of the European powers to keep them isolated and obstruct the flow of European "contagion" into the culture, in places such as Port Arthur (Tsing Tao), Hong Kong, and Macao. Finally, the descent of the "Bamboo Curtain" after the 1947 Communist take-over was designed to keep foreign influence out and perhaps just as much to keep the Chinese in.

Accommodating and incorporating diversity, while maintaining a consistent cosmology, is also an important characteristic of Chinese medicine. Thus new discoveries and ideas about medicine did not supplant the old ones; they were just accommodated alongside. For example, as we present later in this chapter, the older practice of Chinese herbal medicine was not supplanted by the newer discovery of acupuncture; instead, they came to exist side by side in a common Chinese cosmology of medicine.

BIRTH OF CHINESE MEDICINE

The ancient mythology of Chinese medicine attributes the birth of medicine to three legendary, semimythical emperors. The semimythical origins of these three kings are said to extend back in time nearly 5000 years. The first references to medical practices that begin to resemble Chinese medicine as we currently know it do not occur until the end of the 3rd century BC. Acupuncture first surfaces as a documented therapeutic method only in the 1st century BC. Some interpretations of the ancient archeological evidence and texts seek to establish a greater antiquity for acupuncture by drawing inferences between ancient stone artifacts and modern acupuncture needles. In considering the manner in which Chinese medicine is constructed, none of these theories can be discarded.

In addition to their medical revelations, the three divine emperors are also each credited with introducing many other useful practices into the world, placing medicine into a truly holistic context with the development of other critical aspects of Chinese civilization.

Fu Xi, the Ox Tamer (伏羲, c.3000 BCE), Origins of Medicine

Fu Xi, or the Ox Tamer, taught people how to domesticate animals. He also divined the Ba Gua, eight symbols that became the basis for the Yi Jing, or Book of Changes. Fu Xi reveals celestial knowledge of domestication of the main Chinese beast of burden and engine for physical labor (the original and all-time "Year of the Ox"). He illustrates medicine as an intrinsic part of human society, as well as part of the natural order.

Shen Nong, the Divine Husbandman (神農, c.2750 BCE), Origins of Chinese Herbal Medicine

Shen Nong, or the Divine Husbandman, also known as the "Fire Emperor", is said to have lived from 2737 to 2697 BC. He introduced agriculture to the world when he taught the Chinese people how to cultivate plants and raise livestock. Shen Nong, the celestial source for knowledge on agronomy and agriculture, demonstrates that the breeding of animals and plants includes cultivation of plants for medicines, as well as food.

This semimythical sequence of animal domestication ("ox taming"), followed by agriculture and raising livestock ("divine husbandry"), maps to modern archeological interpretations of the development of complex civilizations in such areas as the Yellow River Valley, where peoples first kept nomadic herds of semidomesticated animals on the move, then eventually settled down in fertile areas to raise animals and grow crops in permanent settlements.

Shen Nong, as the originator of Chinese herbal medicine, learned the therapeutic properties of herbs and other substances by tasting them. Later authors would attribute their own works back in time to Shen Nong to indicate the antiquity and importance of their texts. A good example of this tradition is *The Divine Husbandman's Classic of the Materia Medica* (Shen Nong Ben Cao Jing), which was probably written in AD 220 and reconstructed in AD 500 by Tao Hong Jing. When it comes to Chinese antiquity, it is never easy to separate legend from fact, but all historical evidence points to the truly ancient character of herbal medicine in China, so it is appropriate that Shen Nong is considered its originator. This "Classic of Shen Nong" is not a treatise on ancient medical theory but a simple compilation of plant and other material substances and their influences on the body.

Huang Di, the Yellow Emperor (黃帝, c.2650 BCE) Origins of Acupuncture and Qi Manipulation

Huang Di introduced the more spiritual, "heavenly," and less "earthy" (literally, compared with the roots and plants of medicinal plants) approach to balancing vitality, or qi, through application of acupuncture. This comparatively new method does not use material sources and substances, such as medicinal plants, and is literally "immaterial," allowing more direct access to the spiritual, celestial aspects of healing—thus gaining the attribution, the *spiritual pivot*. Nowadays, Huang Di is perhaps the most generally known of the three legendary emperors. Bringing wisdom gained from visiting in the realm of the immortals, this "Father of the Chinese Nation" is also credited with introducing the art of writing, the techniques for making wooden houses, boats, carts, bows and arrows, silk, and ceramics, as well as the practice of Traditional Chinese Medicine. In archeological sequence, this stage represents the later development of complex civilization for which further social organization was required, for example, for irrigation and controlling floods, in peoples who had settled down to raise crops and livestock.

The Yellow Emperor's Inner Classic (Huang Di Nei Jing) is the first document in which Traditional Chinese Medicine was described in a form familiar nowadays. The text is divided into two books. "Simple Questions" (Su Wen) is concerned with medical theory, such as the principles of yin and yang (paired opposites in dynamic equilibrium, which help to define the nature of life), the five phases (which relate to dynamic processes in the body), and the effects of the four seasons.

"The Spiritual Axis" (Ling Shu) or spiritual pivot deals predominantly with acupuncture and moxibustion. Like *The Divine Husbandman's Classic of the Materia Medica*, *The Yellow Emperor's Inner Classic* was not written by the emperor himself but was compiled long after his death, probably around 100 BC. *The Yellow Emperor's Inner Classic* is still revered in modern times both for its legendary context and for its medical contributions to Chinese culture. The text is written as a series of dialogues between the emperor and his ministers, including the legendary Qi Bo, whose excitement about the "new" treatment of acupuncture resonates down through the centuries until the present. He describes to the emperor that acupuncture represents a more "heavenly" spiritual, or immaterial, approach to healing that does not require the use of the older, dirty, smelly, and often bad-tasting formulations of roots, barks, and leaves from medicinal plants. Debates between the effectiveness and appropriateness of acupuncture versus herbal remedies currently continue among Chinese practitioners.

The knowledge revealed to these three emperors as currently recorded was recovered on materials ranging from silk documents excavated from the Mawangdui Han tombs (168 BCE or earlier) to widely translated works, such as the Shen Nong Bencaojing (神農本草經, Divine Farmer's Materia Medica) and the Huangdi Neijing (黃帝內經, Yellow Emperor's Canon of Internal Medicine, or The Yellow Emperor's Inner Classic).

PRESERVATION AND TRANSMISSION

These legendary origins remain diverse with iconic texts, notable practitioners, and concepts that date back millennia. Yet, these medical systems are at the same time characterized as traditional or unchanging, consistent with Chinese cosmology. Each system of knowledge has significantly evolved often with the intervention of state institutions, originating with the pronouncements of these semimythical, demigod rulers of China as the embodiment of the state (see section, "The Middle

Kingdom and the Body Politic"). Furthermore, travel of practitioners, dissemination of classic textual translations, and exchange and trade of the materia medica and pharmacopeia of Chinese remedies across all of Asia contributed to many manifestations of classic forms of medical knowledge.

The transmission of textual sources via translators depended in part on regional proximity and on sharing the same written language, as was the case for ancient China, Japan, and Korea (where classical Chinese characters were in use until the CE 15th century). Another important factor in considering the spread of Chinese medicine is regional ethnomedical practices based on the use of materia medica, or effective herbal remedies common to geographical distributions where they grow. A common property embedded in all medical practices and materials is the role of qi, or vital energy.

VITAL ENERGY

Two important aspects of Chinese medical cosmology that we address here are vital energy, or qi, and the divine origins of medical knowledge and practice. First, health is a result of the proper balance (yin and yang) of vital energy (qi) in the body, and disease is a result of imbalance. The intervention of a Chinese medical practitioner helps to maintain or restore this balance of vital energy, thus maintaining or restoring health. Medicinal herbs, acupuncture, and physical manipulations (tui na) and exercises (qigong) are all different medical modalities for maintaining or restoring health through the balancing of vital energy. This balance of vital energy is the goal of all these different modalities as different paths to the same end and metaphysically working in the same way.

Another important aspect of Chinese medical cosmology is that the knowledge of these medical modalities is divinely revealed to humans. As detailed previously, every major aspect of Chinese medicine had its origin attributed to the writings and teachings of semimythical, divine rulers in the line of Chinese emperors. Thus attributing the heavens as the source of all human knowledge, channeled through demigod rulers to mortal humans forms the basis for Chinese civilization in general, as well as health and healing. Thence comes the iconic Chinese characterization of its own civilization are representing the "Middle Kingdom," half way between heaven and earth. This concept is directly revealed in China's name for itself, Zhong Guo, literally "the land at the middle." The medicine of China is the medicine of this Middle Kingdom.

THE MIDDLE KINGDOM AND THE BODY POLITIC

Although the heavens are attributed as the source of Chinese civilization, including medical knowledge, the political organization of ancient China provided models for how the body functions. It is striking how all of Chinese medicine, anatomy, and pathology (see later) use terms relating to the political governance of society as metaphors for how the human body is regulated—essentially as a description for human physiology. This view is striking to the Western reader because Western biomedicine uses the metaphor of a machine to describe functions of the human body: the mechanical model. Although the human body has been used as a metaphor for the political governance of a human society (e.g., by the English philosopher Thomas Hobbes in his famous treatise, *Leviathan* [1651]), we do not observe the reverse application in Western medicine. *Leviathan* was the body politic made visible—a social body composed of cells of individual men, just as the human body is composed of individual cells. Modern medicine is largely based on the body being essentially made up of populations of cells comprising tissues and organs that work together as regulated by physiology, as populations of individuals can be seen to make up societies and work together under political governance.

The metaphors of Chinese medicine provide another useful way of representing human functional anatomy and physiology. As an empirical system, Chinese medicine is tremendously sophisticated and nuanced in terms of devising treatments tailored to each individual and to his or her specific conditions. The Chinese use metaphors in medicine that describe human physiology in terms relating to human sociopolitical organization. This use may relate to the preoccupation of Chinese civilization with the emperor (as the source of divine knowledge and wisdom), his Mandarins at court, and the disseminated bureaucratic organization that provided the foundation for government administration of complex works, organizations, and operations, such as irrigation agriculture and public waterways and canals for transportation.

One of the great projects of the ancient Chinese civilization was the creation of canals or "waterways" for irrigation agriculture and transportation. The requirements for organization of labor for such projects had a transactional relationship to the development of Chinese social organization and political control. These processes and relationships were described by Wittfogel (1957) in the classic treatise *Oriental Despotism*. The inherent relations of the contours of Chinese society with major public "infrastructure" projects, the political organization of the Chinese government, and the Chinese pictographic language needed and used for communications result in a rich vocabulary of metaphors used in describing medical aspects of the human body as waterways, channels, and the like in the original Chinese language. The Western translations in most books using such words as *meridians* for the acupuncture energy *channels* do not correctly map to these more "fluid" Chinese metaphorical concepts.

FLOOD OF KNOWLEDGE

The divine origins of knowledge, the concept of vital energy, and its character as representing flow, like water, are all illustrated in the following legend:

The demigod Gun (鯀), grandson of Huang Di, the Yellow Emperor, failed to build dams to restrain the great floods that threatened China. In contrast, his son Da Yu (大禹), one of the forefathers of Daoism, managed to control the floods by opening natural pathways along geographical "lines of force" to drain the accumulated waters.

Controlling and directing the flow of water was seen as one of the first steps to a civilized world. In the Lingshu the rivers and streams of qi within the body were originally compared with the natural waterways of China (as with the nadi of Yoga and the sacred rivers of India). After the analogy between qi channels and watercourses had been made, channeling of qi into routes around the body marked a significant way of bringing the body, like the waterways, under control. A similar process may have occurred with qigong, whose traditional postures were probably developed from more spontaneous movements and breathing behavior. The development and application of these ideas about the nature of health and healing are illustrated in the next section on history and concepts of chinese medicine.

HISTORY OF CHINESE MEDICAL PRACTICE

Little is actually recorded about the practice of medicine in China before 200 BC. Ancient Chinese civilization started with nomadic tribes. Originally scattered across Northern China, they eventually established permanent settlements and developed a social and political structure that became the Shang Dynasty (1766 to 1121 BC). Ancestors were venerated and spiritually consulted on a variety of issues, including the causes of illness, through the use of oracle bones. The scapulae and other flat bones of early domesticated animals were boiled in large bronze pots (an achievement of early Chinese Bronze Age metallurgy that predated the more sophisticated metallurgy that allowed the manufacture of filiform acupuncture needles later).

The Zhou overthrew the Shang and established one of China's longest-lasting dynasties (1122 to 221 BC). The Zhou Dynasty continued many of the Shang practices, including consulting tortoise shell oracles with the aid of *wu* (healer/priests). The wu acted as intermediaries between the living and the dead, played important ritual roles in court activities and in divining the weather, and were called upon to combat demons that caused illness. One of the wu's activities, chasing evil spirits away from towns and homes with spears, might have become conceptually transferred to the human body itself, leading to the practice of acupuncture.

Toward the close of the Zhou Dynasty came a time of violent political strife and social upheaval known as the "Warring States period". This era saw the emergence of two philosophers, Kong Fu Zi (Confucianism) and Lao Zi (Daoism), whose ideas about social and natural order were to have a lasting impact on Chinese culture and medicine, together with the influences of Prince Gautama the Buddha (Buddhism) from India. In medicine also a sense of natural order was emerging, and the human body was no longer seen as subject to the whims of spirits and demons, but rather as part of a coherent natural environment. Those ideas, rooted in the Zhou period, would blossom during the Han Dynasty.

DEVELOPMENT OF CHINESE MEDICAL THEORY AND PRACTICE

The Zhou Dynasty ended in 211 BC, after a period of confusion and political instability. The short-lived Qin Dynasty completed the first version of the Great Wall of China but disappeared soon afterward. The Han Dynasty (206 BC to AD 219) reunited the empire, created a stable aristocratic social order, expanded geographically and economically, and spread Chinese political influence throughout the adjacent peninsulas of Korea and Vietnam (Indochina). This dynasty was such a powerful force that the Chinese people still currently refer to themselves as "the Han." Great cultural developments took place during the Han Dynasty, including integration of the Confucian doctrine, elements of yin-yang, and the five-phase theory (see later). Written evidence first reveals the emergence of a medicine with similarities to the traditional Chinese Medicine known in modern times. (Note: The formal term "Traditional Chinese Medicine" [TCM] refers to a system concocted under Maoist Communist China in the mid-20th century, incorporating some aspects of ancient Chinese medicine, with 20th-century Western biomedical theory.)

The earliest medical literature that survives from the Han era consists of three texts discovered in tombs dating to 168 BC, excavated at Ma Wang Dui in Hunan province. These texts discuss demons, magic, and the relation of yin and yang to the body. The writings present an early concept of energy channels in the body, but these ideas remain less developed than they would later become in the *Yellow Emperor's Inner Classic*. The Ma Wang Dui texts mention moxibustion and the use of heated stones, but they do not speak about acupuncture or specific points on the body, suggesting that the idea of acupuncture proper had not yet emerged at this time.

The Divine Husbandman's Classic of Materia Medica (Shen Nong Ben Cao) appears during this era, presenting the first known example of what has become a long line of formal descriptions of individual medicinal substances. This period also saw the publication of *The Yellow Emperor's Inner Classic*, with its detailed descriptions of medical theory and the use of acupuncture and moxibustion. Its knowledge still guides the practice of traditional Chinese Medicine nowadays, still often quoted in contemporary medical texts. *The Classic of Difficult Issues* (Nan Jing) was compiled sometime during the 1st or 2nd century AD, although its authorship is attributed back in time to the legendary physician Bian Qu, who lived in the 5th century BC. It marks a drastic shift in medical thinking away from magical elements and toward systematic organization of acupuncture theory and practice.

Such classic texts reflected the health care available only to the elite rather than the medical traditions of the general population. At that time, approximately 80% of Chinese people were illiterate farmers or peasants scratching out a bare subsistence and still using Stone Age (Neolithic) technology. Their own ethnomedical traditions were oral, locally oriented, and consisted of folk superstition, historical legend, and aspirations expressing hope of survival and still carrying some of the ideas about ancestors and demons from the earlier Shang and Zhou Dynasties.

In AD 220, following 30 years of strife and religious rebellion by Daoist sects, the Han Dynasty fell and there was another long period of division in China. In AD 589 the Sui Dynasty reunified China but was soon succeeded by the Tang Dynasty (AD 618 to 907), considered by many to be the height of China's cultural development. The Tang Dynasty spread greater China's influence as far as Korea, Japan, Mongolia, Central Asia, and Indochina (Vietnam). During this period both Buddhism and Daoism strongly influenced medical thought.

SYSTEMATIC CHINESE MEDICINE

By the time of the Sung Dynasty (AD 960 to 1280), the practice of medicine had become more specialized, and efforts were made to integrate past insights systematically. In AD 1027 Wang Wei Yi designed and oversaw the casting of two bronze figures designed to illustrate the location of acupuncture points. The bronzes were pierced at the location of the acupuncture points, covered with wax, and filled with water. When a student inserted a needle in the correct place, it found the hole under the wax, and water dripped out, confirming that the needle had been properly placed.

During the Sung Dynasty there were also advances in herbal therapeutics with the publication, under imperial decree, of several complete, illustrated herbal texts. During this time, tastes and properties were assigned to herbs according to their yin or yang nature, and functions were assigned that were a result of the herb's nature and its ability to treat specific symptoms.

During the Sung, Jin, and Yuan Dynasties (AD 960 to 1368), medical education became more formal, the Imperial College of Physicians was founded, and specialized medical thought and independent inquiry continued to develop. Much of what we recognize as Chinese medicine nowadays stems from these three dynasties. Physicians of this period revisited some early theories and used them to develop new therapeutic approaches. They espoused the application of five-phase theory (wu xing), in which dynamic processes in the body are defined in terms of the five phases: earth, metal, water, wood, and fire. Each of these phases is related to various organs of the body, the seasons, times of day, tastes, colors, vocalizations, and other factors (see later). During these three dynasties, the five phases were studied most intensively in relation to seasonal influences and as a way of supplementing the body, purging the body of evil influences, and enhancing yin.

MING AND QING DYNASTIES

From the 14th to the early 20th century, Chinese physicians focused on developing lines of inquiry that had been pursued in preceding dynasties. Some scholars consider the Ming Dynasty (AD 1368 to 1644) to be the peak of the cultural expression of acupuncture and moxibustion in China. In 1644 the Ming Dynasty fell to foreigners from Manchuria, who founded the Qing Dynasty (AD 1644 to 1911). Folk herbal and ethnomedical traditions (as opposed to the ancient wisdom of the three emperors) were collected, organized, and published for the first time during the Qing Dynasty. Political, economic, and social changes engulfed the nation. The Chinese were forced to wear pigtails for the first time in history, which the "Han" resented bitterly. New food crops, including maize (corn), sweet potatoes, peanuts, and potatoes, were imported from the Americas and Africa. As cultural horizons broadened, the scope of medical inquiry expanded, shaking the classical underpinnings of Chinese medical thought. In 1822 acupuncture was formally eliminated from the Imperial Medical College. By the close of the Qing dynasty in 1911 political and cultural institutions were in a state of decline. The scattered practitioners of TCM found themselves increasingly under fire from the advocates of a new and modern China. In contrast to the revealed wisdom of the three emperors, then in disrepute, folk remedies were finally extensively explored and recorded in the 20th century under the guidance of the postrevolutionary government of China, resulting in such texts as *The Barefoot Doctor's Manual,* as part of the creation of TCM.

Chinese Medicine in the 20th Century and Today

In China during the 20th century the course of medical practice had been redefined. With the formation of the Republic of China in 1911, reformers attempted to institute sweeping cultural changes, pushing aside remnants of the old empire to make way for the modern age. In medicine, that meant trying to replace traditional practices with contemporary science.

The Imperial Medical College had been closed, and from 1914 to 1936, both Chinese nationalists (under Sun Yat Sen and Chiang Kai Shek) and Marxists (under Mao Tse Tung, or Zedong) sought to "reform" practitioners of traditional medicine. Even the name came under attack. What had always been called simply "medicine" (yi), was now called "Chinese medicine" (zhong yi), and those practices deemed "unscientific" according to new 20th-century medicine were rejected. Zhong yi redefined TCM into the form in which it is currently practiced.

The aspects of traditional medicine that survived as zhong yi were later appropriated by Chinese Communists in an effort to build a strong, low-cost medical infrastructure for the new nation's vast underserved population.

In 1958 Chairman Mao declared, "Chinese medicine is a great treasure house! We must uncover it and raise its standards!" Traditional medicine was to be rehabilitated by Communist modernists who would predictably "discover" a primitive dialectical ("Marxist") logic within the theoretical underpinnings of the traditional system of ancient Chinese medicine. *The Revised Outline of Chinese Medicine* stated, "Yin-yang and the five phases are ancient Chinese philosophical ideas. They are spontaneous, naïve materialist theories that also contain elementary dialectical ideas."

Zhong yi currently exists in China as a parallel medical system, integrating 20th-century Western biomedical elements while retaining fidelity to the traditional concepts of Chinese medicine. Educational programs emphasize acupuncture and herbal medicine, ranging from an undergraduate technical certificate to PhD programs. Most independent practitioners enter the field with a 5-year medical baccalaureate degree (MB/BS) that is earned following high school. In this system both inpatient and outpatient medical care is delivered from large, well-equipped hospitals, as well as from private clinics and pharmacies.

TCM is currently a global entity that is quite distinct from its premodern counterpart. The chief modalities that have come to characterize TCM include acupuncture, moxibustion, herbal medicine, dietary therapy, tui na (massage), and qigong. Concepts of qi, its cultivation, and flow are critical to each of these modalities. The meridians or channels through which qi flows, or can be blocked or become stagnant, are key sites in considerations of pathology and therapeutic intervention.

Although concepts of qi in TCM theory and practice seem similar to those of classical or premodern forms of Chinese medicine, there has been a transition in the definition and uses of qi in contemporary TCM texts. For instance, in the Suwen, qi was defined as both a cosmic force and bodily substance. However, the concept of qi in post-1949 Chinese medical texts tends to reflect solely physiological dimensions and emphasize qi primarily as a bodily substance like blood and other bodily fluids. Such a transition is due in part to the medicalization of practice and the discourses of scientific Marxism where social, environmental, and phenomenological meanings of the body and its forms are reconfigured into more material categories with physical properties. In the Marxist version the body becomes less an energetic, spiritual entity and is reduced to one that is more predictably material, in consort with Marxism, and presumably more controllable, also in concert with Marxism.

CONCEPTS OF CHINESE MEDICINE

Down through the dynasties of the last more than 2000 years, the philosophy of Chinese medicine began with the concept of yin and yang. These two terms can be used to express both the broadest philosophical concepts and the most focused perceptions of the natural world. Yin and yang express the idea of opposing but complementary phenomena that exist in a state of dynamic equilibrium. An ancient metaphor for this idea was the shady and sunny sides of a hill, with the sunlit southern side representing yang and the shaded northern side representing yin. They are part of one whole but fundamentally different in character. On the bright, sunny yang side, plants and animals are seen to be more prevalent, the air is drier, and the rocks are warm. On the dim, shaded yin side, the air is moist and cool. Yet yin and yang are always present simultaneously.

As Lao Zi, the Daoist contemporary of Confucius, described, "The created universe carries the yin at its back and the yang in front." The paired opposites observed in the world give tangible expression to an otherwise incomprehensible Dao (the Way) of ancient Chinese thought. *The Book of Changes* (Yi Jing), which sought to explore the myriad manifestations of yin and yang, put it this way: "That which lets now the dark, now the light, appear is Dao."

Yang	Yin
Light	Dark
Heaven	Earth
Sun	Moon
Day	Night
Spring	Autumn
Summer	Winter
Hot	Cold
Male	Female
Fast	Slow
Up	Down
Outside	Inside
Fire	Water
Wood	Metal

The Yellow Emperor's Inner Classic was the first text to provide a comprehensive discussion of the medical application of yin and yang, stating that "yin and yang are the way of heaven and earth." This text showed how yin and yang are used to correlate the body and other phenomena to the human experience of health and disease.

"As to the yin and yang of the human body, the outer part is yang and the inner part is yin. As to the trunk, the back is yang and the abdomen is yin. As to the organs, the bowels are yang, whereas the [other] viscera are yin. The liver, heart, spleen, lung, and kidney yin; the gallbladder, stomach, intestines, bladder, and triple burner [an organ known only in Asian medicine] are yang."

Yin and yang are used to express ideas about health and disease and also the manner in which the entire cosmos is organized. These correspondences are similar to the classical and medieval European concepts of the four humors. Summer is yang within yang, fall is yin within yang, winter is yin within yin, and spring is yang within yin. The coldest, darkest, and most yin period, winter, was yin within yin, whereas spring, when the yang began to emerge from the yin, was yang within yin (see "The Five-Phase Theory" section later).

Yin and yang illustrate that reality is in a constant process of transformation and that all things are interconnected. A candle provides a useful analogy: consider the wax to be the yin aspect of the candle and the flame to be the yang; see how the yin nourishes and supports the yang, how the yang consumes the yin and in doing so burns brightly. When the wax is gone, so is the flame. Yin and yang exist in dependence upon one another.

The ancient Chinese cosmology understood human beings to have a nature and structure inseparable from yin and yang, and the same rules that guide the cosmos naturally guide the human body. As in Medieval and Renaissance Europe, the microcosm reflects the macrocosm (e.g., as illustrated in the works of Shakespeare and documented in E. M. W. Tillyard's classic study, *The Elizabethan World Picture*).

"To follow [the laws of] yin and yang means life; to act contrary to [the laws of] yin and yang means death."

Within the traditional medical community of contemporary China, there is much debate over the actual nature of yin and yang. Some exponents of a more scientific, less traditional, perspective on Chinese medicine would like yin and yang to be used as concepts to organize phenomena. Others, who express a less modern perspective, emphatically state that yin and yang are actually tangible phenomena. It is probably most useful to think about yin and yang as descriptive terms that help the Chinese physician to organize information. However, in Chinese medicine, especially its use of medicinal substances, the yin and yang constituents of the body are considered material entities that can be reinforced by specific substances or actions.

THE FIVE ELEMENTS OR PHASES: EARTH, METAL, WATER, WOOD, AND FIRE

Another concept that plays a significant role in development and practice of Chinese medicine is the five phases or processes (wu xing): earth, metal, water, wood, and fire. In Chinese, *wu* means five, and *xing* expresses the idea of movement, of "going." For a period of time the wu xing was translated as "the five elements." This translation does not really convey the dynamism of the Chinese concept, instead it focuses on the apparent similarities between wu xing and the elements of medieval European alchemy. Wu xing may include the implication of material elements, but the term in translation of five phases generally better addresses the dynamic relations occurring among phenomena that are organized in terms of these interconnected phases. This cosmological concept can cover almost every aspect of natural phenomena from bodily organs to the weather.

THE FIVE-PHASE THEORY: CONSTITUENTS, ORGANS, AND POWERS

The human body is like an ecologic system. As yin and yang divide the cosmos into two polar forces, five primordial powers differentiate all vital activity as progressing through five phases that correspond to the seasons in nature. The body can be seen as a garden in this human landscape, which encompasses the five primal forces in nature, which in turn correspond to the seasons.

Fire—Yang—Summer
Earth—Yang and yin in balance—Intervals between seasons
Metal—Yin within yang—Autumn
Water—Yin—Winter
Wood—Yang within yin—Spring

The cycle of human lives also corresponds to the seasons of nature.

Water Phase (yin)—Gestation—In utero
Wood Phase—Birth—New life comes forth
Fire Phase (yang)—Maturation—Adulthood
Metal Phase—Aging
Earth Phase—Interval between these stages
Water Phase—Again—Death

The five phase elements correspond to the seasons in the environment (macrocosm). Five functional systems, or "organ networks," govern particular mental faculties, physiological activities, and tissues of the human body (microcosm).

Kidney
Heart
Liver
Lung
Spleen

These organ networks generate and regulate the body's constituents:

Blood—Nourishes—gives solidity to the shape created by qi; connective tissue
Essence—Provides Foundation—fundamental origin (ovum, sperm); genes, DNA

Moisture—Lubricates—fluids: digestive, joints, eyes, cerebrospinal; buffers body

Qi—Moves—vital force, flow, giving shape ("keeping it together"), adaptation

Shen–Embodies—organizing force of the self, immaterial (yang), body-mind-spirit

Blood in itself is inert, passive, and thick and accordingly has a tendency to stagnate, pool, and congeal (clot). Qi is active and warms and moves the blood. Qi by itself has no material expression and no source for renewal. Providing the material basis, blood links qi with physical form. Blood is said to be the mother of qi, and where qi goes, blood flows.

Accordingly, the body's ecology can be related to that of nature and the cosmos.

Shen—Heavens—integrative consciousness of body-mind-spirit, self-awareness

Qi—Air—animating force in all living processes, manifested as human activity

Moisture—Inner Sea—liquid medium that nurtures and lubricates interfaces

Blood—Soil—substances and structures of the body, repository of mental images

Essence—Earth/Seeds—foundations and phenotypic expressions of basic identity

Each organ network embodies a set of functions, psychologic and physiologic, corresponding to channels of influence, emotional states, and sensory activity, as well as specific tissues. Although they are assigned to a named anatomical structure, they are not fixed in location.

Fire—Heart—envelops Shen, propels Blood, perception and intuition

Metal—Lung—governs respiration, circulation of qi, subconscious, defenses

Earth—Spleen—takes in nutrients, supplies Moisture, thought and memory

Wood—Liver—governs Blood, circulating qi, judgment and temperament

Water—Kidney—stores Essence, instincts, impulses, will, and wisdom

Physical processes are not limited to the body, and feelings and thoughts are not assigned to the brain. Each of five networks influences and regulates a set of both bodily and mental activities and processes.

As in the association with the seasons of nature, the five phases interact with each other according to countervailing sequences of generation and restraint, proliferation and limitation, through which balance is maintained. Sheng is the supporting sequence for generation and proliferation, and Ke is the restraining sequence for limitation. Each phase gives birth to the succeeding phase in the Sheng sequence, and each establishes limits on another in the Ke sequence, all in a cycle.

Sheng Supporting Sequence: Fire/Heart supports Earth/Spleen supports Metal/Lung supports Water/Kidney supports Wood/Liver supports Fire/Heart…and continues the cycle.

Corresponding to the elements of nature, Water nourishes Wood, Wood feeds Fire, Fire generates Earth, Earth gives rise to Metal, Metal vitalizes Water.

In the Ke Restraining Sequence, Fire/Heart controls Metal/Lung controls Wood/Liver controls, Earth/Spleen controls Water/Kidney controls Fire/Heart…and continues. In nature, Water quenches Fire, Fire tempers Metal, Metal restrains Wood, Wood covers Earth, Earth dams Water.

Diseases of excess often advance from one organ network to another on the Ke sequence. Deficiency diseases usually develop along the Shen sequence. The gravity of a disease is assessed by how far along each of the sequences it has progressed and thus how many organ networks are affected.

Balancing Vital Energy

The crucial concept of qi, or vital energy, relates to the idea that the body is pervaded by subtle material and mobile influences that cause most physiological functions and maintain the health and vitality of the individual. This idea is not common to biomedical thinking about the body and is not easy for Westerners to grasp. The common translation of qi as "energy" conceals its distinctly material attributes (as when qi flows with blood). In Newtonian mechanics, energy is defined as the capacity of a system to do work. As energy, the character of qi extends considerably further.

The Chinese character for *qi* is traditionally composed of two radicals (word elements); the radical that symbolizes breath or rising vapor is placed above the radical for rice, which in this context has a broader meaning of food, or foodstuff. Qi is linked with the concept of "vapors arising from food." The concept of qi broadened over time but never lost a distinctly material aspect. To make the concept more challenging in translation, some phenomena labeled as qi do not fit conventional definitions of either substance or matter. The phrase "finest matter influences" or even just "influences" may offer a better translation. It is easy to see why many prefer to simply leave the term qi untranslated, as we do in this text.

The idea of qi is extremely broad, encompassing almost every variety of natural phenomena. There are many different types of qi in the body, depending on source, location, and function. There has been much ancient and modern debate, but qi is generally seen as having the functions of activation, warming, defense, transformation, and containment.

The qi concept is important to many aspects of Chinese medicine. Organ and channel qi are influenced by acupuncture. A characteristic feature of acupuncture treatment is the sensation of "obtaining the qi."

Qigong is a general term for the many systems of meditation, exercise, and therapeutics (see later), anchored in the concept of mobilizing and regulating the movement of qi in the body. Qi is sometimes compared with wind captured in a sail; one cannot observe the wind directly but can infer its presence as it fills the sail. In a similar fashion, movements of the body and the movement of substances within the body are all signs of qi's actions.

For the five-phase system, qi conveys blood throughout the body; blood flows through the body with the qi. Blood is understood to have a slightly broader and less-defined range of actions in Chinese medicine than it does in biomedicine. In general, blood is seen as nourishing the body. Blood is produced by construction qi, which in turn is derived from food and water. Within the body, qi and blood are said to be as closely linked, as are a person and his or her own shadow. This relation is expressed by the Chinese saying "qi is the commander of blood, and blood is the mother of qi," using the sociopolitical metaphors common to Chinese medicine.

Body fluids—thin and viscous substances that serve to moisten and lubricate the body—can be conceptually separated into humor and liquid. Humor is thick and related to the body's organs; among its functions is the lubrication of the joints. Liquid is thin and is responsible for moistening the surface areas of the body, including the skin, eyes, and mouth. In relation to qi, blood and fluids constitute the yin aspects of the body.

Qi, Essence, and Spirit

Qi, essence, and spirit are known in Chinese medicine as the "three treasures". Essence is the gift of one's parents (like genes), and spirit is the gift of heaven. Essence is the most fundamental source of human physiologic processes, of the bodily reserves that support human life, and of the actual reproductive substances of the body. It must be replenished by food and rest.

Spirit is the alert and radiant aspect of human life. We observe it in the luster of the eyes and face in a healthy person, as well as in that person's ability to think and respond appropriately to the surrounding world. The idea expressed by spirit, or shen, encompasses consciousness and healthy mental and physical function.

This connection reflects the concept that mind and body are not separated but fully interactive in a complex and dynamic way. Mental and emotional experiences impact the body, and vice versa. Aspects of human experience that are understood as predominantly mental in a biomedical frame of reference are linked to specific organs in Chinese medicine. For example, anger is related to the liver (as in the Medieval European character of choleric), thought to the spleen, and joy to the heart. These anatomical correspondences guide the application of balancing methods used for treatment in acupuncture, tui na, reflexology, qigong, and herbalism.

BODY OF CHINESE MEDICINE

ANATOMY AND PHYSIOLOGY

The ancient Chinese did not focus on anatomical or pathological dissection as a primary means of understanding the body. Their definitions of the organs were made according to function rather than physical structure. The physician of Chinese medicine encounters a body in which 12 organs function. These organs are divided into the viscera, which includes six zang, or solid, organs. They are heart, lungs, liver, spleen, kidneys, and pericardium (sac of membranes around the heart). The viscera also include the bowels, which comprise six fu, or hollow organs—the small intestine, large intestine, gallbladder, stomach, urinary bladder, and the "triple burner" (san jiao). Chinese and Western definitions of these organs and their functions match in many ways, but there are also key differences. In the Chinese system, the liver is said to store blood and distribute it to the extremities as needed, and the spleen is understood as an organ of digestion.

The circulation and elimination of fluids was observed and attributed to an organ that is said to have a name and function but no form—the so-called "triple burner." It is considered to be either the combined expression of the activity of other organs in the body or a group of spaces in the body. The triple burner has always been surrounded by debate within Chinese medicine because it does not have a clear anatomic structure, only a physiologic function.

The viscera and bowels are paired in what is known as the "yin and yang", or interior/exterior relationship. The heart is linked with the small intestine, the spleen with the stomach, and so forth. Each of the viscera—and each bowel—has an associated energy channel (or "meridian") that runs through it, through the paired organ within the body, and across the body's surface, before connecting with the channel of the paired organ.

Historical evidence suggests that the idea of channels is more ancient than the idea of specific acupuncture points. Disagreements continue about the locations of specific points, and efforts have been made to systematize knowledge of them. Recent research in the People's Republic of China has led to the publication of a number of texts dedicated to reconciling historical perspectives, terminology, and anatomic questions about acupuncture points. At this time there are understood to be 12 primary channels and 8 extraordinary channels. Qi is understood to flow in these channels, making a rhythmic circuit.

Along the pathways of 14 of these channels (the 12 regular channels and two of the extraordinary channels) lie 361 specific points. In addition, a large number of "extra" points have been derived from clinical experience but are not traditionally considered part of the major channel systems. Beyond this formulation, various individual acupuncture theories suggest still other points. There are also local microsystems of acupuncture points on the ear (auricular acupuncture; see later), scalp, hand, and foot, corresponding to reflexology, as well as other areas of the body.

Acupuncture points are often located where a gentle and sensitive hand, with slight pressure on the skin surface, detects a small depression or downward slope. Points exist at the margins or bellies of muscles, in between bones, and over distinctive bony features that can be detected through the skin. Methods used to find acupuncture points vary. In general, points are located by seeking anatomic landmarks (considered the most reliable method), by proportionally measuring the body, or by using finger measurements.

As with qi, the actual term and usage of the Chinese expression that is translated as "point" is important to understand. The character *xue*, translated as point, literally means "hole" in Chinese, which may more accurately reflect the clinician's subjective experience of the acupuncture site. Xue are holes where the qi of the channels can be influenced by inserting a needle or by other means, such as acupressure or moxibustion. Imagine the channel system as a vast internal waterway, with caves and springs punctuating its course, and you will have a concept of the xue, or hole, that is not far from the way the Chinese thought of them for many centuries.

Holes, or points along the channels, have been categorized and organized in many ways. One of the oldest and most well known is a system of categories based on the idea of shu, or transport points. This system of point categories applies exclusively to points on the forearm and lower leg, which embody the image of qi welling gently forth from a mountainous source at the tips of fingers and toes, and gradually gaining strength and depth as it flows, reaching the seas located at the elbow and knee joints.

PATHOLOGY

All illness is ultimately a disturbance of qi within the body. Its expression as a particular disorder displaying specific symptoms depends on the location of the disturbance. Three categories of disease causation are recognized: (1) external, (2) internal, and (3) causes that are neither external nor internal. The first category of external includes six influences that are distinctly environmental: wind, cold, fire, dampness, summer heat, and dryness. When they cause disease, these six influences are known as "evils." If the defense qi is not robust, the correct qi is not strong, or if the evil is powerful, then the evil may enter the surface of the body and under certain conditions penetrate to the interior.

The three causes of disease (san yin):

External causes, or the "six evils": wind, cold, fire, damp, summer heat, and dryness
Internal causes, or internal damage by the seven affects: joy, anger, anxiety, thought, sorrow, fear, and fright
Nonexternal, noninternal causes: dietary irregularities, excessive sexual activity, trauma, parasites, and taxation fatigue (too much or too little activity)

The nature of the evil and its impact on the body are understood through the observation of nature and of the body in illness. In this sense the biomedical distinction between cause and disease is somewhat blurred.

For example, the evils of wind and cold are frequently implicated in the sudden onset of symptoms associated with the common cold: headache, aversion to cold temperature, aching muscles and bones, fever, and a scratchy throat. Wind is expressed in the suddenness of the symptoms' onset and in their manifestation in the upper part of the body; cold is displayed in the pronounced aversion to cold and in aching muscles and bones. Whether or not the person had a specific encounter with a cold wind shortly before, the onset of the symptoms is not particularly relevant. Although it is not unusual for people to announce that they had been abroad on a chilly and windy day prior to the onset of a cold, such exposure could also easily result in signs of "wind heat" (i.e., a less marked aversion to cold, a distinctly sore throat, and a dry mouth). The six evils are not the agents of specific diseases but rather the agents of specific symptoms. These ideas developed in a setting where there was no means of investigating a bacterial or viral cause. Careful observation of the body's host response to disease instead provided the information necessary for treatment. Each of the evils affects the body in a similar manner to its behavior in the environment. The human body stands between heaven and earth and is subject to the influences of both. These six evils are identified as environmental influences that attack the body's surface, but they may also occur within the body, causing internal disruption.

Internal damage by the "seven affects" refers to the way in which mental states can influence body processes. However, such a statement implies a separation of mind and body that does not exist in Chinese medicine. Each of the seven affects can disturb the body if it is strongly or frequently expressed or repressed. As was discussed previously, each of the mental states—joy, anger, anxiety, thought, sorrow, fear, or fright—is related to a specific organ.

Nonexternal, noninternal causes encompass the origins of disease that do not arise specifically as a result of environmental influences or mental states. They include dietary irregularities, excessive sexual activity, taxation fatigue caused by overwork or extreme inactivity, trauma, and parasites. The role that most have in producing disease is obvious to us, with the exception of excessive sexual activity and taxation fatigue. Excessive sexual activity suggests the possibility that too frequent emission of semen by the male can cause illness. This can occur because semen is directly related to the concept of essence, which is considered to be vital to the body's function and difficult to replace. This category also includes possible damage to the essence through excessive childbearing or bearing a child at too young or too old an age.

Taxation fatigue expresses the dangers of engaging in a variety of activities for a prolonged period of time. It includes both the idea of overexertion and excessive inactivity as possible causes of disease. All the concepts included within taxation fatigue reflect the essential thought of Chinese medicine that moderation is the key to health. Lying down for prolonged periods damages the qi, and prolonged standing damages the bones. These images have powerfully informed Chinese medicine from the moment that the Yellow Emperor asked Qi Bo, in the *Classic of Internal Medicine*, why people now die before their time and received his answer that balance, harmony, and moderation are key.

QI BO EXPLAINS THE ORDERLY LIFE OF TIMES PAST

In *The Yellow Emperor's Inner Classic* the first book of "Simple Questions" begins with the Yellow Emperor asking his minister, Qi Bo, why life spans are now so short when in the past people lived close to 100 years. Qi Bo explains that in the past people maintained an orderly life. "In ancient times those people who understood Dao [the Way], patterned themselves upon the yin and the yang, and they lived in harmony with the arts of divination."

Each of the causes of disease—from prosaic factors, such as dietary irregularities, to somewhat exotic concepts, such as wind evil—disrupts the free movement of qi and the balance (of yang and yin) within the body. Learning the precise pattern of imbalance is the beginning of the diagnosis process.

DIAGNOSIS

There are four main methods of diagnosis in Chinese medicine: inspection, listening and smelling, inquiry, and palpation. The fundamental goal is to collect information that reflects the status of mind-body processes and then to analyze this information to determine how each process has been affected by a disorder.

Inspection (wang) refers to the visual assessment of the patient, particularly the spirit, form, and bearing; the head and face; and the substances excreted by the body. The color, shape, markings, and coating of the tongue are carefully inspected. For instance, in the case of a person who had been attacked by wind and cold, we would expect to see a moist tongue with a thin white coating, signaling the presence of cold. If heat were present, we might expect a dry mouth and a red tongue. The observation of the spirit, which is considered very important, relies on assessing the overall appearance of the patient, especially the eyes, complexion, and quality of the voice. Good spirit—even in the presence of serious illness—is thought to bode well for the patient.

The second aspect of diagnosis, listening, and smelling (wen) refers to listening to the quality of speech, breath, and other sounds, as well as to being aware of the odors of breath, body, and excreta. As with each aspect of diagnosis, the five-phase theory can be incorporated into the assessment of the person's condition. Each phase and each pair of viscera and bowel have a corresponding vocalization and smell.

The inquiry phase of diagnosis (like listening and smelling, also known as "wen") involves taking a comprehensive medical history. This process has been presented in many ways. Well known is the system of 10 questions described by Zhang Jie Bin during the Ming Dynasty. The questions were presented as an outline of diagnostic inquiry asking the patient about sensations of hot and cold, perspiration, head and body, excreta, diet, chest, hearing, thirst, previous illnesses, and previous medications and their effects. For example, an inquiry of a hypothetical patient suffering from wind and cold symptoms would be likely to reveal an aversion to any sort of exposure to cold, headache, body aches, and an absence of thirst. Inquiry is considered critical to a good diagnosis. Pulse diagnosis is sometimes regarded as a central feature of Chinese medicine and is rightly regarded as an art but should not form the sole basis of a diagnosis.

Palpation (qie), the fourth diagnostic method, involves pulse examination, general palpation of the body, and palpation of the acupuncture points. Pulse diagnosis offers a range of approaches and can provide a remarkable amount of information about the patient's condition. The process of pulse diagnosis is carried out with the patient in a calm state, sitting or lying down. The physician's fingers are placed on the radial arteries of the left and right wrists, approximately where a pulse is normally taken in Western medicine. There are three pulse positions, known as the "inch, bar, and cubit". The inch position, nearest the wrist, indicates the status of the body above the diaphragm. The bar indicates the status of the body between the diaphragm and navel. The cubit indicates the status of the area below the navel. Beyond this simple conceptual structure (and variations in technique), each pulse position can be interpreted to shed light on the status of the various organs and channels.

The pulse allows the practitioner to feel the quality of the qi and blood at different locations in the body. Pulse qualities are organized on the basis of size, rate, depth, force, and volume of the pulse. The practitioner will recognize such pulse qualities as rough, slippery, or bowstring and with many years of experience can find great meaning in overall quality of the pulse and the variations in quality at certain positions. For instance, the hypothetical patient afflicted with a wind-cold evil might display a pulse that was floating and tight, signaling the presence of a cold evil on the surface of the body.

After the practitioner of Chinese medicine has carried out the diagnostic process, he or she constructs an appropriate image of the disease's configuration so that it can be addressed by effective therapy. Central to this process is the idea of pattern identification (bian zheng), gathering signs and symptoms through diagnostic procedures using traditional theory to understand how fundamental substances of the body, the organs, and the channels have been affected.

The first step of pattern identification is localization of the disorder and the assessment of its essential nature, using the eight principles as an expansion of yin and yang correspondences: yin, yang, cold, hot, interior, exterior, vacuity (sometimes translated as deficiency), and repletion (sometimes translated as excess). The five phases may also be used, alone or in conjunction with the yin and yang correspondences.

Like other aspects of contemporary Chinese medicine, the eight principles originated in the Sung Dynasty (AD 960 to 1280). Kou Zong Shi proposed a structure that organized disease into eight essentials: cold, hot, interior, exterior, vacuity, repletion, evil qi, and right qi. These were improved upon in 1732 in the text *Awakening the Mind in Medical Studies* (Yi Xue Xin Wu). The original source was written in the spirit of the times to create a formal diagnostic structure for herbs that could be conceptually integrated with the ideas already in use for acupuncture. This formal structure is currently applied to both acupuncture and herbal medicine.

Say the hypothetical wind-cold patient came to us with these symptoms: a marked aversion to exposure to cold, headache, body aches, an absence of thirst, a moist tongue with a thin white coating, and a floating and tight pulse. In terms of the eight principles, this condition would be an exterior, cold, repletion pattern. The principles of yin and yang would not directly apply.

The eight principles serve fundamentally to localize a condition. When a Chinese physician says that a condition is external, he or she means that it has not yet penetrated beyond the skin and channels to the deeper parts of the body. In this case a cold condition betrays itself through the body's expression of cold signs. To say a condition is replete is to say that the evil attacking the body is strong.

The eight principles are typically the first step in developing a clear pattern identification, especially if there is organ involvement. The eight principles are the application of a yin- and yang-based theoretical structure.

Chinese diagnosis often cannot be related to single biomedical disease. For example, viral hepatitis is associated with at least six distinctive diagnostic patterns, and lower urinary tract infection might be related to one of four particular diagnostic patterns. Each of these patterns would be treated in different ways, as the saying goes, "One disease, different treatments."

There is also the saying, "Different diseases, one treatment," reflecting the concept that many different diseases may be captured within one pattern. One contemporary text lists such diverse entities as nephritis (inflammation of the kidneys), dysfunctional uterine bleeding, pyelonephritis (inflammation of the kidney and its pelvis), and rheumatic heart disease under the diagnostic pattern of "disharmony between the heart and kidney."

Types of diagnostic patterns:
Eight principles
Six evils
Qi and blood and fluids
Five phases
Channel patterns
Viscera and bowels
Triple burner
Six channels
Four levels

TREATMENTS

After a diagnosis has been reached and, when relevant, a pattern has been identified, therapy begins. Treatment in Chinese medicine follows a fundamentally allopathic philosophy (i.e., it addresses the disease with opposing measures). As described in *The Yellow Emperor's Inner Classic,* "Cold is treated with heat, heat is treated with cold, vacuity is treated by supplementation, and repletion is treated by drainage."

Within the realm of acupuncture, moxibustion (heating herbs on or near the skin), and herbal medicine, three fundamental principles of therapy are understood and applied: treating disease at its root, eliminating evil influences and supporting right influences, and restoring the balance of yin and yang. For instance, with our hypothetical wind-cold patient, the practitioner would seek to eliminate the cold evil and support the right qi. Where the symptoms reflect a more complex underlying pattern, the physician might attempt to treat the root of the patient's condition. Functional uterine bleeding due to a disharmony of the heart and kidney would be addressed primarily by harmonizing the heart and kidney; treating the root of the condition would adjust its symptoms at the uterine level. The most common methods for treating health problems include acupuncture, moxibustion, cupping, bleeding, massage, qi cultivation (qigong), herbal medicine, and diet.

Acupuncture and moxibustion can be used independently of each other but are so deeply wedded in Chinese medicine that the term for this therapy is zhen jiu, meaning "needle moxibustion," sometimes translated as "acumoxa therapy." Both techniques are used to provide a focused stimulus to points that lie along channel pathways or to other appropriate sites. The basis of their close linkage lies in ancient origins of the methods and that moxibustion appears to have been the first form of therapy applied to the channels and holes to treat problems on or within the body. We address acupuncture and related practices in detail in Chapter 15.

CHOICES IN CHINESE MEDICINE

There are many choices in Chinese medical concepts and approaches that can be used, and there are many pathways for a traditional Chinese practitioner to learn and practice from among these different concepts. The medicine that works best is often the modality that best meets our cultural expectations and "comfort zone." Understanding acupuncture and other traditional forms of healing begins with the unique cultural environment in which it has been developing for thousands of years.

Medicine is a human endeavor, and as such, it is shaped by human concerns, including economics, politics, and culture. A medical scientist or physician might perceive medicine as a steady march from ignorance to light, but these are typically revisionist histories. In the practice of medicine, ideology, belief, convenience, and even simple ignorance have probably had a greater influence than rationality. For instance, take the choice of how to conduct a medical procedure.

An example is the case of a Chinese patient who chose traditional herbal medicine to manage painful and debilitating kidney stones. Although the treatment ultimately took care of his problem, his choice was less medically based than career driven. He knew that if he had undergone surgery, he would have been classified as an invalid on his work papers and therefore been barred from advancement in his job. Institutions are as culturally biased as are individuals. There remain hospitals that close their doors to the practice of acupuncture despite the fact that acupuncturists are licensed medical practitioners and their services are routinely requested by hospital patients. In each instance, health care choices primarily involved cultural considerations, not medical ones.

Our own definitions of medicine, even of the human body and how it works, are profoundly affected by culture; we carry with us firmly entrenched expectations about our own and other healing systems. For instance, we tend to envision Chinese herbal medicine as a gentle therapy using benign ingredients, overlooking the fact that it also incorporates highly toxic substances and drastic purgative therapies. We are selective in how we explore other medicines. Naturalistic and rational elements intrigue us, but unfamiliar elements tend to make us uncomfortable. The ideas that medical knowledge is revealed from heavenly sources to divine rulers appear nonsensical, so we tend to ignore them.

When we encounter new ideas, we often like to think about them in familiar terms. This tendency can be seen in the use of the word "energy" to express the idea of qi or the word "sedation" as a translation for the therapeutic method of draining "evil influences" from channels in the body. Neither energy nor sedation have much to do with the concepts that underlie qi and draining, but these terms are more familiar to us and help to make Chinese medicine more accessible.

Unfortunately, such expedient translations are inaccurate and can obscure the breadth and depth of meaning in these terms. We have a tendency to think of Chinese medicine as a monolithic structure that has remained essentially unchanged since its origins, which, if legend is to be believed, reach back 5000 years. Instead, we have seen that Chinese medicine includes a tremendously diverse body of knowledge. It is tempting for Westerners to expect medical systems to be possessed of an internal logic that reconciles all of their elements. Although many aspects of Chinese medicine fit together with complete consistency, others appear to be quite contradictory. This trait leads us to what has probably been the most important aspect in understanding Chinese medicine throughout its history. Certain medical practices might have been relegated to the attic, but they remain available if needed.

A striking example is the work of Zhang Zhong Jing (AD 142 to 220), whose system of diagnosis and therapy did not attract much attention during his lifetime but became highly influential centuries after his death. Later Chinese medical practitioners believed his theory to be incomplete and broadened its perspective. However, his theories, and the new theories that emerged in response to them, are still important to the contemporary Chinese practitioner. In the West an incomplete theory is rejected and then disappears. In the history of Chinese medicine, theories, practices, and concepts may fade away, but they do not entirely vanish. A new theory can exist beside the one that it sought to replace. The clinician can choose to apply the perspective that he or she feels is most appropriate. In this way, conflicting concepts, systems of diagnosis, and treatments have continued to exist side by side over many centuries.

THE LOGIC OF INCONSISTENCY

Whereas Western biomedicine believes all theories are proven either right or wrong and should accordingly be retained or eliminated, Chinese medicine embraces multiple theories, like the yin-yang character and the five phases of all things, knowing that each may prove its utility when the right circumstances arise. As the 20th-century philosopher, scholar, and author Lin Yutang explained:

"The temperament for systematic philosophy simply wasn't there, and will not be there so long as the Chinese remain Chinese. They have too much sense for that. The sea of human life forever laps upon the shores of Chinese thought, and the arrogance and absurdities of the logician, the assumption that 'I am exclusively right and you are exclusively wrong,' are not Chinese faults, whatever other faults they may have."

Even in modern China, where the sheer volume of information and size of the population make it necessary to teach a standard curriculum to thousands of students each year, this tolerance for varying clinical perspectives continues. For instance, there are herbal physicians known as "Minor Bupleurum Decoction (Xiao Chai Hu Tang) doctors" because their prescriptions are organized around a single herbal medicinal formula from the *Treatise on Cold Damage* (Shang Han Lun), an early text on diagnosis and herbal therapy written during the Han dynasty (206 BC to AD 220). There also are herbal physicians who reject traditional formulas entirely and use contemporary biomedical research on the Chinese pharmacopoeia to organize their prescriptions.

Within acupuncture there are practitioners whose clinical focus might be dedicated almost entirely to only six acupuncture points and who now use computed tomography (CT) scans to plan interventions. At the same time, two floors down in the same Chinese hospital, physicians may base their selection of acupuncture points on obscure and complex aspects of traditional calendars and systems, such as the "Magic Turtle." In China, although a practitioner might be limited to the use of only six acupuncture points, in the United States, a licensed medical doctor can become an acupuncturist with only 6 weeks of training. Yet in Chinatowns around the world, practitioners must have six generations in their lineage to be trusted.

Any form or choice of health care modality works best when it meets the cultural expectations of the recipient. That is not to say that the powerful effects of the modalities are attributable to the "placebo effect." To the contrary, practitioners of Chinese medicine discovered aspects of human physiology that are not used in Western biomedicine. Although they are expressed in terms that are consistent with Chinese views of the cosmos and conceptualizations of how medical knowledge originates, they are no less valid than Western "scientific" constructs in terms of the empirical evidence for their effectiveness.

SUGGESTED READINGS

Chang, K. C. (Ed.), (1977). *Food in Chinese culture*. New Haven and London: Yale University Press. 429 pp.

Said, E. (1978). *Orientalism*. New York: New World Books.

Wittfogel, K. A. (1957). *Oriental despotism: A comparative study of total power*. New Haven and London: Yale University Press. 556 pp.

Chapter 15

Acupuncture and Moxibustion

The therapeutic goal of acupuncture is to regulate qi. In doing so, chronic pain and many pain conditions can be effectively controlled. In Chinese medicine, when qi and blood flow freely together through the body, the person is in a state of health. When the flow of qi is interrupted by some cause—such as an "evil," a disturbed mental state, or a trauma—illness results and pain can occur. Pain is directly linked to an injury or to the interruption of the flow of qi. Acupuncture is used to remove the obstruction and restore the flow. Needling may be used to remove the evil, to direct qi to places where it is insufficient, or to cause qi to flow where it previously had been blocked.

The "spiritual axis" of *The Yellow Emperor's Inner Classic* described nine needles for use in acupuncture. With the exception of one that appears to have had a specifically surgical application, the remaining eight needle types are still currently in use, either in original or adapted form. Modern acupuncture also includes other tools and methods that have been added over the centuries.

The most common acupuncture tool in use nowadays is the filiform or fine needle, which can vary significantly in terms of structure, diameter, and length. A typical acupuncture needle has a body or shaft 1 inch long and a handle of approximately the same length. The distinctive part of an acupuncture needle is its tip, which is rounded and moderately sharp, much like the tip of a pine needle. Solid and gently tapered, the acupuncture needle does not have the cutting edge of a hollow-point hypodermic needle. Its diameter typically is 0.25 mm (0.01 inch) or less.

STICKING TO IT

After the location for placement has been determined, the needle is inserted rapidly through the skin and then adjusted to an appropriate depth. An AD 12th-century text, *Ode of the Subtleties of Flow*, states, "Insert the needle with noble speed then proceed [to the appropriate depth] slowly; withdraw the needle with noble slowness, as haste will cause injury." Although a substantial number of considerations

Acknowledgments to Kevin V. Ergil and Marnae C. Ergil for prior contributions in Micozzi, M.S. (ed.), (2016). *Fundamentals of complementary and alternative medicine* (5th ed.). St Louis: Elsevier Health Sciences/Saunders.

affect the angle and depth of insertion, methods of manipulation, and length of retention, the following description outlines a basic procedure.

The essential aim is to obtain qi at the needling site, and the acupuncturist seeks either an objective or subjective indication that the qi has arrived, "obtaining qi." The practitioner can sense qi through his or her hands as the needle is manipulated or can determine its presence through observation of its effects or reports from the patient. The practitioner often feels the arrival of qi as a gentle grasping of the needle at the site, like a small fish on the end of a line. The patient may sense the arrival of qi as itching, numbness, soreness, a swollen feeling, a local temperature change, or a distinct "electrical" sensation. Acupuncture points in different areas of the body respond differently, and variations in response can be an important diagnostic indicator. It is not unusual for a clinician to retain a needle in an acupuncture point where the qi has not yet arrived, or been obtained, until the characteristic sensation occurs.

After qi has been obtained, the clinician may choose to manipulate the needle to achieve a desired therapeutic effect. Methods range from simply putting the needle in place and leaving it there to engaging in complex manipulations that involve slow or rapid insertion of the needle to greater or shallower depths. These techniques may create a distinctive sensation along the channel (or "meridian") pathway. The needle may be withdrawn promptly after qi arrives, or a short, fine needle (known as an "intradermal") may be retained in the site for several days. In all instances, the goal of the clinician is to influence the movement of qi.

One simple style of needle manipulation involves adjusting the direction of the needle to supplement or drain the qi at the particular channel point. If the acupuncture point is visualized as a hole where the channel qi can be touched and moved, this operation can either cause the qi to become secure and increase in the channel (supplementing) or cause the qi to spill out (draining).

For the patient who is experiencing the symptoms of "wind cold," an acupuncturist might choose to needle a number of acupuncture points including: Wind Pool (Feng Chi GB 20), located on the back of the neck below the occipital bone; Union Valley (He Gu LI 4), located in the fleshy area between the base of the thumb and forefinger; and Broken Sequence (Lie Que LU 7), on the forearm. These particular points could all be treated with a draining method because in this case the channels are replete with the influences of the external evils of wind and cold. Wind Pool, as its name indicates, is often used to drain wind from the surface of the body, relieving headache and neck pain. Union Valley is an important acupuncture point that is used to influence the upper part of the body and to control pain. In this case the point is used because of its ability to redirect wind, resolve the exterior, and to treat headache and sore throat. Broken Sequence is said to dispel cold and to diffuse the lung. It affects the channels and can be used to treat sore throat and headache.

Another way to choose acupuncture points is based on their associations with the five phases. Each of the phases corresponds to an organ (Box 15.1) (see also Chapter 14).

BOX 15.1 *The Five Phase Correspondences*

Wood to liver
Fire to heart
Earth to spleen
Metal to lungs
Water to kidney

Each phase is also related to a number of other categories, including taste, smell, climate, and time of day. If the patient displayed signs of vacuity of the water phase, a choice of points could be made from the transport points along the kidney channel associated with water, to supplement the water phase.

Points also may be chosen on the basis of the actual anatomic trajectory of the channel upon which they lie on the body. Union Valley is considered an important point for the head and face because the pathway of the large intestine channel on which it lies traverses that area of the body. Similarly, points on the lower extremity that lie on the urinary bladder channel, which traverses the entire back, frequently are used for back pain.

Finally, the practitioner often selects acupuncture points entirely on the basis of their sensitivity to palpation or on the basis of a variation in texture that the practitioner can perceive. Often a number of acupuncture points in a specific area may be assessed to determine which would be most suitable for needling. In some cases, points that do not lie on specific channels, or form part of the collection of recognized extra points, may be identified by their tenderness. These points are known as "ah shi," or "ouch, that's it," points, and are an important part of clinical acupuncture's traditional history and contemporary practice.

With so many acupuncture points from which to choose, and so many methods for choosing them, it is not surprising that many clinicians focus on a few specific methods or a particular collection of points so that they can develop more expertise in the application of those key treatments.

MOXIBUSTION (JIU FA)

Moxibustion refers to the burning of dried and powdered leaves of *Artemisia vulgaris* (ai ye), or wormwood, on or near the skin to affect the movement of qi in the channel. *A. vulgaris* is said to be acrid and bitter and, when used as moxa, to have the ability to warm and enter channels. References to moxa appear in very early materials, such as the texts recovered from excavated tombs at Ma Wang Dui, which date to 168 BC. Moxibustion can be applied to the body in many ways: directly, indirectly, by pole moxa, and by the warm needle method. Direct moxa involves burning a small amount of moxa, approximately the size of a grain of rice, directly on the skin. Depending on the desired effect, larger or smaller pieces of moxa may be used, and the moxa fluff can be allowed to burn all the way to the skin, causing a blister, or it can be removed before it has reached the skin.

These techniques are used to stimulate acupuncture points where the action of moxibustion is traditionally indicated or where warming the point seems to be the most appropriate response.

Indirect moxibustion involves the insertion of a substance between the moxa fluff and the patient's skin. This approach gives the practitioner greater control over the amount of heat applied to the patient's body and offers the patient increased protection from burning, allowing moxa treatments in such delicate areas as the face and abdomen. Popular substances that can be placed between moxa and the skin include ginger slices, garlic slices, and salt. The substance is often chosen because it has medicinal properties of its own that combine well with the properties of moxa. For instance, ginger might be selected in cases in which vacuity cold is present, whereas garlic is considered useful for treating hot and toxic conditions.

During pole moxa, a cigar-shaped roll of moxa wrapped in paper is used to warm the acupuncture points gently without touching the skin. This method is very safe and can be taught to patients for self-application.

The warm needle method is accomplished by first inserting an acupuncture needle into the point and then placing moxa fluff on its handle. After the moxa is ignited, it burns gradually, imparting a sensation of gentle warmth to the acupuncture point and channel. This method is useful especially for people with arthritic joint pain.

Together, acupuncture and moxibustion are used to address a wide range of conditions and symptoms. Based on the basic concept that all disease ultimately involves disruption of the flow of qi and that acupuncture and moxibustion regulate the movement of qi, there is no pain condition that could not theoretically benefit from these methods (Box 15.2).

BOX 15.2 *Common Pain Conditions Most Commonly Treated With Acupuncture*

Disorders of the Mouth
Acute and chronic pharyngitis (sore throat)
Gingivitis (inflammation of the gums)
Toothache, postextraction pain

Gastrointestinal Disorders
Acute and Chronic Gastritis
Chronic duodenal ulcer (used for pain relief)
Duodenal ulcer (without complications)
Gastric hyperacidity

Acute and Chronic Colitis
Acute bacillary dysentery
Constipation
Diarrhea

BOX 15.2 *Common Pain Conditions Most Commonly Treated*
With Acupuncture—cont'd

Spasms of Esophagus and Cardia (Junction of Esophagus and Stomach)
Gastroptosis (downward displacement of stomach)
Hiccups
Paralytic ileus (intestinal obstruction and painful colic)

Neurological and Musculoskeletal Disorders
Cervicobrachial syndrome (disease of neck and arm)
Facial palsy (early stage, i.e., within 3–6 months)
Frozen shoulder, tennis elbow
Headache and migraine
Intercostal neuralgia (pain between the ribs)
Low back pain (acute and chronic)
Meniere disease (auditory vertigo)
Neurogenic bladder dysfunction
Nocturnal enuresis (involuntary urination)
Osteoarthritis
Pareses (paralysis) following a stroke
Peripheral neuropathies (nerve disorders)
Poliomyelitis Complications
Sciatica
Trigeminal neuralgia (shooting pains in the face)

Common Medical Conditions With Pain
Upper Respiratory Tract
Acute rhinitis
Acute sinusitis
Acute tonsillitis
Common cold

Lower Respiratory System
Acute bronchitis
Bronchial asthma

Disorders of the Eye
Acute conjunctivitis
Cataract (without complications)
Central retinitis
Myopia (in children)

Note: The list is based on the scope of pain conditions and disorders that "lend themselves to acupuncture treatment," according to criteria developed in the late 1970s by a World Health Organization (WHO) Interregional Seminar. This list is not based on controlled clinical research, and the specific pathologic names are not meant to indicate acupuncture's efficacy in treating them. The list is not complete but is informative in terms of the routine application of acupuncture in China. The results of contemporary controlled trials on acupuncture treatment of pain are given elsewhere in the chapter.

AURICULAR ACUPUNCTURE

The stimulation of acupoints on the external ear is a style of traditional acupuncture that integrates both Asian and Western approaches to health care. The earliest clinical records of ear acupuncture points can be traced back to ancient Chinese texts written 2000 years ago, the style in which auricular acupuncture is currently practiced in modern China and throughout the rest of the world originated with the work of a French physician in 1957.

Unlike the traditional array of acupuncture points on the ear that had been used by ancient Chinese doctors, Dr. Paul Nogier of Lyons, France, proposed that the auricle can be perceived as an inverted fetus. Medical conditions associated with the head and face are treated by ear reflex points on the lower regions of the auricle. Dysfunctions of the neck and upper back are found on middle regions of the auricle. Pain or pathology in the lower back, leg, and foot are represented on the highest regions of the external ear. Nogier's original report of an inverted, somatotopic pattern on the external ear was first presented at a scientific meeting in France, then distributed internationally by a German publication, next translated into Japanese, and ultimately printed in China. By 1958 the Nanjing Army Ear Acupuncture Research Team had conducted a clinical survey of 2000 patients who had been successfully treated with auricular acupuncture alone.

Many Western scientists remain skeptical of the concept that the organization of auricular acupoints exhibits any somatotopic arrangement. However, human brain imaging studies demonstrate greater responses in the brain's somatic cortex area representing the hand when activated by acupoint stimulation of the hand area of the auricle of the ear.

Classical acupuncture theory attributes health and disease to the blockage of energy flow along acupuncture meridians as invisible lines of force extending over the surface of the body. Classically, only the yang acupuncture meridians directly connect to the acupuncture points on the external ear. As with body acupuncture, the purported ability of auricular acupoints to heal is attributed to the increased flow of qi energetic forces throughout the body. Although Nogier was knowledgeable of the Chinese energetic perspective of the human body, he instead emphasized ontogenetic and neurophysiologic connections between auricular reflex points and the central nervous system to explain the somatotopic relations between auricular regions and body pathology.

In his subsequent writings Nogier proposed three different territories on the external ear that are related to different types of neural innervation, and three different types of embryologic tissues. These three territories of the auricle can be viewed as three concentric circles or rings. The embryologically based endodermal organs are found at the central concha of the ear. The mesodermal tissue that becomes the somatic musculature is represented on the middle ridges of the auricle. The ectodermal skin and nervous system tissue are represented on the outer ridges of the ear. The central concha of the ear is actually innervated by the cranial nerve, the vagus, and serves as the region for autonomic regulation of visceral pain and pathology associated with internal organs.

The surrounding antihelix and antitragus ridges of the ear are innervated by the somatic trigeminal cranial nerve and are used to treat myofascial pain that contributes to headaches, backaches, and body aches in the limbs. The outer rim of the auricle represents central nervous system pathways that affect neuropathic pain, such as peripheral neuropathies and trigeminal neuralgia. The ear lobe, at the bottom of the auricle, corresponds to the brain, whereas the outer helix tail of the auricle represents the spinal cord and spinal nerves. A different, but complementary, perspective to the theory that auricular acupuncture is based upon neurophysiologic reflexes is suggested by the role of endorphin hormones (see later).

AURICULAR MASTER POINTS

Auricular acupuncture treatments are provided by (1) electrical stimulation of low electrical resistance acupoints on the ear, (2) insertion of half-inch needles into ear points based upon established treatment protocols, or (3) application of pressure by small "acubeads" taped to the ear. The first set of ear acupoints considered for stimulation are referred to as master points and supportive points. These auricular points do not correspond to one specific body organ but affect many different medical conditions. The first two master points, Point Zero and Shen Men, are used in most auriculotherapy treatment plans for the alleviation of several health disorders. Point Zero, first described by Nogier, is found in a notch on the Helix Root as it arises from the Concha Ridge. Point Zero functions as a homeostatic balancing point which leads to normalizing of dysfunctional conditions.

The Shen Men point is the most frequently used ear point found in Chinese treatment protocols, serving to alleviate stress, pain, tension, anxiety, depression, and substance abuse disorders. The English translation of this Chinese ear acupuncture point is "Spirit Gate," suggesting that activation of this auricular point connects an individual to one's spiritual essence, enhancing the vital forces of life and one's general well-being. The physical location of this auricular point is toward the tip of the triangular fossa. Detection of auricular points by an electrodermal point finder typically reveals that Point Zero and Shen Men are electrically reactive in most patients.

Two master points used in many neurological conditions and pain disorders are the Autonomic Sympathetic Point, referring to its use in regulating the autonomic nervous system, and the Thalamus or Subcortex Point, representing a brain region that serves as a higher brain center for the control of pain. The Autonomic Sympathetic Point is found on the underside of the internal helix, where it meets the antihelix inferior crus. The Thalamus Point is found on the base of the concha wall, behind the antitragus. The Endocrine Point is a nearby region of the intertragic notch, which represents the pituitary gland, the master control gland for all other endocrine glands. Stimulation of this auricular point affects circulating hormones, such as cortisol and endorphins, whose levels are frequently altered during many conditions associated with pain and stress. At the center of the ear lobe, vertically below Point Zero, is the Master Sensorial Point, which is used to alleviate any disturbing somatic sensations. Central to this point on the ear lobe is the Master Cerebral Point, also referred to as the neurasthenia or "worry point."

Its stimulation is used to control pathological obsessions, unwarranted worry, and generalized anxiety. Above the Master Cerebral point is an auricular point that represents the cingulate gyrus, an area of the paleocortex limbic system that affects emotional aspects and perceptions of pain and suffering.

MUSCULOSKELETAL AURICULAR POINTS

In his original text, *The Treatise of Auriculotherapy,* Nogier focused on auricular representation of the musculoskeletal body in that new practitioners of auriculotherapy could observe for themselves that specific regions of electrical conductivity and tenderness on the external ear correspond to specific areas of the body where the patient feels myofascial discomfort. The cervical vertebrae are represented on the concha side of the antihelix tail, the thoracic vertebrae are represented on the central side of the antihelix body, and the lumbosacral vertebrae are represented on the inferior crus of the antihelix. There are some differences between the somatotopic arrangement shown in many Chinese ear acupuncture charts. With regard to the musculoskeletal system, the European and Chinese charts are relatively similar. The posterior groove behind each level of the antihelix is also stimulated to effectively reduce pain from muscle spasms.

The occiput is appropriately represented on the antitragus region adjacent to the lowest portion of the antihelix tail that corresponds to the upper cervical spine. Toward the middle of the antitragus, the auricular microsystem point for the temples is found. Toward the base of the antitragus, near the intertragic notch, is the Forehead point. The most reactive of these antitragus auricular points is used to treat both tension headaches and migraines. The temporomandibular joint (TMJ) point used for the relief of tight and tense muscles of the lower and upper jaw is located at the junction of the upper regions of the ear lobe and the lower sections of the scaphoid fossa. In Chinese auricular charts, the hip, knee, ankle, and foot are represented in an upside-down perspective on the superior crus of the antihelix. The somatotopic presentation of these same leg points in the European system is also found in an inverted orientation, but they are located in the triangular fossa. As with vertebral points, stimulation of the posterior side of the triangular fossa and superior crus also serves to enhance the relief of myofascial pain in the legs or feet.

There is no discrepancy between European and Chinese ear charts that indicate auricular representation of the upper extremities. Treatment of shoulder problems is achieved by stimulation of a point in the scaphoid fossa peripheral to Point Zero. The shoulder point is logically located next to the junction of auricular representation of the cervical and thoracic spine. The somatotopic system on the ear is an inverted orientation, and the Elbow point is found in the region of the scaphoid fossa above the shoulder point. Ascending higher in the scaphoid fossa, one arrives at the wrist point, and above are several points for the fingers. Both the front and back sides of the ear can be stimulated to relieve tennis elbow, carpal tunnel syndrome, and arthritic pain in the fingers. In addition to auricular points for the arms and legs, there are areas on the external ear used to treat sensory dysfunctions related to the eyes, nose, and inner ears.

Visceral Disorders

Visceral organs derived from endodermal embryological tissue are found in the central valley of the auricle, the concha. The only location on the body where the autonomic vagus nerve reaches the superficial skin is in the region of the concha floor. Near the opening to the actual auditory canal is the opening to the digestive system, the mouth. Extending peripherally from the auditory canal is the esophagus point, which leads to the stomach point found on the concha ridge. Stimulation of the auricular stomach point in animals reduces neuronal firing rates in the feeding center of the hypothalamus, whereas neuronal discharges in the satiety center of the hypothalamus are elevated by auricular stimulation. On the superior concha, auricular representation of the small and large intestines is found. Stimulation of these points relieves physiological dysfunctions in each organ, such as nausea, diarrhea, or constipation, or may alter the energetic function of the corresponding acupuncture meridian named for that organ. Studies have shown that stimulation of ear reflex points for the stomach alter physiological patterns in the nervous connections from the gastrointestinal tract to the hypothalamus in the brain.

The five element theory suggests that five yin organs affect problems of energetic constitution other than the known physiologic functions of that organ. The kidney is energetically related to neurological and hearing disorders, as well as physiological urinary dysfunctions.

Liver can energetically affect tendon and ligament sprains, as well as hepatitis.

Spleen can energetically alleviate muscle spasms, as well as affect lymphatic disorders.

Lung is energetically used to treat skin disorders and drug detoxification, as well as respiratory problems.

Heart is energetically used for mental calming, as well as cardiovascular irregularities.

The auricular point for the heart is found at the very center of the inferior concha, in the deepest region of the concha floor. Nogier demonstrated an additional heart point on the antihelix area where the chest is represented. Coronary heart disease would be treated in both locations.

Nervous system tissue is derived from ectodermal tissues represented on lower regions of the external ear. The ear lobe and antitragus above it represent not only the face and head but also the brain inside the head. Represented at the intertragic notch is the anterior cingulate gyrus, an area of the limbic system found to be very active in human pain patients and suppressed by body acupuncture stimulation. Stimulation of the cingulate gyrus ear point is effective in relieving chronic pain in human patients. Other important auricular points for pain relief are the Thalamus Point and the Brain Point, both found on the concha wall behind the antitragus.

Such simple procedures effectively alleviate pain in many different parts of the body, and practitioners repeatedly observe that specific areas of the auricle are more sensitive to pressure and more electrically active in a predictable pattern that conforms to the inverted fetus perspective that Nogier first proposed. Activation of these auricular points with needle insertion, transcutaneous electrical stimulation, or application of pressure pellets has been shown to alleviate physical symptoms in the corresponding parts of the body. Growing use of auricular acupuncture is being made in China, Europe, and the United States in concert with repeated clinical experience of the effectiveness of this technique. Neurologic reflexes connect distant regions of the body to somatotopic microsystems on the ear. These observations suggest a new kind of neuronal organization that appears to have been discovered and can be applied in practice outside the current boundaries of current Western biomedical science.

RESEARCH ON ACUPUNCTURE FOR PAIN

An important correlate of Chinese medicine coming to the West and spreading globally is that it is being subjected to extensive and intensive Western biomedical scientific testing, which has generated convincing scientific evidence of safety and effectiveness for pain.

A critical component of the modern enterprise of medicine in Europe and North America theoretically involves performing research and obtaining regulatory approval on every treatment in practice. This expectation has the effect of constraining "freedom of choice" and places control of medical practice ultimately in the hands of medical research elites and those who have money (e.g., pharmaceutical industry) and/or control (e.g., government bureaucracies using taxpayers' money) over the tens of billions of dollars required each year to perform acceptable research studies. Although Western biomedicine has been quick to require the highest standards of research evidence when it comes to alternative therapies, such as Chinese medicine and acupuncture, for example, the former US Congressional Office of Technology Assessment (since conveniently abolished) estimated as of the 1990s that 80% of mainstream medicine as practiced in the United States was in fact not based upon acceptable standards of research evidence.

Substantial research efforts have taken place in Asia since the early 20th century and during the latter part of that century in North America and Europe as well. Research approaches and standards vary widely and like medicine itself are subject to cultural influences. Although the West recognizes the randomized, placebo-controlled, and double-blinded clinical trial as the definitive standard for an unambiguous biomedical answer, other societies do not require or encourage their medical communities to secure knowledge in this fashion. In addition, much of the research data that have been gathered remains inaccessible in the West due to language differences and difficulty of obtaining publications despite the public investment in institutions like the National Library of Medicine. As one result, the scientific communities of China, Japan, Europe, North America, and Australia do not all have access to the same set of information and are not influenced by the same body of research.

Problems surrounding research design and methods have come into focus as the Chinese medicine communities of North America and Europe have conducted more research, and as the biomedical community has become better educated about Chinese medicine. For example, in 1991 the US Congress required the National Institutes of Health (NIH) to create an Office of Alternative Medicine (OAM), which co-hosted several conferences dealing with the issue of research study design in the complementary and alternative medicine (CAM) fields, including Chinese medicine. The OAM also funded numerous small research grants, many of which have been in the area of Chinese or Oriental medicine.

In 1994 the OAM sponsored a workshop in cooperation with the US Food and Drug Administration (FDA). Members of the acupuncture, allopathic medical, and Western scientific communities gave presentations detailing the safety and effectiveness of acupuncture needles. These presentations became the core of a petition that led in 1996 to the FDA reclassifying acupuncture needles from a class III, or experimental device, to a class II, or medical device, for use by qualified practitioners with special controls (sterility and single use).

THE FDA: NOT SO FAST...

During the early 1990s one of the important aspects of acupuncture under consideration by the FDA was the safety and effectiveness of acupuncture for asthma. The potent drug bronchodilator inhalers developed for asthma were having severe problems with safety of the drugs and the propellants used, leading to many deaths in young people with asthma. Ironically these drugs were originally based on the traditional Chinese herb, ma huang, or ephedra, researched by Carl Schmidt at the University of Pennsylvania in the 1930s. Ephedra was later to run into its own safety problems with the FDA with its inappropriate use for weight loss, and athletic performance, associated with several deaths in young athletes in the early 2000s. This led to a temporary ban and the placing of related "over-the-counter" products currently back behind the pharmacist counter.

Regarding asthma, the FDA was appropriately concerned with finding other treatments that were effective but also safe. As founding editor of the first medical journal on complementary and alternative medicine in 1995, an author of this book (Micozzi) was impressed by the effectiveness of acupuncture for asthma and other respiratory diseases (challenging the notion that acupuncture was useful only for pain) and had compiled hundreds of references on the use of acupuncture in asthma. Meanwhile, the reclassification of the acupuncture needle had come up at the FDA for reclassification from an experimental device (approved for use only in accepted research protocols) to a therapeutic device (approved for use in regular clinical practice).

Several dedicated officials at the FDA, including a number of Vietnamese-Americans, obtained permission to work on this approval action on their own time, during evenings and weekends, to speed the approval process. Hundreds of references from the author's (Micozzi) office were sent over on a computer disk so that FDA doctors would not need to have their government clerical staff (who are not known for their accuracy, speed, precision, or command of the English language) to re-enter these technical references. The result was a victory for science, health, and the long pain and suffering of millions of Americans.

The NIH (1997) convened a Consensus Development Conference on acupuncture. For 2 days, experts in the field presented evidence on the safety and effectiveness of acupuncture in treating specific pain and other conditions. The scientific panel that reviewed the presentations noted in the NIH Consensus Statement of 1997 that, although acupuncture was widely practiced and studied in the United States, much of the research was inconclusive due to problems in design, sample size, and other factors. One particular difficulty involved finding appropriate controls, such as placebos and sham acupuncture groups, because inserting a needle into the skin is not the same as taking a drug or placebo orally. The report's authors concluded,

"promising results have emerged, for example, showing efficacy of acupuncture in adult postoperative and chemotherapy nausea and vomiting and in postoperative dental pain. There are other situations such as addiction, stroke rehabilitation, headache, menstrual cramps, tennis elbow, fibromyalgia, myofascial pain, osteoarthritis, low back pain, carpal tunnel syndrome, and asthma, in which acupuncture may be useful as an adjunct treatment or an acceptable alternative or be included in a comprehensive management program. Further research is likely to uncover additional areas where acupuncture interventions will be useful."

Considering that less than 2 years earlier acupuncture needles had been considered experimental devices in the United States, this finding marked a significant degree of progress.

In late 1998 the OAM was renamed as the National Center for Complementary and Alternative Medicine and provided by Congress with an increase in funding. Since its inception this organization has continued to refine and develop its approach to fostering research into complementary therapies and in the process has involved various established institutions in research projects. Two such institutions, the Center for Addiction and Alternative Medicine Research at the University of Minnesota Medical School & Hennepin County Medical Center, and the Center for Alternative Medicine Pain Research and Evaluation at the University of Maryland School of Medicine, have built their centers around long-term and sustained research efforts in specific areas, which has allowed them to make substantial strides as funding became available.

Other national and international organizations, such as the Society for Acupuncture Research (SAR), have emerged out of the broad-based community of acupuncturists, physicians, and researchers interested in the range of research issues posed by this field. SAR holds annual meetings and publishes its proceedings. Among its objectives are scholarly exchange between researchers in the area of acupuncture, as well as other therapies related to Asian medicine, the encouragement of research activities by acupuncturists, and the clarification of research issues, such as study design. In 1996 two SAR officers, Richard Hammerschlag (author Micozzi's former mentor during a college research fellowship at City of Hope National Medical Center in Duarte, CA) and Stephen Birch, compiled a summary of the most successful and well-designed controlled clinical trials.

Researchers have been successful in obtaining measurable results when exploring such fundamental concepts as qi, channels, acupuncture points, pulse diagnosis, and pattern diagnosis. However, these studies are difficult to design in ways that remain true to the traditional Chinese system, while obtaining data recognized by the world's scientific community.

For example, Chinese researchers have been pursuing questions about the physiologic basis of Chinese medical concepts. One such study examined the nature of kidney yang and reached the conclusion that patients displaying a diagnostic pattern associated with kidney yang vacuity showed low levels of certain steroids (17-hydroxy cortical steroids) in their urine, suggesting a relationship between the concept of kidney yang and the adrenal cortical system.

The study of pulse patterns has been pursued for some time in North America and Europe, as well as China, Japan, and Korea. This research typically includes applying pressure sensors over the radial artery, mimicking the way a clinical practitioner holds his or her fingers during a pulse reading. Pulse patterns are then recorded and correlated to determine the physical foundation of the diagnostic information the practitioner obtains from the pulse. Initial results are intriguing, but too many questions remain about the size and design of the study to make hard data available.

Research concerning channels and acupuncture has relied on a variety of techniques, including the measurement of electrical resistance, thermography, tracing the pathways of injected radioisotopes, and anatomical dissection (although dissection has proved disappointing in this area). Some interesting work is being done to determine how the body's bioelectrical properties transmit information. This approach relates to earlier studies demonstrating that the skin, at many acupuncture points, has a measurably lowered electrical resistance.

Yoshio Manaka, the Japanese surgeon and acupuncturist who accomplished pioneering work in this field during and after World War II, hypothesized the presence of a signaling system he calls the X-signal system. This concept was drawn from biological theories, such classic texts as *The Yellow Emperor's Inner Classic*, and observations in his acupuncture clinic. His perspective grew out of exploration of both Chinese and Japanese needling methods, including the gentler needling techniques associated with the school of meridian therapy that had arisen in Japan.

These discussions remain preliminary because, even in those areas that have generated solid, reproducible results (such as lowered electrical resistance over acupuncture points), they raise as many questions as they answer. Scientific research may simply not prove to be the best vehicle for understanding the fundamental principles of Traditional Chinese Medicine. It may be that the genius of Chinese medicine in these areas lies in its empirical ability to generalize about the manifestations of incredibly complex biologic phenomena in an articulate, internally consistent, and clinically useful fashion.

Despite the early and widespread interest in acupuncture, comparatively few studies have been designed in a fashion that renders their results useful to other researchers, clinicians, or policymakers. Rather than focusing on useful observations, many of these investigations (some conducted by the first tenured professor in Complementary/Alternative Medicine in the United Kingdom) have the character of "debunking" experiments, perhaps more suitable to the former magicians, such as the self-styled "Amazing Randi," whose agenda appears to be a blind attempt to disprove rather than attempt to understand this ancient, safe, and effective therapy that has already been recognized by the FDA, NIH, and leading academic medical centers.

Many of the most solid studies from North American and Europe were presented at the OAM's Workshop on Acupuncture and Consensus Panel of Acupuncture. The clinical work presented was primarily done in five areas: antiemesis (antivomiting) treatment, the management of acute and chronic pain, substance abuse treatment, treatment of paralysis due to stroke, and the treatment of respiratory disease. Good clinical results were also shown in treatment of female infertility, breech presentation, menopause, depression, and urinary dysfunction.

RESEARCH EVIDENCE ON PAIN CONTROL

Pain control is the most universal application of acupuncture, but it is also one of the most problematical to research. Some of these problems are illustrated by the results of two meta-analyses of studies examining acupuncture in the management of chronic pain. (A meta-analysis is a research method that pools the results of many different studies in an effort to reach conclusions more powerful than those generated by a smaller, individual study.) The first meta-analysis combined data from 14 studies that used randomized and controlled trials of acupuncture as a treatment for chronic pain, measuring outcomes in terms of the number of patients whose condition was improved. This study reached a number of conclusions about the relations of study design to research outcomes and determined that acupuncture compares favorably with placebo and conventional treatment.

A second meta-analysis reviewed more than 50 studies and compared the quality of published, controlled, clinical trials on the basis of research design and such specific factors as randomization, single and double blinding, and numbers of subjects. Investigators found studies showing the effectiveness of acupuncture but then determined that the studies favorable to acupuncture were less well designed than those that associated negative results with acupuncture. Their conclusion was that evidence suggested that the effectiveness of acupuncture as a treatment for chronic pain remained doubtful.

A third meta-analysis reviewed this second meta-analysis and found that the authors of the second analysis had included studies that did not meet appropriate standards and criteria, such as a study that was not controlled and one in which laser light was used instead of needles. The authors of this third meta-analysis observed a trend toward improvement of studies over time, suggesting that many poorly designed studies should be viewed as preliminary efforts by nonexpert investigators who were not sufficiently familiar with acupuncture to be able to design an appropriate study in the first place. This observation points out another problem with research on CAM: many Western scientists who have access to powerful methods and research funding do not have sufficient knowledge of the historic use of CAM remedies to be able to design useful studies (Micozzi & Cassidy, 2015). In contrast, in Germany, long known for the high quality of research, the first criterion considered by regulators and scientists is the historic use of CAM treatments.

Acupuncture and Chronic Pain Conditions

The control of pain is considered to be a major area for the clinical application of acupuncture. As we have seen, one of the conclusions of the Consensus Development Conference on Acupuncture was that acupuncture could be demonstrated to be efficacious for reduction of postoperative dental pain. One study showed that patients receiving acupuncture required less postoperative analgesia after oral surgery than a group receiving a sham acupuncture treatment (Lao, Bergman, Langenberg, Wong, & Berman, 1995).

Low Back Pain

Although patients frequently seek out acupuncture for low back pain, and acupuncturists regard *low back pain* as an area in which they provide effective treatment, the research evidence produced over the years has remained equivocal. A systematic review of randomized controlled trials determined that "acupuncture for acute back pain has not been well studied" and that the value of acupuncture in treating chronic back pain "remains in question" (Cherkin, Sherman, Deyo, & Shekelle, 2003). Birch's review of reviews found that only two out of the seven reviews examined indicated that acupuncture had been shown to be effective for low back pain. The remaining reviews found promising or contradictory results (Birch, Hesselink, Jonkman, Hekker, & Bos, 2004).

A 2005 meta-analysis concluded that acupuncture provided short-term relief of chronic low back pain (Manheimer, White, Berman, Forys, & Ernst, 2005). In addition, it was concluded that true acupuncture worked better than sham acupuncture. The authors also stated that they could not reach a conclusion about the effectiveness of acupuncture compared with other active treatments.

Against this background, published results of the findings of the German acupuncture trials were particularly striking (Haake et al., 2007). These trials were conducted from 2001 through 2005 and involved 340 outpatient practices. In all, 1162 patients were treated for low back pain and received ten 30-minute sessions of acupuncture each week. The study offered acupuncture delivered according to Traditional Chinese Medicine principles (administered by physicians trained in acupuncture) and two control treatments. One of the control treatments was sham acupuncture, which was provided by needling areas that were identified as "nonacupuncture points" (Molsberger, et al 2006), and the other was conventional therapy consisting of drugs, physical therapy, or exercise.

At the end of the study, when patients were assessed 6 months after concluding treatment, the response rate for acupuncture was 48%, whereas the response rate for conventional therapy was 27%. These statistically significant results demonstrated unequivocally that acupuncture could be more effective than conventional therapy in the treatment of low back pain. The greatest surprise lay in the patient response to sham acupuncture, which was 44%, almost as high as the response to true acupuncture treatment. These results, although substantiating acupuncture's claim to therapeutic effectiveness, have raised significant questions about the importance of specific point locations in effective acupuncture treatment of low back pain.

Because the points chosen for sham acupuncture were typically 5 cm away from any described acupuncture points and were needled shallowly (only 3 mm), the results of this study strongly suggest that there may be little importance to needling at traditionally described needling sites or that at least the degree of specificity implied by traditional locations is not relevant to this acupuncture effect.

Arthritis

Over the years, a number of studies have suggested that the *joint pain of osteoarthritis* seems to respond well to acupuncture (Dickens & Lewith, 1989; Junnila, 1982; Thomas, Eriksson, & Lundeberg, 1991), and one study suggested a significant cost benefit when the use of acupuncture eliminated the need for surgical intervention (Christensen et al., 1992). The implications of these studies led to the increased investigation of the potential role of acupuncture in the management of osteoarthritis and the production of promising clinical data (Berman et al., 1999). This work culminated in 2004 with publication of the results of a large-scale trial of acupuncture involving 570 subjects who received acupuncture, sham acupuncture, or patient education. The study's authors concluded that acupuncture provided improvement in function and pain relief when used as an adjunctive therapy for osteoarthritis (Berman et al., 2004).

Headache

Headache pain is often treated with acupuncture. In 1989 a controlled trial of the use of acupuncture in the management of migraines was conducted that enrolled 30 patients who had chronic migraine headaches. Acupuncture was significantly effective in controlling the pain of migraine headaches (Vincent, 1989). A more recent pragmatic trial of acupuncture for chronic headache and migraine demonstrated clinical benefits for patients and low costs (Vickers et al., 2004).

Mechanism of Actions of Acupuncture in Pain

What might be termed the "modern" history of acupuncture research in the West has a scope of just under 40 years (and perhaps 60 years in East Asia). Earlier efforts were distinct, isolated, and comparatively limited and certainly not part of the system of internationalized research communication that constitutes what scientists term "modern."

Ongoing lines of scientific inquiry into acupuncture have focused primarily on three specific types of questions: (1) Are there physiological processes that can at least partially explain acupuncture effects, such as pain control? (2) Is acupuncture safe? (3) Can acupuncture be shown to treat specific clinical conditions effectively?

One of the advantages of acupuncture is that its primary therapeutic tools and methods are not abstract in any sense. The acupuncture needle is a tangible object that is introduced into or adjacent to tissue. That simple physical reality has formed the basis for many intriguing ideas and investigations into the basic physiology of acupuncture. Acupuncture has become among the most credible of complementary therapies in terms of acceptance by the medical community. This greater acceptance may be the result of the existence of a substantial body of data showing that acupuncture in the laboratory has measurable and replicable physiological effects that can begin to offer plausible mechanisms for the presumed actions. This point was echoed by Filshie and White (1998): "Acupuncture owes much of its respectability to the discovery that it releases opiate peptides." That acupuncture can point to a body of basic research provides a number of scientifically derived hypotheses for many of its clinically observed effects and has been helpful in supporting its acceptance in a variety of medical settings.

The contrast between ancient and traditional models of acupuncture and contemporary biomechanistic models is quite distinct. The classical constructs of acupuncture theory model a system that has been described through the observation of the body in health and disease and the body's response to stimulus. Although these models are explanatory, they were not developed in the context of the linearity and reductionism of the currently popular positivist, reductionist scientific enterprise. Instead they were developed on the basis of empirical observation and an effort to describe observed relations systematically. They capture a diverse range of information in very broad and general terms.

Biomechanical Models

Contemporary biomechanistic models are constructed on the basis of currently established understandings of anatomy and physiology. The most prevalent models apply concepts derived from studying the neurophysiology of pain and accordingly seek to explain acupuncture in terms of what is already "known" about the body. Newer models have actually used traditional descriptions of physical responses to acupuncture stimulation to develop experiments that have led to new understandings of the way the body, particularly connective tissue, responds to acupuncture. From an acupuncturist's perspective, 30 years of basic science research into acupuncture using a biomechanistic model has furnished valid and valuable insight into many acupuncture phenomena but cannot yet adequately explain the full range of observed acupuncture phenomena. There is no reason that it should be expected to do so. Science consists of a rigorous process of investigation and explanation that relies on careful descriptions of observable processes. The methodology of science derives its power from the strict limitations placed upon its methods. Scientific knowledge is continually developing, and so we should expect two things from proposed scientific models of acupuncture: (1) that they will be limited or incomplete because the current state of our knowledge about the body is incomplete and (2) that they will continue to develop as our understanding develops.

Bioelectrical Models

Acupuncture theories are based on observations of the results of processes that are then organized in very general terms and in terms that make sense of observable results but not the underlying processes. It should not come as a surprise when acupuncture theories are not entirely captured by current scientific models or, to put it another way, when scientific models fail to capture all aspects of acupuncture theory and observations in practice.

When investigating some of the basic science underlying our understanding of acupuncture, we observe that acupuncture exploits a wide range of bodily responses to stimulation in a systematic fashion. No single physiological process fully explains all of acupuncture's effects, and at this time, acupuncture theory may offer a more coherent model for organizing and using (although not describing the causes of) acupuncture effects.

For instance, there are now two very suggestive theories concerning the significance of channels from a scientific point of view. One theory suggests that there is a detectable difference in the electrical impedance of channels compared with that of surrounding tissue. Another suggests that described channels may correspond to the distribution and spatial organization of fascia (connective tissue) and that the network formed by interstitial connective tissue throughout the body may form the basis of the communicating channels and networks described by acupuncture (Langevin & Yandow, 2002). Both theories are highly suggestive, but neither has been completely demonstrated to be correct, nor would they fully explain all of acupuncture's observed effects.

Acupuncturists have been thinking about acupuncture for more than 2000 years, whereas scientists have been thinking about it for perhaps 100 years. This circumstance is not to imply that all acupuncture theory is "true" in scientific terms but that a rush to reduce its meaning to a few very basic physiological processes may ultimately limit, and even prohibit, understanding of both acupuncture and a more complete or holistic view of human physiology.

ROLE OF CHANNELS AND POINTS

The contrast between scientific understanding and the traditional forms of knowledge associated with acupuncture becomes vividly clear when analyzing two well-known acupuncture concepts: points and the external pathways of the regular channels. Depending on the approach guiding the research—and perhaps the disposition of the researcher or the interpreter of the data—it can be concluded that either there is no such thing as an acupuncture point or channel at all or that channel theory represents a reasonably accurate description of a collection of interacting structures and processes.

From a reductionistic point of view, the impulse is to clearly establish an absolute physical structure that correlates precisely to all aspects of the acupuncture model. This impulse led to the tragedy and travesty of the Korean researcher Bong Han, who became a virtual cultural hero in Korea during the 1960s because of his reported discovery of Bong Han corpuscles, distinct tissue structures that were found only at acupuncture points and along channels. These were later shown to be artifacts of microscopic slide preparation, and Bong Han committed suicide. Of course, the entire modern practice of surgical pathology, for example, is based on the systematic artifacts introduced when devitalized tissues removed from the living body are manipulated by chemical and mechanical processes and rendered in a two-dimensional plane of microscopic slide preparations of a vanishingly small subsample of tissue cells.

Although there is research suggesting that the areas defined as acupuncture points and external channels may have features associated with them that are distinctive (and that distinguish them from other areas of the body's surface), there is nothing to suggest that there are any specific physical structures corresponding precisely and uniquely to points and channels. Instead there is research indicating that (1) the regions described by acupuncture points are particularly rich in nerve bundles and small blood vessels, (2) the tissues specified by channels and points may have different electrical characteristics than surrounding tissues, and (3) the organization of fascia shows distinctive characteristics underlying many acupuncture points and along channel pathways (Langevin, Churchill, & Cipolla, 2001; Langevin, Churchill, Wu, et al., 2002).

ELECTRICAL POTENTIAL

The idea that there are differentials in the electrical resistance of acupuncture points and channels is a comparatively old one, dating to research efforts as far back as 1950 (MacPherson et al., 2008). The works of Becker (1985) and Tiller (1997) have been very influential in suggesting that the activity of acupuncture channels and points may be closely related to their electrical properties. It is hypothesized by clinicians applying these ideas that variations in the electrical activity of acupuncture points and channels in disease states may aid in diagnosis of those disease states or that variations among acupuncture points, channels, and surrounding skin surface can be detected by measuring differences in electrical resistance. Although these concepts have given rise to the production, sale, and use of a vast array of electrodiagnostic devices and "point detectors," the present state of the science does not support their clinical use.

All these devices work by measuring galvanic current, the standing current produced by the normal skin surface. The measurement of galvanic current is achieved with what is essentially an ohmmeter. The subject holds an electrode in one hand and a probe is applied to a desired area of the skin surface. Direct current is typically supplied through the probe and measured by the meter. However, even slight variations in the pressure with which the probe is applied can cause significant fluctuations in current flow (resistance), which essentially causes a point to be detected wherever the probe is pressed firmly against the skin. For this reason, although the few well-designed studies of these phenomena are very suggestive, conclusive statements about the electrodermal properties of acupuncture channels and points remain elusive.

The idea that fascia might have a distinctive role in acupuncture phenomena has become very well established as a consequence of the work of Helene Langevin and her research team at the University of Vermont Medical School. Langevin began with a question concerning the physical basis of de qi, the sensation of the needle's being "grabbed" on insertion that is associated in many acupuncture traditions with the arrival of qi. She asked if there could be an actual anatomical-physiological event associated with the sensation reported by practitioners over centuries of acupuncture practice. Her initial hypotheses were that the "needle grasp," or the gripping associated with de qi phenomenon, was caused by the winding of connective tissue around the needle during rotation. The manipulation of the needle, now coupled with connective tissue, "transmits a mechanical signal to connective tissue cells via mechano-transduction" (Langevin, Churchill, & Cipolla, 2001).

She was able to demonstrate that the increased pull-out force associated with rotated needles was 18% greater at acupuncture points than at control points (Langevin, Churchill, Fox, et al., 2001). She simultaneously proposed a mechanism through which the physical stimulation of connective tissue at the needling site might produce a variety of "downstream" changes in interstitial connective tissue that might be implicated in acupuncture effects. A later paper demonstrated a close relation between channel pathways and connective tissue and between acupuncture points and areas where intermuscular and intramuscular connective tissue was particularly dense (Langevin & Yandow, 2002).

Her work demonstrates the potential existence of a non-neural signaling system, the course and structure of which parallels ancient observations concerning channels and networks. At present the data are only suggestive. Langevin's work substantially supports the ideas of other authors who have proposed that acupuncture effects not attributable to neural events may be related to connective tissue signaling systems (Oschman, 1993).

TRIGGER POINTS AND PAIN

Intriguingly, the concept of trigger points (MTrPs) is often presented as a science-based and medically established version of the idea of acupuncture points. MTrPs have a long history of conceptual development based on the palpation of tender regions in the musculature of patients with pain. Travell and Simons (1983) substantially organized the concept and coined the term, which is applied to points that are located on palpation and are exquisitely tender on palpation (and are typically found in areas where the patient is experiencing pain). Unlike the locations of channel and extra points, which are substantially fixed, the described locations of MTrPs are areas where MTrPs may be found if they are present. The presence of an MTrP is evidenced by acute tenderness on palpation and, in the case of an active MTrP, by local pain as well.

As is the case with acupuncture points, there is no clear evidence of any distinctive anatomic features specific to MTrPs. However, because they were conceptualized within the biomedical model and because there are bioscience-based hypotheses concerning their production and action, MTrPs are considered to be a scientifically developed idea. The publication in 1977 by Melzack (of the Melzack-Wall gate theory of pain) of a paper claiming a 71% correlation between acupuncture points and these "trigger points" seemed to suggest that acupuncture points formed part of a well-described domain in the neurobiology of pain (Melzack, Stillwell, & Fox, 1977). Since publication of this paper, MTrPs originally described in relation to the diagnosis and treatment of myofascial pain are frequently invoked to explain or dismiss effects or models described in traditional acupuncture theory (Baldrey, 1993, 1998; Bowsher, 1998).

Ironically, as Steve Birch has been careful to point out, some 6 years after the publication of Melzack's article, Travell and Simons's textbook on MTrPs contained an analysis of the Melzack et al. study. Their conclusion: "Acupuncture points and trigger points are derived from vastly different concepts. The fact that a number of pain points overlap does not change that basic difference. The two terms should not be used interchangeably" (Travell et al., 1983, cited in Birch, 2008).

Although it is clear from our earlier discussion that a region that is tender on palpation, or an ah shi point, is an important category of point in acupuncture therapy, it is not clear that all or even a majority of acupuncture points used in the treatment of pain are equivalent to MTrPs. This issue has been well demonstrated. A careful analysis of Melzack's assertions (Birch, 2003; Birch & Felt, 1999) suggests that the actual correlation between MTrPs and the acupuncture points examined by Melzack that are actually used for the treatment of pain is approximately 18%.

However, as suggested by Birch, the desire to establish that acupuncture points fall fully within the domain described by MTrPs seems to be deeply compelling to segments of the medical community. The unsuccessful attempt by Dorsher (2008) to rebut Birch's analysis of Melzack et al. by insisting that the majority of acupuncture points are directly equivalent to MTrPs is an example of this determination.

It is important to remember that acupuncture points may be channel points, extra points, or ah shi points. It is clear that the ah shi point and the MTrP are almost exactly equivalent in concept if not in location. They both are evanescently present when they elicit pain on palpation and are not present when they do not. Channel points or extra points may be painful on palpation and may even act as ah shi points, but their clinical application is not limited to pain, nor are they present only when painful. From this point of view, acupuncture and trigger point therapy exploit similar physical observations with regard to exceptionally tender myofascial points. The close agreement of the trigger point theory and the theory of ah shi points suggests that an equivalent physiologic phenomena has been independently observed by two very different traditions of clinical practice. However, the conceptualization of acupuncture points as purely MTrPs limits the complete understanding of acupuncture channels, channel points, and extra points.

Although it is very clear that acupuncture channels and points as traditionally described do not define new or distinct structures unknown to science, it is quite likely that they describe relations among existing tissue and processes that may cooperate and interact in ways that are not presently completely understood.

Splinter Effect Theory

Acupuncture, like any therapy, must interact with existing anatomy and physiology to produce its effects. There are a number of well-described and scientifically demonstrated models of the way in which acupuncture might achieve its effects. It is very clear that acupuncture effects are not the consequence of any single physiologic process but rather of a complex dynamic of local tissue, vascular, and CNS-mediated neuroendocrine events.

Birch's description of the "splinter effect" (Birch & Felt, 1999) illustrates the complex range of vascular events that occur when the body encounters a common injury. This model suggests that many of the physiologic responses to acupuncture are quite common to the body's response to injury with any sharp object, hence the splinter effect. The splinter effect captures the potential complexity surrounding such an obviously "simple" event as insertion of an acupuncture needle. Birch presents his concept of the splinter effect to illustrate a range of local and regional vascular effects that can occur with acupuncture (Box 15.3). The splinter effect involves a series of vascular responses to acupuncture that are equivalent to the changes provoked by any tissue damage with a sharp object. Local vascular effects are only one set of the many changes provoked by acupuncture (see Box 15.3).

Local and Central Nervous System Responses

Based on his interpretation of the research data, Ma has created a useful description of seven specific events or "chain reactions" that acupuncture activates in both local tissue and the central nervous system (CNS) (Ma, Ma, & Cho, 2005). Although most of these are local, central responses are also described because Ma inherently considers local and central responses to be "physiologically inseparable" (Box 15.4). Ma's outline captures the elements of Birch's splinter effect and points out some additional interesting features of the physiological events provoked by acupuncture. His observations capture complex local effects, such as "current of injury," which refers to the creation of a current flow produced by any lesion in tissue. In this case

---

BOX 15.3 *The "Splinter" Effect*
Splinter or Needle Pierces Skin

Vasoconstriction commences to halt blood loss and prevent circulation of any microorganisms carried on the object (duration 20 min).

Slightly later vasodilation increases local circulation to allow white blood cells and other cells to enter the area to assist in infection control and tissue repair (duration 2 to 3 h).

Vasomotion begins after 1 h. This is the pumping of microscopic vessels to allow flushing away of damaged cells and blood (duration 1 h).

Birch's splinter effect (Birch & Felt, 1999) describes a series of vascular changes that support defensive, tissue repair, and metabolic processes that are typical of the body's response to a wound and illustrate the immediate vascular changes associated with acupuncture.

BOX 15.4 *Seven Local and Central Reactions to Needling an Acupuncture Point*

---

1. Skin and tissue reactions at needle site, including induction of "current of injury"
2. Interaction between needle shaft and connective tissue
3. Relaxation of contracted muscle, increased circulation to site
4. Nociception and motor neuronal activation, neuroendocrine activation via central nervous system, segmental, and nonsegmental pathways
5. Blood coagulation, lymphatic circulation
6. Local immune response
7. Tissue repair (DNA synthesis) at site of injury (needling)

---

the acupuncture needle produces a very focused lesion with a small current (10 mA) that supports tissue growth and healing (Ma et al., 2005).

Ma's inclusion of nociception and motor-neuronal activation and neuroendocrine activation via CNS, segmental, and nonegmental pathways captures the central idea: acupuncture needling that provides a detectable level of stimulus (some styles do not) invokes a complex of neurophysiologic responses that diminish pain. In particular, acupuncture is considered to invoke descending pain regulation by stimulating the production of the body's own chemical messengers for pain control (see Box 15.4).

ENDOGENOUS OPIATES OR ENDORPHINS

The Nobel Prize–winning discovery in 1975 by the late Solomon Snyder and Candace Pert of opiate neuropeptides, which have come to be known as endorphins, shed a great deal of light on certain aspects of the process of pain control. This discovery occurred coincident with recently emergent medical interest in acupuncture and acupuncture effects in pain control. By 1977 published studies strongly suggested that acupuncture effects in pain control or acupuncture analgesia might be linked to the activity of endorphins (Mayer, Price, & Rafii, 1977; Pomeranz & Chiu 1976). These studies showed that the effects of acupuncture analgesia, induced both by manual stimulation of acupuncture needles and by electrical stimulation, could be blocked by the administration of the opiate antagonist naloxone. This finding suggested that acupuncture's ability to control pain relied, at least in part, on its ability to trigger the release of endogenous opiates. Responding later to criticism that the reversal of acupuncture analgesia by the administration of naloxone was insufficient to validate the hypothesis that acupuncture analgesia was produced by endorphins, Pomeranz (1988) provided a list of 17 distinct lines of experimental evidence that support the acupuncture analgesia–endorphin hypothesis. Six examples of these lines of experimentation are provided in Box 15.5.

Based on these data, it is conventionally accepted that many of acupuncture's perceived effects in the direct reduction of pain are likely mediated by the production of endogenous opiates. This conclusion may be overly general in light of the

BOX 15.5 *Examples of Experimental Evidence Supporting the Endorphin Hypothesis for Acupuncture Analgesia*

- Different opiate antagonists block acupuncture analgesia.
- Rats with endorphin deficiency show poor acupuncture analgesia.
- Mice with genetic deficiency in opiate receptors show poor acupuncture analgesia.
- When endorphins are protected from enzymatic degradation, acupuncture analgesia is enhanced.
- Transference or cross-circulation of cerebrospinal fluid from an animal with induced acupuncture analgesia to a second animal will produce acupuncture analgesia, and this effect is blocked by naloxone.
- Lesions of the periaqueductal gray, an important endorphin site, eliminate acupuncture analgesia.

Adapted from Pomeranz and Stux (1998).

specific nature of the evidence that supports it. However, the assertion that endorphin secretion lies at the root of acupuncture effects is still a popular one.

STIMULATION OF BRAIN CENTERS

Functional magnetic resonance imaging (fMRI) has been applied to the investigation of acupuncture since the late 1990s. Within the limitations of the technology, which includes limited access to the body and the need for the subject to remain immobile during data collection, fMRI studies of acupuncture have produced intriguing results. One of the earliest studies presented the dramatic conclusion that there might be a direct correlation between the stimulation of an acupuncture point and cortical activation (Cho et al., 2006). What appeared initially to be evidence of the specificity of the action of acupuncture points, as demonstrated by regional neural activation, was later seen to be a comparatively typical response to needling. Over the years, the preponderance of evidence has suggested that acupuncture effects revealed by fMRI need to be understood in terms of the role of the CNS in processing the signals produced by the acupuncture stimulus.

Other research has suggested that traditional Chinese needling techniques that elicit de qi can create neural deactivation of the limbic system in a way that can benefit patients with chronic pain (Hui et al., 2000, 2005).

This line of inquiry has produced research showing that patients with *carpal tunnel syndrome*, for example, respond to acupuncture very differently than do healthy subjects. Patients experiencing the pain of carpal tunnel syndrome have been shown to respond to acupuncture stimulation with neural deactivation of the limbic system, which can be hyperactivated in chronic pain conditions (Napadow et al., 2007). Concurrent activation of the lateral hypothalamic area, a region critical to the release of endogenous opiates (a pain control system), also occurs. This information has been interpreted to suggest that patients with pain respond differently to acupuncture than do healthy individuals.

Evaluating Acupuncture Research

These studies highlight some key problems in acupuncture research. For example, should the investigator be trained in acupuncture? Is acupuncture treatment appropriate for the condition being studied? Does the study allow for adjusting treatment to the individual patient's needs according to traditional diagnostics? Are outcome measures clear? Will placebo or sham acupuncture be used, and, if so, how will it be administered? Unlike herbal medicine studies, in which a placebo capsule can be administered, subjects in acupuncture studies always know when they have been stuck with a needle, so the concept of "blinding" the participants to the treatment is not valid. Various solutions have been proposed, including comparing acupuncture to other treatments or selecting acupuncture points that are, by traditional standards, irrelevant to the condition being treated. But, so far, no well-accepted study design has emerged from the discussion.

Despite these difficulties, effective studies can be cited. In one, acupuncture patients demonstrated a lower need for postoperative anesthesia for pain following oral surgery compared with a group receiving sham acupuncture treatment, harkening back to the dramatic experiences of James Reston during President Nixon's diplomatic mission to China in 1971. Another study tracked 43 women with menstrual pain; those receiving acupuncture experienced considerably less pain than the placebo and control groups. When 30 migraine headache sufferers participated in a controlled trial, acupuncture was significantly effective in controlling the pain. A number of other studies demonstrated the effectiveness of acupuncture for back pain and for osteoarthritis. One study suggested the use of acupuncture may produce a considerable cost benefit by eliminating the need for surgery.

Research in the area of postoperative nausea and vomiting revolves around the use of the acupuncture point Inner Gate, which has also been shown to control the nausea of pregnancy and chemotherapy. Other fruitful areas of study include management of substance addiction; pulmonary disease, such as asthma; and pain and paralysis following stroke.

Looking back, as of 1995, there had been approximately 200 randomized controlled trials, 42 review articles, and 4 meta-analyses performed just in the United States alone. The amount of research conducted in China and Japan is vast, and translations are becoming more numerous; one English compilation contains 117 Chinese studies on acupuncture and moxibustion. Improvements in study design are occurring in both the East and West, bringing these two bodies of knowledge closer together.

Like acupuncture research, the field of Traditional Chinese Medicine in general is plagued with difficulties in designing effective studies. The cultivation of qi, such as qigong, is highly personal and does not lend itself to standardized studies (see Chapter 16). The challenge is developing an effective control and ruling out other variables that may influence the results. However, a number of intriguing investigations have been conducted in China and more recently in the United States.

Promising areas of study include the use of qigong for managing gastritis and hypertension and for increasing immune competence. On the other hand, attempts to study the effects of externally transmitted qi have encountered problems with measurement. Some researchers believe qi involves measurable portions of the electromagnetic spectrum, whereas others hypothesize that qi exists but cannot be measured by currently available technology, only by its effects on the human body. Qi cultivation remains a challenging part of the broad fabric of China's traditional medicine.

OUTLOOK FOR SAFE AND EFFECTIVE TREATMENTS

Forty years ago, few non-Asians had ever heard of acupuncture or Chinese medicine. Currently, it is well known throughout the West and has become a staple of our cultural vocabulary. Initially opposed by the medical establishment, it has gained legal and professional acceptance, which has led to government funding for research at respected academic institutions worldwide. Much about Traditional Chinese Medicine and acupuncture remains a mystery. However, it is clear that this ancient form of health care is moving into the world's medical mainstream. It offers tremendous potential health benefits to those many millions suffering with chronic pain and conditions for which modern Western biomedicine has had little to offer, as well as far-reaching possibilities for affordable, effective, and sustainable health care that represent true "health care reform."

This most ancient but influential form of medicine has extended beyond the time and space of China and Asia to represent a worldwide resource for health and healing in the 21st century using medical practices and technologies that are accessible to everyone, everywhere.

REFERENCES

Baldrey, P. E. (1993). *Acupuncture, trigger points and musculo-skeletal pain.* London: Churchill Livingston.

Baldrey, P. E. (1998). Trigger point acupuncture. *Filshie and White's medical acupuncture.* London: Churchill Livingston.

Becker, R. O. (1985). The body electric. *Electromagnetism and the foundation of life.* New York: Quill/William Morrow.

Berman, B. M., Lao, L., Langenberg, P., Lee, W. L., Gilpin, A. M., & Hochberg, M. C. (2004). Effectiveness of acupuncture as adjunctive therapy in osteoarthritis of the knee. *Annals of Internal Medicine, 141*(12), 901–910.

Berman, B. M., Singh, B. B., Lao, L., Langenberg, P., Li, H., Hadhazy, V., et al. (1999). Randomized trial of acupuncture as an adjunctive therapy in osteoarthritis of the knee. *Rheumatology (Oxford), 38*(4), 346–354.

Birch, S. (2003). Trigger point-acupuncture point correlations revisited. *Journal of Alternative and Complementary Medicine, 9*(1), 91–103.

Birch, S., Hesselink, J. K., Jonkman, F., Hekker, T. A., & Bos, A. (2004). Clinical research on acupuncture. Part 1. What have reviews of the efficacy and safety of acupuncture told us so far? *Journal of Alternative and Complementary Medicine, 10*(3), 468–480.

Birch, S. (2008). Trigger points should not be confused with acupoints. *Journal of Alternative and Complementary Medicine, 14,* 1184–1185.

Birch, S. & Felt, R. (1999). *Understanding acupuncture*. London: Churchill Livingston.

Bowsher, D. (1998). Mechanisms of acupuncture. *Filshie & White's medical acupuncture*. London: Churchill Livingston.

Cherkin, D. C., Sherman, K. J., Deyo, R. A., & Shekelle, P. G. (2003). A review of the evidence for the effectiveness, safety, and cost of acupuncture, massage therapy, and spinal manipulation for back pain. *Annals of Internal Medicine, 138*(11), 898–906.

Cho, Z. H., Hwang, S. C., Wong, E. K., et al. (2006). Neural substrates, experimental evidences and functional hypotheses of acupuncture mechanisms. *Acta Neurol Scand, 113*(6), 370.

Christensen, B. V., Iuhl, I. U., Vilbe, K. H., Bülow, H. H., Dreijer, N. C., & Rasmussen, H. F. (1992). Acupuncture treatment of severe knee osteoarthritis. *Acta Anaesthesiologica Scandinavica, 36*, 519–525.

Dickens, W. & Lewith, G. (1989). A single-blind, controlled and randomised clinical trial to evaluate the effect of acupuncture in the treatment of trapeziometacarpal osteoarthritis. *Complementary Medical Research, 3*, 5.

Dorsher, P. T. (2008). Can Classical acupuncture points and trigger points be compared in the treatment of pain disorders? Birch's analysis revisited. *Journal of Alternative and Complementary Medicine, 14*(4), 353–359.

Filshie, J. & White, A. (1998). *Medical acupuncture: A Western scientific approach*. London: Churchill Livingston.

Haake, M., Muller, H., Schade-Brittinger, C., Basler, H. D., Schäfer, H., Maier, C., et al. (2007). German Acupuncture Trials (GERAC) for chronic low back pain: Randomized, multicenter, blinded, parallel-group trial with 3 groups. *Archives of Internal Medicine, 167*, 1892–1898.

Hui, K. K., Liu, J., Makris, N., Gollub, R. L., Chen, A. J., Moore, C. I., et al. (2000). Acupuncture modulates the limbic system and subcortical gray structures of the human brain: Evidence from fMRI studies in normal subjects. *Human Brain Mapping, 9*(1), 13.

Hui, K. K., Liu, J., Marina, O., Napadow, V., Haselgrove, C., Kwong, K. K., et al. (2005). The integrated response of the human cerebro-cerebellar and limbic systems to acupuncture stimulation at ST 36 as evidenced by fMRI. *NeuroImage, 27*(3), 479.

Junnila, S. Y. T. (1982). Acupuncture superior to piroxicam in the treatment of osteoarthritis. *American Journal of Acupuncture, 10*, 341.

Langevin, H. M., Churchill, D. L., & Cipolla, M. J. (2001). Mechanical signaling through connective tissue: A mechanism for the therapeutic effect of acupuncture. *FASEB Journal, 15*(12), 2275.

Langevin, H. M., Churchill, D. L., Fox, J. R., Badger, G. J., Garra, B. S., & Krag, M. H. (2001). Biomechanical response to acupuncture needling in humans. *Journal of Applied Physiology, 91*, 2471.

Langevin, H. M., Churchill, D. L., Wu, J., Badger, G. J., Yandow, J. A., Fox, J. R., et al. (2002). Evidence of connective tissue involvement in acupuncture. *FASEB Journal, 16*(8), 872. http://www.fasebj.org/cgi/reprint/16/8/872.

Langevin, H. M. & Yandow, J. A. (2002). Relationship of acupuncture points and meridians to connective tissue planes. *The Anatomical Record, 269*(6), 257.

Lao, L., Bergman, S., Langenberg, P., Wong, R. H., & Berman, B. (1995). Efficacy of Chinese acupuncture on postoperative oral surgery pain. *Oral Surgery, Oral Medicine, Oral Pathology, Oral Radiology, and Endodontics, 79*, 423.

Ma, Y., Ma, M., & Cho, Z. (2005). *Biomedical acupuncture for pain management: An integrative approach*. London: Churchill Livingston.

MacPherson, H., Thomas, K., Armstrong, B., De Valois, B., Relton, C., Mulilnger, B., et al. (2008). Developing research strategies in complementary and alternative medicine. *Complementary Therapies in Medicine, 16*, 359–362.

Manheimer, E., White, A., Berman, B., Forys, K., & Ernst, E. (2005). Meta-analysis: Acupuncture for low back pain. *Annals of Internal Medicine, 142*, 651–663.

Mayer, D. J., Price, D. D., & Rafii, A. (1977). Antagonism of acupuncture analgesia in man by the narcotic antagonist naloxone. *Brain Research, 121*(2), 368.

Melzack, R., Stillwell, D. M., & Fox, E. J. (1977). Trigger points and acupuncture points for pain: Correlations and implications. *Pain, 3*, 3.

Micozzi, M. S. & Cassidy, C. M. (2015). Issues and challenges in integrative medicine. In M. S. Micozzi (Ed.), *Fundamentals of complementary and alternative medicine*. Philadelphia: Elsevier Health Sciences/Saunders.

Molsberger, A. F., Boewing, G., Diener, H. C., Endres, H. G., Kraehmer, N., Kronfeld, K., et al. (2006). Designing an acupuncture study: The nationwide, randomized, controlled, German acupuncture trials on migraine and tension-type headache. *Journal of Alternative and Complementary Medicine, 12*, 237–245. 2006.

Napadow, V., Kettner, N., Liu, J., Li, M., Kwong, K. K., Vangel, M., et al. (2007). Hypothalamus and amygdala response to acupuncture stimuli in carpal tunnel syndrome. *Pain, 130*(3), 254.

National Institutes of Health. (1997). Acupuncture. *NIH Consensus Statement, 15*(5), 1.

Oschman, J. (1993). *A biophysical basis for acupuncture* (p. 141). Boston: Society for Acupuncture Research.

Pomeranz, B. (1988). Scientific basis of acupuncture. In G. Stux (Ed.), *The basics of acupuncture* (p. 4). New York: Springer-Verlag.

Pomeranz, B. & Stux, G. (1998). *Basics of acupuncture*. Berlin, Heidelberg: Springer-Verlag.

Pomeranz, B. & Chiu, D. (1976). Naloxone blockade of acupuncture analgesia: Endorphin implicated. *Life Sciences, 19*, 1757–1762.

Thomas, M., Eriksson, S. V., & Lundeberg, T. (1991). A comparative study of diazepam and acupuncture in patients with osteoarthritis pain: A placebo controlled study. *American Journal of Chinese Medicine, 19*, 95.

Tiller, W. A. (1997). Science and human transformation. *Subtle energies, intentionality and consciousness*. California: Pavior.

Travell, J. G. & Simons, D. G. (1983). Myofascial pain and dysfunction. *Trigger point manual*. Philadelphia: William & Wilkins. 1983.

Vickers, A., Rees, R., Zollman, K., McCarney, R., Smith, C. M., Ellis, N., et al. (2004). Acupuncture for chronic headache in primary care: Large, pragmatic, randomized trial. *British Medical Journal, 328*, 744.

Vincent, C. A. (1989). A controlled trial of the treatment of migraine by acupuncture. *The Clinical Journal of Pain, 5*, 305.

Suggested Readings can be found on the companion website, http://www.micozzipainconditions.com.

Chapter 16

East Asian Manual and Movement Therapies Part One: Acupressure, Jin Shin Do, Qigong, Reflexology, T'ai Chi, and Tui Na

There are a number of manual and movement techniques within classic Chinese and East Asian medical practice, or derived from them, that make use of the knowledge of vital energy and acupuncture points and meridians—but without using acupuncture needles to influence them. These may be particularly appealing to those aforementioned who are "needle phobic" or in situations in which sterile needles are not available.

TUI NA: MANUAL POINT STIMULATION (CHINESE MASSAGE)

Tui na, literally "pushing and pulling," refers to a system of massage, manual acupuncture point stimulation, and manipulation that is vast enough to warrant a modality of its own. These methods have been practiced at least as long as acupuncture and moxibustion, if not longer, but the first formal massage training class was not held until 1956 in Shanghai. Nowadays this field of study can serve as a minor component of a traditional medical education or as an area of extensive clinical specialization. A distinctive aspect of tui na is the extensive training necessary for clinical practice. The practitioner's hands are taught to accomplish focused and forceful movements that can be applied to various areas of the body. Techniques such as pushing, rolling, kneading, rubbing, and grasping are repeated until they become second nature. Students practice on a small bag of rice until their hands develop the necessary strength and dexterity.

Tui na is often applied to highly localized areas of the body, and the techniques can be quite forceful and intense. Conditions routinely treated with tui na include orthopedic and neurological pain conditions, asthma, dysmenorrhea

Acknowledgment to Amy L. Ai for prior contributions in Micozzi, M.S. (ed.), (2011). *Fundamentals of complementary & alternative medicine* (4th ed.). St Louis: Elsevier Health Sciences/Saunders.

(menstrual pain), and chronic gastritis. Tui na is used as an adjunct to acupuncture treatment to increase the range of motion of a joint or instead of acupuncture, when needles are uncomfortable or inappropriate, such as when the patient is very young or old or is "needle phobic." As with all aspects of Chinese medicine, there are many regional styles and distinctive family lineages of practice. The formal curriculum available in Chinese programs is extensive but still does not cover all the possibilities.

ACUPRESSURE AND JIN SHIN DO

Acupressure is the application of the fingers to acupuncture points on the body, also "acupuncture without needles." It is based on the meridian or channel system, which informs other Chinese medical practices. According to this system there are 12 major channels through which vital energy, or qi, flows. Although most of the channels are named for specific organs, they do not necessarily correspond to the anatomical body part but rather are more functional in nature. Interruptions in the flow of qi cause functional aberrations associated with that particular channel. These interruptions can be released by specific application of needles or fingers.

Jin shin do, or the "way of the compassionate spirit," was developed by psychotherapist Iona Teeguarden. It is a form of acupressure in which the fingers are used to apply deep pressure to hypersensitive acupuncture points. Jin shin do represents a retrospective synthesis of Daoist philosophy, psychology, breathing, and acupressure techniques. In accordance with this philosophy the body is linked to the mind and spirit, and tender points found in the body can represent expressions of emotional trauma or locked memories (somatoemotional component).

The theory of jin shin do states that various stimuli cause energy to accumulate at acupuncture points. Repeated stress in turn causes a layering of tension at the point, known as "armoring". The most painful point is termed the local point as a frame of reference. Other related tender points are referred to as distal points. Deep pressure applied to the point ultimately causes a release, and the tension dissipates. The overall effect is to re-establish flow in the channel and balance body energy. The context of the jin shin do treatment is as much psychological as physical and reiterates the importance of the body-mind-spirit philosophy of this treatment form.

During the treatment session the practitioner identifies a local point and "asks permission," nonverbally, to treat it. A finger is placed on the local point while another finger is applied to a distal point. Gradually increasing pressure is applied to the local point. After 1 or 2 minutes the practitioner feels the muscle relaxing, followed by a pulsation (practitioners of craniosacral therapy refer to this phenomenon as the "therapeutic pulse"). When the pulsing stops, the patient usually reports a decreased sensitivity at the point, indicating a successful treatment. Myofascial (muscle-connective tissue) releases are sometimes accompanied by emotional releases as painful memories are brought to the surface of consciousness.

REFLEXOLOGY

In the Chinese meridian system of the body, the major meridians or channels are represented in the hands and feet. Acupuncture is usually not performed on the soles of the feet because of their sensitivity (the feet, hands, and face are very dense in sensory nerves). Thus a system of foot massage was developed in China.

Later, William Fitzgerald (1872 to 1942), who called it "zone therapy," introduced this Chinese system to the West in 1913. Now referred to as reflexology the technique involves the application of deep pressure to various points on the hands and feet by the thumbs and fingers of the practitioner. The feet receive the preponderance of attention in this method, with various identified points corresponding to the energy channels of the body and also to specific organs and systems. When treatment is given, areas of tenderness or skin texture changes are identified and pressure is applied. This maneuver has the effect of opening that channel and allowing body energy to flow unimpeded through the entirety of the channel and to effected organs. When all points are successfully treated, the energy system is flowing and balanced. Stimulation of these reflex areas helps the body to correct, strengthen, and reinforce itself by returning to a state of homeostasis. In Asian countries, some reflexologists also use electrical or mechanical devices. However, these approaches are discouraged in Europe and North America.

Fitzgerald found that application of pressure to various locations on the body also deadened sensation in definite areas and relieved pain. These findings led to the development of zone therapy. In the early years Fitzgerald worked mainly on the hands. Later the feet became very popular as a site for treatment. In his book on zone therapy, in 1917 Fitzgerald spoke about working on the palmar surface of the hand for any pains in the back of the body and working on the dorsal aspect of the hands and fingers for any problems on the anterior (front) part of the body. Joe Shelby Riley was taught zone therapy by Fitzgerald. He developed the techniques on to finer points and created detailed diagrams and drawings of the reflex points located on the feet and hands in 1924. As noted earlier, reflexology is based on the premise that there are zones and reflexes in different parts of the body that correspond to all parts, glands, and organs. Manipulating specific reflexes removes stress, activating a parasympathetic nerve response to enable the blockages to be released by a physiological change in the body. With stress removed and circulation enhanced, the body is allowed to return to a state of homeostasis.

Conventional zone theory (CZT) is the foundation of hand and foot reflexology. Zones represent a system for organizing relations among various parts, glands, and organs of the body and the nervous reflexes. There are 10 equal longitudinal or vertical zones running the length of the body from the tips of the toes and the tips of the fingers to the top of the head. From the dividing center line of the body, there are five zones on the right side of the body and five zones on the left side. These zones are numbered 1 to 5 from the medial side (inside) to the lateral side (outside). Each finger and toe falls into one of the five zones (e.g., the left thumb is in the same zone as the left big toe, zone 1). The reflexes are considered to pass all the way through the body within the same zones. For example, the same reflex can be found on the front and also on the back of the body and on the top and on the bottom of the hand or foot. Reflexology zones, as developed in this system, are not the same as acupuncture or acupressure meridians.

Pressure applied to any part of a zone affects the entire zone. Every part, gland, or organ of the body represented in a particular zone can be stimulated by working any reflex in that same zone. In addition to the longitudinal zones of CZT, reflexology also uses the transverse zones (horizontal zones) on the body and feet or hands. The purpose is to help to fix the image of the body by mapping it onto the hands or feet in proper perspective and location. Four transverse zone lines are commonly used: transverse pelvic line, transverse waistline, transverse diaphragm line, and transverse neck line. These transverse zone lines create five areas: pelvic area, lower abdominal area, upper abdominal area, thoracic area, and head area. Internal organs layer on top, over, behind, between, and against each other in every possible configuration. The reflexes on the hands and feet corresponding to the parts, organs, and glands also overlap.

A basic premise of CZT is that the right foot or hand represents the right side of the body, and the left foot or hand, the left side. However, in the nervous system, the right half of the brain controls the left side of the body and vice versa. In any disorder that affects the brain or the central nervous system, a reflexologist will emphasize the reflexes or areas of the disorder on the opposite hand or foot. For example, the brain reflexes are worked on the left foot or hand for strokes that caused paralysis on the right side of the body. Although it is commonly assumed that the hands and feet are the only areas to which reflexology can be applied, there are reflexes throughout the 10 zones of the body that may present seemingly unlikely relations within these zones. For example, there is a zonal relationship between the eyes and the kidneys because both lie in the same zone. Working the kidney reflexes can affect the eyes. If there is an injury on the foot, the area should be avoided and should not be worked, and alternate parts of the body in the same zones may be worked instead. For example, the arm is a reflection of the leg, the hand of the foot, the wrist of the ankle, and so forth. If any part of the arm is injured, the corresponding part of the leg can be worked and vice versa. Common problems, such as varicose veins and phlebitis in the legs, can be helped by working the same general areas on the arms.

This approach can be used to find other referral areas by identifying the zone(s) in which an injury has occurred and tracing it to the referral area. Tenderness in the referral area will usually help to locate it. Referral areas can give insights into problem areas by showing the relations to the areas in the same zone(s) that may be at the root of the problem. For example, a shoulder problem may be caused by a hip problem because the shoulder lies in the same zone as the hip. These relations may also be understood biomechanically, as well as energetically. A reflexology session usually begins on the right foot or hand and finishes on the left foot or hand. In addition, the reflexes on both feet and hands are worked from the base of the foot or hand up to the top, with the toes or fingers worked last.

FEEDBACK CONTROL

For self-regulation of the body, a highly complex and integrated communication control system or network operates as a "feedback control loop." Different networks in the body control diverse functions, such as blood carbon dioxide levels, temperature, and heart and respiratory rates. Homeostatic control mechanisms are categorized as negative or positive feedback loops. Many of the important and numerous homeostatic control mechanisms are negative feedback loops.

Negative feedback loops are stabilizing mechanisms. For example, they maintain homeostasis of blood carbon dioxide concentration. As blood carbon dioxide increases, the respiration rate increases to permit carbon dioxide to exit the body in increased amounts through expired air. Without this homeostatic mechanism, body carbon dioxide levels would rapidly rise to toxic levels, and death would result.

The blood circulation loop is from the left side of the body to the right side—fresh oxygenated blood enters the aorta from the left ventricle of the heart and travels to the body, and venous blood with carbon dioxide enters the vena cava on the right side of the heart. By beginning a reflexology session on the right foot or hand, the reflexologist is helping to boost the loop by pushing venous or deoxygenated blood into the heart and lungs so that fresh oxygenated blood will be available to the body cells. The same rationale applies to the direction that the reflexologist works on the foot or hand—from the bottom of the foot upward, to bolster the homeostatic loop.

Reflexology demonstrates four main benefits: (1) it promotes relaxation with the removal of stress; (2) it enhances circulation; (3) it assists the body to normalize the metabolism naturally; and (4) it complements other healing modalities. When the reflexes are stimulated, the body's natural energy works along the nervous system to clear any blockages in the corresponding zones. A reflexology session seems to break up deposits (felt as a sandy or gritty area under the skin), which may interfere with the flow of the body's electrical energy in the nervous system.

In clinical studies reflexology has been found to be effective in reducing pain in women with severe premenstrual symptoms and in patients with migraine and tension headaches. It has also demonstrated benefit in alleviating motor, sensory, and urinary symptoms in patients with multiple sclerosis. Recent reviews on the efficacy of reflexology in cancer patients found positive improvements in anxiety and pain. The adverse effects of reflexology are minor and may include fatigue (increase in parasympathetic activity), headache, nausea, increased perspiration, and diarrhea.

For practitioners, certification is provided by certain educational institutions. There are many schools of reflexology that can provide adequate training, ranging from 100 to 1000 hours of instruction. The interested individual should look for a school that is established and, if possible, recognized by a local governing body. In the United States and Canada there are regulations for practicing reflexology, and individual states and provinces (though not all) have their own sets of educational or licensing requirements.

Reflexology impacts the autonomic nervous system directly, balancing the parasympathetic nervous system and the sympathetic nervous system, the two subdivisions of the autonomic nervous system that exert opposite effects on the end organs, to maintain or restore homeostasis (see Fig. 4.1).

The well-known homeostasis of Western scientific medicine and physiology is reflected in the ancient concept of balance as the goal of Chinese medical therapies.

QIGONG AND T'AI CHI (QI CULTIVATION)

Vital energy, or qi, may also be influenced by other means without specific reference to acupuncture points, channels, or meridians, as in the practice of qigong (QG).

QG, or qi cultivation, encompasses a broad range of practices and activities including the meditative systems of Daoist and Buddhist practitioners, the health-giving exercises developed by ancient physicians, and the martial arts traditions of China. The common feature of these practices is the intention of enhancing qi—by allowing the individual to increase its quantity, smooth its flow, and place it under a greater degree of conscious control—thereby strengthening the body, energy, mind, and spirit.

While Daoist and Buddhist QG focus on spiritual realization, medical qi cultivation addresses three areas. The first is self-cultivation or the development of the practitioner's own health and stamina. The second involves the cultivation of the practitioner's ability for safely transmitting qi to the patient, either by means of needles or directly through the hands. The third is teaching patients to perform specific QG practices that may address particular health issues or generally strengthen their qi.

How Qigong Works

"Flowing water will never turn stale, the hinge of the door will never be eaten by worms," explains Lu's Spring and Autumn Annals. "They never rest in their activity: that's why."

Qi cultivation is a very ancient part of Traditional Chinese Medicine (TCM). The texts recovered at Ma Huang Dui include illustrated guides to therapeutic properties and physical practices of a form of QG known as "conduction" (dao yin). In the 2nd century Hua Tou created a series of exercises based on the movements of the tiger, deer, bear, monkey, and bird, which were practiced to ward off disease. Zhang Zhong Jing in his Golden Cabinet Prescriptions recommended treating disease with dao yin and tui na (exhalation and inhalation breathing exercises fundamental to QG). QG has many forms of practice, which can be performed standing, sitting, or lying down but always involves relaxation of the body, regulation of the breath, and calming of the mind. One form of QG involves visualizing internal and external pathways of the channels and imagining qi moving along them in concert with the breath (like guided imagery; see Chapter 7). As the practice develops, the practitioner begins to experience the sensation of qi traveling along the channel pathways. The mind guides qi to a specific area of the body, then the qi guides blood to that same area, improving circulation. This exercise is designed to train qi and blood to move freely along the channel pathways, leading to good health.

Another exercise, often recommended for people with bronchitis, emphysema, or bronchial asthma, involves the use of breath, visualization, and simple physical exercises to benefit the qi of the lungs. Assuming a relaxed posture, the practitioner begins by breathing naturally and allowing the mind to become calm. The upper and lower teeth are then clicked together gently 36 times. As saliva is produced, it is retained in the mouth, swirled with the tongue, then swallowed in three parts while imagining that it is flowing into the middle of the chest and then to an area about three finger widths below the navel (the dan tian or cinnabar field, as related to the chakras of Ayurvedic medicine; see Chapter 18). At this point the practitioner imagines that he or she is sitting in front of a reservoir of white qi, which enters the mouth on the inhale and is transmitted through the body on the exhale, first to the lungs, then to the dan tian, and finally out to the skin and body hair. This process of visualization is repeated 18 times.

These exercises have been used for many centuries to enhance breathing, circulation, and other vital bodily functions, as well as to address the individual's mental and spiritual state.

UNDERSTANDING QIGONG

To understand the rationale for QG requires knowledge of its primary guiding philosophy, Daoism (Taoism). In its Chinese character, *dao* refers to the way, or the universal order, to be followed in life and in nature. In a cosmic sense, dao refers to the ultimate, indefinable principle underlying all movements—the process involving every aspect in the universe. QG is the phonetic juxtaposition of two Chinese characters: *qi,* meaning "flow of air" in a more literal sense or "vital energy" in a more symbolic sense, and *gong,* meaning "perseverant practice." Chinese teachers referred to "working with the life energy, learning how to control the flow and distribution of qi to improve the health and harmony of mind and body." Shen considered QG as an ancient therapeutic martial art. Qian, an advocate of the scientific study of QG in China and the leading Western-trained biophysicist there, defined QG as an ancient system for self-development that involves movement, breathing exercises, and conscious control of body energy, integrating these perspectives.

Notably, the idea of flowing vital energy is shared by non-Western healing, as well as shamanic traditions. Some indigenous people in Africa call it "num," whereas Native American and Southeast Asian groups speak of the "Holy Wind." Indians term it "prana," and modern Russians name it "bioplasma" in contemporary technical terms. The uniqueness of the Chinese concept of qi lies in (1) its focus on holistic health in terms of multilevel energy patterns rather than solely on the physical body or on an external divinity or spirit, (2) its pathway of qi circulation (i.e., the acupuncture channel system consisting of several hundred points), and (3) its rationale, which resembles accepted tenets of quantum theory in modern physics. In this view, relations and activities of energy patterns are seen as fundamental in both human nature and the universe. The term qi refers not only to the essence of all material objects but also to their interactions in terms of the rhythmic alternation of two fundamental forces, yin and yang, similar to positive and negative charges in modern chemistry.

FORMS OF QIGONG

The role of qi in health and healing was first described 2000 years ago in *The Yellow Emperor's Inner Classic* (Hung De Nei Jing Su Wen). The Inner Classic system viewed the human in both cosmological and geographical terms. It explicitly went beyond earlier supernatural and magical healing and instead described illness and therapies in terms of pernicious influences and emotional disturbances. The Inner Classic recommended the earliest documented form of QG, Dao Yi, as a healing exercise to cure chills and fevers and to achieve a state of tranquility, contentment, and sage-like spirit, yet full of vital energy.

In many early forms of QG, slow-moving dance reproducing animal postures was used to promote animal-like vitality, balance, grace, and strength. The founder of Daoist philosophy, Lao Zi (Lao Tzu), first described basic QG principles that had been followed by practitioners for centuries, such as concentration, emptiness of desire, quiescence, flexibility, and infant-like breath. In the 4th century BC, Zhuang Zi, Lao Zi's follower, wrote about the role of infant-like breathing and physical exercise in promoting longevity and described a sage intent on extending his life. In the AD 2nd century, Hua Tuo was known for both his famous anesthetic herb formula, Ma Fu San, and his QG practice, Five Animal Plays, based on the movements of the tiger, deer, bear, monkey, and bird. Throughout Chinese history, many forms of QG have been developed among Daoists, Buddhists, TCM practitioners, and martial artists.

QG first reached Europe in the late 18th and early 19th centuries. In 1779 the Jesuit missionary Cibot translated Daoist QG exercise and respiratory techniques in terms of the martial art, cong-fou (kung fu, kong-fu, gongfu) into French with illustrations. His translated text later became influential for Per Henrik Ling (1776 to 1839), who founded medical gymnastics on the basis of a vital energy theory to promote health. Ling's theory and practice laid a foundation for contemporary massage and physical education (see Chapter 13). However, the idea of vital energy was dropped in the late 19th century in the West in the clash with modern materialistic science.

In contrast, in China the culturally rooted legacy of qi has never been abandoned despite the rapid changes in political regimes in China during the 20th century. The initial use of QG in the formal Chinese medical profession began in the 1950s, when some QG rehabilitation institutes established by the Chinese government demonstrated the therapeutic effects of internal QG in treating hypertension and "neurasthenia." The late 1970s witnessed a true renaissance in the practice of medical QG or QG therapy for the purpose of medical care and rehabilitation. An influential advocate was Guo Lin, an elderly master who had persistently practiced Daoist QG after she developed advanced uterine cancer in her 30s. She and her students used QG to heal diseases with diagnoses in Western medicine, especially cancer. Since then, numerous styles of QG therapy have been invented, all of which share the essential principles of ancient Daoism and its expression in TCM.

QIGONG PRACTICE

In practice, QG consists of two foundational forms: (1) dynamic or active QG, which involves visible movement of the body, typically through a set of slowly enacted exercises, and (2) meditative or passive QG, which entails still positions with inner movement of the diaphragm. (To some extent, this distinction mirrors Yoga as a meditative practice with both more contemplative forms and more physical forms, such as Hatha-Yoga, popular in the West, see Chapter 19). Essential to both are precise control of abdominal breathing, alert concentration, and a tranquil state of mind. The most well-known dynamic QG in the Western world is t'ai chi (tai ji). Dynamic QG also includes varied forms of martial QG (kung fu), which focus on the development of physical capacity. However, in contrast to Western exercise, dynamic QG centers on flexibility and inner strength rather than masculinity and body size. Based on different philosophical foundations, affiliated intentionality, and spiritual goals, QG can also be classified intellectually and spiritually into Daoist, Buddhist, and Confucianist forms (Dao Jia Gong, Fa Jia Gong, and Ru Jia Gong).

From a clinical perspective, classification of QG therapy into two systems is proving useful. Internal QG aims to control internal qi flow, to promote one's own health, or to self-heal illness through an individual's own practice. External QG attempts to achieve healing by manipulating or transmitting another's qi, based on the idea that energy can be led outside or travel through a therapist's body and be conducted to other living and nonliving systems. This form of therapy is performed by a QG master whose practice has reached an advanced level or who has an inherent talent in this respect. A healer can provide qi through projection without direct contact or through other methods with contact, such as touching of acupoints, massage, and osteopathic adjustments. Diseases treated by internal QG in China include cardiovascular diseases, such as essential hypertension, coronary heart disease, heart arrhythmia, rheumatic heart disease, and stroke, as well as other functional and organic diseases.

QIGONG OBSERVED

Public interest in QG spurred basic and clinical research in China during the 1980s and some international interest in its role and mechanisms in the 1990s. However, relatively few clinical studies on QG's efficacy have been conducted outside China. Moreover, little documentation has been found, even in China, regarding research on external QG, except for a single case report on its experimental use as anesthesia, although the effectiveness of t'ai chi and QG in the treatment of psychosomatic disorders has been discussed in Germany.

The practice of QG became known in the United States during the 1990s. *New York Magazine* reported Dr. Mehmet Oz's experiments using American therapists during open heart surgery at Columbia-Presbyterian Medical Center. An acupoint known as "Yong Quan" (Bubbling Spring or KI1), at the beginning part of the kidney meridian located on the soles of the feet, was used in the application of "energy medicine." At the dawn of the new millennium, the National Institutes of Health began to fund scientific investigations of QG efficacy.

Because of the different cosmology underlying Chinese medicine versus modern biomedical sciences, conducting research is not an easy task. For the most part the operative philosophy of science is embodied in Aristotelian empirical materialism. The formulation of a Cartesian mind-matter *(res cogitans-res extensa)* dualism in the

17th century helped to bring about the birth of modern science. In this paradigm, matter as the observed object is seen as completely separated from the scientist as an observer. Biomedicine, as an offspring of this outlook, focuses primarily on the material structure of the body, which is further broken down into systems, organs, tissues, cells, chromosomes, genes, and molecules. For example, in this biomedical model, the heart is treated as a pump, a mechanical organ with regular outputs. The diagnosis and treatment of heart disease are centered on aspects of the material organ or other levels of structure: physical, physiologic, biochemical, and genetic.

However, in Chinese medicine, the heart signifies more than an anatomical organ. Strangely, the energetic concept of heart, which is reflected in everyday experiences of Western cultures, often referred to as "heart qi" in China, also contains some function of the mind. In a modern view, this involves the brain-heart relationship, which is explainable in terms of the heart-related functions involving neuroendocrinology, immunology, and the pituitary-hypothalamic-adrenal axis. Even without these scientific concepts, the ancient Chinese perspective organized all these phenomena in a system of vital energy movement. The circulation of qi within the human body and its interactions thus became essential to theory. Accordingly, QG was built on an energy-centered worldview, a Daoist view that differs remarkably from that supporting contemporary Western medicine.

Daoist Dialectic

More than 2000 years ago Daoism crystallized one of many ancient intellectual legacies of the Chinese culture. The emergence of Daoism echoes the historical environment of its founder, Lao Zi, who is believed to have lived between 571 and 471 BC during the spring and autumn period of the late Zhou dynasty, which lasted for 242 years. This historical period was marked by chaotic and ceaseless battles among hundreds of warring dukes and by schools of varied philosophies. Reality was perceived by Daoists in complex relations; the truth in human nature and in universal phenomena was nothing short of ambiguity, paradox, and contradiction. Ancient Daoists sought to achieve a conscious awareness and philosophical understanding of universal principles or the manner and process of change that underlies all cosmological processes. By embodying the invisible but perceivable image of "flow of air," the word qi was used as a vivid metaphor to illustrate the changing energy patterns in universal processes.

In ancient Greece, Aristotle had described the world as a systematic structure, and Democritus pioneered the concept of atoms as the basic unit of natural substances. These philosophical perspectives established the fundamental materialistic worldview underlying modern Western sciences, in particular classic physical theory. However, ancient Daoists were more interested in mastering the order of ever-changing patterns that explained the interactive phenomena at multiple levels in nature, including humans. Concurrently, they observed that the transformation of energy is the unifying principle or force among all beings (anticipating Albert Einstein in the 20th century). The ontological difference between the outlooks of the Greek and Chinese traditions was noted by a modern physicist, Fritjof Capra. In The Tao of Physics (1999), he suggests that the Daoist ontology resembles that of quantum physics. Both traditions propose that all forms of substance are nothing but the materialization of energy. Both view the dynamic patterns of energy as the primary and continual forces in nature, whereas substantive aspects are secondary.

Without scientific terminology, Lao Zi had used nonbeing, or wu in Chinese, and being, or yu, to summarize the energetic and substantive aspects of all things. An original energy in the pure form of nonbeing was considered as the primary force that generated the materialistic universe, the sum of all being. In his world-famous Dao De Jing (Tao Te Ching), Lao Zi wrote: "All things are born of being; being is born of nonbeing. All living things are formed by being, and shaped by their environment, growing if nourished well by virtue, the being from nonbeing." In other words, an invisible energetic force as the origin of the world existed before all material substances emerged. Accordingly the Daoist worldview considers invisible energy movements as constant, ultimate reality, whereas visible materialistic aspects of the world are transient phenomena in a cosmic sense. For example, each human body has its circle between life and death, but the energetic movement of its particles continues at different levels beyond this circle. The Chinese character *yu* can be translated as something exists. In contrast, *wu* can be translated or interpreted as nothing exists, or nothingness. The latter interpretation is somewhat similar to the Buddhist nothingness or emptiness. Both concepts refer to images of reality, mean that "nothing exists," and are perceived through intuition rather than empirical observation. However, the Daoist nonbeing tends to differ from the Buddhist emptiness in both perspective and content. The Daoist concept concerns the nature of ultimate reality itself. It conceptualizes the origin of the universe or all objective being in the form of energetic nonbeing, or wu, or in modern terms, a void field filled with energetic movement. The Buddhism concept of emptiness involves subjective reflection to that ultimate reality. It offers a cognitive solution as detachment to human suffering through the emptiness of the mind. Taking Lao Zi's dialectic view, therefore, nothingness could imply something within, such as moving energy, or Daoist qi, or the awareness of spiritual truth through Buddhist liberation, or Nirvana, and enlightenment. This ontologic difference shapes the different focus of meditative QG.

The being versus nonbeing relation of Lao Zi implies not only the Daoist ontology concerning the nature of the universe, including humans, but also its dialectical epistemology. Fritjof Capra noted that the Chinese tradition appreciates intuitive thinking above rational thinking more than its Western counterpart. Despite their basic outlook shared with modern physicists, Daoists do not use formal logic, empirical observation, and deductive reasoning. Rather, their way of knowing is based on dialectical thinking, intuitive imagery, and cyclical patterning. Because of their puzzling dialectics and multiplicity of meanings, some Daoist passages seem to be logically incomprehensible. As Lao Zi said in Dao De Jing:

"When living by the Tao, awareness of self is not required, for in this way of life, the self exists, and is also non-existent, being conceived of, not as existentiality, nor as non-existent." Stated abstractly in this passage, fact A holds with both B and non-B. Seemingly contradictory arguments such as this are expressed throughout his book, as object lessons, because paradox and mutuality are a part of truth in the Daoist philosophy.

The Daoist dialectic way of circular reasoning presents a stark contrast to the laws of formal logic tracing back to ancient Greece, and particularly Aristotle. Central to the latter are three laws: identity, noncontradiction, and the excluded middle. The first law claims that everything must be identical with itself. The second law insists that no statement can be both true and false. The third law declares that A is either B or non-B. For example, in *The Republic*, Plato recorded a conversation about beauty and ugliness with Socrates that clearly differs from the previous Lao Zi passage: "Since fair is the opposite of ugly, they are two." "Of course." "Since they are two, isn't each also one?" "That is so as well." The same argument also applies then to justice and injustice, good and bad, and all the forms. Accordingly, at least until recently, the order of the world in the Western perspective has tended to follow a path of certainty, specification, and a linear logic that links cause to effect. (For example, if A leads to B and B leads to C, then A also leads to C.) Formal logic defines the relative truth concerning the contingent reality in structures, which allows natural law to be comprehensible within specified domains. It eventually paved a way to the emergence of modern science that informs current medicine.

Change, Contradiction, and Holism

By contrast, central to Daoist dialectics are three different but interrelated principles: change, contradiction, and holism. The first principle claims that reality is in constant flux. The second principle states that reality is full of paradoxes. The last principle declares that all things are interdependent and interactive. The order of the world, including human health, therefore tends to follow a path of uncertainty, mutuality, and the circular logic that links an individual part to the whole. This last principle is the essence of dialectical thinking as the consequence of the first two. The truth thus is often presented in a liquid sense in reference to its context, or as opposite but related aspects, rather than in an isolated and absolute stage. As Lao Zi said, "We cannot know the Tao itself, nor see its qualities directly, but only see by differentiation, which it manifests. Thus that which is seen as beautiful is beautiful compared with that which is seen as lacking beauty."

Corresponding to this last principle, holism, Daoists believe that all things in the world are interrelated and affect every other thing in mutually interactive and cyclical ways. The parts become meaningful only in relation to the whole context. Accordingly, ancient Daoists summarized the absolute truth concerning the ultimate reality in a mysterious web of complex energy systems, which appears to be incomprehensible as the whole. However, its manifestation in the form of changing patterns, such as health, is perceivable in comparison to and in connection with opposing and multiple aspects within all phenomena. Daoist dialectics do not lead to classic science or its structurally detailed modern medical diagnosis and intervention. However, it can be a helpful lens in comprehending dynamic energetics in totality, such as with Chinese medicine and modern physics. Daoist energy systems are shown in interactive images, symbols, and metaphors. To demonstrate the universal part-whole dynamics of energetic patterns, the Daoist tai ji symbol is shown in a half-black and half-white round pattern, a sign of two interactive cosmic forces, yin and yang, or a dynamic union of two forces generating the vital energy, qi.

Corresponding to the second principle, contradiction, the polarized yin and yang aspects define each other in all paradoxical relations, such as being and non-being, energy and substance, spirit and matter, or mind and body. The sigmoid or "S curve" dividing line between the yin-yang halves in the tai ji symbol implies the constant cyclical movement in contradictive pairs, mutually creating, controlling, and penetrating. Both sides can influence and transform into each other in certain ways, such as in the relationship between health and illness. From this relativist perspective, the metaphor of the qi and the yin-yang relation can be used to describe the energetic and functional relationship of both physical nature and human phenomena. Metaphorically, at an atomic level, this relation can be understood as one between positive and negative particles. At a physical and physiological level each person has both yin and yang sides at multiple levels, such as the relation of invisible functions to solid organs. At the basic neuropsychological level all humans have both a rational left hemisphere and an intuitive right hemisphere.

Daoism respects nature and emphasizes a harmonic relationship with nature, as do many ancient traditions, such as Buddhism, Hinduism, and Native American thought. Yet in keeping with the first principle, change, Daoists were uniquely interested more in the constant movements in the nonbeing aspect of nature rather than the visible (e.g., physical landscape) or invisible (e.g., the spirit) properties in its being aspects. The universal principle of all change is presented by a single word, dao, the law inherent in nature rather than that created by a creator. The law of nature is not perceived in fixed order but in continuous flow in the constant movement of both nonbeing and being aspects within a hierarchical system (e.g., from a higher level of the universe to a lower level of humans). This basic idea is stated by Lao Zi in Dao De Jing: "When the consistency of the Tao is known, the mind is receptive to its states of change. Man's laws should follow natural laws, just as nature gives rise to physical laws, whilst following from universal law, which follows the Tao." The law of the universe, not of human logic, is what Daoism comprehends philosophically, appreciates aesthetically, and acknowledges spiritually.

The I Ching: A System for Comprehending Change

Daoism uniquely uses mathematics to predict changing patterns in nature and humans. However, unlike for scientists, even the mathematical patterns of such principles are displayed in symbolic ways. This method can be traced back 5000 years to an ancient book, I Ching (Yi Jing), or the Book of Changes, which had profound influence on Chinese healing traditions. The book is entirely devoted to the basic ordering principles and was used to calculate predictable changing patterns in ancient times. The 64 hexagrams of the I Ching are considered an oracle. Each of these 64 figures is composed of six lines, as shown in Fig. 16.1. A line disconnected in the middle, "– –," represents yin, and a complete line, "—," represents yang. The 64 hexagrams register the maximum possible combinations of yin and yang in six lines. Therefore yin and yang are the two basic codes in this complex

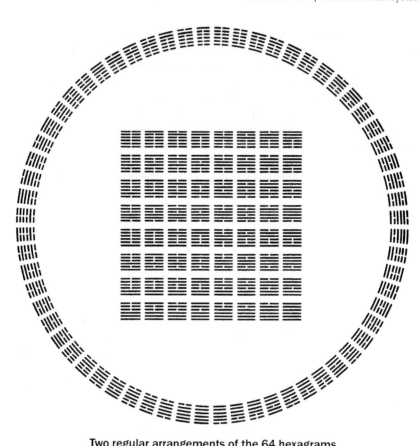

Two regular arrangements of the 64 hexagrams

FIG. 16.1 | The 64 hexagrams of the I Ching.

patterning system, including human health. This dichotomized coding system resembles, but emerged thousands of years before, the digital, mathematical base one, or "zero-one," language used in computer science. Capra praises the I Ching in *The Tao of Physics*: "Because of its notion of dynamic patterns, the I Ching is perhaps the closest analogy to S-matrix theory in Eastern thought. In both systems the emphasis is on the process rather than object."

Throughout Chinese history Daoism has been the most influential intellectual tradition underlying the development of QG. Like Daoist ontology QG in theory becomes a function and health-centered system, rather than a structure and disease-oriented system. Each person is considered as an energetic cosmos in miniature. Health phenomena are viewed in light of a complex hierarchical web of qi, rather than as merely isolated physical matters. One's energy movement manifests the same pattern as does the universe. In antiquity the physical parts and major acupoints of a human body in practice were illustrated and described in accordance with moon images and other symbols, which indicates that qi patterns in humans correspond to those in seasonal changes and cosmic movements.

Because the energetic nonbeing is more fundamental than the substantive being, QG focus primarily on the holistic processes of multilevel energy patterns and their interrelations rather than on the material structure of body parts, as does Western medicine. Even organs (zhang fu) are primarily described in terms of qi, with reference to interactive functions within each one and among all, rather than in terms of their exact anatomical structures, because organs are the reservoir of qi. Likewise, QG exercise places more emphasis on the internal movement via breath technology to cultivate essential qi, rather than on external movement via muscular training to build up body size, as do Western physical exercises. However, Daoist healing systems do not deny physical aspects of human health. Instead, these phenomena are integrated into the primary energetic process.

Identified in their physical structures, the 12 organs are not too distant from their placement by European contemporaries in biomedical anatomy. These organs are divided into the viscera, including six zang or solid organs, and the bowels, including six fu or hollow organs. The organs of the viscera (heart, lungs, liver, spleen, kidneys, pericardium) and bowel (small intestine, large intestine, gallbladder, stomach, urinary bladder, "triple burner" [san jiao]) are paired in terms of their interior-exterior (yin-yang) relationship. Aside from the triple burner, in TCM the major physiological functions of these organs are close to those associated with organs similarly named in biomedicine.

However, unique to this system are two energy-oriented concepts essential to QG practice. One is san jiao, which has no corresponding anatomical structure. This concept refers to the three energetic locations at the middle of the chest, diaphragm, and abdomen, which express the functional connection and interaction among paired organs. Another concept relates to acupuncture meridians (or channels), a circulation system of qi, which also has no identifiable physical anatomical structure. It consists of 12 primary channels corresponding to the six pairs of yin-yang organs and an additional set of eight extraordinary vessels. Along the pathways of 14 of these channels (the 12 regular channels and two of the extra channels) lie 361 specific acupuncture points. Qi flows along these channels, making a rhythmic circuit over 24 hours daily. Each channel has its own peak energetic time in a daily circle, which can be correlated to the fluctuation of the immune and neuroendocrinology systems over 24 hours. To cultivate vital energy, some Daoist QG styles emphasize meditation on certain acupoints and qi pathways at certain times every day according to the temporal order of daily qi flow (zi wu liu zu).

In principle, health and illness conditions in QG theories follow the coding system in the I Ching by matching multilevel energetic components of each individual. Ancient Greeks used four elements—water, fire, earth, and air—to represent the basic qualities of natural phenomena. Similarly in the Han Dynasty approximately 2000 years ago, a five-element system—wood, fire, earth, metal, and water—was introduced. The energetic interaction among the five elements follows the mutual generating and controlling processes. The five-element theory was combined with the yin-yang system in the I Ching to register the complex energetic interplay among multilevel phenomena that are associated with health. Paired organs, tissues, meridians, some acupuncture points, pulse, tongue status, sounds, tastes, colors, time, seasons, directions, planets, temperament, herbs, food, and external pathogens are all coded by these integrated categories along with interconnected relations. Organized by the five-element theory, seven emotions or psychic elements (joy, anger, anxiety, concentration, grief, fear, fright) are also linked with the energetic patterns of all functional organs.

Based on this system, the "qi flow of the human" becomes a relatively predictable phenomenon, corresponding to the similarly ordered energetic phenomena in the universe. Consistent with Daoist epistemology, QG theory is literally a systematic elaboration on the changing patterns of qi with respect to the inter-relations of body, mind, and spirit, as well as their interactions with the energetic environment, in terms of nature, society, and cosmos. Health is maintained only in the internal and external energetic qi contexts of each individual and is perceived with constant changes, contradictions, and holism. Because of the principle of holism, illness conditions are often individually assessed and addressed using multiple principles concerning the whole energy system rather than using a standardized diagnosis and assessment for structural abnormality. Because of the principle of contradiction, health is not viewed as the state of opposition to or absence of disease but rather as an uncertain process of constantly balancing normal and abnormal qi patterns. Because of the principle of change, health and illness can be transformed into each other, depending on the interaction between the ailment stage and health practice by an individual. Accordingly, QG practice should be integrated into one's lifestyle, which then can boost overall energy, balance the effect of illness, and allow the natural healing capacities to prevail constantly and to transform an ill state into a healthy process.

Back in the Middle

Daoist essence is reflected in the Chinese character *zhong yi*. *Yi* means "medicine," and *zhong* usually means "middle." As discussed at the beginning of this book this character represents the "medicine of the land at the middle," or the Middle Kingdom of China, half-way between heaven and earth. In Daoism and QG it also refers to the internally balanced "golden medium." In this perspective zhong yi does not only mean the "medicine of middle kingdom" or of China but refers to the "medicine for inner balance." Inner balance lies in the harmonic pattern of ever-changing qi in relation to the interplay between ying and yang at all levels of human function, as well as in one's habits and environment. This perspective enables QG practice to focus on the prevention of illness conditions through sensitive recognition and management of qi and to emphasize the treatment of pre-illness stages (e.g., functional disorders) before ailments are manifest as pathologic changes in tissues, organs, and cells. A classic text of TCM, the Classic of Difficult Issues (Nan Jing), compiled more than 2000 years ago, presented many therapeutic principles for becoming an excellent doctor who can prevent substantive illnesses from progressing to a state of pathology and mortality.

Each individual therefore must take the responsibility for his or her own healthy lifestyle, harmonic attitude, and energy exercise, QG. In keeping with its preventive orientation, QG as an energy-oriented practice becomes an art of health, healing, and holistic life, integrating body, mind, and spirit, not a "magic bullet" for treatment of specific diseases.

Now, Take a Breath

The spirit of Daoism also guides QG practice with a heavy emphasis on breathing technique as one approach to holistic health. Lao Zi stated in Dao De Jing:

Maintaining unity is virtuous, for the inner world of thought is one with the external world of action and of things. The sage avoids their separation, by breathing as the sleeping babe, and thus maintaining harmony. From constancy, there develops harmony, and from harmony, enlightenment. It is unwise to rush from here to there. To hold one's breath causes the body strain; exhaustion follows when too much energy is used, for this is not the natural way.

Held in the posture of standing, sitting, or lying, the meditative Daoist QG practice appears to be similar to the Zen Buddhist approach. Both emphasize deep breathing, concentration, and relaxation. However, these two approaches differ from each other in terms of goals and techniques. The name of Buddha is "he who woke up," and Buddhism stresses the experience of awakening from the illusion of life (enlightenment). Daoism emphasizes a more muscular practice (literally, in the example of QG), cultivating energy and spirit (shen), as well as promoting health and longevity. Buddhist practice tends to center on the emptiness of mind (detachment), whereas some Daoist practices guide consciousness to follow the flow of qi passively along a certain meridian system, such as "heavenly circulation" (zhou tian) around the middle line in front and back of the body. Daoist QG practice also tends to concentrate on the most important energy center, the cinnabar field (dan tian), at about three finger widths below the navel. This area is considered to be the "ocean of qi," where the root of vital energy and longevity reside. (This location also represents an important Chakra in Vedic traditions.)

In modern terms, QG is essentially a mind-body practice and also a spiritual cultivation. As with early Hippocratic medicine, the approach of QG is psychosomatic and does not follow a soma and psyche dualism. Physical health and ailments are seen not only as inseparable from, but also as internal responses to, emotional stimuli and environmental stress. When any type of affect becomes overwhelming, emotions become internal agents of illness. Conversely, the dysfunction of organs will be manifested not only in somatic symptoms but also in certain types of emotional distress. For example, the heart is classified as the "fire" element—an "emperor" organ that houses the individual's spirit (shen) and mental energy, with a tendency to be excessive. It is related to the color red and the emotion of joy. Indeed, in light of modern neuroendocrinology, the heart beats faster because of the increased secretion of adrenal hormones in an ecstatic emotional state, whereas many patients with cardiovascular disease also experience depression and anxiety.

Interestingly, some American physicians also speak of this mind-body aspect of the heart in terms of "dual hearts" in a human: first a pulsating of muscle in the chest and then a precious second cable of communicating neurons that create feeling, longing, and love. This view recognizes the important role of neuroendocrinology and the immune system in organ-brain or body-mind communication, reflecting an ancient idea essentially expressed in the concept of qi and QG practice.

QG practice thus emphasizes the guidance of mind for the flow of qi through constant meditative breathing exercise, which in turn spontaneously affects bodily function. Following Daoist dialectics, no type of emotion is seen as absolutely positive or completely negative. For example, excessive joy is believed to cause harm to one's energetic balance, as do negative emotions, such as anger. This situation can be understood in modern terms. For example, a person with coronary heart disease can experience sudden cardiac arrest when attending holiday festivities, a family gathering, or a birthday party. This heart attack may result from excessive joy or excitement that in turn leads to extra stress. To protect well-being, the QC emphasis is on zhong (i.e., balancing mood, in relation to organ health) rather than positivity per se (i.e., pursing happiness to its extreme end). The key to health in this QG perspective lies in the integration and balancing of overall energetic functions rather than in the pursuit of extremity.

Likewise, Daoist QG practice does not deny sexuality as a sinful desire, nor does it encourage extreme sexual play in the spirit of hedonism. Rather, sexual energy and behaviors are inseparable parts of health, emotion, and longevity, but they may also be associated with certain illnesses when badly practiced. Some QG support techniques promote healthy sexuality in relation to physical and emotional heath. Returning to the fire organ example, the qi of the pericardium, a parallel fire organ to the heart, acts to facilitate sexual functioning. A defective pericardium function is believed to affect human activity in varied ways, ranging from hyposexuality to hypersexuality, as well as impacted joy. Currently, this conception may also be explainable by neuroendocrinology and psychology. QG practice helps to maintain the tranquil qi balance in these fire organs, readjust dysfunction of both organs and emotions, and restore healthy energetic patterns in related sexuality. In these ways QG, is one of the most ancient yet modern, profound yet simple applications of the spiritual healing and vital energy of Chinese medicine.

QIGONG IN THE 21ST CENTURY

During the late 20th century, QG, or the practice of breath work and healing through cultivating one's qi, became an immensely popular form of exercise and healing in crowded, urban areas, especially in China itself. Throughout major cities and towns one could always find practitioners in the early dawn in parks, on sidewalks, near public buildings, on campuses, and even in streets participating in daily regimens of QG exercise. Broad social awareness of this practice was reflected in mainstream state newspapers and popular novels.

QG was understood as fostering the movement of qi through the body either by internal visualization and meditation or through external bodily practices involving physical movement. Rather than being viewed merely as a physical substance, qi was embraced as cosmologic energy by practitioners and masters. Such popular views of qi as a healing force seemed to return to earlier, more "traditional" notions of qi according to which individuals could draw upon or embody its transformative powers present in the environment and cosmos rather than merely in a body confined by everyday spaces.

Most QG manuals nonetheless tend to echo traditional medical texts in the discussion of yin-yang and how qi is manifest with these dual qualities. Experiencing qi was a central component of practice that all QG practitioners encountered and discussed on a daily basis. However, because there are multiple forms of qi, the ways in which qi was invoked to describe practice varied widely.

Despite the multitude of styles and practice, QG can be distinguished into two types: external and internal. The external form, based on waidan (外丹) cultivation principles, tends to emphasize "hard" qi and "hard" bodies that can withstand much force and perform superhuman powers. This martial arts form tends to be practiced not so much in public parks but in arenas, such as acrobatic troupes, or military compounds (and more by men).

The internal and meditative form, based on neidan (內丹) cultivation, was pursued by practitioners of all backgrounds (particularly women) as such forms helped to promote the circulation and transformation of qi as crucial steps towards enhancing vitality.

QG had emerged during the 1980s (the initial post-Mao period prior to the formation of a massive market economy and global pharmaceutical industry later in the 1990s) simultaneously as a private act for individuals, as well as a public performance for masters. In contrast to previous decades in which socialized medicine attended to the masses with a focus on public health, the re-emergence of QG was linked to the desire for self-care and individualized forms of healing and daily practice. Elderly people could address their complaints of rheumatism or arthritis, sufferers of neurasthenia or chronic pain could seek relief, and parents of children with congenital disorders could seek help when no other options could be found in either TCM or biomedicine. QG became a practice that promised release and hope. Whether in parks or in stadiums, it became accepted to cry openly or express fervent belief in something that was not state ideology. As some forms of QG began to overlap with Daoist, Buddhist, and other spiritual practices, references to QG as a religion or New Age spiritualism also appeared.

During the 1990s official state debates about traditional QG situated it clearly apart from popular QG. Although testimonial accounts of QG healing continued, there were calls to differentiate between "real" (zheng, char) and "false" (jia, char) QG. There was an attempt to separate those individuals who claimed to be masters and healed for lucrative purposes from those with "true" abilities, practicing "more orthodox and uniform" forms. A state-appointed bureau to regulate QG used scientific discourse about QG (kexue de QG, char) as a means to cleanse and discipline the ranks of "false" masters. QG, like many practices in Chinese medicine, has been described as based on a "philosophy of balance whereas biomedical science is based on the western philosophy of conquest" (Jonas, 1999). This view is in keeping with a natural, ecological interpretation of qi, but given the plurality of QG forms, it may be a somewhat romantic view. Taken out of context QG could be considered essentially apolitical in nature, but as in the West, the Chinese sociopolitical body has at times unconsciously expressed what is not culturally or politically acceptable. This manifestation has arguably been the case with QG (the word itself, as having a standardized meaning, was actually created by government in 1953).

With the lifting of many restrictions in China in the 1990s, more elaborate spontaneous forms of QG enabled expression of much that had remained repressed under Mao (in a culture that is not overly given to emotional self-expression). In the words of one commentator, QG practice became "a symptom of repressed desires" [Xu]. With rise of the falun gong (法輪功) protest movement, QG was very definitely politicized as had been the Boxer uprising of 1900. The body politic has influenced the understanding of the effects of medical practices on the human body from ancient times to the present. Medical practices, east and west, reflect the cultural, economic, political, and social contexts in which they arise. This ancient and rich mixture in China has given rise to a much fuller and comprehensive practice of qi manipulation, including acupuncture, than what has generally been accounted for, or rendered, in Western interpretations.

Qigong as a Bioenergy Modality

QG as a bioenergy modality originating in Asia, more specifically ancient China, and has been used for many years to aid healing. The term QG itself can be parsed to help to explain its use. In China, qi is considered the universal life force described sometimes as energy. Gong refers to the training and cultivating of qi (Guo, Zhou, Nishimura, Teramukai, & Fukushima, 2008). Therefore QG is the practice of cultivating the universal life force. QG is thought to be made up of two different types of qi: internal and external. Internal QG refers to a self-practice (typically involving stereotypical movements) to restore qi. External qi is practitioner-based, in which QG masters exude their "qi" onto their patients to foster healing (Jahnke, Larkey, Rogers, Etnier, & Lin, 2010). There is no agreed-upon physical evidence to show the qi is ever emitted or even that it exists at all.

The gentle movements, meditation, and controlled breathing of internal QG exercises have evidence to support their use in physiologic and psychologic ailments. In a comprehensive review of t'ai chi (an ancient Chinese practice to improve internal qi) and QG, evidence was evaluated for cardiopulmonary conditions, as well as its effects on bones, physical function, quality of life, self-efficacy, psychologic functioning, and immune function (Jahnke et al., 2010). The studies varied with regard to population under investigation, intervention length, and intervention goal. One study showed a positive effect on bone density. As other reviews have reported, there were consistent findings for reducing blood pressure. When used in conjunction with antihypertensive medication, the effect is greater than just the use of medication alone (Drukteinis et al., 2007). The evidence for QG on lipid profiles and ejection fraction were inconclusive. Cardiopulmonary fitness outcomes varied based on the study population and the outcome measures used. Physical function outcomes were inconclusive, and improvements in two quality-of-life studies were not statistically significant, whereas psychological evidence was positive and promising.

Three studies showed significant decreases in anxiety when compared with active exercise. One study included in the review showed a significant decrease in depression symptoms compared with newspaper reading. Biomarker studies were also examined, and QG significantly decreased blood catecholamines and cortisol. Three studies examined immune function and inflammation, and these studies showed positive effects on these systems. Antibody levels increased after influenza vaccinations in an aging study group compared with usual care. Another study showed positive modulation of interleukin-6. The review concluded by noting that overall there appear to be positive benefits of QG in health outcomes.

There are a number of systematic reviews supporting this conclusion. Drukteinis et al. (2007) reviewed the literature on QG for hypertension, and although they conclude that many of the studies are of poor methodological quality, they performed a meta-analysis on a subset of the better-quality studies. This analysis indicates that QG plus antihypertensive drugs results in significantly lower blood pressure than antihypertensive drugs alone. Another review (Guo et al., 2008) examined the effectiveness of internal QG and its clinical effectiveness in essential hypertension. Nine studies were extracted from their search for randomized controlled trials evaluating clinical effectiveness of QG on hypertension (stages I and II). The studies reported varied in their comparators and had other differences in methodologies. Nonetheless, the authors declare QG to be better than nontreatment, equal or less effective compared with active controls, and has the greatest effect when used in conjunction with medication.

QG has been shown to be of benefit for anxiety and depression in a systematic review and meta-analysis of randomized controlled trials (Wang et al., 2013). Twelve randomized controlled trials were evaluated, and although QG showed no difference when compared with cognitive-behavioral therapy, when QG and usual care were compared to wait-lists or usual care, the high-quality studies included had results supporting the benefit of QG for depressive symptoms. As is the case for much of the research in these areas, the authors conclude that most of the studies have a number of methodological errors. The benefits are often associated with specific populations, such as cancer patients and patients suffering with Parkinson's disease. Reviews typically explicitly state that no adverse events resulted from QG in any of the included studies in their review (Oh, Choi, Inamori, Rosenthal, & Yeung, 2013). Although these reviews, like many other CAM studies, report methodological weaknesses in the underlying studies, the overall conclusion is that QG has benefit for some people and in some conditions. Application of psychometric evaluation to better match individual to these kinds of treatments should be warranted.

REFERENCES

Capra, F. (1999). *Tao of physics: An exploration of the parallels between modern physics and Eastern mysticism* (4th Ed.). Shambhala Publications, Inc.

Drukteinis, J. S., Roman, M. J., Fabsitz, R. R., Lee, E. T., et al. (2007). Cardiac and systemic hemodynamic characteristics of hypertension and prehypertension in adolescents and young adults: the strong heart study. *Professional Heart Daily*. http://dx.doi.org/10.1161/CIRCULATIONAHA.106.668921.

Guo, X., Zhou, B., Nishimura, T., Teramukai, S., & Fukushima, M. (2008). Clinical effect of qigong practice on essential hypertension: A meta-analysis of randomized controlled trials. *Journal of Alternative and Complementary Medicine, 14*, 27–37.

Jahnke, R., Larkey, L., Rogers, C., Etnier, J., & Lin, F. (2010). A comprehensive review of health benefits of qigong and tai chi. *American Journal of Health Promotion, 24*(6), e1–e25.

Jonas, W. B. (1999). One kind of medicine or many? The view from the NIH. In M. S. Micozzi & A. N. Bacchus (Eds.), *The physician's guide to alternative medicine* (pp. 367–369). Atlanta, GA: American Health Consultants.

Oh, B., Choi, S. M., Inamori, A., Rosenthal, D., & Yeung, A. (2013). Effects of qigong on depression: A systemic review. *Evidence-based Complementary and Alternative Medicine*, Article 134737.

Wang, F., Man, J. K. M., Lee, E. K. O., Wu, T., et al. (2013). The effects of qigong on anxiety, depression, and psychological well-being: A systematic review and meta-analysis. *Evidence-based Complementary and Alternative Medicine*, Article 152738.

Suggested Readings can be found on the companion website, http://www.micozzipainconditions.com.

Chapter 17

East Asian Manual and Movement Therapies Part Two: Reiki and Shiatsu

This chapter addresses two therapies involving manual therapy and bodywork, as well as energy manipulation and hand movements, respectively. As discussed in Section III, hand-mediated healing modalities may involve physically touching the patient or may literally take a "hands-off" approach relying on movements of the practitioners to influence vital energy, or qi. Reiki and shiatsu also have in common some semimythical, retrospective origins in China via Japan and have become widely popular in recent years.

REIKI

Despite granting itself great antiquity, reiki is similar to the dietary practices of macrobiotics in having originated in 1920s Japan, having then been organized in the United States in the mid-20th century, and having an alarming lack of research for a practice that is so widespread and popular. However, like ancient Chinese medicine, it is said to have originated in earlier times. Reiki is also ascribed semimythical origins, which are projected back onto historically ancient practices. However, unlike Chinese medicine, reiki is very much in its entirety a product of the 20th century whose popularity has been bolstered by the New Age. Reiki is translated from Japanese as *universal life energy*. A method of hands-on healing, it is handed down in oral tradition from master to student. Thus many different schools, or *streams*, as they are described in the present-day Japanese view, developed from the original teachings of Mikao Usui in the early 1920s.

RETROSPECTIVE SHINTO ROOTS

The roots of the 20th-century Usui System of Natural Healing for reiki have been interposed onto those of Shintoism, which is said to be a religion of Japanese

Acknowledgments to Kerry Palanjian for prior contribution in Micozzi, M.S. (ed.), (2011). *Fundamentals of complementary & alternative medicine* (4th ed.). St Louis: Elsevier Health Sciences/Saunders.

peoples, prior to acculturation to China. However, even Shintoism itself had no formal organization until it was used as a political tool to enhance the lineage of the 19th-century Meiji Emperors and Meiji Restoration of 1868, in turn, projecting backwards in time to ascribe itself greater antiquity. As practiced in its earliest form (200 BC), Shintoism included belief in spirit beings and the energy of every living or inanimate object in nature, such as stones and waterways. Reiki can be understood in its fullest capacity when linked with the Shinto worldview, which recognizes elemental spiritual forces and energy. However, the system is also said to rely on Buddhist tradition, introduced from China, in some of its practices, which regards the world and its elements as transient. Furthermore, there are Christian charismatic elements that might be seen as appropriate to the cultural era of 1920s Japan as it emerged into the 20th-century world prior to becoming isolated again in the militarism of the 1930s and World War II.

As told in the "creation myth" of modern reiki, Dr. Mikao Usui was searching for concrete ways in which both Jesus and the Buddha had been able to heal with the "laying on of hands." Oral histories agree that the point of origin for this system occurred when Dr. Usui undertook a lengthy meditation and fast on Mount Kuriyama outside Kyoto, Japan, and received information, guidance, and initiation into this healing modality. Dr. Usui began teaching his method in 1920, and 1 year later opened a reiki practice in Harajuku, Tokyo, appropriately enough, close to the Meiji Jinju. Dr. Usui developed and taught five spiritual precepts as guidelines for everyday living and foci for personal meditation. Followers disagree about the basis of these precepts. Some believe they are based on the Meiji Emperor's five rules of life. Others believe these writings were developed as positive reflections of the five hindrances to spiritual enlightenment presented by the Buddha.

Several reiki lineages have grown out of the original teachings of Dr. Usui. A Hawaiian-born, Japanese-American woman, Hawayo Takata, began teaching reiki in the West in the 1970s. Her story is widely known among aficionados and has been rendered in many books and retold throughout the world. Many schools have developed with varying requirements in training, but all hold that transfer of energy, or reiki, from one human being to another living being is real. There is a growing number of anecdotal accounts regarding the rebalancing of mind, body, and spirit and the release of disease or pain.

The Usui system of reiki is being taught to nurses in hospitals and nursing schools. Some doctors, dentists, psychologists, and other health care providers are learning this technique to add a "hands-on" dimension of healing touch to their practices. There are manuals and written texts, cassettes, and videos, discussing a wide array of personal interpretations of this system. Techniques of application are diverse because they depend on the oral teachings of each "master" as he or she initiated and instructed students. Not until the Usui system itself faced competition from other emerging reiki schools and styles was there any attempt by a professional organization to establish a systematic application. The Reiki Alliance was originally formed to support the teachings of Hawayo Takata through her granddaughter Phyllis Furumoto. In 1993 it began to define qualifications and ethical standards for reiki practice. Several organizations have subsequently developed their own criteria to promote wider acceptance.

Healing What Is Needed

Most reiki practitioners are not qualified to deal with a client's medical diagnosis and do not concern themselves with it, unless they are coordinating with a doctor or other medical provider. Reiki is said to support healing only of "what needs to be healed" rather than what the practitioner conceptualizes or intends to be healed. Reiki practitioners generally do not promise any specific symptom improvement or "cure." Sometimes only one session is needed and sometimes multiple sessions are needed for clients to begin to realize they are experiencing shifts in their perspectives of life, disease, attitudes, and the nature of the symptoms that brought them to the session in the first place.

Part of the approach can be attributed to the body's response to gentle, appropriate contact between practitioner and client. The practitioner gains permission to touch the client, then places his or her hands in a prescribed pattern on the client's body. The client is clothed and may be standing, sitting, or reclining on a bed, massage table, or the floor. Several nursing observations have shown that this gentle act of appropriate touch can help a person to make a profound shift, from the tense response of the fight-or-flight pattern of the sympathetic autonomic nervous system to the healing response of the relaxation pattern of the parasympathetic autonomic nervous system.

In her early diary Hawayo Takata, the "energetic" woman who brought the teaching and use of the Usui system out of Japan, stated that "this power [reiki] is unfathomable, immeasurable, and being a universal life force, it is incomprehensible to man. Yet, every living being is receiving its blessings daily, awake and asleep." Many compare the feeling of receiving reiki to the sensation felt when praying, meditating, singing, walking in the woods, or in any other way actively seeking the deity. Many reiki practitioners believe these sensations are physical responses to making a connection with a power greater than themselves. Students are assisted in becoming aware (again) of a life force that abounds in everything and from which human beings benefit when they remain open to it.

The body autonomically directs healing energy to wounds, strain, tension, and other ailments. It is believed that the receiver of reiki draws energy through the hands of the practitioner, who is open to its universal availability.

The hands are simply placed over an area of pain, infection, or tension; the mind is opened; and energy is allowed to flow. There is no manipulation of muscles or of the "electromagnetic field" of a client. The only method is to apply touch to a client's body in the prescribed hand positions or to be guided by an intuitive force. Some schools of reiki do not allow the practitioner's hands to touch the client's body. The origin of this no-hands practice is not clear. Traditional practitioners use this "hands-off" technique only when treating open or fresh wounds caused by accident or surgery. Some schools of reiki teach that the practitioner's hands should remain in place for a period of 3 to 5 minutes. The traditional practitioner leaves the hands in position until the flow of energy is no longer felt.

For any condition, the basic routine is to offer a complete treatment session and then return to the sites of the original pain, stress, or tension. However, there have been case reports indicating that after applying the full body treatment, a practitioner feels no need to return to the original areas of complaint.

When a practitioner places hands on a client, both the practitioner and the client observe sensory changes around or under the hands of the practitioner. These changes include the sensations of warmth, tingling, cold, extra fullness, and electrical charge. These sensations can change from one day to the next, from one client to the next, and can be experienced differently by the practitioner and the client. These sensory changes indicate that something is passing between the practitioner and client. When the sensation dissipates after a time of holding the hands in one position, it signals the practitioner to change hand positions, in other words, to move on.

There is no conscious effort needed on the part of a practitioner to "turn reiki on." When the body is in pain, has sustained a wound, or is beset by an unbalanced glandular, metabolic, or enzymatic process, it is thought to give out an electromagnetic, neural, atomic, or vibrational alarm. There is stimulation of a healing response from the rest of the body. How does the body's immune system send its cells to determine the form of an intruding bacteria or platelets to a wound to help to stop bleeding? There are chemotactic factors and cellular gradients that send molecular signals. Reiki posits that if such a signal could be detected with sensitive diagnostic equipment, it could be understood as a call of the body for internal or external energy. The sensation of reiki energy flow dissipates after a time, which tells the practitioner that the particular need has been satisfied for the time being. The time frame for this shift may be as little as a few seconds or as long as 45 minutes or until the practitioner tires of holding the position.

The phenomenon of energy exchange can also explain the intuitive experience of many practitioners who find their hands drawn to a particular part of the client's body. The practitioner has no conscious knowledge of where the client is holding tension. It has been explained that the energy itself, meaning reiki, feels the call of the body and is pulled to the need.

Intentionality in Healing

In the proliferation of anecdotes in books and on the Internet, no harmful effects of reiki have been reported. One of the issues frequently discussed is the role of the intent of the practitioner. It is most often agreed that the only necessary intent is to be available to channel the energy rather than the intent "to heal" a certain symptom or condition. Clients are often healed in unexpected ways. For this reason, traditional reiki practitioners make no promises regarding the efficacy of treatment. Many practitioners, seeking to avoid any promise of therapeutic value, refer to the hour-long applications of energy simply as "sessions" or "appointments."

The many anecdotal testimonies show reiki to support the natural healing process of the body to such an extent that it can stimulate what is called a "healing crisis" (a term originally coined in homeopathy [e.g., bringing a boil to a head, thus allowing the wound to be cleaned], or a quick rise in temperature in someone with an infection, followed by a gradual return to normal). Some practitioners have reported that cuts, surgical wounds, and broken bones healed faster than expected after application of reiki (see Chapter 8). There is also anecdotal evidence of reiki resulting in a reduction of the side effects of chemotherapy and radiation treatment.

Reiki is often described as working on the root cause of a disease or imbalance. If a mental, emotional, or spiritual disturbance is a major factor in a physical impairment, the client often recognizes the disturbance during a reiki session. How to deal with a painful relationship or a financial problem can be revealed during a session. When practitioners or others who have been attuned to reiki regularly apply this energy to themselves, they experience a dramatic reduction in daily stress levels. When energy application is coupled with focused attention, through "processing work," or meditation, on the five precepts, personal understanding and an increase in compassion and openness to life can also occur.

People who have attended classes describe personal experiences that defy logical explanation. These experiences are designated as mystical, synchronistic, or even cosmic. They are often very personal, and they are not referred to in medically oriented classes so as not to put off clinicians who require concrete explanations.

TREATMENT STYLES

European treatment styles differ from those taught in American schools. Some teach more hand positions and often offer the application of reiki to clients who are covered with only a sheet or blanket. Other styles of reiki applications are not described in relationship to body organs. Traditional Japanese anatomy, like Chinese, is based on energetic relationships and not based on anatomical dissection with the physical locations of the organs as known to Western medicine. For example, one school of reiki designates a series of hand positions in relation to chakras, or energy centers (see Chapters 18 and 19), in a line from the pubic bone to the crown of the head. This chakra system is derived from Vedic philosophy and was not in the original teachings of the Usui system.

Three Degrees of Reiki

Traditionally there have been three levels or degrees in the Usui system:

First degree (reiki I) is often called "beginning reiki." This label may lead a person to believe that he or she has to have a complete understanding of reiki or to be able to completely use it. In the traditional system, reiki I is sufficient to become a reiki practitioner or to offer reiki to oneself and family members for health maintenance and stress prevention. This class is taught in three 4-hour sessions and includes four initiations or "attunements"; which are the methods of connecting an individual with the source of energy. During this class students are taught the history of reiki, observe the hand positions, and are invited to give and experience a full body application. Discussion of the five precepts is encouraged. Students are also encouraged to experience self-treatment and to investigate the application of reiki in emergencies, in hospices or hospitals, and to clients with acute or chronic conditions. Many case studies are reviewed, and the dynamic potential of having access to this energy is outlined. Often students experience changes in their health, their relationships, or other human conditions during this training. The only prerequisites for learning are openness, a desire to learn, and a commitment to use reiki regularly.

Second degree (reiki II) in some schools, is referred to as "advanced training". It involves instruction in additional applications of reiki through the use of symbols or energy patterns. These additional applications include being able to offer reiki to a person who is not in the room. This person can be next door or on the other side of the globe. The technique is called "sending reiki" or "distant reiki" and is akin to distant healing. Another application is that of mental rebalancing, which involves a specific hand position and techniques to help to relieve addictions and habits and also to improve mental clarity. A third application is the ability to focus reiki into a laser-like beam or to intensify its concentration. This class is taught over 2 days or a minimum of two sessions. Often a reiki master asks a student to return in a month to share experiences regarding practice at this level of application.

Third degree reiki (reiki III), or "master training", may last as long as a year. Other schools have divided this training into two additional levels, third degree and master teacher training, whereas others have consolidated this training into a 1-day experience. Many agree that this level of training can be taxing on the person who wishes to pursue this degree of commitment. According to the Reiki Alliance, a student of reiki should have been actively working with reiki for 3 to 10 years before moving into this level of training. A person who completes this training has the knowledge and technique with which to educate and open others to reiki. How to initiate others into all three degrees is only one part of this mastery. Several organizations have developed teaching protocols for all levels of training. Each master may add his or her own requirements.

All three levels are taught by a master who has fulfilled all training requirements. They are known as reiki masters, not because they have mastered the energy, but because they have made a commitment to "stand in the light of reiki" and allow their lives to "exemplify the qualities described in the five precepts." This commitment is made on many levels, including financial, political, emotional, and spiritual (Box 17.1).

BOX 17.1 *Practice and Self-Practice*

Reiki was originally intended as a self-practice. Nowadays it is often performed by practitioners to help their clients to strengthen their wellness, cope with symptoms (such as pain or fatigue), or support their medical care, sometimes in the case of chronic illness or at the end of life. Reiki was developed by Mikao Usui in Japan in the 1920s as a spiritual practice. One of his master students, Chujiro Hayashi, with Usui's help, extracted the healing practices from the larger body of practices. Hayashi began to teach these practices and opened a clinic to treat patients. Reiki practice itself is extremely passive. Practitioners lay their hands gently on the patient or hold them just above the body without moving their hands except to place them over another area. The reiki practitioner does not attempt to adjust the patient's energy field or actively project energy into the patient's body. In addition, unlike other forms of energy medicine and more like meditation, reiki does not involve an assessment of the patient's energy field or an active attempt to reorganize or adjust the patient's energy field. Instead, reiki practitioners believe that healing energy arises from the practitioner's hand as a response to the patient's needs. It is in this way customized to the patient's needs and condition.

RESEARCH

In one study, 23 reiki-naïve, healthy volunteers participated in standardized 30-minute reiki sessions. They often reported experiencing a "liminal state of awareness." This state is characterized by novel and paradoxical sensations, often symbolic in nature. The experiences run the gamut from disorientation in space and time to altered experience of self and the environment, as well as relationships with people, especially the reiki master. In another study, quantitative measures of anxiety and objective measures of systolic blood pressure and salivary immunoglobulin A were altered significantly by the reiki experience; anxiety and systolic blood pressure were lowered, whereas immunoglobulin A level was increased. Skin temperature, electromyographic readings, and salivary cortisol level were all lowered but not significantly (Engebreston & Wardell, 2002). When these results are taken together, it is apparent that in this study reiki induced states of lowered stress and anxiety and should be considered salutogenic in nature. The authors concluded that the liminal state and paradoxical experiences are related to the ritual and holistic nature of this healing practice (Engebretson & Wardell, 2002).

SHIATSU

The literal meaning of the Japanese word shiatsu is finger pressure or thumb pressure. Over the centuries, Chinese and East Asian medicine and massage therapy, as well as 20th-century advancements, combined to yield "modern" shiatsu. The practice of massage dates back 3000 years in China. The actual word massage comes from the Arabic word for stroke. Shiatsu is seen to have antecedents in Chinese medicine (e.g., in the 2000-year-old *Yellow Emperor's Classic of Internal Medicine*, as discussed in Oliver Cowmeadow's *The Art of Shiatsu*).

Shiatsu is within the touch and massage therapies and in juxtaposition to ancient and modern Japanese culture. As a healing art or treatment it grew from earlier forms of anma in Japan and Tuina in China (see Chapter 16). *An* denotes "pressure," and *ma* means "rubbing." This method, well known in China, found its way to Japan and became recognized as a safe and easy way to treat the human body. In Japan a tradition developed for shiatsu to be used and taught by blind practitioners who relied on their hands to diagnose a patient's condition (see later).

Anma was recognized as a medical modality in Japan during the Nara period (710 to 784) but subsequently lost its popularity before gaining more widespread use in the Edo era (1603 to 1868), prior to the Meiji Restoration, during which doctors were required to study anma. During the Edo period most practitioners were blind and provided treatments in their patients' homes. An extensive handbook on anma was published in 1793. Anma's understanding and assessment of human structure and meridian lines were and are believed to be important distinctions that separate shiatsu therapy from other healing modes and massage therapies. When Western massage was introduced to Japan in the late 1880s, the many vocational schools that taught anma were dominated by blind instructors. However, this very limitation stopped the further development of anma and led to the evolution of what we recognize today as shiatsu therapy.

Modern shiatsu, as noted previously, is a product of 20th-century refinements and evolution that produced the form of therapy used today. Shiatsu, like reiki and macrobiotics, began its modern evolution in the 1920s (the Taisho period), when anma practitioners adopted some of the West's hands-on techniques, including those of chiropractic and occupational therapy.

The practice of shiatsu received support from studies conducted after World War II when US Military Governor General Douglas McArthur directed the Japanese Health Ministry. There were more than 300 unregulated therapies in Japan at that time. McArthur ordered all 300 to be researched by scientists at the universities, to document which ones had scientific proof of merit and which did not. At the end of 8 years, the universities reported back that "shiatsu" was the only therapeutic practice to receive scientific approval at that time. In 1955 the Japanese parliament adopted a bill on "revised anma," which gave shiatsu official government endorsement. This endorsement allowed shiatsu to be legally taught in schools throughout Japan. Shiatsu received further official Japanese government recognition as a therapy in 1964. In the early 1970s shiatsu began spreading to the West and rapidly gained widespread acceptance.

Although shiatsu and its distant cousin acupuncture are now considered medically sound and are accepted methods of treatment for more than one quarter of the world's population, the United States and many other Western nations still consider both techniques as quasi-experimental. However, many US hospitals now allow the use of acupuncture, and medical students are taught the theories and practice of acupuncture, shiatsu, and macrobiotics as part of exposure to what is called "complementary and alternative medicine." Shiatsu is now part of the growing trend and movement toward integrative medicine.

Everything Is Energy

Many followers of Asian health traditions believe that the natural state of humanity is to be healthy. The simple understanding that humans are equipped to heal themselves and that they can also help others forms the underlying philosophical foundation of shiatsu. Shiatsu acts like a spark or catalyst to the human body, and a combination of treatment and healthy lifestyle form the basis of total care. The major underlying principles of shiatsu are derived from the tenets of Asian medicine but may actually be seen as a reflection of modern scientific thought. Simply stated, "Everything is energy." When considered in the context of molecular structure, all matter is a manifestation of energy. Shiatsu interacts directly with this energy and therefore with life itself.

From the perspective of classic Chinese medicine, energy moves along distinct pathways, meridians, or channels (kieraku in Japanese). Accounts in the shiatsu tradition posit that meridians were discovered when certain acupoints (specific locations along the meridians) were stimulated and beneficial results were observed. For example, asthma-like symptoms caused by certain types of battle wounds were relieved when the corresponding acupoint was touched, and menstrual pain was reduced when a heated rock from a fireplace brushed against a point on the inner thigh.

Studies have been conducted by biophysicists in Japan, China, and France. They postulate that measurement of acupoint electrical potential provides a biophysical marker that illustrates the objective existence of the meridian system. They found that acupoints have a lower skin resistance. When an electrical current is passed through a classical acupoint, it has higher electrical conductance and lower resistance than the surrounding area. They also discovered that when disease or illness is present, pathological changes take place in the body, whereas changes are found in the resistance of relevant meridians and acupoints. Researchers also found that the external environment, such as temperature, season, and time of day, changed the resistance of acupoints.

At the Lanzhou Medical College in China, a test of the acupoints of the stomach meridian showed significant variations in conductance when the stomach lining was stimulated by cold or hot water, either before or after eating. In Beijing, ear acupoint research reported that low resistance points on the outer rim of the ear were elevated either in the presence of disease or following long-term stimulation of a corresponding internal organ. In addition to scientific theory the effects of shiatsu are reported by the experiences of clients and practitioners. Asthmatic clients experience volatility (pain and sensitivity) along their lung meridian. Clients with lower digestive track symptoms, such as constipation, experience this same sensitivity along their large intestine meridians. When clients experience the connection with the body's own level of pain along related organ meridian lines, it makes shiatsu therapy evident.

Some shiatsu practitioners believe that meridians develop from energy centers in the body called "chakras" and that organ systems develop guided by the meridian network. There is some support for this belief among theories regarding development of the embryo along energetic lines. In shiatsu, there are 10 meridians seen directly related to internal organs, 2 indirectly related, and 2 related to systems not recognized by Western medicine.

Along the meridian lines are points called "tsubos" (SUE-bows). The word Tsu-bo derives from the Oriental characters meaning hole or orifice and position, the position of the hole. Traditionally the word hole was combined with other terms, such as hollow, passageway, transport, and ki, or qi (vital energy). This usage suggests that the holes on the surface of the body were regarded as routes of access to the body's internal cavities. The acupoints are spots where ki or qi is accessed.

Shiatsu recognizes three phases in the historical development of the concept of these holes or acupoints. In the earliest phase people would use any body location that was painful or uncomfortable. Because there were no specific locations for the points, they had no names. In the second phase, after a long period of practice and experience, certain points became identified with specific diseases. The ability of distinct points to affect and be affected by local or distant pain and disease became predictable. In the final phase, many previously localized points, each with a singular function, became integrated into a larger system that related and grouped diverse points systematically according to similar functions. This integration is called the "meridian" or "channel" system.

Acupuncture without Needles?

Although the analogy is not completely accurate, shiatsu is often called "acupuncture without needles." To alter a client's internal energy system or pattern, an acupuncturist inserts needles in the same tsubos as used by a shiatsu practitioner. The most significant difference between the two disciplines is that whereas acupuncture punctures the skin and is performed by extensively trained doctors, shiatsu is noninvasive and can be practiced by either a professional therapist or a layperson. Shiatsu is also a whole-body technique versus one that is defined by the insertion of needles at specific tsubos. Acupuncture is considered more symptom-oriented in that people are unlikely to go to an acupuncturist without a specific complaint, whereas clients often equate shiatsu with health maintenance and go for treatments without particular "problems." Although some consider shiatsu a close cousin to acupuncture, others suggest a more "distant cousin" relationship. The distinctions between the two disciplines are worth noting. It is also important to note here that simple shiatsu can be practiced with little or no understanding of the underlying principles. The practitioner (or patient) does not have to agree with the principles or understand them to provide shiatsu. However, the techniques are part of a more complicated healing system that, when adhered to and studied, provides more effective results.

A simple analogy for understanding the meridian pathways and tsubos in relation to the body's internal organ systems is that tsubos can be compared with a system of volcanoes on the earth's surface. We know that a volcano's real energy is not at the surface but is found deep inside the earth. A volcano is a superficial manifestation of the underlying energy. In a similar fashion a tsubo can be thought of as a manifestation of the underlying energy of the organ system. This relationship does not imply that the therapist should ignore the area of pain a shiatsu client may describe. However, a classically trained shiatsu practitioner looks past sore shoulders, ligaments, and tendons (unless the cause of the pain is trauma to these structures) and focuses on the related organ system via the meridian network. Philosophically, shiatsu practitioners relate health to the condition of the related "vital" organs (i.e., those associated with the meridian system). Although shiatsu is noninvasive and appears to deal with external or surface pain, according to shiatsu theory, it stimulates, sedates, and balances energy inside the body as a way to address the root causes of surface and bodily discomfort.

Principles

The principles of Asian medicine evident in shiatsu theory and practice posit that there are two fundamentals states existing in the universe. These two states, called "yin" and "yang", exist side by side and are considered both complementary and opposing (see Chapter 14). Asian medicine looks at health more as a manifestation of balance between yin and yang and how an imbalance may allow pain, infection, or disease to manifest. When a person's health and metabolism adjust to universal cosmic guidelines, natural harmony occurs from the inside out. Varying states of yin and yang are experienced.

In defining yin and yang, a continuum exists between the extremes of each. In shiatsu major organs are paired together under one of the five major elements, or phases. Each pair has both a yang and yin organ. One organ is more compact and tighter (yang), whereas the other is more open and vessel-like (yin). The five elements, wood (tree), fire, earth (soil), metal, and water, proceed in a clockwise manner within the five-element wheel used in Asian medicine.

According to shiatsu principles an organ is fed by its opposite energy. For the shiatsu practitioner, pressing and rubbing movements proceed in the direction energy travels along each respective meridian. Shiatsu texts often use the term structure to describe an organ, whereas acupuncture texts may describe the same organ in terms of the energy that feeds it through the meridian. A yang organ is fed by yin energy. A shiatsu practitioner generally describes the compact kidney as yang because of its structure (compared with its paired, more hollow and open yin organ, the bladder). A classically trained acupuncturist generally describes the kidney as yin because it is fed by yin energy that flows up the body on the kidney meridian. Such differences between the two disciplines in terms of descriptive language can be confusing, although little if any differences in application of goals, practice, or theory really exist.

Another major principle applied to the practice of shiatsu involves the concepts of kyo (KEY-o) and jitsu (JIT-sue). Kyo is considered empty or vacant, whereas jitsu is considered full, excessive, or overflowing. A jitsu condition along the gallbladder meridian may be a manifestation of a gallbladder imbalance, resulting perhaps from recent consumption of a large pizza and two dishes of ice cream. A kyo or empty condition along the lung meridian (and within the lung itself) may exist in an individual who does not exercise and rarely expands his or her chest cavity or heart. Understanding and finding these energy manifestations is critical to diagnosis in shiatsu practice and is an ongoing, lifelong learning experience for the serious shiatsu practitioner. Although it is generally easy to find jitsu, or excess, it is much harder to find emptiness or vacancy (kyo) within the meridian network. One of the keys to doing highly successful or refined shiatsu is the ability to find specific kyo within the body or the organ's meridian network and then to manipulate it effectively.

SCOPE OF PRACTICE

Shiatsu massage is not viewed by its practitioners as a panacea. Shiatsu philosophy is very clear in reinforcing the need for dietary and lifestyle guidance and changes to complement and support a shiatsu session (or series of sessions). The choices made by the recipients of treatment are theirs. Many recipients are content to stay at the level at which shiatsu is simply used for pain reduction and for producing a "calmed sense of revitalization." However, others who are open to the underpinnings of shiatsu philosophy may be willing to take additional steps suggested by a classically trained shiatsu practitioner regarding diet and behavior modification.

With sufficient training, the shiatsu practitioner learns to view the energy manifesting at major tsubos on the surface of the skin as indicative of the underlying condition of the organ to which the tsubo is related and connected. For instance, a client may think shoulder pain is caused by how he or she sleeps or sits at a desk. A classically trained shiatsu practitioner does not ignore these factors but looks beyond to the underlying organ system and the foods that affect that organ system. The practitioner attempts to change the energy pattern not just by working at the proximate points of client complaint and distress but also along the entire meridian (or set of meridians).

Shiatsu training touches on the principles of Asian medicine because the nature of the organ systems and their related energy should be understood for effective treatment to occur, although, as mentioned previously, this knowledge is not an absolute requirement to practice shiatsu. How far this education goes, particularly in relation to the underlying effects of specific foods and their yin and yang effects on various organs and the body as a whole, depends on the quality of the school, knowledge of the instructor, and interest of the students.

The Art of Diagnosis

The art of shiatsu diagnosis is a lifelong learning process. Subtle yet specific, diagnosis is an ongoing and evolving pursuit, in which a practitioner is continually mastering and learning. Modern diagnostic techniques are a relatively recent development in the history of medicine. Powerful, precise, and accurate to a large extent, their contribution to the improvement of the human condition cannot be denied. However, diagnostic procedures in Western medicine use a disease-oriented model and tend to focus on parts (e.g., cells, tissues, organs) rather than on the whole organism. For example, Louis Pasteur (1822 to 1895) believed that microbes were the primary cause of disease. Although this theory has proved correct and is applicable to a large number of cases, germs are not the sole cause of disease. Although Asian diagnosis has been practiced for thousands of years, Western medicine has largely ignored its value.

In shiatsu there are two underlying levels of diagnosing human beings: constitutional and conditional. Simply stated, an individual's constitution is what he or she was born with. Along with inherited traits, the quality of life, energy, and food intake experienced by the mother while a person is in utero are all considered factors that make up a person's constitution. A person's condition is the sum of his or her experience, which includes diet. In classical shiatsu diagnosis both constitution and condition are assessed according to the methods listed next.

Four methods of observing "phenomena" are used:
1. Bo-shin: diagnosis through observation
2. Bun-shin: diagnosis through sound
3. Mon-shin: diagnosis through questioning
4. Set su-shin: diagnosis through touch

Each day, whether we realize it or not, we use the first three methods of observation extensively in our interactions with others and the environment. We all have experienced a funny feeling in our stomachs when we enter a room that has recently been the site of some tension related to human interaction. We choose partners based on some innate sense of energy recognition we find compatible with our own. Although we are unaware that we use aspects of Asian diagnosis in our everyday lives, we nonetheless make assessments and judgments based on these principles. Without these "diagnostic skills," we would not survive. Shiatsu uses the first three methods liberally and also relies heavily on the fourth.

In traditional shiatsu, diagnosis begins with the first contact between client and practitioner, whether in person or on the telephone. The client's tone of voice, speed of delivery, and choice of words give clues to the trained ear regarding the condition and constitution of the shiatsu client.

On meeting a client for the first time, constitutional and conditional assessments are made. How did the client enter the room? Did she walk upright? Did he smile or frown? Was her handshake strong or weak? Was his hand wet, damp, dry, hot, cold? The client is often unaware that a classically trained shiatsu therapist begins work with the first contact and continues the assessment the minute a face-to-face meeting begins. Visual diagnosis and verbal questioning continue as the first meeting between client and therapist proceeds.

To arrive at a constitutional diagnosis, the therapist looks at various physical attributes. No single factor observed gives a total picture, but a macro assessment takes the various micro elements into account. Size of ears, shape and size of head, distance between the eyes, size of mouth, and size of hands are fundamental observations made in constitutional diagnosis before any physical treatment begins.

Factors considered in conditional assessment are slightly different but work in tandem with the overall assessment. The stated reason for the visit is a factor. In addition, tone and volume of the client's voice, pupil size, eye color, color and condition of the tongue, condition of the nails, and response to palpation along specific points on the hands and arms may be used. Pulse diagnosis (the act of reading distinctly differently levels of heartbeats near the wrists on both hands) may be used, depending on the practitioner's level of training. Generally speaking, pulse diagnosis is more the tool of an acupuncturist, but it has been and can be used by a properly trained shiatsu provider.

These four diagnostic methods (observation, sound, questioning, and touch) are used to develop a singular yin-yang analysis. At its basic level Asian diagnosis sets out to determine whether a person is vibrationally, or energetically, more yin or more yang because these two opposing but complementary states of energy affect each of us.

The diagnostic assessment process continues along specific lines:

Yang diagnosis: Excess body heat and desire for coolness; great thirst and desire for fluids; constipation and hard stools; scanty, hot, dark urine.

Yin diagnosis: Cold feeling and desire for warmth; lack of thirst and preference for hot drinks; loose stools; profuse, clear urine; flat taste in mouth; poor appetite.

The key is determining what tendency within an individual may be contributing to his or her state and also the particular organ or organs that have a jitsu or kyo condition and then working those organs' meridians to change that state.

At this point the practitioner's hands become the primary diagnostic tools. Although diagnosis is an ongoing process during treatment, traditional shiatsu first assesses by palpation the major organs located in the client's hara, or abdomen. Alternatively, some styles of shiatsu begin a treatment session with touch diagnosis on the upper back, an area that also yields a vast amount of information regarding a person's condition. Assessment and diagnosis include palpatory observations that describe the following physical properties: tightness or looseness, fullness or emptiness, hot or cold, dry or wet, resistant or open, stiff or flexible.

Diagnosis in a shiatsu session does not cease after an initial assessment but is an ongoing process of observation, listening, feeling, and changing focus based on continuously revealed information. The ability to quickly make an accurate diagnosis can be extremely helpful to a practitioner and client in their mutual attempt to create energetic change for the receiving partner. However, shiatsu can be effective in the hands of a relatively unskilled diagnostician. By following the simple concept of paying attention to what is going on underneath one's hands, a layperson with relatively little training can provide an effective, relaxing, and enjoyable shiatsu treatment for family and friends in a nonprofessional setting.

Learning Shiatsu

Unlike some disciplines, shiatsu is easy to learn. It is not possible for a layperson to practice chiropractic, acupuncture, or osteopathy because medical professionals need not only training but also time and continuing education to master techniques and improve skills. Shiatsu also requires a disciplined approach, constant practice, and continuing study to develop in-depth understanding. However, the practice remains simple, effective, and safe. Shiatsu techniques can be learned and safely applied by anyone, typically resulting in positive effects for both the recipient and provider. It can be performed anywhere, takes place fully clothed, and requires no special tools, machines, or oils.

Although ki may indeed emanate from the giver's fingertips, it may not be in this way or only in this way that shiatsu works. More than 150 years ago, Shinsai Ota, in a book on Ampuku (hara, or abdominal) shiatsu, emphasized that "honest, sincere, and simple Shiatsu is much better than merely technique-oriented professional Shiatsu." Indeed, shiatsu training often emphasizes that the most important element is to be in touch with what is going on right under one's hands. Experts agree, indicating that when a practitioner applies pressure and stimulation, he or she should then react and follow up based on an intuitive sense of and reaction to internal changes within the recipient. A traditionally trained shiatsu practitioner, knowledgeable in the energy fundamentals of yin and yang and applying those principles in his or her life, is arguably better suited to respond intuitively to the client. It is believed that intuition is enhanced by being in harmony with nature, a condition achieved by following the guidelines of living within nature's principles and the earth's rhythms of yin and yang. Harmony in the body is achieved by being in harmony with the universe.

Relaxed and Revitalized

Because shiatsu can yield a "calmed sense of revitalization," the combination of being both relaxed and energized is an experience that may be savored throughout the day. Americans often equate "calm and relaxed" with an inactive state. Although shiatsu yields different results for different people, one of the most unique effects experienced by most clients is indeed this calmed sense of revitalization. It is not uncommon for a new shiatsu client to report, when treated by a competent practitioner, that he or she has "never felt this way before."

One reason for the difference in the energetic effects of shiatsu as opposed to other techniques (usually called "regular massage" by the general public) is easy to explain. In many forms of therapeutic massage a technique described as effleurage or stroking (sweeping the skin with the hands) is used. The benefits of this type of movement on the skin are many, including stimulation of blood flow and the movement of lymph. Although this technique is beneficial, one of its effects is often a feeling of lethargy. Because the effects of shiatsu are realized more on the underlying blockage of energy related to the body's organ systems than on the lymphatic system, a shiatsu session can yield a feeling of increased short- and long-term energy. This is why chair massage using shiatsu techniques is so appropriate and why many consider it superior to other techniques in the corporate setting. Employees do not experience the short-term negative energetic effects (lethargy) of effleurage, but rather the energetic boost, the calmed sense of revitalization so often associated with effective shiatsu technique.

Both anma and European massage directly stimulate blood circulation, emphasizing the release of stagnated blood in the skin and muscles and tension and stiffness resulting from circulatory congestion. On the other hand, shiatsu emphasizes correction and maintenance of bone structure, joints, tendons, muscles, and meridian lines, whose malfunctioning distort the body's energy and autonomic nervous system causing disease.

Like other methods, shiatsu is best received with an empty stomach. This may not always be possible, and recent food consumption is certainly no bar to receiving shiatsu. However, practitioners and recipients should bear in mind that when the body's energies are focused inward toward digestion, a shiatsu session, with its attempt to change the body's energies, is compromised and less effective.

In some ways the beginning of a shiatsu session is similar to other massage styles. The room used should be simple, clean, and quiet. A thorough history of the client and his or her concerns should be taken. Questions regarding sleep patterns, lifestyle, eating habits, and work history are not uncommon. A high level of trust should be established quickly. Often a client is seated in a chair or on a floor mat as the shiatsu practitioner observes and asks questions regarding the client's expectations and level of understanding. Diagnostic techniques to determine the client's constitution and condition are undertaken. The hands, eyes, tongue, and coloration along the upper and lower limbs may be examined. Several deep breaths to begin the process may be suggested. A well-trained shiatsu practitioner obtains a complete history to uncover any risk factors affecting the appropriateness of shiatsu treatment. Clinical experience and training, coupled with good references regarding a therapist's skills and practice, should be the determining factors in selecting a shiatsu practitioner. There are many variations to the basic techniques, and numerous schools that teach specific shiatsu practices offer more distinct focus to the underlying themes presented earlier. The American Organization of Body Therapies of Asia (AOBTA) notes 12 specific areas of Asian technique. The six major schools of Asian practice generally regarded as shiatsu are described in the following sections, as shown on the AOBTA website.

FIVE ELEMENT SHIATSU

The primary emphasis of five element shiatsu is to identify a pattern of disharmony through use of the four examinations and to harmonize that pattern with an appropriate treatment plan. Hands-on techniques and preferences for assessment vary with the practitioner, depending on their individual background and training. The radial pulse usually provides the most critical and detailed information. Palpation of the back and/or abdomen and a detailed verbal history serve to confirm the assessment. Considerations of the client's lifestyle and emotional and psychological factors are all considered important. Although this approach uses the paradigm of the five elements to tonify, sedate, or control patterns of disharmony, practitioners of this style also consider hot or cold and internal or external symptoms and signs.

JAPANESE SHIATSU

Although shiatsu is primarily the application of pressure, usually with the thumbs along the meridian lines, extensive soft-tissue manipulation and both active and passive exercise and stretching may be part of the treatments. Extensive use of cutaneous-visceral reflexes in the abdomen and on the back are also characteristics of shiatsu. The emphasis of shiatsu is the treatment of the whole meridian; however, effective points are also used. The therapist assesses the condition of the patient's body as treatment progresses. Therapy and diagnosis are one.

MACROBIOTIC SHIATSU

Founded by Shizuko Yamamoto and based on George Ohsawa's philosophy that each individual is an integral part of nature, macrobiotic shiatsu supports a natural lifestyle and heightened instincts for improving health. Assessments are through visual, verbal, and touch techniques (including pulses) and the five transformations.

Treatment involves noninvasive touch and pressure using hand and barefoot techniques and stretches to facilitate the flow of ki and to strengthen the bodymind. Dietary guidance, medicinal plant foods, breathing techniques, and home remedies are emphasized, and corrective exercises, postural rebalancing, palm healing, self-shiatsu, and qigong are included in macrobiotic shiatsu.

Shiatsu Anma Therapy

Shiatsu anma therapy uses a unique blending of two of the most popular Asian bodywork forms practiced in Japan. Dr. Kaneko introduces traditional anma massage therapy based on the energetic system of Traditional Chinese Medicine in the long form and contemporary pressure therapy, which is based on neuromusculoskeletal system in the short form. Ampuku, abdominal massage therapy, is another foundation of anma massage therapy in his school.

Zen Shiatsu

Zen shiatsu is characterized by the theory of Kyo-Jitsu, its physical and psychologic manifestations, and its application to abdominal diagnosis. Zen shiatsu theory is based on an extended meridian system that includes and expands the location of the traditional acupuncture meridians. The focus of a zen shiatsu session is on the use of meridian lines rather than on specific points. In addition, zen shiatsu does not adhere to a fixed sequence or set of methods that are applied to all. It uses appropriate methods for the unique pattern of each individual. Zen shiatsu was developed by Shizuto Masunaga.

The extended meridian network described and taught by Masunaga is a highly regarded part of shiatsu education. It is taught in quality schools as an integral part of shiatsu theory, diagnosis, and style. It is common for a practitioner to learn the extended meridian network toward the end of his or her shiatsu education as an extension to the classical meridian network, in the same manner that Master Masunaga explored this expansion in shiatsu thinking, theory, and practice.

Research

The results of a number of clinical trials have been published. What follows is a brief listing of these studies, grouped by category. A study in a university-affiliated hospital documented a decrease in systolic, diastolic, and mean arterial pressure, as well as heart rate and skin blood flow, when acupressure points were stimulated by pressure. Researchers concluded that acupressure can significantly and positively influence the cardiovascular system. A crossover design study in which patients were taught how to self-administer acupressure concluded that real acupressure was more effective than sham acupressure for reducing shortness of breath.

Finger pressure applied bilaterally to two "major" acupressure points during the first 10 days of a chemotherapy cycle reduced the intensity and experience of nausea among women undergoing therapy. The use of acupressure at the P6 acupoint was shown to reduce the incidence of nausea and vomiting within 24 hours of anesthesia from 42% to 19% compared with placebo. The use of acupressure at the P6 point was shown to reduce the incidence of nausea and vomiting after Caesarean section compared with placebo. Acupressure bands placed at the P6 points on subjects receiving general anesthesia for ambulatory surgery experienced less nausea (23%) versus the control group (41%), suggesting this method as an alternative to conventional antiemetic treatment. The incidence of postoperative vomiting in children was significantly lower (20%) than in the placebo group (68%) when stationary acupressure was applied to the Korean K-K9 point for 30 minutes before and 24 hours after undergoing strabismus surgery. The stimulation of the P6 (Neiguan) acupoint was determined to prevent nausea and vomiting in adults, although no antiemetic effects were noted in children undergoing strabismus surgery. However, it was determined that prophylactic use of bilateral acuplaster in children reduced the incidence of vomiting from 35.5% to 14.7% in the early emesis phase, 58.1% to 23.5% in the late emesis phase, and 64.5% to 29.4% overall. Researchers concluded that the use of acupuncture plaster reduced vomiting in children undergoing strabismus correction.

Finding a Practitioner

There are currently no government regulatory standards in the United States for shiatsu practitioners, while the American Massage Therapy Association (AMTA) cites 30 states that have regulations governing massage therapy. There are more than 100,000 credentialed practitioners at this writing. Numerous schools of massage offer certificate programs in shiatsu or more broad-based programs that include shiatsu massage. These programs may be weekend seminars of 1 or 2 days or may provide 600 or more hours of training particular to shiatsu. It is not uncommon for schools to offer 350 to 500 hours of training in classical shiatsu with an additional 150 hours in anatomy and physiology. There appears to be a growing trend for internships in all schools of massage.

The AOBTA (formerly the American Asian Body Therapy Association) is the largest and most prevalent organization particular to the practice of shiatsu. Certified practitioner applicants must complete a 500-hour program, preferably at a school or institution recognized by AOBTA. The AMTA is a general association of massage practitioners; it does not actively focus on shiatsu therapy. It is a highly respected association that meets with the AOBTA as a federated massage-supporting organization. The AMTA's mission is to develop and advance the art, science, and practice of massage therapy in a caring, professional, and ethical manner to promote the health and welfare of humanity.

The American Bodywork and Massage Professionals (ABMP) is another highly respected association of massage professionals. Unlike the AOBTA and the AMTA, the ABMP is a for-profit organization.

The National Certification Board for Therapeutic Massage and Bodywork (NCBTMB) is a nationally recognized credentialing body formed to set high standards for those who practice therapeutic massage and bodywork. It accomplishes this through a nationally recognized certification program that evaluates the competency of its practitioners. Since 1992 more than 40,000 massage therapists and bodyworkers have received their certification. The NCBTMB examination is now legally recognized in most states and in many municipalities. The NCBTMB represents a diverse group of massage therapists, not just shiatsu practitioners. A minimum of 500 hours of formal massage education and successful completion of a written exam are the basic requirements for certification. Practitioners must be recertified every 4 years.

A person considering the use of any massage therapy as an adjunct to health maintenance should carefully select the provider of that therapy. In addition to personal references, it is important to evaluate the practitioner's training, experience, professional affiliations, and certification.

Although shiatsu, like reiki, has not been subjected to extensive research scrutiny, its clear effects on stress reduction and relaxation, as well as influences on breathing and respiration, can be used to help anxiety and lessen perception of pain, as well as bringing healing attention, intention, and benefits to specific painful locations of the body.

REFERENCE

Engebretson, J. & Wardell, D. W. (2002). Experience of a reiki session. *Alternative Therapies in Health and Medicine, 8*(2), 48–53.

Suggested Readings can be found on the companion website, http://www.micozzipainconditions.com.

Chapter 18

Ayurveda and Traditional Treatments of India

Three traditional medicinal systems predominate in modern India: Ayurveda, Siddha, and Unani. Ayurveda is found mostly in northern India and in Kerala in the south. Siddha medicine is found mostly in Tamil Nadu and in parts of Kerala. Unani is found throughout India and Pakistan, mainly in the urban areas, and actually derives from ancient Persian and Greco-Arabic medicine, or *Tibb'*, rather than Vedic or Hindu Indian sources.

This chapter describes Ayurveda (and other, related traditional systems), Siddha medicine, and the contemporary development of Maharishi Ayurveda in India and the West. Yoga is a meditative and devotional practice that originated in India. It is not formally part of Ayurveda, and its focus in the West is primarily through physical aspects as expressed in Hatha-Yoga, for example, as described in Chapter 19.

Traditional medicine, in addition to being a highly developed and complex form of ethnomedicine, remains in living use as an available form of primary health care in India. It is also becoming more available in the West as a "complementary and alternative" medical system that is sometimes accessed in the practice of "integrative medicine."

AYURVEDA: THE SCIENCE OF LIFE

Ayurveda is literally the science of life, or longevity. As with any popular development, aspects of this Indian medical system and its cures have sometimes been appropriated by individuals (such as popular "gurus" in the West) not wholly familiar with the basic assumptions of Ayurveda as a science of longevity. However, scholars have undertaken serious study of this ancient healing tradition. The fundamental principles and practices of traditional Ayurveda may be understood from their work on the classical Sanskrit sources and from accounts from traditional Indian practitioners.

On the basis of available literary sources, the history of Indian medicine generally occurred in four main phases (Zysk, 1991, 1993). The first, or Vedic, phase dates from 1200 to 800 BCE. Information about medicine during this period is obtained from numerous curative incantations and references to healing that are

Acknowledgments to Marc Micozzi and Julie Staples for prior contributions in Micozzi, M. S. (ed.), (2016). *Fundamentals of complementary and alternative medicine* (5th ed.). St Louis: Elsevier Health Sciences/Saunders.

found in the Atharvaveda and the Rigveda, two religious scriptures that reveal a "magicoreligious" approach to healing (Zysk, 1993). The second, or classical, phase is marked by the advent of the first Sanskrit medical treatises, the Caraka.

Samhita (Sharma, 1981–1994) and Sushruta Samhita (Bhishagratna, 1983), which probably dates from a few centuries before to several centuries after the start of the common era. This period includes all medical treatises dating from before the Muslim invasions of India at the beginning of the 11th century. These works tend to follow the earlier classical compilations closely and provide the basis of traditional Ayurveda. The third, or syncretic, phase is marked by clear influences from Unani, Siddha, and other nonclassical medical systems in India. Bhavamishra's 16th-century Bhavaprakasha text shows results of these influences, such as diagnosis by examination of pulse or urine (Upadhyay, 1986). This phase extends from the time of the Muslim incursions to the present era.

The fourth phase may be phrased as "New Age Ayurveda," wherein the classical paradigm is being adapted to the world of modern science and technology, including quantum physics, mind-body science, and advanced biomedical science. This recent manifestation of Ayurveda is most visible in the Western world, although there are indications that it is filtering back to India in its worldwide reach. These four phases of Indian medical history provide a simple chronological grid for understanding the development of this ancient system of medicine. A more comprehensive chronology of historical developments relating to traditional Indian medicines in the region of Middle Asia is given in Table 18.1.

From its beginnings during the Vedic era, Indian medicine has adhered closely to the fundamental connection between the microcosm and macrocosm as in Western traditions until the modern era. Human beings are seen as minute representations of the universe and contain within them everything that also makes up the surrounding world. Comprehending the world is crucial to comprehending the human, and, conversely, understanding the world is necessary to understanding the human.

FIVE ELEMENTS

According to Ayurveda, the cosmos consists of five basic elements: earth, air, fire, water, and space. Certain forces cause these elements to interact, giving rise to all

TABLE 18.1 *Medical Traditions of South Asia and the Middle East*

Phase	Dates	Sources	Modalities
I. Vedic	1200-800 BCE	Atharvaveda, Rigveda	Magicoreligious
II. Classic	700 BCE-AD 400	Sanskrit texts: Caraka, Sushruta, Samhita	Herbal medicines
III. Syncretic	1000-1980	Muslim influences, Unani, Siddha, Bhavaprakasha	Pulse, urine diagnosis
IV. New Age	1980-2010	Maharishi Ayurveda	Quantum physics

that exists. In human beings these five elements occur and combine as the three *doshas,* forces that, along with the seven *dhatus* (tissues) and three *malas* (waste products), make up the human body.

THREE DOSHAS

When in equilibrium the three *doshas* maintain health, but when an imbalance occurs among them, they defile the normal functioning of the body, leading to the manifestation of disease. An imbalance indicates an increase or decrease in one, two, or all three of the *doshas.* The three *doshas* are *vata, pitta,* and *kapha* (Svoboda, 1984; Table 18.2).

TABLE 18.2 *The Three Doshas: Vata, Pitta, Kapha*

Dosha	Effect of Balanced Dosha	Effect of Imbalanced Dosha	Factors Aggravating
Vata	Exhilaration	Rough skin	Excessive exercise
	Clear and alert mind	Weight loss	Wakefulness
	Perfect functioning	Anxiety, worry	Falling, bone fractures
	of bowels and urinary	Restlessness	Tuberculosis
	tract	Constipation	Suppression of natural
	Proper formation of all	Decreased strength	urges
	bodily tissues	**Arthritis**	Cold
	Sound sleep	Hypertension	Fear or grief
	Excellent vitality and	Rheumatic disorder	Agitation or anger
	immunity	Cardiac arrhythmia	Fasting
		Insomnia	Pungent, astringent, or
		Irritable bowel	bitter foods
		syndrome	In the United States: Late
			autumn and winter
			In India: Summer and
			rainy season
Pitta	Lustrous complexion	Yellowish complexion	Anger
	Contentment	Excessive body heat	Strong sunshine
	Perfect digestion	Insufficient sleep	Burning sensations
	Softness of body	Weak digestion	Fasting
	Perfectly balanced heat	Inflammation	Sesame products, linseed
	and thirst mechanisms	Inflammatory bowel	Yogurt
	Balanced intellect	diseases	Wine, vinegar
		Skin diseases	Pungent, sour, or salty
		Heartburn	foods
		Peptic ulcer	In the United States:
		Anger	Summer and early
			autumn
			In India: Rainy season
			and autumn

TABLE 18.2 *The Three Doshas: Vata, Pitta, Kapha—cont'd*

Dosha	Effect of Balanced Dosha	Effect of Imbalanced Dosha	Factors Aggravating
Kapha	Strength	Pale complexion	Sleeping during daytime
	Normal joints	Coldness	Heavy food
	Stability of mind	Laziness, dullness	Sweet, sour, or salty foods
	Dignity	Excessive sleep	Milk products
	Affectionate, forgiving nature	Sinusitis	Sugar
	Strong and properly proportioned body	Respiratory diseases, asthma	In the United States: Spring
	Courage	Excessive weight gain	In India: Late winter and spring
	Vitality	Loose joints	
		Depression	

Entries in **bold** type indicate pain and pain-related conditions.

Vata or *vayu*, meaning "wind," is composed of the elements air and space. It is like the principle of kinetic energy and is responsible for all bodily movement and nervous functions. It is located below the navel, in the bladder, large intestines, nervous system, pelvic region, thighs, bone marrow, and legs; its principal seat is the colon. When disrupted, its primary manifestations are gastrointestinal gas and muscular or nervous energy, leading to pain.

Pitta, or bile, is made up of the elements fire and water. It governs enzymes and hormones, and is responsible for digestion, pigmentation, body temperature, hunger, thirst, sight, courage, and mental activity. It is located between the navel and the chest, in the stomach, small intestines, liver, spleen, skin, and blood; its principal seat is the stomach. When disrupted, its primary manifestations are acid and bile, leading to inflammation, also associated with pain.

Kapha, meaning "phlegm," is made up of the elements of earth and water. It connotes the principle of cohesion and stability. It regulates *vata* and *pitta* and is responsible for keeping the body lubricated and maintaining its solid nature, tissues, sexual power, and strength. It also influences patience. Its normal locations are the upper part of the body, the thorax, head, neck, upper portion of the stomach, pleural cavity, fat tissues, and areas between joints. Its principal seat is the lungs. When it is disrupted, its primary manifestations are liquid and mucus, leading to swelling, with or without discharge, also associated with pain.

The attributes of each *dosha* help to determine an individual's basic bodily and mental makeup and to isolate which *dosha* is responsible for pain and disease. *Vata* is dry, cold, light, irregular, mobile, rough, and abundant. Dryness occurs when *vata* is disturbed and is a side effect of motion. Too much dryness produces irregularity in the body and mind. *Pitta* is hot, light, intense, fluid, liquid, putrid, pungent, and sour. Heat appears when *pitta* is disturbed and produces irritability in the body and mind. *Kapha* is heavy, unctuous, cold, stable, dense, soft, and smooth. Heaviness occurs when *kapha* is disturbed and produces slowness in body and mind.

Seven Dhatus

The seven *dhatus*, or tissues, are responsible for sustaining the body. Each *dhatu* is responsible for the one that comes next in the following order, according to Zysk (1993).

1. Rasa, meaning sap or juice, includes the tissue fluids, bile, lymph, and plasma and functions as nourishment. It comes from digested food.
2. Blood includes the red blood cells and functions to invigorate the body.
3. Flesh includes muscle tissue and functions as stabilization.
4. Fat includes adipose tissue and functions as lubrication.
5. Bone includes bone and cartilage and functions as support.
6. Marrow includes red and yellow bone marrow and functions as filling for the bones.
7. *Shukra* includes male and female sexual fluids and functions in reproduction and immunity.

The Three Malas

The *malas* are the waste products of digestion. Ayurveda delineates three principal *malas*: urine, feces, and sweat. A fourth category of other waste products includes fatty excretions from the skin and intestines, cebum (ear wax), mucus of the nose, saliva, tears, hair, and nails. According to Ayurveda, an individual should evacuate the bowels once a day and eliminate urine six times a day.

Importance of Diet and Digestion

Ayurveda considers digestion to be the most important function that takes place in the human body. It provides all that is required to sustain the organism and is the principal cause for all maladies from which an individual suffers. The process of digestion and assimilation of nutrients is discussed under the topics of the Agnis (enzymes), Ama (improperly digested food and drink), and Srotas (channels of circulation).

Three Agnis

The Agnis, or enzymes, assist in the digestion and assimilation of food and are divided into three types according to Zysk (1993).

1. Jatharagni is active in the mouth, stomach, and gastrointestinal tract and helps to break down food. The waste product of feces results from this activity.
2. Bhutagnis are five enzymes located in the liver. They adapt the broken-down food into a homologous chyle in accordance with the five elements and assist the chyle to assimilate with the corresponding elements in the body. The homologous chyle circulates in the blood channels as rasa, nourishing the body and supplying the seven *dhatus*.
3. Dhatvagnis are seven enzymes that synthesize the seven *dhatus* from the assimilated chyle homologized with the five elements. The remaining waste products result from this activity.

Ama

Ama is the chief cause of disease and is formed when there is a decrease in enzyme activity. A product of improperly digested food and drink, it takes the form of a liquid sludge that travels through the same channels as the chyle. However, because of its density, it lodges in different parts of the body, blocking the channels. It often mixes with the *doshas* that circulate through the same pathways, and it gravitates to a weak or stressed organ or to a site of a disease manifestation. Because all diseases invariably come from Ama, the word Amaya, meaning "coming from Ama," is a synonym for disease. Internal diseases begin with Ama, and external diseases produce Ama. In general, Ama can be detected by a coating on the tongue, turbid urine with foul odor, and feces that is passed with undigested food, an offensive odor, and abundant gas. The principal course of treatment in Ayurveda involves the elimination of Ama and the restoration of the balance of the *doshas*.

Thirteen Kinds of Srotas

The Srotas are the vessels or channels of the body through which all substances circulate. They are either large, such as the large and small intestines, uterus, arteries, and veins, or small, such as the capillaries. A healthy body has open and free-flowing channels. Blockage of the channels, usually by Ama, results in disease (Zysk, 1993).

1. Pranavahasrotas convey vitality and vital breath *(prana)* and originate in the heart and alimentary tract.
2. Udakavahasrotas convey water and fluids and originate in the palate and pancreas.
3. Annavahasrotas convey food from the outside and originate in the stomach.
4. Rasavahasrotas convey chyle, lymph, and plasma and originate in the heart and in the 10 vessels connected with the heart. Ama primarily accumulates within them.
5. Raktavahasrotas convey red blood cells and originate in the liver and spleen.
6. Mamsavahasrotas convey ingredients for muscle tissue and originate in the tendons, ligaments, and skin.
7. Medovahasrotas convey ingredients for fat tissue and originate in the kidneys and fat tissues of the abdomen.
8. Asthavahasrotas convey ingredients for bone tissue and originate in hipbone.
9. Majjavahasrotas convey ingredients for marrow and originate in the bones and joints.
10. Shukravahasrotas convey ingredients for the male and female reproductive tissues and originate in the testicles and ovaries.
11. Mutravahasrotas convey urine and originate in the kidney and bladder.
12. Purishavahasrotas convey feces and originate in the colon and rectum.
13. Svedavahasrotas convey sweat and originate in the fat tissues and hair follicles.

BODY CONSTITUTION

This broad outline presents the Ayurvedic view that the human body's anatomical parts are composed of the five basic elements, which have undergone a process of metabolism and assimilation in the body. Human beings differ in their normal bodily constitution *(prakriti)*, which is determined at the moment of conception and remains so until death. The four factors that influence constitutional type include the father, the mother (particularly her food intake), the womb, and the season of the year. A large imbalance of the *doshas* in the mother will affect the growth of the embryo and fetus, and a moderate excess of one or two of the *doshas* will affect the constitution of the child.

Prakriti

There are seven normal body constitutions *(prakriti)* based on the three *doshas*: *vata, pitta, kapha, vata-pitta, pitta-kapha, vata-kapha*, and *sama*. The latter is triple balanced, which is best but extremely rare. Most people are a combination of *doshas*, in which one *dosha* predominates. The classic characteristics of *doshas* are outlined in Box 18.1 and Table 18.2. In general, *vata*-type people tend to be anxious and fearful, exhibit light and "airy" characteristics, and are prone to *vata*-diseases. *Pitta*-type people are aggressive and impatient, exhibit fiery and hot-headed characteristics, and are prone to *pitta*-diseases. *Kapha*-type people are stable and entrenched,

---

BOX 18.1 *Classic Characteristics of Vata, Pitta, and Kapha*

Vata (Ectomorphic Constitution)
Light, thin build
Performs activity quickly
Tendency to dry skin
Aversion to cold weather
Irregular hunger and digestion
Quick to grasp new information, also quick to forget
Tendency toward worry
Tendency toward constipation
Tendency toward light and interrupted sleep

Pitta (Mesomorphic Constitution)
Moderate build
Performs activity with medium speed
Aversion to hot weather
Sharp hunger and digestion
Medium time to grasp new information
Medium memory
Tendency toward irritability and temper
Enterprising and sharp in character
Prefers cold foods and drinks
Cannot skip meals
Good speakers
Tendency toward reddish complexion and hair, moles, and freckles

BOX 18.1 *Classic Characteristics of Vata, Pitta, and Kapha—cont'd*

Kapha (Endomorphic Constitution)
Solid, heavier build
Greater strength and endurance
Slow, methodical in activity
Oily, smooth skin
Tranquil, steady personality
Slow to grasp new information, slow to forget
Slow to become excited or irritated
Sleep is heavy and for long periods
Hair is plentiful, tends to be dark color
Slow digestion, mild hunger

---

exhibit heavy, wet, and earthy characteristics, and are prone to *kapha*-diseases (Svoboda, 1984).

These are the principal factors that help the Ayurvedic physician to determine the correct course of treatment to be administered to a patient for a particular ailment.

MENTAL STATES

In addition to physical constitution, Ayurveda understands that an individual is influenced by three mental states based on the three qualities *(gunas)* of balance *(sattva)*, energy *(rajas)*, and inertia *(tamas)*. In the state of balance, the mind is in equilibrium and can discriminate correctly. In the state of energy, the mind is excessively active, causing weakness in discrimination. In the state of inertia, the mind is excessively inactive, also creating weak discrimination.

Ayurveda always has recognized that the body and the mind interact to create a healthy, normal *(prakriti)*, or unhealthy, abnormal *(vikriti)* condition. A good Ayurvedic physician will determine both the mental and physical condition of the patient before proceeding with any form of diagnosis and treatment.

NAMING DISEASE

Aspects of the Ayurvedic understanding of disease have been mentioned earlier. These understandings provide a basis for the Ayurvedic classification of disease, the naming of disease, and the manifestations of disease (Dash, 1980; Dash & Kashyap, 1980).

Ayurveda identifies three broad categories of disease, on the basis of causative factors (Zysk, 1993).

1. Adhyatmika diseases originate within the body and may be subdivided into hereditary diseases, congenital diseases, and diseases caused by one or a combination of the *doshas.*

2. Adhibhautika diseases originate outside the body and include injuries from accidents or mishaps, and, in the terminology of the modern era, from germs, viruses, and bacteria.

3. Adhidaivika diseases originate from supernatural sources, including diseases that are otherwise inexplicable, such as maladies stemming from providential causes, planetary influences, curses, and seasonal changes.

A six-step process determines the manner by which a *dosha* becomes aggravated and moves through the different channels to produce disease. An accumulation of a *dosha* leads to its aggravation, which causes it to spread through the channels until it lodges in a particular organ of the body, bringing about a manifestation of disease. After a general form of the disease appears, it progressively divides into specific varieties. As in systems of medicine worldwide, many patients consult the Ayurvedic physician only after the disease appears.

Ayurveda delineates seven basic varieties of disease on the basis of the *doshas:* diseases involving a single *dosha,* diseases involving two *doshas,* and diseases involving all three *doshas* together.

In Ayurveda, diseases receive their names in one of six ways. A disease is named for the condition it produces (fever or Jvara), its chief symptom (diarrhea or Atisara), its chief physical sign (jaundice or Pandu), its principal nature (piles or Arshas), the chief *dosha*(s) involved (wind-disease or *vata*-roga), or the chief organ involved (disease of the duodenum or Grahani). Regardless of its given name, most diseases are understood to involve one or more of the *doshas.*

During the course of a disease an Ayurvedic physician seeks to identify its site of origin, its path of transportation, and its site of manifestation. The site of manifestation of a disease usually differs from its site of origin. Recognizing this distinction enables the physician to determine the correct course of treatment.

Ayurveda describes the manifestation of all diseases in the same fundamental way. Causative factors (e.g., food, drink, regimen, season, mental state) suppress digestive (enzyme) activity in the body, leading to the formation of Ama. The circulating Ama blocks the channels. The site of the disease's origin is where the blockage occurs. The circulating Ama, often combining with one or more of the *doshas,* then takes a divergent course, referred to as the path of transportation. Finally, the *dosha(s)* and Ama mixture comes to rest in and afflicts a certain body part, which is known as the site of disease manifestation. Treatment entails correction of all the steps in the process resulting in disease manifestation, thus restoring the entire person to his or her particular balanced state (Zysk, 1993).

DIAGNOSIS AND TREATMENT

In Ayurveda, restoring a person to health is not viewed simply as the eradication of disease. It entails a complete process of diagnosis and therapeutics that takes into account both mental and physical components integrated with the social and physical worlds in which the patient lives. It begins with Ayurvedic diagnosis, examination of the disease, and types of therapeutics (Jolly, 1977; Lad, 1990; Sen Gupta, 1984).

Ayurveda uses a detailed system of diagnosis, involving examination of pulse, urine, and physical features.

After a preliminary examination by means of visual observation, touch, and interrogation, the Ayurvedic physician undertakes an eightfold method of detailed examination to determine the patient's type of physical constitution and mental status and to get an indication of any abnormality.

FEELING THE PULSE: SNAKE, FROG, AND BIRD

The first mention of pulse examination is in a medical treatise from the late 13th to early 14th century. It is a highly specialized art, and not all Ayurvedic physicians use pulse examination. The diagnostic process involves evenly placing the index, middle, and ring fingers of the right hand on the radial artery of the right hand of men and the left hand of women, just at the base of the thumb. A pulse resembling the movement of a snake at the index finger indicates a predominance of *vata*. A pulse resembling the movement of a frog at the middle finger indicates a predominance of *pitta*. A pulse resembling the movement of a swan or peacock at the ring finger indicates a predominance of *kapha*. A pulse resembling the pecking of a woodpecker in all three fingers indicates a predominance of all three *doshas*. To get an accurate reading, the physician must keep in mind the times when each of the *doshas* are normally excited and should take the pulse at least three times, making sure to wash his or her hands after each reading. Optimum timing for the reading is early in the morning when the stomach is empty or 3 hours after eating in the afternoon (Upadhyay, 1986).

URINE EXAMINATION

Like pulse examination, urine examination probably was formalized in the syncretic phase (see Table 18.1). After collecting a midstream urine evacuation in a clear glass container, after sunrise, the physician submits the urine to two kinds of examination. First the physician studies it in the container to determine its color and degree of transparency. Pale-yellow and oily urine indicates *vata*; intense yellow, reddish, or blue urine indicates *pitta*; white, foamy, and muddy urine indicates *kapha*; urine with a blackish tinge indicates a combination of *doshas*; and urine resembling lime juice or vinegar indicates Ama. The physician also puts a few drops of sesame oil in the urine and examines it in sunlight. The shape, movement, and diffusion of the oil in the urine indicate the prognosis of the disease. The shape of the drops also reveals which *dosha(s)* is involved. A snakelike shape indicates *vata;* umbrella shape, *pitta;* and pearl shape, *kapha*.

EXAMINING THE BODY

The physician concludes his diagnostic examination with careful scrutiny of the tongue, skin, nails, and physical features to determine which *dosha(s)* is affected. Using the basic characteristics of each of the *doshas,* the physician will examine the different parts of the body. Coldness, dryness, roughness, and cracking indicate *vata;* hotness and redness indicate *pitta;* and wetness, whiteness, and coldness indicate *kapha*.

Having completed this phase of the diagnosis, the Ayurvedic physician proceeds to examine any malady present.

FIVEFOLD STEPS

A detailed examination of the disease involves a five-step process, leading to a complete understanding of the abnormality (Zysk, 1993).

1. Finding the cause. A disease is caused by one or several of the following factors: mental imbalances resulting from the effects of past actions (karma); unbalanced contact between the senses and the objects of the senses affecting the body and the mind; effects of the seasons on the mental and doshic balance; the immediate causes of diet, regimen, and microorganisms; *doshas* and Ama; and the interaction of individual components such as *doshas* and tissues or *doshas* and microorganisms.
2. Early signs and symptoms appear before the onset of disease and provide clues to the diagnosis. Proper diet and administration of medicine can avert disease if it is recognized early enough.
3. Manifest signs and symptoms. The most crucial step in the diagnostic process involves determining the site of origin, site of disease manifestation, and the path of transportation of the Ama and *dosha(s)*. Most signs and symptoms are associated with the site of manifestation, from which the physician must work his or her way back to the site of origin to affect a complete cure. Although symptomatic treatment was largely absent in traditional Ayurveda, modern medicine in India has introduced Ayurvedic physicians to techniques of symptomatic treatment in cases of acute disease.
4. Exploratory therapy. This step involves 18 different experiments that use herbs, diet, and regimens to determine the precise nature of the malady and suitable therapy by allopathic and homeopathic means.
5. Prognosis. Because Ayurvedic physicians traditionally did not treat persons with incurable diseases, it was important for the physician to know precisely the patient's chances of recovery. Therefore a disease is classified as one of three types: (1) easily curable, (2) palliative, or (3) incurable or difficult to cure.

The three categories of prognosis are similar to those described in ancient Egyptian medicine as laid out in the Edwin Smith papyrus, for diseases of the head and neck, as "diseases I will treat," implying the expectation of cure, "diseases with which I will contend," implying the expectation to alleviate pain and suffering, and "diseases I will not treat," implying the untreatable or incurable (van Houten & Micozzi, 1981).

In general, if the disease type *(vata, pitta, kapha)* is different from the person's normal physical constitution, the disease is easy to cure. If the disease and constitution are the same, the disease is difficult to cure. If the disease, constitution, and season correspond to doshic type, the disease is nearly impossible to cure (Singhal, 1972–1993).

Having determined the patient's normal constitution, diagnosed his or her illness, and established a prognosis for recovery, the Ayurvedic physician can begin a course of treatment.

Continuous Healing

Ayurveda recognizes two courses of treatment on the basis of the condition of the patient. The first is prevention, for the healthy person who wants to maintain a normal condition based on his or her physical constitution and to prevent disease. The second is therapy, for an ill person who requires health to be restored. Once healthy, Ayurveda recommends continuous prophylaxis based on diet, regimen, medicines, and regular therapeutic purification procedures. When a person is diagnosed with a doshic imbalance, either purification therapy, alleviation therapy, or a combination of these is prescribed.

Purification: Five Actions

Purification therapy involves the fundamental five actions, or *Pañchakarma*, treatment. This fivefold process varies slightly in different traditions and regions of India, but a standard regimen generally is followed. All five procedures can be performed, or a selection of procedures can be chosen on the basis of different factors, such as the physical constitution of the patient, his or her condition, the season, and the nature of the disease.

Before any action is taken, the patient is given oil internally and externally (with massage) and is sweated to loosen and soften the *dosha(s)* and Ama.

An appropriate diet of food and drink is prescribed.

After this two-part preparatory treatment, called "Purvakarma," the five therapies are administered in sequence over the period of approximately a week.

The patient is advised to set aside time for treatment in light of the profound effects on the mind and body. First, the patient might be given an emetic to induce vomiting until bilious matter is produced, thus removing *kapha*. Second, a purgative is given until mucus material appears, thus removing *pitta*. Third, an enema, either of oil or decocted medicines, is administered, flushing the bowels, to remove excess *vata*. Fourth, head purgation is given in the form of smoke inhalation or nasal drops to eradicate the *dosha(s)* that have accumulated in the head and sinuses. Fifth, leeches may be applied and bloodletting performed to purify the blood. Some physicians do not consider bloodletting in the five therapies of *Pañchakarma*, instead counting oily and dry (decocted medicine) enemas as two separate forms (Singh, 1992).

Alleviation therapy uses the basic condiments honey, butter or ghee, and sesame oil or castor oil to eliminate *kapha, pitta,* and *vata,* respectively. This therapy and *Pañchakarma* are often used in conjunction with one another. It is becoming increasing difficult to find ghee (or clarified butter).

Herbal Remedies

Ayurveda prescribes a rich store of natural medicines that have been collected, tested, and recorded in medical treatises from ancient times. The tradition of collecting and preserving information about medicines in recipe books, called "Nighantus," continued to the 20th century (Nadkarni, 1908). The most traditional source of

Ayurvedic medicine is the kitchen garden. From an early stage of development, Indian medical and culinary traditions worked hand in hand with each other.

In light of the close association between food and medicine, Ayurveda classifies foods and drugs (usually vegetal) by the taste on the tongue, potency, and taste after digestion (Tables 18.3 and 18.4).

Rasa, taste by the tongue, is categorized into six separate tastes, with their individual elemental composition and energetic effects on the three *doshas* (Zysk, 1993):

1. Sweet, composed of earth and water, increases *kapha* and decreases *pitta* and *vata*.
2. Sour, composed of earth and fire, increases *kapha* and *pitta* and decreases *vata*.

TABLE 18.3 *Tastes and Food Qualities: Effects on the Doshas*

Tastes	
Decrease Vata	**Increase Vata**
Sweet	Pungent
Sour	Bitter
Salty	Astringent
Decrease Pitta	**Increase Pitta**
Sweet	Pungent
Bitter	Sour
Astringent	Salty
Decrease Kapha	**Increase Kapha**
Pungent	Sweet
Bitter	Sour
Astringent	Salty
Major Food Qualities	
Decrease Vata	**Increase Vata**
Heavy	Light
Oily	Dry
Hot	Cold
Decrease Pitta	**Increase Pitta**
Cold	Hot
Heavy	Light
Oily	Dry
Decrease Kapha	**Increase Kapha**
Light	Heavy
Dry	Oily
Hot	Cold

TABLE 18.4 *Common Examples of the Six Tastes and Major Food Qualities*

Six Tastes	Common Examples
Sweet	Sugar, milk, butter, rice, breads
Sour	Yogurt, lemon, cheese
Salty	Salt
Pungent	Spicy foods, peppers, ginger, cumin
Bitter	Spinach, other green leafy vegetables
Astringent	Beans, pomegranate
Six Major Food Qualities	**Common Examples**
Heavy	Cheese, yogurt, wheat products
Light	Barley, corn, spinach, apples
Oily	Dairy products, fatty foods, oils
Dry	Barley, corn, potato, beans
Hot	Hot (temperature) foods and drinks
Cold	Cold foods and drinks

3. Saline, composed of water and fire, increases *kapha* and *pitta* and decreases *vata*.
4. Pungent, composed of wind and fire, increases *pitta* and *vata* and decreases *kapha*.
5. Bitter, composed of wind and space, increases *vata* and decreases *pitta* and *kapha*.
6. Astringent, composed of wind and earth, increases *vata* and decreases *pitta* and *kapha*.

Virya, potency, is composed of eight types of taste or sensation in total, divided into four pairs: hot-cold, unctuous-dry, heavy-light, and dull-sharp.

Vipaka, postdigestive taste, identifies three kinds of after taste: sweet, sour, and pungent.

Contrary foods and drugs are always to be avoided. For instance, clarified butter and honey should not be taken in equal quantities, alkalis and salt must not be taken for a long period, milk and fish should not be consumed together, and honey should not be put in hot drinks.

COMPOUNDING

Four important criteria are considered when compounding plant substances and other ingredients into medical recipes. The substances that make up the recipe should have many attributes that enable it to cure several diseases; they should be usable in many pharmaceutical preparations, they should be suitable for the recipe and not cause unwanted side effects, and they should be culturally appropriate to the patients and their customs. Every medicine should be able to treat the disease's site of origin, site of manifestation, and its spread simultaneously.

A brief survey of the different kinds of medical preparations indicates the depth and content of Ayurvedic pharmaceuticals. The botanically based medicines derive largely from the Ayurvedic medical tradition, whereas the mineral and inorganic-based drugs derive from the Indian alchemical traditions, called "Rasashastra" (Zysk, 1993).

Juices are cold-presses and extractions made from plants.

Powders are prepared from parts of plants that have been dried in the shade and other dried ingredients.

Infusions are parts of plants and herbs that have been steeped in water and strained. Cold infusions are parts of plants and herbs that were soaked in water overnight and filtered the next morning. Decoctions are vegetal products boiled in a quantity of water proportionate to the hardness of the plant part and then reduced by a fourth. It is then filtered and often used with butter, honey, or oils.

Medicated pastes and oils. Often the plant and herbal extracts are combined with other ingredients and formed into pastes, plasters, and oils. Used externally, pastes and plasters are applied for joint, muscular, and skin conditions, and oil is used for hair and head problems. Medicated oils also are used for massages and enemas.

Large and small pills and suppositories. Plant and herbal extracts are also formed into pills and suppositories to be used internally.

Alcoholic preparations are made by fermentation or distillation. Two preparations are delineated: one requires the drug to be boiled before it is fermented or distilled, and in the other, the drug is simply added to the preparation. Fifteen percent is the maximum allowable amount of alcohol content in a drug.

Several Ayurvedic medicines are prepared from minerals and metals ultimately derived from ancient traditions (Zysk, 1993). Sublimates are prepared by an elaborate method leading to the sublimation of sulfur in a glass container. They are found in recipes (Rasayanas) used in rejuvenation therapies.

Bhasmas are ash residues produced from the calcination of metals, gems, plants, and animal products. Most are metals and minerals that are first detoxified and then purified. An important bhasma is prepared from mercury, which undergoes an 18-stage detoxification and purification process. Ayurveda maintains that bhasmas are quickly absorbed in the blood and increase the red blood cells.

Pishtis are fine powders made by trituration of gems with juices and extracts.

Collyrium is made from antimony powder, lead oxide, or the soot from lamps burned with castor oil. Collyrium is used especially to improve vision.

Of the hundreds of plants, minerals, and metals mentioned in various Ayurvedic treatises, only a small selection are commonly used by the typical Ayurvedic physicians today. Similar emphasis and some shared traditions are illustrated in the practices of Siddha medicine in Southern India, the subject of the next section of this chapter.

SIDDHA MEDICINE OF SOUTH INDIA

Unlike Ayurveda, which has a long and detailed textual tradition in Sanskrit dating from thousands of years ago, Siddha medicine's textual history, in the Tamil language of South India, remains vague and uncertain until approximately CE 13th century, when there begins evidence of medical treatises. Most of our knowledge about Siddha medicine comes from modern-day practitioners, who often maintain an unverified history of the development of their own tradition, and who, in light of the modern upsurge of Tamil pride, make fantastic claims about the age and importance of Siddha medicine vis-à-vis its closest rival in India, Ayurveda.

Based on the evidence of written secondary sources and the reports of field-workers in Siddha medicine, Siddha and Ayurveda share a common theoretic foundation but differ in their respective forms of therapy. This disparity suggests an original form of Siddha medicine may have consisted primarily of a series of treatments for specific ailments. These individual therapeutic prescriptions were then later overlaid with a theoretical component from Ayurveda. In addition, diagnosis by pulse and urine, based on Ayurveda and perhaps also Unani, could well have been the source, in turn, for the same means of pulse and urine diagnosis.

The same pattern of medical development, which involves empirical practice first, followed by theory, may also apply to other forms of Indian medicine, beginning with Ayurveda itself, and including the more recent Visha Vaidya tradition of Kerala.

Siddha medicine is also distinctive in its use of alchemy, with fundamental principles that conform to the alchemical traditions of ancient Greece and China, and of Arabic alchemy, as reflected, for example, in Unani medicine. Siddha alchemy might well have been derived from one or a combination of these older traditions.

Just as Ayurveda eventually left India and found fertile ground in the West and where alternative and complementary forms of healing have become popular in recent decades, there are signs on the horizon that Siddha medicine may follow the same course. Indian systems of medicine must undergo changes and adaptations to be accommodated in a foreign environment, as in the case of Maharishi Ayurveda in the West. Some of these modifications find their way back to India, where they become integrated into the indigenous systems. Such has been the pattern of traditional medicine in most parts of the world so that the final chapter on the history of a particular medical system can never be written. An understanding of Siddha's medical history can only be revealed in light of change and adaptation over time.

SOUTHERN SOURCES

Looking into Siddha medicine in Tamil Nadu, South India, presents challenges to understanding this medical system and its history. A central problem lies with the limited availability of primary sources (akin to the "classics" of traditional Ayurvedic or Chinese medicine) and the reliability of secondary sources prepared primarily by modern Tamil Siddha doctors. Little research on the subject has been carried out by Western students and scholars of India and Indian medicine. Even in the 21st century, much of this mysterious medical tradition remains to be discovered.

Along with increased awareness of the Tamil language's Dravidian roots, in the second half of the 20th century, a strong nationalist movement has grown up in Tamil Nadu. Tamils consider their cultural and linguistic heritage to be older and more important than that of the Indo-Aryans of northern India; some even claim their ancestors comprised the first civilization on the planet. This controversy has recently been kindled by a debate centering on the still-to-be-deciphered script of the so-called Indus Valley Civilization. This ancient urban culture, which predated the Hindu civilization of the Ganges River valley, extended along the Indus River and its tributaries in what is now Pakistan. It resembled the great civilizations of ancient Egypt and Mesopotamia in size, development, and age. One side of the debate maintains that the script represents a language probably of Dravidian origin, whereas the other side claims that it does not represent a language at all. Tamils, whose language is Dravidian, are anxiously following the debate, for if the former side prevails, it would confirm their antiquity on the Indian subcontinent. The lens through which Tamils look at their own history influences the image in favor of Tamil superiority and antiquity.

References to Ayurveda occur early in Tamil literature. Already in the CE mid-5th-century text, Cilappatikara, there is reference to Ayurveda (Tamil: *āyulvetar*). Mention of the three humors (Tamil: *tiritocam*, Sanskrit: *tridosha*) occurs in the Tirukural, a collection of poems that dates from approximately CE 450 to 550.

MIDDLE EASTERN CONNECTIONS

The first Tamil Siddha text is the *Tirumandiram* written by Tirumular and dated probably to around CE 6th or 7th century. There is mention of alchemy used to transform iron into gold, but no specific references to Tamil medicinal doctrines. The major sources of Siddha medicine belong to religious groups called "Kayasiddhas." They seek the "perfection of the body" by means of yoga, alchemy, medicine, and certain types of Tantric religious rituals. Their works date from approximately CE 13th to 14th century and are attributed to numerous authors, including Akattiyar (Sanskrit: *Agastya*), the traditional founder of Siddha medicine and Teraiyar (c. late 17th century), who is said to have written 12 works on medicine. His famous disciple, Iramatevar, traveled to Mecca in the late 17th or early 18th century where he studied, converted to Islam, and took on the name Yakkopu (i.e., Jacob). The numerous texts on Siddha medicine, which present it as a system of healing, are probably not older than the 16th century. Therefore Tamil Siddha medicine, as it now exists in both theory and practice, began in Tamil Nadu around the 16th century, but elements of healing practices that became part of Siddha medicine, including those they hold in common with Ayurveda, came from an earlier period.

BUDDHIST CONNECTIONS

Tamil folklore surrounding healing shares a common origin with Buddhism from northern India. Legend holds that Akattiyar performed a trephination on a sage to remove a toad (terai) from inside his skull. Akattiyar's disciple made the toad jump into a bowl of water. Because of his skill in removing the toad, Akattiyar gave the disciple the name Teraiyar (who is a different person from the late 17th-century medical author of the same name).

This legend is interesting because there is a similar account in Buddhist literature, and the legend of the toad and the cranium is a popular motif of Buddhist art and sculpture. In its earliest version found in the Pali texts of the Buddhist Canon, a skilled physician opened the cranium of a merchant from Rajagriha and removed two centipedes by touching them with a hot poker. The merchant made a full recovery. Versions of this folk story also occur in the Sanskrit literature of later Mahayana Buddhism and were translated into Tibetan and Chinese. The uniqueness of the story and its spread throughout Buddhist Asia demonstrates the influence of Buddhism in the dissemination of medical knowledge in premodern India.

SPIRITUAL SOURCES

Like all systems of Hindu knowledge, Siddha medicine attributes its origin to a divine source; hence its knowledge is sacred and eternal, passed down to humans for the benefit of all humanity. According to Hindu tradition, the god Shiva transmitted the knowledge of medicine to his wife Parvati, who in turn passed it on to Nandi, from whom it was given to the first practitioners of Siddha medicine. Tradition lists a total of 18 Siddha practitioners, beginning with Nandi and the legendary Akattiyar through to the final Siddhar, Kudhambai.

They are the acknowledged semimythical transmitters of Siddha medical doctrines and practices. By attributing a divine or extrahuman origin to its medicine, the Tamil Siddhars have assured Siddha medicine a legitimate place in the corpus of Hindu knowledge. Although the transmission begins with Nandi, who in the form of a bull is Shiva's mode of transportation, tradition attributes the origin of medicine as well as of the Tamil language to Akattiyar.

SHIVA AND SHAKTI

According to Siddha cosmology, all matter is composed of two primal forces of matter (shiva) and energy (shakti). These two principles of existence operate in humans, as well as nature, and connect the microcosm with the macrocosm. This connection is expressed by the association between the human body and the signs of the zodiac in Indian astrology, or jyotish. The formulation of the sequence of body parts is interesting because it follows a Babylonian and Greco-Roman system of head-to-toe correspondence rather than an Indian one, which begins from the earth at the toes and moves upwards. This formulation is illustrated in the following list, using Latin-based zodiac names, according to Zysk (2000):

♈ Áries (0 degrees) = the neck
♉ Taurus (30 degrees) = the shoulders
♊ Gémini (60 degrees) = the arms and hands
♋ Cancer (90 degrees) = the chest
♌ Leo (120 degrees) = the heart and the stomach
♍ Virgo (150 degrees) = the intestines
♎ Libra (180 degrees) = the kidneys

♏ Scórpio (210 degrees) = the genitals
♐ Sagittárius (240 degrees) = the hips
♑ Capricornus (270 degrees) = the knees
♒ Aquárius (300 degrees) = the legs
♓ Pisces (330 degrees) = the feet

In addition to this cosmic connection, which occurs in all traditions of Indian astrology (or *djoytish*), Siddha medicine relied on Ayurveda for medical doctrines that bridge the natural world and the human body. In modern-day Siddha practice, evidence of that genealogy is not always acknowledged.

There are five elements (pañcamahabhutam), which make up the entire natural world: solid/earth, fluid/water, radiance/fire, gas/wind, and ether/space. These elements combine in specific ways to grant the three bodily humors, called "muppini" in modern Tamil. They are said to be in the proportion of 1 part wind to ½ part bile to ¼ part phlegm, according to Zysk (2000):

1. Wind (Tamil: *vatham,* Sanskrit: *Vata*) is a combination of space and wind, and is responsible for nervous actions, movement, activity, sensations, and so on. It is found in the form of the five bodily winds.

2. Bile (Tamil: *pittam,* Sanskrit: *pitta*) is made up of fire alone and governs metabolism, digestion, assimilation, warmth, and so on. Its principal seat is in the alimentary canal, from the cardiac region to small intestines. Some Ayurvedic formulations state that bile is a combination of the elements fire and water.

3. Phlegm (Tamil: *siletuman,* Sanskrit: *shleshman, Kapha*) is a combination of earth and water and is responsible for stability in the body. Its principal seats are in the chest, throat, head, and joints.

Next, there is the shared doctrine of the seven tissues (Tamil: *dhatu*) of the body: lymph/chyle, blood, muscle, fat, bone, marrow, and sperm and ovum. Finally, there are the five winds (Tamil: *vatham,* Sanskrit: *prana*), which circulate in the body and initiate and carry out bodily functions: *pranam* is the inhaled breath and brings about swallowing; *apanam* is the exhaled breath and is responsible for expulsion, ejection, and excretion; *samanam* helps digestion; *vyanam* aids circulation of blood and nutrients; and *udanam* functions in the upper respiratory passages. There are also five secondary winds: *nagam,* the air of higher intellectual functions; *kurmam,* the air of yawning; *kirukaram,* the air of salivation; *devadhattham,* the air of laziness; and *dhananjayam,* the air that acts on death.

Like Ayurveda, Siddha medicine maintains that the three humors predominate in humans in accordance with their nature and stage of life and that they vary with the seasons. Every individual is born with a unique configuration of the three humors, which is called the "individual's basic nature" (Sanskrit: *prakriti*). It is fixed at birth and forms the basis of his or her normal, healthy state. However, during the three different stages of life and during the different seasons, one humor usually predominates. This pattern is normal, but domination by a humor must be understood in relation to the person's fundamental nature to maintain the balance that is the individual's basic natural state. The classification of the humors according to stages of life and seasons in Siddha differs from that found in Ayurveda. In the case of the seasons, the variation is attributed simply to the different climatic conditions that occur in the different parts of the year in the northern inland areas and the southern, Tamil coastal and inland environment (Table 18.5).

According to Siddha, wind predominates in the first third of life, bile in the second third, and phlegm in the last third of life, whereas in Ayurveda, phlegm dominates the first third and wind the last third of life. In terms of climate in the Indian subcontinent, the north is colder in the winter (December and January) than is the south, and the west coast has rain in June and July (with prevailing westerly winds in the Northern Hemisphere), when the east coast is extremely hot. A dry, cold climate is rare in the south, but it is precisely that climate which increases wind. In contrast, bile and phlegm are increased when it is hot and wet.

Diagnosis: Eight Features

The diagnosis of disease in Siddha medicine relies on the examination of eight anatomical features *(envagi thaervu)*, which are evaluated in terms of the three humors, according to Zysk (2000):

1. Tongue: black indicates wind, yellow or red bile, and white phlegm; an ulcerated tongue points to anemia.
2. Complexion: dark indicates wind, yellow or red bile, and pale phlegm.
3. Voice: normal indicates wind, high-pitched bile, and low-pitched phlegm.
4. Eyes: muddy colored indicates wind, yellowish or red bile, and pale phlegm.
5. Touch: dryness indicates wind, warmness bile, and cold, clammy phlegm.
6. Stool: black indicates wind, yellow bile, and pale phlegm.
7. Pulse: a complex system described later.
8. Urine: also described in detail later.

TABLE 18.5 *Times of Day, Seasons, and Life Cycle Classified According to the Doshas*

Kapha time	Approximately 6 a.m. (sunrise) to 10 a.m. and 6 p.m. to 10 p.m.
Kapha season	In the United States, spring; In India, late winter and spring
Kapha period in life cycle	Childhood
Pitta time	Approximately 10 a.m. to 2 p.m., and 10 p.m. to 2 a.m.
Pitta season	In the United States, summer and early autumn; in India, rainy season and autumn
Pitta period in life cycle	Adulthood
Vata time	Approximately 2 a.m. to 6 a.m. (sunrise), and 2 p.m. to 6 p.m.
Vata season	In the United States, late autumn and winter; in India, summer and rainy season
Vata period in life cycle	Old age

Pulse examination is the most emphasized diagnostic approach for modern Siddha doctors. Both diagnosis and prognosis can be obtained through this one process. These methods of diagnosis also occur in Ayurveda but only after the 14th century, perhaps influenced by the introduction of Unani medicine with the arrival of the Mogul (Persians converted to Islam) in northern India. Prior to this time, and in the Ayurvedic classical literature, diagnosis of disease was determined by vitiation of one or more of the humors based on observation, touch, and interrogation.

Siddha pulse diagnosis (Tamil: *natiparitchai,* Sanskrit: *nadipariksha*), like that found in Ayurveda, probably owes it origins to Unani medicine. It requires a highly developed sense of touch and refined subjective awareness. According to Siddha, the following conditions must not be present in the patient when doing a reading of the pulse: emotional distress, exhaustion, full stomach or hunger, or oily hands.

If readings cannot be taken on the hand, other arterial points may be used, such as the ankle, neck, or ear lobes. It is also advised to read the pulse at different times of the day and during different seasons of the year because the body and mind change during the course of the day and climatic conditions affect the person's psychological and physiological states.

The pulse is felt on the female's left and male's right hand by the doctor's opposite hand, a few centimeters below the wrist joint, using the index, middle, and ring fingers. Pressure should be applied by one finger after the other beginning with the index finger. Each finger detects a particular humor, which in normal conditions has a movement representative of certain animals. The index finger feels the windy humor, which should have the movement of a swan, a cock, or a peacock; the middle finger feels the bilious humor, which should have the movement of a tortoise or a leach; and ring finger feels the phlegmatic humor, which should have the movement of a frog or a snake. Any deviation from these normal movements indicates which humor or humors are disturbed. If all humors are affected, the pulse is usually rapid with a good deal more volume than normal. After long periods of practice under the guidance of a skilled teacher, a student can begin to detect subtle differences in the flow, volume, and speed of the pulse at the point of each of the three fingers. These changes correspond to abnormalities in particular parts of the body, which the skilled Siddha doctor can pinpoint and for which the appropriate cure can be prescribed (Zysk, 2000).

Urine examination (muthira paritchai) is another form of diagnosis in Siddha medicine. Not an original part of Ayurveda, urine examination probably derived from Unani medicine, in which this form of diagnosis is described in early Arabic and Persian medical literature; it is also important in Tibetan medicine. Siddha practice examines the urine for its color, smell, and texture and further uses a technique for determining the vitiated humor by reading the distribution of a drop of gingili (sesame) oil added to the urine. The meaning of the drop's configuration is as follows: longitudinal dispersal indicates windy humor, dispersal in a ring indicates bilious humor, and lack of dispersal points to phlegmatic humor. A combination of two types of dispersal means that two humors are involved. Prognosis is determined by such reading as well: A slow dispersal of a drop in a circular form, or a drop that forms the shape of an umbrella, a wheel, or a jasmine or lotus blossom indicates positive prognosis. A drop that sinks, spreads rapidly with froth, splits into smaller drops and spreads rapidly, mixes with the urine, or spreads so that its pattern is that of an arrow, a sword, a spear, a pestle, a bull, or an elephant indicates a poor prognosis.

Finally, as in Ayurveda and Unani, the conditions of the eyes show which of the humors is vitiated, as well as the patient's mental and emotional state: shifty, dry eyes point to wind; yellow eyes with photophobia indicate bile; watery, oily, eyes devoid of brightness reveal that phlegm is effected; and red, inflamed eyes show that all three humors are vitiated.

TREATMENT

According to traditional Siddha, a physician must be knowledgeable in alchemy, astrology, and philosophy. He must be able to apply intuition and imagination. He must not seek fame or fortune from healing. He must not treat a patient before a proper diagnosis has been reached. And he must use only medicines that he has prepared himself.

Treatment and pharmaceutics are two areas in which Siddha differs considerably from Ayurveda. As in yoga (see later), the principal aim of Siddha medicine is to make the body perfect, not vulnerable to decay, so that the maximum term of life can be achieved. Like Ayurveda, Siddha places emphasis on positive health so that the object of the medicine is disease-prevention and health promotion.

Traditional Ayurveda lists the following eight branches of medicine: general medicine, pediatrics, surgery, treatment of ailments above the neck, toxicology, treatment of mental disorders due to seizure by evil spirits, rejuvenation therapy, and potency therapy. Siddha medicine developed expertise in five particular branches of medicine: general medicine, pediatrics, toxicology, ophthalmology, and rejuvenation. Further, Ayurveda prescribes a therapeutic regimen involving the *Pañchakarma*, purification, or "five purifying actions," including emetics, purgative, enemas, and bloodletting. (These same approaches were also independently used in the practice of "regular medicine" in the West up to the 20th century.) Siddha uses only purgation for purification purposes.

GENERAL MEDICINE

In Ayurveda, surgical practice forms a separate school of medicine, but surgery per se is not a significant part of Siddha medicine. Medicated oils and pastes are applied to treat wounds and ulcers, but the use of a knife is rarely encountered at all.

Closely connected with the tradition of the martial arts in South India there developed a type of acupressure treatment based on the vital points in the human body, known as "varmam" (Sanskrit: *marman*). There are 108 points mentioned in the Ayurvedic classics, which identify them and explain that if they are injured, death can ensue. In Siddha medicine, the number of important varmam points is also 108 (some say 107) out of a total of 400. Siddha doctors developed techniques of applying pressure to special points, called "Varmakkalai," to remove certain ailments and of massaging the points to cure diseases. They also specialized in bone setting and often practiced an Indian form of the martial arts, called "cilampam" or "silambattam," which involved a kind of dueling with staffs.

According the French Institute in Pondicherry, India, the art of varmam is particularly widespread among the hereditary Siddha practitioners belonging to the Natar caste in the district of Kanyakumari in Tamil Nadu. The development of this special form of healing appears to have evolved naturally because the men of this caste, while carrying out their task of climbing coconut and borassus trees to collect the fruits and sap for toddy, occasionally fell from great heights. To repair the injury or save the life of a fall victim, skills of bone setting and reviving an unconscious patient by massage developed among certain families within the caste, who have passed down their secret art from generation to generation by word of mouth. In the past, rulers used members of this caste to cure injuries incurred in battle and to overpower their enemies by their knowledge of the Indian martial arts.

TOXICOLOGY

Toxicology as part of Siddha medicine seems to be closely linked to indigenous systems of treating snake bites and other forms of poisoning. It may have some affinity to the Visha Vaidya (poison-doctor) tradition practiced by certain Nambudiri Brahmins of Kerala. Similar to this Kerala toxicological tradition, Siddha has adopted the Ayurvedic system of the three humors to explain the different effects of poisons, but it remains fundamentally an indigenous and local toxicological tradition. It classifies the severity and cure by means of the number of teeth or fang marks left in the victim. Four, the most severe, is incurable; it implies two complete bites. One fang mark, the least severe, is cured by cold water baths and fomentation on the site of the bite. Even the bite of a venomous snake may not carry venom; the more fang marks the greater likelihood that venom was injected.

OPHTHALMOLOGY

Siddha medicine excels in ophthalmology. It has two separate treatises devoted to the treatment of 96 different eye diseases. This focus may be related to the strength of Arabic optics from the Unani tradition that was evidently introduced.

REJUVENATION THERAPY (HEALTHY AGING)

Closely connected with Siddha Yoga, the Siddha system of rejuvenation therapy, known as *Kayakalpa* (from Sanskrit, meaning "making the body competent for long life"), marks a distinctive feature of Siddha medicine. It involves a five-step process for rejuvenating the body and prolonging life.
1. Preservation of vital energy via breath control (Tamil: *vasiyogam* or Sanskrit: *pranayama*) and yoga.
2. Conservation of male semen and female sexual secretions.
3. Use of muppu, or rare earth salts.
4. Use of calcinated powders (Tamil: *chunnam,* Sanskrit: *bhasma*) prepared from metals and minerals.
5. Use of drugs prepared from plants special to each Siddha doctor.

The esoteric substance called "muppu" is particular to Siddha medicine. It may be considered Siddha's equivalent of the "philosopher's stone." Its preparation is hidden in secrecy, known only by the guru, and taught only when the student is deemed qualified to accept it. It is generally thought to consist of three salts (muuppu), called "puniru," "kallupu," and "vediyuppu," which correspond respectively to the sun, moon, and fire. Puniru is said to be a certain kind of limestone composed of globules that are found underneath a type of clay called "Fuller's Earth," which contains heavy metals. In early Europe, Fuller's Earth was used by fullers, or those who prepared and preserved wool to weave into cloth. It is collected only on the full-moon night in April, when it is said to bubble out from the limestone. It is then purified with the use of a special herb. Kallupu is hard salt or stone salt (i.e., rock salt) that is dug up from mines under the earth, obtained from saline deposits under the sea, or gathered from the froth of sea water that carries the undersea salt. Kallupu is considered to be useful in the consolidation of mercury and other metals. Finally, vediyuppu is potassium nitrate, which is cleaned seven times and purified with alum.

This magical-religious form of therapy is a common component of Siddha alchemical practice and provides a basis for the rich assortment of alchemical preparations comprising the pharmacopoeia of Siddha medicine.

PHARMACOPOEIA

The precise origin of the system of Siddha pharmacology is not known, but it seems to have been closely linked to the Tantric religious movement, which can be traced back to CE 6th century of in North India, and influenced both Buddhism and Hinduism. It was strongly anti-Brahmanical and stressed ascetic practices and religious rituals that involved "forbidden" foods and sexual practices and often included the use of alchemical preparations.

The alchemical part of Siddha is present from at least the time of Tirumular's Tirumandiram (CE 6th or 7th century). Alchemy is also found in Sanskrit texts from North India but only from approximately CE 6th or 7th century. It later became an integral part of Ayurvedic medicine, called "Rasashastra," "traditional knowledge about mercury." However, in the classical treatises of Ayurveda mention of alchemy is absent, and only certain metals and minerals are mentioned in late classical texts from CE 7th century. Because alchemy reached a far greater level of development in Siddha medicine than in Ayurveda, it is believed that medical alchemy may well have begun in South India among the Siddha yogins and ascetics and was later assimilated into Ayurveda.

There are three groups of drugs in Siddha medicine: (1) inorganic substances (*thatuvargam*); (2) plant products (*mulavargam*); and (3) animal products (*jivavargam*). These drugs are all characterized by means of taste (rasa), quality (*guna*), potency (*virya*), postdigestive taste (*vipaka*), and specific action (*prabhava*).

Siddha has further classified the inorganic substances into the following six types, according to Zysk (2000):

1. Uppu: 25 or 31 varieties of salts and alkalis, which are water soluble and give out vapor when heated;

2. Pashanam: 64 varieties (32 natural, 32 artificial) of non–water-soluble substances that emit vapor when heated;
3. Uparasam: seven types of non–water-soluble substances that emit vapor when heated, including mica, magnetic iron, antimony, zinc sulfate, iron pyrites, ferrous sulfate and asafetida *(hingu);*
4. Loham: six varieties of metals and metallic alloys that are insoluble but melt when heated and solidify when cooled, including gold, silver, copper, iron, tin, and lead;
5. Rasam: drugs that are soft and sublime when heated, transforming into small crystals or amorphous powders, such as mercury, amalgams and compounds of mercury, and arsenic;
6. Gandhakam: sulfur that is insoluble in water and burns off when heated.

Rasam and gandhakam combine to make kattu, which is a "bound" substance (i.e., a substance whose ingredients are united by a process of heating).

In addition, there are 13 varieties of gems and minerals, 16 varieties of mud and siliceous earth, 35 varieties of animals, and 24 varieties of rocks. This variety resembles in some respects the remedies of homeopathic medicine as developed in Europe during the 18th century.

The cornerstones of Siddha pharmacology are mercury and sulfur, which are equated to the deity Shiva and his consort, Parvati, and are combined to make mercuric sulfide. Mercury, or quicksilver, is the crucial ingredient in almost every Siddha alchemical preparation. It is used in five forms *(panchasthuta):* pure mercury *(rasa),* red sulfide of mercury *(lingam),* mercuric perchloride *(viram),* mercurous chloride *(puram),* and red oxide of mercury *(rasacheduram).* Although mercury plays a key role in both the Siddha and Ayurvedic forms of medical alchemy, mercury in its pure form is not found in India and, therefore, must have become available through trade with the Roman and Byzantine Empires and, subsequently, the Italian city-states of the Middle Ages. As an aside, mercury was a popular remedy in Europe until the middle of the 19th century when its German name "quacksalber" gave origin to the term "quack" for those who practiced dangerous and ineffective medicine.

Siddha pharmacology combines substances that from a natural affinity to each other, such as borax and ammonia sulfate, to create a compound greater than the sum of the individual parts. This combination is called "nadabindu," where nada is acidic and bindu is alkaline, or, in the Siddha cosmology, the female Shakti mated with the male Shiva. The most important mixture of this kind is alkaline mercury and acidic sulfur. Similarly, Siddha medicine has devised a classification of drugs as friends and foes. The former increase the curative effect, whereas the latter reduce it.

Six pharmaceutical preparations are common to both Siddha and Ayurveda. They can be administered internally or on the skin. They include: calcinated metals and minerals *(chunnam),* powders *(churanam),* decoctions *(kudinir),* pastes *(karkam),* medicated clarified butter *(nei),* and medicated oils *(ennai).* However, particular to Siddha medicine are three special formulations: *chunnam,* metallic preparations that become alkaline, yielding calcium hydroxide, which must always be taken with another more palatable substance (*anupana*, "after drink"); *mezhugu*, waxy preparations that combine both metals and minerals; and *kattu*, inextricably bound preparations, which are impervious to water and flame. Sulfur and mercury or mercuric salts are combined to make them resistant to heat. While on the fire, certain juices are added by drops to empower the substance. The drug can be kept for long periods and given in small doses once a day. However, it should not be completely turned into a powder but should be rubbed on a Sandal stone so as to yield only a few grains of the powerful substance (Zysk, 2000).

Both Ayurveda's Rasashastra, or traditional knowledge of mercury, and Siddha's alchemy have devised different methods for purifying or detoxifying metals and minerals, called "shodhana" in Sanskrit, and "suddhi murai" in Tamil, before they are reduced to ash (Sanskrit: *bhasman*, Tamil: *chunnam*). Purification is accomplished by one of two methods. One involves repeatedly heating sheets of metal and plunging them into various vegetable juices and decoctions. The other method, called "killing" *(marana)*, entails destroying the metal or mineral by the use of powerful herbs so that it loses its identity and becomes converted into fine powders with the natures of oxides or sulfides, which can be processed by the intestinal juices. After this purification procedure, the metal or mineral is combined with its appropriate acid or alkaline and is prepared for its final transformation into an ash or "bhasman" by incineration in special furnaces made of cow-dung cakes (replaced by electric ovens in modern establishments!).

According to Zysk (2000), there are nine principles that must be followed in the calcination of metals and minerals:
1. There is no alchemical process without mercury.
2. There is no fixation without alkali.
3. There is no coloring without sulfur.
4. There is no quintessence without copper sulfate.
5. There is no animation without conflagration.
6. There is no calcination without corrosive lime.
7. There is no compound without correct blowing.
8. There is no fusion without suitable flux.
9. There is no strong fluid without sal ammoniac.

The traditional incineration process may vary slightly among different Siddha doctors, but all procedures require repeated heating in a fire fueled by dung patties. The number of burnings can reach 100 for certain preparations. In traditional Ayurveda, the duration and intensity of the heat is regulated by the size of the pile of dung, called a *puta* in Sanskrit. Siddha medicine devised a method with a special substance made of inorganic salts, in Tamil called *jayani*, which reduces the number of burnings to only three or four. To increase the potency of the ash *(chunnam)*, Siddha practitioners add the esoteric substance *muppu*, which seems to vary in individual composition from one Siddha doctor to another. Other ingredients added to increase a chunnam's potency are healthy human urine *(amuri)* or urine salts *(amuriuppu)* obtained from the evaporation of large quantities of urine. Neither of these additives is found in Ayurveda's Rasashastra.

According to Zysk (2000), in modern Siddha medicine, different metals have different healing effects:

Mercury is antibacterial and antisyphilitic (and was used for this purpose in the West until the early 20th century).

Sulfur is used against scabies and skin diseases, rheumatoid arthritis, spasmodic asthma, jaundice, blood poisoning, and internally as a stool softener.

Gold is effective against rheumatoid arthritis, and as a nervine tonic, an antidote, and a sexual stimulant.

Arsenic cures all fevers, asthma, and anemia.

Copper is used to treat leprosy, skin diseases, and to improve the blood.

Iron is effective against anemia, jaundice, and as a general tonic for toning the body.

This kind of knowledge about the healing properties of various minerals was ultimately carried into the use of mineral baths, spas, and water therapies in the West.

Despite the scientific evidence that shows many of these inorganic substances—minerals and metals—to be toxic to the human body, both Siddha and Ayurvedic practitioners continue to use them in their everyday treatment of patients. They claim that their respective traditions have provided special techniques to detoxify the metals and minerals and to render them safe and extremely potent. Again, as in the practice of homeopathy, certain biologically active substances that are toxic in one form or dose may be prepared so that its beneficial effects predominate.

PLANT PRODUCTS

In terms of herbal drugs, Siddha practitioners draw upon a *materia medica* of more than 100 plants and plant products, some of which are imported from as far away as the Himalaya. These herbal remedies are used for three purposes in Siddha medicine. First, as mentioned earlier, certain drugs purify the minerals and metals before they are transformed into ash. Second, many plants and plant substances are used to eliminate waste products from the body through a process of body purification involving purgation of the nose and throat, enemas and laxatives, and the removal of toxins from the skin by the application of medicated pastes. This procedure resembles the process of the five methods of purification (Sanskrit: *pañchakarman*) in Ayurveda. Third, plants are used to treat specific ailments and for the general toning or tonification of the body.

ANIMAL PRODUCTS

Siddha doctors also used animal products, such as human and canine skulls and bones, in the preparation of a special "ash" or *chunnam* (Tamil: *peranda chunnam*), which is said to be effective against mental disorders. The preparation of bone ash would serve to alkalinize (make basic vs. acidic) any mixtures and unbind various active principles that might otherwise not be metabolically available. A clear example from American Indian ethnomedicine is the use of ash, or mineral lime from seashells, to alkalinize maize, allowing the B vitamins (such as niacin) to become unbound and available for metabolism when ingested.

Ayurvedic pharmaceutical manufacturers in India have begun to adopt the Western system of "good manufacturing procedures" and to resort to Ayurveda's rich pharmacopoeia of plant-based medicines to make their products more accessible to a Western clientele. Such is not the case with Siddha medicine, which has yet to experience the financial rewards that come from serving Western markets.

Both Siddha and Ayurveda are sophisticated systems of medicine practiced in India for more than 2500 years. Traditional medicine in India focuses on the whole organism and its relation to the external world to re-establish and maintain the harmonious balance that exists within the body and between the body and its environment. Few reliable sources for traditional Ayurveda have been available in English. Most of the accurate works are by and for specialists and are virtually inaccessible to the reader without knowledge of Sanskrit (e.g., Meulenbeld, 1974; Srikanta Murthy, 1984). This circumstance suggests that many of the mysteries of Ayurvedic and Siddha healing are yet to be uncovered and may hold yet greater promise than has yet been realized.

HERBS FOR PAIN AND INFLAMMATION USED IN SOUTH AND SOUTHEAST ASIA

The use of many versatile herbs included in Ayurvedic and Siddha traditions spread throughout the ancient historical region of "Further India." The "Spice Islands" of Southeast Asia are within the ancient realms of Further India and were also a valuable source of many medicinal plants that were used as and considered spices in indigenous and European food preparation (and preservation). In present day their medicinal properties are commonly available today in the West.

The plant chemicals present in herbs and spices are able to protect the plant from the oxidizing effects of the sun, from microbes, and from insect and animal predators, as well as allowing them to compete with other plants for soil, water, and nutrients. The biologically active plant chemicals in turn have properties as antioxidants, antibiotics, and other medicinal activities. These properties made spices invaluable in being able to preserve meats and foods, making them precious to Europeans in the era before refrigeration or canning of foods. They offer many of the same properties that make them safe and effective herbal remedies today. See Table 18.6 for a summary of herbal remedies useful in the management of pain and pain conditions.

Boswellia serrata (Frankincense)

Boswellia is a commonly used ingredient in herbal preparations. It comes from a gum tree that grows in South and Middle Asia and was probably carried over land on the ancient Silk Route to ancient Greece and Rome. In Christian belief it was one of the traditional gifts brought from the East by the Three Magi at Epiphany. During the Crusades it was also brought back to Europe, including by the famous Germanic (Frankish) crusader, Frederick Barbarossa (or "Red Beard"), thus acquiring the common name, "frank incense," or frankincense. Its immune effects are

TABLE 18.6 *Summary of South and Southeast Asian Herbal Remedies*

Genus, Species (common English name)	Conditions and Results
Allium sativum (garlic)	Hyperlipidemia: results in improved levels of lipids (lipid lowering, antithrombotic, antihypertensive, immunomodulatory)
Boswellia serrata (frankincense)	Arthritis: solid reports of beneficial effects (anti-inflammatory)
Capsicum annuum (chili pepper, paprika)	Cluster headaches, neuropathy, and arthritis: improvement reported in several studies External: rubifacient, blocks pain neurotransmitter-substance P, depletes substance P, desensitizes the sensory neurons Internal: reduces platelet aggregation and triglycerides, and improves blood flow
Curcuma longa (turmeric)	Functional gall bladder problems (increase in secretin and bicarbonate output), hyperlipidemia: studies report improvement in cholesterol levels (fatty acid metabolism alteration and decrease in serum lipid peroxide levels) Osteoarthritis: studies report positive results (anti-inflammatory)
Commiphora guggulu (guggul lipid)	Hyperlipidemia: improved lipid levels noted (antagonist of farnesoid X receptors)
Withania somnifera (winter cherry)	Arthritis: studies report improvement (anti-inflammatory)
Zingiber officinale (ginger)	Antiemetic (carminative, local effect on stomach): reduces nausea Osteoarthritis: studies report benefit (anti-inflammatory, inhibits cyclo-oxygenase pathways, prostaglandin [PGE2], and leukotriene [LTB4] synthesis)

similar to those of corticosteroid anti-inflammatory drugs but without the side effects. Boswellic acids are reported to have significant analgesic, anti-inflammatory, and complement-inhibitory properties. In one study involving 30 patients with osteoarthritis of the knee, those who received *Boswellia* tree extract reported a significant improvement in their knee pain, range of motion, and walking distance. In another study of rheumatoid arthritis patients, a special gum extract of *Boswellia serrata,* resulted in a significant improvement of symptoms of pain and swelling. These results are promising for safe and effective relief of joint pain.

Capsicum annuum (Chili Pepper)

Common names of this plant/herb include cayenne pepper, paprika, red pepper, bird pepper, and Peruvian pepper. The preparations of this plant are used in topical creams and ointments. Of course, it is also commonly taken internally as a frequent component of spicy food preparations. It is commonly used for pain related to herpes zoster and diabetic neuropathy. Many use it for osteoarthritis pain. Some basic science studies have shown that it reduces pain by depleting substance P, a chemical pain transmitter. There are also reports of the herb acting by desensitizing neurons thus ameliorating pain.

Curcuma longa (Turmeric)

The active ingredient, curcumin, in this commonly used spice in South and Southeast Asian curry dishes has anti-inflammatory and lipid-lowering effects. It is one of the three components of traditional curry spices, together with coriander and cumin and sometimes chili pepper (see previous). Curcumin's lipid-lowering effects observed in animal experiments are attributed to changes in fatty acid metabolism and facilitating the conversion of cholesterol to bile acids. There are also reports of its strong benefit in patients with osteoarthritis and joint pain. The many other health benefits of turmeric for both body and mind are also being actively studies. Its use as a spice in an overall healthy diet is prudent, and it is also available as an ingredient in dietary supplements.

Withania somnifera (Winter Cherry)

Basic science studies suggest that this herb has anti-inflammatory, antioxidant, immune-modulatory and hematopoietic, as well as "antiaging" properties. It may also have a positive influence on the endocrine and central nervous systems. The mechanisms of these proposed actions require additional clarification. Several observational and randomized studies have reported its usefulness in the treatment of arthritic conditions and joint pain.

Zingiber officinale (Ginger)

Ginger is widely used throughout Asia and the Middle East, most commonly for control of nausea and osteoarthritis pain. Several studies have shown its benefit in controlling nausea associated with pregnancy, motion sickness, and anesthesia, and some studies have demonstrated its usefulness in the treatment of osteoarthritis.

CLINICAL PAIN TREATMENTS

There are clinical protocols available from traditional Indian medicine useful for many of today's common pain problems. Approaches derived directly from the ancient Sanskrit texts of Ayurveda are provided here for allergies and asthma, arthritis, fever and headache, and peptic ulcer that can help to prevent the development of these pain disorders and provide relief for those already suffering from these painful conditions.

Furthermore, they offer help without the risks of side effects and complications that are unfortunately common with high-powered drugs, surgery, and medical procedures of mainstream treatments. These remedies also offer natural health enhancements that help to improve quality of life, longevity, and perhaps less painful relationships with fellow human beings.

Such approaches treat the causes and not just the symptoms of diseases, and they are effective at preventing and treating these problems. In addition to what is offered here, ancient Sanskrit remedies are available for many other medical problems, such as diabetes mellitus, high blood pressure, and viral hepatitis, but require treatment with complex herbal preparations (available today from trusted sources) that are beyond the scope of this book.

ALLERGIES AND ASTHMA

Astyma is the Sanskrit term for allergies, from which the English word asthma is derived. Ayurveda views allergies as altered reactivity caused by weakened metabolism in one or more of the seven tissues of the body. They are categorized according to the three constitutional types: *vata, pitta,* and *kapha.*

Immediate allergic reactions (anaphylactic reactions, from the Greek *ana*, not or without; *phylaxis*, defense or protection) are seen as related to *pitta*. Intermittent allergies (pets, foods) are *vata-pitta* or *vata-kapha* types, and delayed allergies (seasonal) are *kapha.*

Vata allergic symptoms include aches and pains, coughing, gas, sneezing, and sensitivity to dirt, dust, and pollens. Symptoms may also include heart palpitations, muscle allergies, and wheezing (a symptom associated with the constriction of the airways found in asthma). People having these *vata*-type allergies may find they are sensitive to plants from the *Solanacea* family, for example, eggplant, potato, tomato, and deadly nightshade (the source of the drug atropine, or bella donna, from the Italian meaning, "beautiful woman," because women during the 1700s, a time when Italy was a "fashion capital" of Europe, placed atropine in their eyes to cause dilation of the pupils, producing that "doe-eyed" look, due to the toxic effects on the autonomic nervous system effecting the ciliary muscles of the eyes). Other *vata*-type food sensitivities may include black beans, chickpeas (garbanzo beans, for making houmus), and other beans. These allergies can often be managed with a *vata*-pacifying diet and *vata*-reducing herbs.

Pitta-type allergic symptoms include acne, contact dermatitis, eczema, and sensitivity to heat and light, insect bites, foam (as in pillows and mattresses), formaldehyde, and preservatives. Food sensitivities include bananas, eggs, carrots, grapefruit, garlic, pork, onions, and certain cheeses and spicy foods. A *pitta*-pacifying diet and herbs are recommended.

Kapha-type allergies include asthma, allergic rhinitis, hay fever and pollen sensitivities, and latent spring fever, causing symptoms of colds, runny nose and teary eyes, as well as laryngeal edema (swelling of the throat), and possibly generalized edema. Food sensitivities may include avocado, bananas, beef, dairy, cucumbers, lemons, lamb, pork, peanuts, and watermelon. A *kapha*-reducing diet with hot, green teas (with methyl xanthenes, such as caffeine and theophylline, which are natural treatments for decongestion and expansion of airways) and herbal teas are recommended.

The thymus gland and spleen are seen in Ayurveda as important to the immune system. The thymus gland, which is active in childhood and shrinks at adulthood, is important in development of the "T-cell" lymphocytes, or white blood cells, as part of the immune system. The spleen has an important role in filtering the blood and houses large numbers of white blood cells, as well as a reserve of red blood cells. The heating factor of the thymus helps to maintain immunity in proper balance, and weakness may be a cause of *kapha*-type allergy. The spleen is understood as the root of the blood-forming system of the body and as a reservoir for blood (indeed it has this role during fetal development and early childhood and acts as a reserve for blood cells during adulthood). The spleen also is said to contain components that destroy foreign particles and microbes, which is indeed an important function of the spleen as part of the immune system. Weakness in the spleen is detectable in the pulse and likely present in individuals prone to allergies.

ARTHRITIS

Arthritis is known as *amavata* in Sanskrit, which implies the involvement of Ama in the digestion and the *vata dosha* (wind). No distinction is made between rheumatoid arthritis (rheumatism) and osteodegenerative arthritis. The cause is seen as all factors leading to poor digestion, with formation of Ama: poor digestive function, excessive intake of fatty foods and meats, insufficient exercise, and generally unhealthy foods and habits. In arthritis, Ama is said to build up and leave the digestive tract, spilling over and accumulating in the joints and the heart (which are indeed involved in acute rheumatic fever). As implied by the name, *vata* is the principle *dosha* effected, aggravation of which causes indigestion, joint pain, and rough skin. If *pitta* is also involved, a burning sensation, especially in the joints, may spread throughout the body (like some of the complaints in the mysterious modern syndromes of chronic fatigue and fibromyalgia, thought to be a rheumatoid illness, or a disorder of central nervous system pain processing). If *kapha* is further involved, the victim gradually becomes crippled. Less pain is experienced in the morning because at that time, Ama is just beginning to move.

Treatments involve using diet, herbal remedies, and physical modalities and procedures to reduce Ama and alleviate *vata*. The first line of treatment is:
Mild fasting.
Herbs with bitter taste, hot potency, and pungent, post-digestive aftertaste for stimulation of the digestion (bitter-tasting herbs stimulate release of bile from the gallbladder into the intestines—a powerful digestive).
Sweating.

The second line then proceeds to the formal purification therapy of *Pañchakarma*.

Preparation with oleation (oil treatments) and sweating.

Comprehensive, five-part, classic purification therapy protocol over 5 days, including enema, herbal decoctions, and oil.

Third, the patient should then adopt a healthy regimen:

Avoid sleep during the day and after meals (to help to stimulate digestion).

Avoid heavy foods.

Regular massage.

Modern medical research has also shown the importance of meditation and yoga at increasing movement and reducing symptoms in arthritis (see Chapters 5 and 19). These steps are also generally helpful at preventing the development of arthritis. Effective ongoing treatments of arthritis, including childhood arthritic conditions (juvenile arthritis), involve wet massages in conjunction with enemas for digestion and detoxification. Affected joints can be given tapotement (massage term for light tapping or patting) with a cloth bag filled with warm sand or rice cooked with milk and herbs—delivering heat and physical therapy to the joints. Simple massage with oils is also helpful.

One of the reasons Western biomedicine is so often ineffective at treating arthritis may be related to missing the insight into the digestive system and missing the connection to diet and digestion (or the rheumatologist sending the patient to the gastroenterologist—and never "putting it together"). The importance of exercise and physical activity may or may not be addressed, and ignoring the importance of sleep patterns can generally be assumed in Western medicine.

HEADACHE AND FEVER

The common complaint of headache (or head pain; Sanskrit, *Shira Shula*), according to Ayurveda, has many different causes, including cold and flu, indigestion, lack of sleep, muscle tension, overwork, and stress. Migraine headaches specifically are thought to relate to inborn constitutional factors and are most commonly caused by *vata* and/or *pitta* imbalances.

Diagnosis is based upon presence of symptoms associated with each of the three *doshas*.

Vata: extreme pain, constipation, dry skin, and depression and anxiety; worsens with excessive activity, irregular lifestyle, stress, and worry.

Pitta: anger, burning sensation, irritability, light sensitivity, redness of eyes and face, nosebleeds; may be accompanied by liver problems, or blood toxicity.

Kapha: dull ache, heaviness, fatigue; may be accompanied by excess phlegm and salivation, or nausea and vomiting, or lung problems; accumulation of *kapha* in the head.

Treatments for both general headache and migraine are similar.

Sinus and congestive headaches (*vata* and *kapha* types) are usually associated with allergies, common colds, and coughs due to colds. They are given decongestant and expectorant herbs: angelica, bayberry, calamus, ginger, and wild ginger (see previous).

Effective soothing volatile oils are provided by camphor, holy basil (also as tea), eucalyptus, tulsi, and wintergreen.

In addition, therapies are added depending upon the *dosha* type:

Vata: purgation, herbal sedatives for restorative sleep.

Pitta: liver cleansing with aloe powder or rhubarb root, cooling the head with sandalwood oil and avoiding heat and sun, internal gotu kola, inhalation of aromatic oils of rose or lotus.

Application of medicated oils to the head and in the nose is recommended for all forms of headache, including migraine.

Meditation and yoga (see Chapter 19) are also helpful for tension headaches and migraine. In addition, Ayurvedic Marma therapy provides 107 points on the body that are sensitive to touch and may be stimulated to restore balance among the *doshas.* These points are accessed on the skin and specifically associated with enhancing immunity, raising serotonin levels, and increasing secretion of hormones associated with the pineal gland (the vestigial "third eye" sometimes associated with the chakra in the head). Five sets of points are specifically used in the treatment of headache:

Base of eyes (above the tear ducts, at the medial epicanthal folds)

Either side of the nose (one-third of the way down from bridge to nostrils)

Above the upper lip (midway between the margin of the upper lip and the base of the septum)

Top of the head (crown)

At the pineal gland (third eye).

Fever in Ayurveda is seen (Jwara Roga) as both a disease and a symptom. Fever is simply a physiologic response by the body to arrest the multiplication of infectious disease-causing microbes, until the immune system can naturally overcome the infection. Accordingly, fever is viewed as a positive sign in Ayurveda because it is said to loosen and release Ama, the cause of illness. Therefore, it is often allowed to run its course, letting the fever "break," unless one or more of the following danger signs are present:

Both high and prolonged elevation in body temperature

History of prior seizure due to fever in a child

Rapid "depletion" of patient.

In addition to infection, causes are seen to be wrong combinations of food (e.g., mixing hot with cold [fruit with starch, bananas with milk—a typical Western breakfast]) or excessive emotion, such as anger, fear, or stress from overwork. Fever is classified according to the three *doshas:*

Vata: during *vata* time of day (dawn or dusk), or season (fall), begins in colon, pushes digestive fire into channels for transporting lymph, chyle and plasma, and heating the blood:

primary: body ache, headache, shivering, tremors

secondary: backache, constipation, fatigue, insomnia

Pitta: mid-day and midnight, and during summer, onset like *vata* fever:

primary: diarrhea, nausea and vomiting, rash, red eyes, perspiration, sensitivity to light

secondary: severed dehydration and reduction in blood pressure (e.g., fever with severe dehydration is typical of cholera, which has been a historic problem in India and persists to this day in areas like Calcutta)

It may also be caused by alcohol abuse, very sour foods, or fermented beverages. Aspirin is not given because it may damage the stomach, which is already involved in this condition

Kapha: morning and evening, and late winter and spring, production of excessive secretions, which dampen digestive fires and causes undigested food to accumulate, increasing Ama and forcing it out into the body:

primary (prodromal): cold, congestion, runny nose

low-grade fever, chest pain, cough, shortness of breath

laryngitis, sinusitis, sinus congestion, and sinus headache

loss of appetite, cold and clammy skin, heavy and dull feeling

causes may be overexposure to cold, improper combinations of foods, especially involving milk.

Ayurveda is able to make further distinctions among fevers caused by intestinal parasites, and continuous versus fluctuating, or remittent, fevers (such as malaria, another historic problem in India).

Peptic Ulcer (Stomach and Duodenum)

Peptic ulcers (*Parinama Shula,* in Ayurveda) and associated pain are associated with excess stomach acid and have been linked with stress, as well as presence of specific bacteria in the stomach. Ulcers also appear in patients who have suffered shock, severe burns, and head injuries. The following prodromal symptoms are addressed in Ayurvedic texts:

Belching of sour taste

Heartburn

May be accompanied by nausea and vomiting.

Symptoms are brought on by overeating, alcohol, or greasy, sour, or spicy foods. Hyperacidity may be accompanied by migraine headache.

Vomiting may alleviate symptoms. With a gastric ulcer, there is more pain between meals, which is alleviated by eating and neutralizing excess acid. A duodenal ulcer is painful after eating as acidic stomach contents are emptied into the intestines.

Each of the three *doshas* is associated with stomach ulcers:

Vata: excessive mental activity and nervousness lead to stress and overwork, causing ulcer; more gas in the stomach with radiating pain outward.

Pitta: anger, aggression, frustration and anger cause high acid secretion in stomach and lead to ulcers; localized, sharp, penetrating pain, can cause waking in the middle of the night; more likely to lead to perforated ulcer.

Kapha: deficiency of protective mucus secretions of stomach permit stomach acids to burn through the lining of the stomach, even in the presence of normal or low stomach acidity; deep, dull but bearable pain.

For all types of ulcers, a *pitta*-pacifying diet is given, excluding citrus, sour and spicy foods, and including ghee (clarified butter), milk, and whole grains, such as basmati rice. Alcohol and smoking is avoided.

Specific herbal compounds are recommended before (Avipattikara) and after (Jatamamsi, Kamadudha, Shatavari) meals. For a bleeding ulcer the remedy Sat Isabgol is taken with milk before sleep. If blood is seen passing into the stool (duodenal ulcer) other specific herbal remedies may be applied.

INDIVIDUALIZED MEDICAL PROFILE ACCORDING TO AYURVEDA

We will describe the use of modern psychometric profiling to match personality types to susceptibility to diseases and to treatments in Appendix I (pp. 572–579). Ayurveda also uses constitutional types on an empirical basis to match personalities, propensities, susceptibilities, and treatments. The information in this section on medical conditions can be used with the tables in this chapter. Ayurvedic therapies are designed to rebalance and reintegrate the individual based upon constitutional type and the type of the disorder from which patients suffer or are at risk. Every remedy is seen as either tonifying (or nourishing) a deficiency or a weakness in the organ(s) involved, and/or to detoxify (or reduce) aggravation of the *doshas*. Reducing the specific problem usually comes first, followed by rejuvenation to generally rebuild strength. Reduction of the condition usually consists of palliation, followed by purification.

Palliation involves strengthening the digestive fires, reducing Ama, and calming excess *dosha*. Purification involves the five-step classic therapy of *Pañchakarma*. All these approaches emphasize the natural, self-healing abilities of the patient while providing individually tailored treatments for the person and the disorder.

REFERENCES

Dash, B. (1980). *Fundamentals of Ayurvedic medicine*. Delhi, India: Bansal & Co.

Dash, B. & Kashyap, L. (1980). *Basic principles of ayurveda based on ayurveda saukhyam of todarananda*. New Delhi, India: Concept Publishing Company.

Meulenbeld, G. J. (1974). *The Madhavanidana and its chief commentary*. Leiden, Germany: EJ Brill.

Nadkarni, A. K. (1908). *Dr. K. M. Nadkarni's Indian materia medica* (3rd ed.). Bombay (Mumbai), India: Popular Prakashan.

Sen Gupta, K. N. (1984). *The Ayurvedic system of medicine*. 1906, Reprint, New Delhi, India: Logos Press.

Singh, R. H. (1992). *Pañchakarma therapy*. Varanasi, India: Chowkhamba Sanskrit Series Office.

Singhal, G. D., et al. (Trans.). (1972–1993). *Ancient Indian surgery. [Sushruta Samhita]* (10 Vols.). Varanasi, India: Singhal Publications.

Srikanta Murthy, K. R. (Ed.), (1984). *Sharngadharasamhita of Shrangadhara*. Varanasi, India: Chaukhamba Orientalia.

Svoboda, R. E. (1984). *Prakruti. Your Ayurvedic constitution*. Albuquerque, New Mexico: Geocom.

Upadhyay, S. D. (1986). *Nadivijana (Ancient Pulse Science)*. Delhi, India: Chaukhamba Sanskrit Pratisthan.

van Houten, T. & Micozzi, M. S. (1981). *The Edwin Smith Papyrus, Museum Applied Science Center for Art and Archaeology (MASCA)*. Philadelphia: University of Pennsylvania.

Zysk, K. G. (1991). *Asceticism and healing in ancient India. Medicine in the Buddhist monastery*. New York: Oxford University Press.

Zysk, K. G. (1993). *Religious medicine. The history and evolution of Indian medicine*. New Brunswick, New Jersey: Transaction Publishers.

Zysk, K. G. (2000). *Asceticism and healing in ancient India*. 1991, Reprint, Delhi: Motilal Banarsidass.

Chapter 19

Yoga and Breathing

Like Ayurveda, but not a formal part of it, yoga is a textual and practical tradition that developed in India with origins in classic writings and traditions passed down over time. In the traditional Indian context, yoga is first and foremost a philosophical system the purpose of which is spiritual development and devotion leading to the full realization of the spirit.

A wide range of modalities and techniques of yoga have developed to facilitate this journey on life's path. These techniques may include meditation, devotional practice, postural stretching and exercise, diet and nutrition, sound, and sexual exercises. Yoga can be used as complementary medicine, but as with the practice of Ayurveda, it encompasses a broader philosophical system and lifestyle, in addition to those modalities that may represent specific therapies.

Traditional Ayurveda developed separately from the tradition of yoga in India, each coming down through the centuries with perceivable influences of one upon the other. It may be observed that yoga practice has incorporated aspects of Ayurvedic medicine to help to maintain the healthy bodily condition necessary for spiritual development.

In the current environment, there may be special teacher-student relationships in which the yogi (one who knows yoga) acts as the mentor (or literally the guru) to impart knowledge of philosophy and technique to the pupil. Formulary versions of Hatha-Yoga, for example, in which the physical postures and techniques are taught without the philosophical basis would not be properly considered yoga but rather physical training and physical therapy, which nonetheless may be beneficial in its own right.

THE YOKE IS ON YOU

Yoga is a common word in Sanskrit, the ancient Indo-European language. It has a range of meanings: conjunction, constellation, team, or union. The term is related to words in other Indo-European languages, including the Latin *iugum,* German *joch,* and English *yoke,* all of which share meanings. According to the Advaita

Acknowledgments to Marc Micozzi for prior contributions in Micozzi, M. S. (ed.), (2005). *Fundamentals of complementary and alternative medicine* (3rd ed.). St Louis: Elsevier Health and Sciences/Saunders and Julie Staples in Micozzi, M. S. (ed.), (2016). *Fundamentals of complementary and alternative medicine* (5th ed.). St Louis: Elsevier Health and Sciences/Saunders.

Vedanta, yoga is characteristic of philosophical teachings that subscribe to a nondualist metaphysical reality in which the self is the ultimate being underlying all phenomena. However, there is also a dualist school, known as "Raja-Yoga", or "Classical Yoga", founded by the semimythical Patanjali. In this case yoga represents not so much the union with an ultimate reality but disunion or separation from the ego. The ultimate outcome is similar because when the yoga practitioner succeeds in transcending the ego, he or she simultaneously realizes the true essence of the self or soul. Thus yoga comprises different schools that (1) embrace total renunciation of the world *(samnyasa)*, (2) encourage proper performance of one's worldly obligations *(karma)*, (3) regard dispassionate wisdom *(jnana)* as the means to spiritual enlightenment, or (4) place love and devotion above all else *(bhakti)*. One may observe these same ranges of expression within other spiritual traditions, such as Judaism, Islam, and with various orders in Roman Catholicism. Although different versions of yoga are more or less religious and ritualistic, all are spiritual, and yoga may even be regarded perhaps as India's common brand of spiritualism.

The Vedas

Evidence of yoga beliefs and practices may be observed in the ancient *Rigveda* (or knowledge of praise), which serves as a source of the sacred heritage of Hinduism. It is the oldest of the four Vedas (knowledge), dating back to about 1200 BCE, the others being the Samaveda, Yajurveda, and Atharvaveda. The *Veda* is comprised of classic Sanskrit texts said to have been heard *(shruta)* by and thereby revealed to seers *(rshi)* in the form of poems or hymns based on their mystical visions, ecstasies, and insights and traditionally regarded as "revealed wisdom." Yogins within the Hindu tradition based themselves on this Vedic revelation *(shruti)*. Those who did not, such as Gautama the Buddha and Mahavira, the founders of Buddhism and Jainism, respectively, deviated from these revealed teachings.

The *Bhagavad-Gita* (Lord's Song), the most popular and treasured of all yoga scriptures, dates to approximately 2500 years ago. Mahatma Gandhi referred to it as "my mother." It is embedded in the *Mahabharata,* one of two Hindu epics (the other being the *Ramayana*). It tells the story of a great war between two ancient Indian peoples: the Kurus and the Pandavas. Its mythical author Vyasa weaves spiritual teachings into the account of the events leading up to the war, the 18-day war itself, and its aftermath. The tale of the *Bhagavad-Gita* begins on the morning of the first battle, when the Pandava prince Arjuna refuses to fight because he finds teachers and friends among the ranks of the enemy. Krishna, appearing in a divine incarnation as Arjuna's charioteer, encourages to him to do his duty because this is a "just war" to restore moral order.

Yoga teachings are also given elsewhere in the *Mahabharata*.

During the period 500 BCE to approximately 100 CE, many *Upanishads* containing yoga teachings were composed. "Classical" yoga emerged in approximately 200 CE, as codified by Patanjali in the famous *Yoga-Sutra*, or aphorisms of yoga. In Patanjala's text, yoga is defined as the stopping of the endless series of thoughts *(yogah cittavrittinirodhah)*.

Later (post-Classical) sources of yogic knowledge are the *Tantras* (or webs), which belong to the tradition of Shiva-Shakti worship. Shiva manifests the universal male principle and is usually worshiped as a Hindu god; Shakti, meaning "power," refers to female principle or energy in the world, usually visualized as a goddess. Tantric yoga is concerned with enlisting this goddess energy in the yogic process.

Yoga is also an integral part of Shiva worship, as given in the Agamas (traditions).

Hatha-Yoga (or forceful yoga) is an important tradition that emerged in the 11th century under the influence of Tantrism and has its own scriptures, including the *Geranda-Samhita* and the *Shiva-Samhita*.

The classic texts and history of yoga cover many traditions within Hinduism and can also be found within the tradition of Buddhism and Jainism. The Buddha's "noble eightfold path" presents an early form of non-Vedic yoga.

The *Upanishads* are esoteric and philosophical scriptures describing the way to self-understanding, transcendence, and union with the universe. Wisdom is seen as the supreme means to this goal. Wisdom is distinct from knowledge, which relies empirically on the senses, and grasps knowledge from the outside. The spiritual discipline of wisdom is represented in Jnana-Yoga.

Swami Vivekananda, a 19th-century yogin in the Hindu tradition of Advaita Vedanta, represented Hinduism at the World Parliament of Religions in 1894:

Every particle in the body is continually changing; no one has the same body for many minutes together, and yet we think of it as the same body. So with the mind: one moment it is happy, another moment unhappy; one moment strong, another weak— an ever changing whirlpool. That cannot be the Spirit which is infinite…Any particle in this universe can change in relation to any other particle. But take the universe as one; then in relation to what can IT move? There is nothing besides IT. So this infinite unit is unchangeable, immovable, absolute, and this is the Real Man [sic].

The Real Man (or Woman) of Vivekananda is the eternal gender-transcending subject, the essential self of all beings and things. The insights of 20th-century fundamental physics, as well as much of the knowledge of human physiology, biology, and pathology, came in large measure after Swami Vivekananda's insights of 1894.

Since the beginning, practitioners of yoga have cultivated the ideal of "renunciation" (*samnyasa*). Some interpret this practice to imply abandoning worldly life altogether. Others take renunciation primarily as an inner attitude. To the practitioner of Jnana-Yoga, renunciation comes naturally as a realization of the true pattern of life and nature of reality.

HUMAN PAIN, SUFFERING, AND SPIRIT

Yogic philosophy holds that human pain and suffering is caused by *kleshas*, which are the following:
1. Ignorance, or unawareness of reality
2. Ego
3. Attraction toward objects
4. Repulsion from objects
5. Fear of death

At the same time, it realizes that these kleshas are not independent but that one leads to the next, the root cause being ignorance. Being unaware of the ultimate reality of connectedness gives rise to a separate identity or ego. Objects or people who strengthen the ego are found attractive. Those that weaken the ego are considered repulsive or unattractive; and the ego or sense of identity leads to a deep aversion to death because it seems a loss of identity.

Reduction of the kleshas is also an aim of yoga as a predominance of kleshas is detrimental to meditation and progress on the spiritual path. As one progresses and evolves along the spiritual path, one realizes that one's view of life in the present state of consciousness is far inferior to the more subtle essence, which slowly reveals itself.

KARMA

Traditional ancient Vedic spirituality was based on the ideal of outward sacrifice combined with inward meditation. The later *Upanishads* prescribed meditation as an inner sacrifice. This distinction was traditionally couched in terms of wisdom *(jnana)* versus action *(karma)*. To the Jnana-yogin, the greater wisdom may be in nonaction. The growth of the attractiveness of nonaction as a path began to concern social leaders in India by the middle of the first millennium. They argued that a person first should wait until his or her social duties were fulfilled to household and family before retiring to the mountaintop (an early and literal form of retirement). Indian lawgivers favored a lifestyle unfolding in four phases *(ashrama):* student, householder, forest-dweller (late maturity), and freely wandering ascetic (in old age).

The follower of Karma-Yoga acts in daily life so as to lessen lawlessness and restore virtue *(dharma)* or harmony. Like Mahatma Gandhi, the Karma-yogin works for the welfare of others. Devotionally this practice may focus on the worship of the deity in personal form, notably Lord Krishna. Although love and devotion are central to Krishna's message, it is unthinkable without the corollaries of action and wisdom.

As a divine incarnation, Krishna is born whenever the moral order has collapsed and the world is enveloped in spiritual darkness. Krishna's Karman-Yoga is sometimes used to justify military action. It must be remembered that the war Krishna encouraged Arjuna to fight against the Kurus had the specific purpose of restoring moral order. The Karman-yogin may be seen as a "warrior" in this sense, whose good fight is manifest in the material world.

The link between Karman-Yoga and meditation is the loss of identification with the self while performing one's karma as the instrument of the supreme consciousness. When the individual no longer considers the self to be the actor, but merely the instrument, the work becomes spiritualized. Desires and mental problems automatically disappear, as do likes and dislikes, which otherwise create obstacles to meditation. In addition, Karman-Yoga further develops the faculty of concentration and the will. Briefly, the will can be defined as the ability to harmonize, motivate, and mobilize all one's abilities and actions to achieve a definite aim.

BHAKTI: DEVOTION

Bhakti means "devotion," generally devotion to God or the supreme consciousness in one of its manifestations. These manifestations may be one of numerous avatars or divine incarnations or may be one's guru or anyone or anything that evokes strong emotional feelings. Instead of directing the attention to an impersonal form of consciousness, as in Raja-Yoga and Jnana-Yoga, one's love is directed to something more tangible and concrete.

It is generally accepted that individuals are continually trying to find someone or something to which they can totally direct their emotion and devotion and that this search carries on continually through life. In Bhakti-Yoga, the state of meditation arises because a person who feels devotion automatically concentrates her or his mind, depending on the degree of devotion. This also results in the person losing awareness of "I-ness," or ego. Ideally Bhakti-Yoga alone can be sufficient to bring about higher states of meditation, and no other practice is necessary.

Although a devotional attitude in spiritual life was originally reflected in the writings of the seers of the Vedas, the independent path of Bhakti-Yoga emerged in the middle of the first millennium and centered on the theistic religions worshiping Krishna (a divine incarnation of Vishnu) and Shiva. Bhakti-Yoga draws from verses of the *Bhagavad-Gita*. Shiva worshipers in the same era created the *Shvetashvatara Upanishad* as a devotional text. The Bhakti-Yogin devotes himself or herself to the constant remembrance of the divine in all things, whether known as Krishna, Rama, Sita, Parvati, or other god or goddess. As mentioned, this worship takes the form of rituals, love-intoxicated chanting, singing, dancing, and meditation.

Raja-Yoga (or Classical Yoga) was formulated by Patanjali in the Yoga-Sutra around 200 BCE. This school is considered one of the six orthodox systems of Hindu philosophy. Raja-Yoga provides the most systematic access to the practical dimensions of Yoga. Patanjali enumerated eight principal limbs of yogic practice, as follows:

Moral restraint: gentleness, truthfulness, honesty, chastity, and generosity (*Yama*, or social code)

Discipline: purity, contentment, asceticism, study, and devotion (*Niyamas*, or observances)

Posture (*asana*)

Breathing (*pranayama*)

Withdrawal of the senses (*pratyahara*)

Concentration (*dharana*)

Meditation (*dhyana*)

Ecstasy (*samadhi*)

These eight limbs are seen as stages for progressive steps toward attainment of successful meditation and indicate how obstacles on the spiritual path can be overcome.

The social and personal codes of conduct (*Yama* and *Niyamas*) prepare the mind and body for the higher stages of meditation by reducing attachment and inducing tranquility. *Asanas*, or yogic postures, provide steady and comfortable positions for the body to facilitate practice concentration and meditation without physical disturbance. Any position of the body that is even slightly uncomfortable will result in preoccupation of the mind with the body. At the same time other asanas are more therapeutic than meditational. These therapeutic asanas are helpful in treatment and prevention of certain diseases of both body and mind. They also help to induce tranquility of mind, thereby encouraging successful meditation practice.

The word *prana* is often used in yoga and is often misunderstood to mean only "breath." Prana denotes "life force" or vital energy. It is also the medium through which matter and mind are linked to consciousness. The aim of *pranayama* is control over the flow of prana, which is intimately linked to the breathing process. Pranayama results in redistribution of prana in the body, enabling the mind to ascend to the next stages of concentration.

Pratyahara is a method to withdraw the mind from association with the external world so that it can go to the stage of dharana and dhyana. This detachment is accomplished by reducing to zero the selection of sense impressions that are communicated to the mind. The mind is often likened to a naughty child, who does the opposite of what one wants the child to do. This idiosyncrasy of the mind is used for pratyahara, in which the mind is forced to think of external things with the eyes closed; in time, the mind tends to lose interest in the external sounds and does not associate with sense impressions. (Like the childlike lack of mental discipline reflected in the aphorism, "out of sight, out of mind.") "Antarmouna" is a pratyahara technique that specifically exploits this behavior of the mind. Pratyahara also requires that the sitting position, or asana, be comfortable. Many techniques involve a systematic rotation of the awareness around different parts of the body, awareness of the breathing process, and awareness of sounds uttered either mentally or verbally. This satisfies the wandering tendency of the mind in a controlled manner.

Dharana, or concentration, is the method to eliminate memories of the past and projections of future events by concentrating totally on one object to the exclusion of all others. In yogic concentration the mind is not held completely rigid; the processes of the mind are not curtailed. The mind is held so that it is aware of one object, but it should move in the sense that it realizes deeper aspects of the object not perceivable earlier.

Dhayana is an extension of dharana and has been defined by Patanjali as the uninterrupted flow of concentration of mind on the object of meditation or concentration. The difference between dharana and dhyana is that the practitioner has to bring back the awareness to the object of concentration while in dhyana; the mind has been subjugated and is totally and continually absorbed in the object.

Samadhi is the fullest extension of dhyana and is the climax of meditation. Patanjali has defined Samadhi as that state in which there is only consciousness of the object and no concurrent consciousness of the mind.

The stages from dharana to samadhi are really different names for different degrees of attainment. One automatically and spontaneously leads to the next; these are not totally different practices as are the lower five stages. However, it is at these stages that the master or "guru" becomes a necessity for guiding the aspirant safely. Safety is also a concern in practicing and accessing the potency of the next form of yoga, kundalini.

KUNDALINI

In accordance with ancient writings, kundalini yoga was designed to awaken the "serpent power" or spirit within the body. At present, kundalini awakenings are grouped under the medical category of "spiritual emergence," which is considered a psychologic crisis. In *Kundalini Experience* (1976), American psychiatrist Lee Sannella argued that such "awakenings" should be considered spiritual rather than psychiatric in nature.

The Sanskrit word *kundalini* is the feminine form of *kundala,* meaning "ring" or "coil." It thus means "she who is coiled," like a serpent. This is an appropriate metaphor for its psychospiritual potential. Its power is conceived as the goddess counterpart of Shiva, which is pure consciousness.

Each level of the mind is associated with a psychic center, or chakra. The aim of kundalini yoga is to overcome usual inactivity of the higher chakras so that they are stimulated and the individual is able to experience higher levels of the mind. The basic method of awakening these psychic centers in kundalini yoga is deep concentration on the centers and willing their arousal.

A fully awakened kundalini is said actually to restructure the body, leading to a reordering of control over vital functions, such as pulse, intestinal contractions, and brain activity. In Hatha-Yoga (see later), various techniques are used to accomplish these results by focusing the life breath or life force *(prana)* through mental concentration and controlled breathing. Because kundalini is thought to be dormant in the lowest chakra of the energetic body, effort is concentrated on that particular spot.

CHAKRAS

The energetic body in yoga is thought to consist of five to seven energy centers, or *charkas* (literally, "wheels"). In Hatha-Yoga and many Tantric schools of yoga, the seven energy centers are, in ascending order, as follows:

Muladhara: "root-prop wheel," situated in the perineum (yoni), corresponding to the sacrococcygeal nerve plexus, associated with the earth element—the resting place of dormant kundalini.

Svadhishthana: "own-base wheel," located in the genitals, corresponding to the sacral plexus at the fourth lumbar vertebra, associated with the water element.

Manipura: "jewel-city wheel," located at the navel, corresponding to the solar plexus, associated with fire.

Anahata: "wheel of the unstruck," located at the heart, corresponding to the cardiac plexus, associated with the air element.

Vishuddhi: "wheel of purity," located at the throat, corresponding to the laryngeal plexus, associated with the ether element.

Ajna: "command wheel," located in the brain, corresponding to the vestigial third eye (known as the eye of Shiva, or the pineal gland in Western medicine), associated with the mind.

Sahasrara: "thousand-spoked wheel," located at the crown, associated with nonlocal consciousness (Fig. 19.1).

These chakras as conceptualized here may be seen as illustrating two fundamental insights of yoga: matter is a low-velocity form of vibrational energy that exists in states of high velocity elsewhere, and consciousness is not inevitably bound in matter but is inherently free. Kundalini yoga is a method for finding that freedom of consciousness.

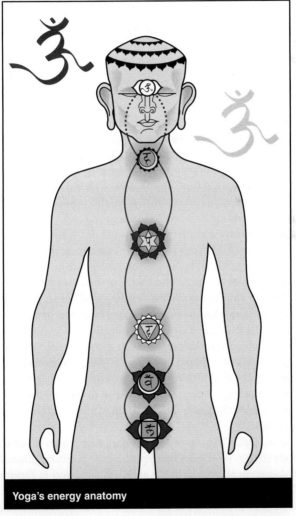

Yoga's energy anatomy

FIG. 19.1 | Symbolic representation of the yogic *nadi* and chakra model.

NADIS

The word *nadi* means a "current," or "flow," connecting the different charkas and other psychic centers. There are said to be 72,000 such nadis; those of particular importance are the Sushumna, pingala, and ida nadis.

Sushumna is by far the most important nadi, with its base at the mooladhara chakra and traveling through the spinal column and terminating at the center of the Sahasrara chakra via the swadhishthana, manipura, anahata, and vishuddhi chakras. It is in this nadi that the kundalini flows when it is awakened.

The pingala and ida nadis start at the mooladhara and terminate at the ajna chakra, crossing the sushumna at the swadhishthana, manipura, anahata, and vishuddhi chakras in a serpent-like fashion, forming semicircular curves between two consecutive chakras. The pingala or "solar nadi" starts with a right curve from the mooladhara; the ida or "lunar nadi" starts with a left curve from the mooladhara.

HATHA-YOGA

Hatha means "force" or "forceful" and refers to the practice of yoga that uses physical purification and body strengthening as an arduous means of self-transformation and transcendence. A frail or diseased body may prove an obstacle on the path to enlightenment of the spirit and therefore must be properly trained.

Physical and mental training and fitness are important because at the core of Hatha-Yoga is the potentially dangerous process of awakening the kundalini-shakti. This arousal of the power of consciousness at the lowest psychospiritual center *(chakra)* of the body and transmission to the highest center in the crown is tremendously powerful, physically and mentally. Historically, Hatha-Yoga is based on the development of Tantrism (Tantra-Yoga). The awakening of kundalini-shakti was central to Tantric esotericism, long before the emergence of Hatha-Yoga, as a practice for the preparation of the mind and body for this awakening.

Another school of thought holds that in the word hatha; *ha* stands for the ida (lunar) nadi, and *tha* stands for the pingala (solar) nadi. It is held that when the flow of prana in ida is equal to the flow of prana in pingala, kundalini automatically starts to rise. Therefore Hatha-Yoga is concerned with the two nadis, ida and pingala, and its aim is balancing the flow of prana in each nadi. When the kundalini is activated in this way, it stimulates the chakras, and meditation automatically takes place.

Many of the Hatha-Yoga practices also attempt to directly stimulate the chakras and to clean and generally improve the condition of various physical organs that are linked to the chakras.

In preparation, Hatha-Yoga incorporates many techniques for cleansing and stabilization of body energy. It includes many postures or positions *(asanas)* to maintain or restore well-being, to improve vitality and flexibility, and to facilitate prolonged meditation. The basis is breathing and breath control *(pranayama),* and various techniques are used to modulate the body's vital winds *(prana)* through the breath. This form of yoga is best known in the West, although its deeper philosophical foundations are rarely understood or practiced. It is widely reduced to another form of "fitness training."

The 20th-century Hatha-Yoga master B.K.S. Iyengar trained many American Hatha-Yoga teachers. He said, "The original idea of yoga is freedom and beatitude, and the by-products...including physical health, are secondary for the practitioner."

Hatha-Yoga entails a complex program of physical cleansing *(shodhana)*. The *Geranda-Samhita* describes six acts, as follows:

Dhauti (cleansing), consisting of four techniques: inner, dental, "heart" or chest, and "base" purification. "Inner cleansing" uses four exercises: swallowing the breath and expelling it through the anus, filling the stomach with water, stimulating the abdominal "fire" by repetitions of contracting the navel against the spine, and washing the prolapsed intestines (not medically recommended). "Dental cleansing" covers the teeth, tongue, ears, and frontal sinuses. "Heart cleansing" consists of induced or self-induced emesis. "Base cleansing" is manual cleansing of the anus with water or other solution.

Vasti or *Basti:* bladder cleansing by contracting the urinary sphincter, usually while standing in water.

Neti: threading a thin cloth through the nostril and out the mouth to remove mucus and "open up the third eye."

Lauli or *nauli:* rolling the abdominal muscles sideways to massage the inner organs.

Trataka: gazing steadily at a small, close object, such as a candle flame, until tears flow, to develop the powers of concentration.

Kapala-bhati: three practices involving breathing in through the right nostril and out through the left (and vice versa), drawing water through the nostrils and expelling it through the mouth, and sucking water up through the mouth and expelling it through the nose. This is done to purify the frontal portion of the brain.

Relaxation, as with purification, is another important preparatory aspect involving the postures *(asanas)* of Hatha-Yoga. Relaxation applies not only to the body but also to the mind. When posture is cultivated properly, it creates the sensation that the body is loosening up and widening out. Thus, posture is more than gymnastics or acrobatics; it is the art of relaxation to the point of meditation and beyond. Following are some postures for meditation:

- *Siddha-asana,* the "successful posture," is achieved by pressing the left heel against the perineum and placing the right foot above the genitals.
- *Padmasana,* the "lotus posture," is achieved by placing the right foot on the left thigh and the left foot on the right thigh. The classic texts also teach crossing the arms behind the back and grasping the left toe with the left hand and the right toe with the right hand, called the "bound lotus". The lotus posture, in addition to promoting relaxation, is said to alleviate a number of diseases. It often is seen in depictions of the Buddha.
- *Sukhasana,* the "happy posture," favored by many Americans, is widely known as the "tailor's seat".

Other well-known postures are the tree, triangle, hands-to-feet, adamantine, cow-face, back-stretching, serpent (cobra), all-limb, plow, and head postures.

In addition to the postures, Hatha-Yoga has a series of bandhas (bonds or locks) and mudras (seals). There are three principal types of locks, in which the life force is forcibly retained in the body: The root lock is the contraction of the anal sphincter. The upward lock is executed by pulling the stomach up until there is a hollow below the rib cage, said to force the vital energy upward "like a great bird." The throat contraction lock is done by placing the chin down against the collarbone, stopping the downward flow of ambrosial fluid (possibly a reference to hormonal secretions). It prevents the life force (and the vital breath) from escaping through the nose or mouth.

The Hatha-Yoga seals consist of the following eight most important techniques:

Space-seal: turning the tongue back and inserting it in the nasopharynx (cavity at the back of the mouth leading to the nose), possible only if the frenulum underneath the tongue has been deliberately cut. This mudra is said to satisfy hunger, quench thirst, cure disease, and postpone death.

Power-stirring: contracting the anus and forcing the vital energy into the central channel at the lowest chakra, the seat of the kundalini.

Shambu: a meditation technique more than a physical exercise, it requires a wide-eyed, unfocused gaze. Shambu, another name for Shiva, is regarded as the revealer of the secrets of Tantrism.

Vajroli: sucking released semen back into the urethra. Females also learn this technique so as not to waste the valuable hormonal and chemical properties of semen.

Sahajoli: rubbing ejaculated semen into the skin.

Amaroli: drinking the midflow of the urine, thought to have certain healing properties.

Womb: while seated in the siddha-asana posture, with eyes, ears, and nostrils closed with the 10 fingers, the body's energy is forced through the six chakras by means of breath control, mantra, and visualization.

Six-openings: placing the thumbs on the two ears, the index and middle fingers on the two eyes, and the ring and the little fingers on the two nostrils.

Similarly, there are eight major breathing techniques *(pranayama)* for modulating the flow of vital energy into the body. Incorrect *pranayama* may cause hiccups, asthma, headache, and other ailments.

MENTAL IMAGERY

Similar to many mind-body interventions (see Chapter 7), yoga uses visualization as one of the traditional forms of meditation. Visualization has been practiced particularly in the Tantric Buddhism of Tibet (see also Section II of this book). *Deity yoga* involves the visualization of deities and is the essential practice of what is called "Highest Yoga Tantra". Deities are usually visualized together with their respective environments, known as "mandalas", or "circles."

MEDITATION

It is important to meditate in a secure environment where interruptions can be minimized. Having a usual location reserved for meditation and yoga is helpful. Repeated meditation in the same location may help to develop an energetic environment (or imprint) that facilitates the meditative state.

Time of day is important. As with location, it is useful to meditate at a consistent time regardless of which time is chosen. Most traditions indicate that early morning is the best time to meditate. Yogins in India typically meditate at sunrise, known as the "hour of Brahma". Meditation at noon, sunset, and midnight is also recommended.

It is advised at the outset to sit in meditation for no more than 15 minutes at a time. Initially the desire for sleep or mental indulgence in fantasies or daydreaming may tend to replace the meditative state. Being well rested is also important for meditation, as it is for general health, because tiredness merely invites sleep or daydreaming. Sexual activity should be avoided shortly before meditation because it may deplete the psychoenergetic centers *(chakras)*.

MANTRAS

The consciousness-altering effects of sound are well known and probably belong to the earliest expression of human culture. Sacred sounds preceded yoga and were most likely part of the early Vedic rituals and religion.

Some of the mystical insights and writings of the ancient Vedic sages have been reinterpreted in light of modern understanding of fundamental physics, for example, that the universe is "an ocean of vibrations." According to the schools of Siddha-Yoga, also known as "Mantra-Yoga", all perceptible sounds ultimately derive from a universal matrix of sound. This expression has been translated as "sonic absolute," which is typically articulated as the monosyllabic sound "OM (A-U-M)." Classic physics states that sounds are waves of consecutive compressions and rarefactions of air or other fluid.

Mantra-Yoga uses the vehicle of sonic vibration to unify consciousness through recitation and contemplation of special numinous sounds such as OM. In addition, the monosyllables HAM, YAM, RAM, VAM, LAM, AH, HUM, and PHAT are also used.

Few mantras have a denotative meaning but rather are used to produce specific states of energy and consciousness. After continuous and dedicated practice, the mantra is repeated automatically without strain or effort. The mantra spontaneously manifests itself and becomes an integral part of the mind. The mind vibrates with the sound of the mantra. This approach provides a powerful means of attaining meditational states, since the mind is rendered calm and concentrated. The mantra acts as a pathway between normal states of consciousness and superconsciousness.

TANTRA

Tantric yoga posits that sexual energy is an important reservoir that should be used wisely to facilitate the spiritual process rather than block it through orgasmic release.

There are right-handed and left-handed practices of Tantric yoga. In left-handed Tantra, sexual union is a central ritual. In many countries throughout the Middle East and South Asia, the left hand is the taboo hand used for private bodily functions, not for eating or greeting. (The Latin term *sinister* also means "left.") In left-handed Tantra, things that are taboo are charged with energy because of the constant, negative attention they receive. This yoga makes a point of breaking with established norms by using taboo functions, such as sexuality in the service of spiritual transformation.

At the center of left-handed Tantra are the five prohibitions: sex, wine, meat, fish, and parched grain. In the West a tantric ritual involving all five taboos includes random sexual coupling. The sexual union itself is accomplished according to strict ritual and with great dignity and meditative visualization. In general, the purpose of sexual union is the healthy circulation of vital energy between the male and female partners.

Tantrism is neither orgiastic nor hedonistic in principle on the one hand, so to speak, nor is it ascetic, on the other. Discipline is essential to Tantric practice. For example, semen is equated with the impulse toward enlightenment and should not be discharged. Orgasm does not lead to bliss but merely to pleasurable sensations. Thus the earnest practitioner must forgo orgasm. Men are advised to apply pressure to the perineum to prevent ejaculation. Some practitioners learn to control their genital functions to the point in which they can suck the ejaculated semen back through the penis.

The same consideration applies to women, although, for example, in Chinese Taoism, orgasm is not seen to have the same depleting effect as in men. The female sexual secretions, or equivalent of semen, are called "rajas", which may refer to the hormone-rich vaginal secretions released during sexual arousal. In some schools, men are urged to absorb the female rajas into their own bodies.

In Tantrism and yoga, sexual activity is not a moral matter, and sexual drive is considered inherently divine. The only reason for suggesting chastity is purely a matter of economics: conservation of energy.

PHYSIOLOGY OF YOGA PRACTICE AND BREATHING

As mentioned previously, Hatha-Yoga is the most widely practiced branch of yoga in the West. There are, in turn, many styles within Hatha-Yoga itself, including Ananda, Ashtanga, Bikram, Integral, Iyengar, Kripalu, Kundalini, Sivananda, Viniyoga, and Vinyasa. These styles range from vigorous to gentle, with varying degrees of emphasis on the precision of the postures. Some styles still maintain a stronger emphasis on psychologic and spiritual growth. Brief descriptions of these styles, as well as their developers and centers, are provided on the Yoga Journal website (Yoga Journal Editors, 2013a) and in the book *Your Brain on Yoga* (Khalsa & Gould, 2012). Although some styles may place more emphasis on one element of yoga or another, the elements of an authentic Hatha-Yoga practice include physical postures, breathing techniques, deep relaxation, and meditation.

Postures (*Asanas*)

There are several categories of physical postures performed in yoga. They include seated, standing, twisting, and arm balance postures; backbends and forward bends; side stretches; inversions; core-strengthening; and restorative postures (McCall, 2007; Yoga Journal Editors, 2013b). Most of the physical postures are labeled with original Sanskrit names and are consistent as practiced across the different yoga styles. Performing these postures provides a systematic way to take the body through various ranges of motion. Obvious physical benefits include increasing flexibility and muscle strength and improving balance and posture. Specific postures also direct the flow of prana and apana and asanas are part of the eight limbs of yoga on the path to self-transcendence. Therefore taken as a comprehensive system, these postures have more far-reaching benefits according to the yogic tradition than simply increasing flexibility and strength.

Breathing Practices (*Pranayama*)

As described previously, prana is the life force in the yogic anatomy. Pranayama is the control of the movement of prana through the use of breathing techniques. There are many kinds of yogic breathing techniques, each with specific effects.

Long Deep Breathing

One of the simplest techniques is long deep breathing. This breath uses the full vital capacity of the lungs; inhaling and (1) letting the belly expand and the air move into the lower portion of the lungs, then (2) expanding the chest to fill the middle part of the lungs, and (3) finally, lifting the chest to fill the upper part of the lungs. The exhale is done in reverse order: releasing the air from the top, then middle, then bottom of the lungs. One of the benefits of long deep breathing is that it is calming and relaxing as accompanied by an increase in parasympathetic nervous system dominance. This type of pranayama is commonly performed during the practice of yoga. Beneficial effects on lung physiology can carry over even when the practitioner returns to breathing normally as demonstrated in a study on the chemoreflex response.

Chemoreflex receptors trigger breathing and chemoreflex sensitivity is often increased in individuals with chronic heart failure, resulting in dyspnea and reduced tolerance to exercise. Therefore decreasing chemoreflex sensitivity is beneficial for these patients. To determine the role of long deep breathing and yoga practice on the chemoreflex response, yoga practitioners were compared with non-yoga practitioners. Long deep breathing (six breaths per minute) decreased chemoreflex sensitivity in both yoga practitioners and nonpractitioners. But yoga practitioners (only) appeared to have a longer-term benefit in that chemoreflex sensitivity remained lower even during spontaneous breathing or breathing at 15 breaths per minute (Spicuzza et al., 2000). Yoga practitioners had a baseline of decreased chemoreflex sensitivity, which persisted even when not actually performing long deep breathing.

Individual Nostril Breathing and Alternate Nostril Breathing

Individual nostril breathing stimulates the ida and pingala energy channels and has effects related to the qualities of these channels. The ida is associated with the "moon energy." It has cooling and receptive characteristics and is associated with calmness, sensitivity, empathy, and synthesis. The pingala is associated with the "sun energy." It has warming and projective characteristics and is associated with vigor, alertness, will power, concentration, and a readiness for action. As mentioned earlier, the ida and pingala are subtle energy structures and have no currently detectable physical structures in the human body. However, they resemble the characteristics of the sympathetic and parasympathetic nervous systems, or the "yin" (moon, etc.) and "yang" (sun, etc.) phases in Chinese cosmology and constitutional medicine. Because the ida ends at the left nostril, breathing through the left nostril is a calming breath. Left nostril breathing may result in a reduction of sympathetic activity, as demonstrated by an increase in volar galvanic skin resistance (Telles, Nagarathna, & Nagendra, 1994). Because the pingala ends at the right nostril, breathing through the right nostril is an energizing breath that also improves alertness and focus. Right nostril breathing has been shown to stimulate the sympathetic nervous system, as measured by increased heart rate and peripheral vasoconstriction, resulting in decreased digit pulse volume (Shannahoff-Khalsa & Kennedy, 1993; Telles, Nagarathna, & Nagendra, 1996).

Another regulated yoga breathing technique is alternate nostril breathing that can be performed by inhaling through the left, exhaling through the right, then inhaling through the right, exhaling through the left *(Nadi Shodhana)*. As part of a more advanced practice, certain breath retentions and breath ratios are added. According to yogic theory, alternate nostril breathing is said to purify the ida and pingala and to balance the right and left hemispheres of the brain.

From the yogic perspective, breathing through the right nostril stimulates the left side of the brain, and breathing through the left nostril stimulates the right side of the brain. Research studies support these effects of individual nostril breathing. There is a natural nasal cycle related to relative congestion and decongestion of the nasal passages, which in turn results in more predominant airflow in one nostril versus the other at a given point in time. The nasal mucosae are densely innervated with autonomic fibers, and it is the autonomic nervous system that regulates the congestion and decongestion. Sympathetic dominance in one nostril produces vasoconstriction and decongestion, allowing for greater airflow. Simultaneous parasympathetic dominance occurs in the contralateral nostril, resulting in vasodilation and congestion, which restricts airflow. The hypothalamus is believed to be responsible for regulating the nasal cycle. The length of the cycle varies and may be from 25 minutes to 8 hours. However, in general, the average cycle lasts approximately 1.5 to 4 hours and takes place 24 hours per day.

The natural nasal cycle has been shown to have a direct relationship to the cerebral hemispheric activity, as measured by electroencephalogram (EEG) (Werntz, Bickford, Bloom, & Shannahoff-Khalsa, 1983). During the portion of the nasal cycle when airflow is predominantly through the right nostril, EEG activity is greater in the left hemisphere; and when airflow is predominantly through the left nostril, the EEG activity was greater in the right hemisphere. By performing forced nostril breathing through one nostril at a time, the ability to shift the contralateral dominance in hemispheric activity was measured. In this study, participants were asked to close off the more open nostril and breathe through the opposite, more closed nostril, and then alternate sides for 11 to 20 minutes. As predicted, while breathing through the right nostril, the EEG amplitude in the left hemisphere is enhanced; then, upon changing to the left nostril, the enhanced EEG activity switches to the right hemisphere (Werntz, Bickford, & Shannahoff-Khalsa, 1987).

Another study was performed to assess whether there is any change observed in functional activities among the two cerebral hemispheres when forced nostril breathing is applied (Shannahoff-Khalsa, Boyle, & Buebel, 1991). Verbal and spatial tests were administered before and after breathing though the right nostril, the left nostril, and both nostrils for 30 minutes. The results showed that right nostril breathing results in higher verbal scores; left nostril breathing results in higher spatial test scores; there were no significant changes while breathing through both nostrils. The greatest improvements were observed in the groups with the forced nostril breathing through the nostril that was initially dominant. These studies suggest that the nasal cycle and alternating cerebral dominance are closely correlated; and by using forced nostril yogic breathing techniques, it is possible to influence cognitive performance. A proposed mechanism for these findings is that decreased cognitive performance is related to decreased cerebral blood flow caused by vasoconstriction of the cerebral blood vessels. Because the majority of autonomic nerve fibers travel ipsilaterally and do not cross over (Saper, Loewy, Swanson, & Cowan, 1976), enhanced sympathetic activity on one side of the body would result in increased airflow in that nostril and decreased cerebral blood flow with diminished cognitive function in the ipsilateral hemisphere (Shannahoff-Khalsa et al., 1991).

The nasal cycle is also a marker for various physiologic states, and one theory is that the hypothalamus not only regulates the nasal cycle but also regulates the coupled ultradian rhythms of the other body systems, including the neuroendocrine, cardiovascular, and immune systems (Shannahoff-Khalsa, Kennedy, Rancisf, & Ziegler, 1996). There is a resting phase and activity phase of these cycles, originally proposed as the basic rest-activity cycle (BRAC). Because of the association of the ida and pingala to the right and left nostrils and the nasal cycle in being tied to multiple body rhythms, the resting phase may be the equivalent of the *ida* and the activity phase may be the equivalent of the *pingala* (Shannahoff-Khalsa, 2007).

Fast Breathing

Depending on the style of yoga practiced, different types of fast breathing may also be incorporated. These types of breathing include Bhastrika, Breath of Fire, and Kapalabhati. Both Bhastrika (bellows) and Breath of Fire consist of breathing with rapid and forceful inhalation and exhalation through the nose. Both breaths are stimulating, raise vital energy levels, and increase alertness, and according to yogic teachings, both balance the nervous system. Breath of Fire is less forceful than

Bhastrika. In Kapalabhati, the inhalation is long and mild and the exhalation is forceful and rapid. Kapalabhati can be done at either a slow speed of 60 exhales per minute or a fast speed of 240 exhales per minute (Sturgess, 1997). Kapalabhati is considered a cleansing breath.

Other Breathing Techniques

The long deep breathing, alternate nostril breathing, and fast breathing techniques represent main types of pranayama. There are also additional breathing techniques observed to have specific benefits. Some brief explanations and examples include a common breath known as ujjayi pranayama. During ujjayi breath, the glottis, above the trachea, or airway, is partially closed, and the breath becomes audible to produce a balancing and calming effect. Sitali pranayama is another type of breath that has a cooling effect on the body. It is performed with the tongue sticking out (like panting) and curled and inhaling through the curled tongue. Bhramari pranayama (humming bee breath), a breath that calms the mind, is performed by closing off the ears with the fingers and making a high-pitched humming sound on the exhale.

PAIN TREATMENT

Although yoga historically is known as a path to spiritual enlightenment, the physical and mental benefits of yoga are becoming widely recognized. Yoga is being incorporated in places such as cancer centers throughout the United States, as well as in institutions, such as the Department of Veteran's Affairs (VA) posttraumatic stress disorder (PTSD) treatment programs (Libby, Reddy, Pilver, & Desai, 2012). Yoga therapy, as a professional practice, is in a relatively early stage in the United States. The International Association of Yoga Therapists (IYTA) published Educational Standards for the Training of Yoga Therapists in 2012 and is beginning the process of accrediting yoga therapy programs that meet these standards. However, yoga therapy is not new, and the clinical application of yoga as a therapeutic intervention first began in 1918 at the Yoga Institute at Versova in Mumbai, India (Khalsa, 2004). The Kaivalyadhama Yoga Institute in Lonavala, Maharashtra India, under Swami Kuvalayananda was established a few years later (Khalsa, 2004). Kuvalayananda began the first research on the psychophysiologic effects of yoga in the 1920s and published the first yoga specialty journal in 1924 called *Yoga Mimamsa.* Yoga research has since spread to the United States, and there are now studies supporting the use of yoga for various physical and mental diseases and pain disorders. Table 19.1 shows a list of the most widely researched pain conditions.

According to the conclusions of the review articles and meta-analyses cited in Table 19.1, the health problems with the strong research evidence for the benefits of yoga include pain and pain conditions. Some of the studies involve a more "holistic" approach that also included a dietary modification and an exercise program in addition to a yoga component. Conditions that are likely to be benefitted by yoga based on reasonably strong research evidence include *back pain, chronic pain,* diabetes,

TABLE 19.1 *Pain Conditions Improved by Yoga*

Rheumatoid Arthritis	1 Meta-analysis (Ward, Stebbings, Cherkin, & Baxter, 2013)
	2 Reviews (Cramer, Lauche, Langhorst, & Dobos, 2013a; Haaz & Bartlett, 2011)
Back Pain	2 Meta-analyses (Cramer, Lauche, Haller, & Dobos, 2013b; Ward et al., 2013)
	1 Systematic review (Posadzki & Ernst, 2011)
	2 Reviews (Hill, 2013; Kelly, 2009)
Osteoarthritis	1 Meta-analysis (Ward et al., 2013)
	3 Reviews (Haaz & Bartlett, 2011; Raub, 2002; Cramer et al., 2013a)
Fibromyalgia	1 Meta-analysis (Ward et al., 2013)
	1 Systematic review (Cramer et al., 2013a)
Chronic Pain Syndrome	1 Meta-analysis (Bussing, Michalsen, Khalsa, Telles, & Sherman, 2012)
	1 Systematic review (Posadzki, Ernst, Terry, & Lee, 2011)

Adapted from Bussing A., Ostermann T., Lüdtke R., Michalsen A. et al. (2012). Effects of yoga interventions on pain and pain-associated disability: a meta-analysis. *J Pain*, 13(1), 1 (Table 1) with updates.

depression, high blood pressure and heart disease, *fibromyalgia, osteoarthritis,* and *rheumatoid arthritis.*

Studies of yoga with pain in cancer patients have shown improvements in quality of life, sleep, anxiety, depression, perceived stress, and psychologic distress. In women with breast cancer, yoga practice has also resulted in improved quality of life, as well as daily functions, and social, spiritual, end emotional well-being. Short-term positive psychologic effects of yoga have also been measured for women in menopause. For a variety of illnesses involving fatigue, yoga has been most beneficial for fatigue related to cancer or cancer treatment. Positive results have been reported for yoga using anxiety as an outcome measure in a variety of health conditions (Sharma & Haider, 2013; Sharma, Haider, & Knowlden, 2013), but the use of yoga for anxiety disorders, per se, has not been widely studied. However, there has been recent interest in the use of yoga for one particular anxiety disorder, PTSD, and several research studies are being performed. The results of one pilot study provides evidence that yoga may be helpful for reducing the hyperarousal symptoms of PTSD and for improving sleep quality (Staples, Hamilton, & Uddo, 2013). Finally, research on asthma to date has shown mixed results on the effectiveness of yoga for symptom improvement and further studies are needed.

MECHANISMS OF ACTION

There are several proposed mechanisms on how yoga may benefit health. Stress is an underlying factor in many diseases and disorders. The cost to the body for maintaining stability and coping in the presence of chronic stress is termed "allostatic load"

(Streeter, Gerbarg, Saper, Ciraulo, & Brown, 2012; Taylor, Goehler, Galper, Innes, & Bourguignon, 2010). One theory on the benefits of yoga is that it reduces allostatic load and restores optimal homeostasis (Streeter et al., 2012). Stress is associated with decreased activity of the neurotransmitter gamma aminobutyric acid (GABA) and just 1 hour of yoga practice increased thalamic GABA levels compared with 1 hour of reading (Streeter et al., 2007). Increased GABA production by yoga may be a mechanism for benefiting such conditions as major depressive disorder, PTSD, and chronic pain, which are characterized by low GABA activity.

Oxidative stress has also been linked to several diseases, such as heart disease, cancer, rheumatoid arthritis, hypertension, Alzheimer's disease, and Parkinson's disease (Martarelli, Cocchioni, Scuri, & Pompei, 2011). Increased oxidative stress also leads to increased inflammation and the production of proinflammatory cytokines, which also play a role in most of the diseases above in addition to osteoporosis and diabetes (Kiecolt-Glaser et al., 2010). Yoga, including yogic breathing practices, have been shown to increase antioxidant formation (Martarelli et al., 2011; Sharma et al., 2003; Sinha, Singh, Monga, & Ray, 2007) and decrease the production of proinflammatory cytokines (Kiecolt-Glaser et al., 2010), suggesting that these may be other mechanisms by which yoga helps to protect against disease and pain. Other possible mechanisms by which yoga may improve health include increasing melatonin production, decreasing cortisol levels, decreasing sympathetic activity, and increasing parasympathetic activity, as well as regulating the hypothalamic-pituitary-adrenal axis (McCall, 2013) (Table 19.1).

Yoga as Therapy

As age-old traditions of yoga and meditation enter contemporary health care, they represent ways to help to manage stress, pain and suffering, and chronic diseases, as well as promoting good health. The health benefits of yoga have been demonstrated by scientific research. There is much research on related practices of hypnotherapy, biofeedback, and relaxation techniques (see Section II of this book), independent of yoga, as well as research specifically associated with yoga. The biofeedback technique in particular has great promise for beginners and for those who are not making discernible progress in meditation, even after constant practice.

The practice of yoga produces physiologic changes in the body, as discussed previously. The monitoring and understanding of these changes have led to a greater understanding of the human body, particularly with regard to its bioenergetic aspects. Basic research has also been done on the psychologic aspects of yoga practice. Personal psychology has methods for assessing states of consciousness, and alterations in consciousness through yoga practice have also been demonstrated. For example, Psychosynthesis has the same aims as yoga: integration of the whole being of an individual and eventual self-realization. Both modern psychology and yoga emphasize the importance of evolution and growth from "less wholeness" to "more wholeness."

Yoga has been studied as part of traditional scientific research in physiology and psychology to gain a better understanding of the human body and mind and also now forms a part of research specifically on complementary medicine as an aid to good health.

Clinical studies as above have shown that yoga is effective therapy for several chronic pain conditions, as well as for stress management.

As with many other natural and complementary therapies using mechanisms of action not fully understood, yoga is helpful in the management of asthma and other breathing disorders, high blood pressure, and heart disease. It also helps to improve mood and counter mild-moderate depression.

Yoga is helpful in the management of a number of musculoskeletal disorders, such as carpal tunnel syndrome and osteoarthritis, and of common occupational health problems, such as low back pain. Evidence also indicates that yoga can be helpful in disorders of the immune system, such as rheumatoid arthritis and lupus. Yoga has also been seen to improve academic and physical performance in school-children, potentially contributing to healthy growth and development.

One of the most important changes that takes place in the body during meditation is the slowing down of the metabolism, resulting in a sharp reduction in oxygen consumption and carbon dioxide output by up to 20%. Although blood pressure and heart rate decrease overall, peripheral blood flow increases during meditation; activities of the sympathetic nervous system are reduced; and constriction of the blood vessels is relaxed. This peripheral blood flow ensures the oxygen is more efficiently delivered to the muscles and that lactate and lactic acid is more quickly and effectively removed. Reduction of lactate levels has a direct effect on reduction of blood pressure and anxiety levels.

The quality of relaxation produced by yoga and meditation may be deeper than that produced by sleep, allowing recuperation of the body from the damaging effects of overproduction of adrenaline and activity of the sympathetic nervous system. Through meditation, the septal region of the limbic system in the base of the brain may become operational for the predominant part of our lives. Ideally, proper activation of the brain leads to a life of relaxation, which at the same time, is more efficient and disease-free.

Yoga practice involves the total body and total mind. Yoga and meditation act as a holistic treatment concerning the whole mind-body complex. Yoga provides a powerful way of controlling physiologic processes and also of controlling physiologic reactions to psychologic events.

In yoga, individual consciousness is thought to be connected with the physical body at the heart. This kind of consciousness, in an "unenlightened" individual, is labeled "self-contraction." This contraction is felt at the level of the heart as a sense of separation, isolation, loneliness, fear, and uncertainty. At the level of the mind, this contraction manifests itself as doubt. Yoga endeavors to expand this contraction.

In the West, yoga often is reduced to fitness training bereft of the consciousness and spirit that can be brought to heart and mind. Although reductionist yoga practice helps many people to maintain and restore physical health, it does not provide the full potential benefits of yoga. Many practitioners of yoga in India and the West know only this reductionist form of yoga.

Yoga was never intended for quick fixes or as a cheap service to the ego. Promises of enlightenment over a weekend or a week are blatant misconceptions. Like anything in life, the benefits from yoga are commensurate with the attention, discipline, and effort put into it. Yoga must be learned from a knowledgeable master. A mature student will have no difficulty in learning from a master in any given field. However, we must, examine our teachers carefully. As proven constantly in our daily experience, neither education nor age is any guarantee of wisdom.

The mass media has profitably manipulated public opinion by confusing the guru tradition with the vexing issues of cult leadership and brainwashing. As more flamboyant and questionable gurus are replaced through experience with true spiritual masters, the practice of yoga should gain in strength as a means of undertaking the journey from body to spirit.

REFERENCES

Bussing, A., Michalsen, A., Khalsa, S. B. S., Telles, S., & Sherman, K. J. (2012). Effects of yoga on mental and physical health: A short summary of reviews. *Evidence-based Complementary and Alternative Medicine, 2012*, 165410. Article ID 165410.

Cramer, H., Lauche, R., Langhorst, J., & Dobos, G. (2013a). Yoga for rheumatic diseases: A systematic review. *Rheumatology (Oxford)*. ahead of print.

Cramer, H., Lauche, R., Haller, H., & Dobos, G. (2013b). A systematic review and meta-analysis of yoga for low back pain. *The Clinical Journal of Pain, 29*(5), 450.

Haaz, S. & Bartlett, S. J. (2011). Yoga for arthritis: A scoping review. *Rheumatic Diseases Clinics of North America, 37*(1), 33.

Hill, C. (2013). Is yoga an effective treatment in the management of patients with chronic low back pain compared with other care modalities—A systematic review. *Journal of Complementary and Integrative Medicine, 10*(1), 1.

Kelly, Z. (2009). Is yoga an effective treatment for low back pain: A research review. *International Journal of Yoga Therapy, 19*(1), 103.

Khalsa, S. B. (2004). Yoga as a therapeutic intervention: A bibliometric analysis of published research studies. *Indian Journal of Physiology and Pharmacology, 48*(3), 269.

Khalsa, S. B. S., & Gould, J. (2012). *Your brain on yoga*. New York: RosettaBooks.

Kiecolt-Glaser, J. K., Christian, L., Preston, H., Houts, C. R., Malarkey, W. B., Emery, C. F., et al. (2010). Stress, inflammation, and yoga practice. *Psychosomatic Medicine, 72*(2), 113.

Libby, D. J., Reddy, F., Pilver, C. E., & Desai, R. A. (2012). The use of yoga in specialized VA PTSD treatment programs. *International Journal of Yoga Therapy*, (22), 79.

Martarelli, D., Cocchioni, M., Scuri, S., & Pompei, P. (2011). Diaphragmatic breathing reduces exercise-induced oxidative stress. *Evidence-based Complementary and Alternative Medicine, 2011*, 932430.

McCall, T. (2007). Yoga as medicine. In *Yoga as Medicine*. New York: Bantam Dell.

McCall, M. C. (2013). How might yoga work? An overview of potential underlying mechanisms. *Journal of Yoga and Physical Therapy, 3*(1), 130.

Posadzki, P. & Ernst, E. (2011). Yoga for low back pain: A systematic review of randomized clinical trials. *Clinical Rheumatology, 30*(9), 1257.

Posadzki, P., Ernst, E., Terry, R., & Lee, M. S. (2011). Is yoga effective for pain? A systematic review of randomized clinical trials. *Complementary Therapies in Medicine, 19*(5), 281.

Raub, J. A. (2002). Psychophysiologic effects of Hatha Yoga on musculoskeletal and cardiopulmonary function: a literature review. *Journal of Alternative and Complementary Medicine, 8*(6), 797.

Saper, C. B., Loewy, A. D., Swanson, L. W., & Cowan, W. M. (1976). Direct hypothalamo-autonomic connections. *Brain Research, 117*(2), 305.

Shannahoff-Khalsa, D. S. (2007). Yogic insights into mind-body medicine and healing. In *Kundalini yoga meditation: Techniques specfic for psychiatric disorders, couples therapy, and personal growth*. New York: W.W. Norton & Company.

Shannahoff-Khalsa, D. S., Boyle, M. R., & Buebel, M. E. (1991). The effects of unilateral forced nostril breathing on cognition. *International Journal of Neuroscience*, *57*(3–4), 239.

Shannahoff-Khalsa, D. S. & Kennedy, B. (1993). The effects of unilateral forced nostril breathing on the heart. *International Journal of Neuroscience*, *73*(1–2), 47.

Shannahoff-Khalsa, D. S., Kennedy, B., Rancisf, E. Y., & Ziegler, M. G. (1996). Ultradian rhythms of autonomic, cardiovascular, and neuroendocrine systems are related in humans. *American Journal of Physiology*, *270*(4 Pt 2), R873–R887.

Sharma, M. & Haider, T. (2013). Yoga as an alternative and complementary therapy for patients suffering from anxiety: A systematic review. *Journal of Evidence-Based Complementary and Alternative Medicine*, *18*(1), 15.

Sharma, M., Haider, T., & Knowlden, A. P. (2013). Yoga as an alternative and complementary treatment for cancer: A systematic review. *Journal of Alternative and Complementary Medicine*. ahead of print.

Sharma, H., Sen, S., Singh, A., Bhardwaj, N. K., Kochupillai, V., & Singh, N. (2003). Sudarshan Kriya practitioners exhibit better antioxidant status and lower blood lactate levels. *Biological Psychology*, *63*(3), 281.

Sinha, S., Singh, S. N., Monga, Y. P., & Ray, U. S. (2007). Improvement of glutathione and total antioxidant status with yoga. *Journal of Alternative and Complementary Medicine*, *13*(10), 1085.

Spicuzza, L., Gabutti, A., Porta, C., Montano, N., Bernardi, L., et al. (2000). Yoga and chemoreflex response to hypoxia and hypercapnia. *Lancet*, *356*(9240), 1495.

Staples, J. K., Hamilton, M. F., & Uddo, M. (2013). A yoga program for the symptoms of post-traumatic stress disorder in Veterans. *Military Medicine*, *178*(8), 854.

Streeter, C. C., Gerbarg, P. L., Saper, R. B., Ciraulo, D. A., & Brown, R. P. (2012). Effects of yoga on the autonomic nervous system, gamma-aminobutyric-acid, and allostasis in epilepsy, depression, and post-traumatic stress disorder. *Medical Hypotheses*, *78*(5), 571.

Streeter, C. C., Jensen, J. E., Perlmutter, R. M., Cabral, H. J., Tian, H., Terhune, D. B., et al. (2007). Yoga Asana sessions increase brain GABA levels: A pilot study. *Journal of Alternative and Complementary Medicine*, *13*(4), 419.

Sturgess, S. (1997). Pranayama. In *The yoga book: A practical guide to self-realization*. Rockport, MA: Element Books Limited.

Taylor, A. G., Goehler, L. E., Galper, D. I., Innes, K. E., & Bourguignon, C. (2010). Top-down and bottom-up mechanisms in mind-body medicine: development of an integrative framework for psychophysiological research. *Explore (NY)*, *6*(1), 29.

Telles, S., Nagarathna, R., & Nagendra, H. R. (1994). Breathing through a particular nostril can alter metabolism and autonomic activities. *Indian Journal of Physiology and Pharmacology*, *38*(2), 133.

Telles, S., Nagarathna, R., & Nagendra, H. R. (1996). Physiological measures of right nostril breathing. *Journal of Alternative and Complementary Medicine*, *2*(4), 479.

Ward, L., Stebbings, S., Cherkin, D., & Baxter, G. D. (2013). Yoga for functional ability, pain and psychosocial outcomes in musculoskeletal conditions: A systematic review and meta-analysis. *Musculoskeletal Care*, *11*(4), 203–217. ahead of print.

Werntz, D. A., Bickford, R. G., Bloom, F. E., & Shannahoff-Khalsa, D. S. (1983). Alternating cerebral hemispheric activity and the lateralization of autonomic nervous function. *Human Neurobiology*, *2*(1), 39.

Werntz, D. A., Bickford, R. G., & Shannahoff-Khalsa, D. (1987). Selective hemispheric stimulation by unilateral forced nostril breathing. *Human Neurobiology*, *6*(3), 165.

Yoga Journal Editors. (2013a). *Which yoga is right for you?*

Yoga Journal Editors. (2013b). *Yoga poses*. http://www.yogajournal.com/poses/finder/browse_categories.

Section V

NATURAL AND NUTRITIONAL REMEDIES FOR PAIN, INFLAMMATION, AND DISEASES OF CHRONIC INFLAMMATION

The prior four sections have addressed how to work with the mind-body connection to influence the body through the mind and the mind through the body, with benefits to both for treating pain and inflammation. The next five chapters in Section V add discussions of the many natural constituents that can be introduced into the body through ingestion, absorption, or inhalation and have profound effects on mind and body for treatment of pain and inflammation.

Chapter 20

Nutrition and Hydration
Part One: Water, Vitamin, and Mineral Micronutrients

Efficacy of Vitamin Supplementation, Nutrients Found in Food and Water, and Preventative Actions

No evidence compels the conclusion that the minimum required intake of any vitamin comes close to the optimum intake that sustains good health.

Linus Pauling

INTRODUCTION TO VITAMIN AND MINERAL MICRONUTRIENTS

Micronutrient is a collective term to describe vitamins and minerals that are present in smaller quantities and concentrations and typically taken in the diet in milligram (mg) or microgram (μg) daily doses. In contrast, **macronutrients** ("macro" derive from the Greek word "makro" or large) refers to nutrients that provide the body with calories or energy and structural requirements, called carbohydrates, proteins, and fats. These macronutrients are consumed in food quantities typically measured in grams.

Vitamins are organic molecules essential for normal health and growth obtained by the human diet and through exceptionally graded supplementation. Vitamins are also plant and food chemical constituents (substances found in foods) necessary for proper functionality of the brain and body. The lack of any one vitamin, or many vitamins, may cause pain, inflammation, disease, illness, and general disability. The food substances (carbohydrates, fats, and proteins) are referred to as macronutrients. These macronutrients have the ability to convert food into much needed energy and structural requirements on which the brain and body rely.

Organic growth factors are vitamins that must be directly obtained from the environment. Natural vitamins found in the environment may act as liaisons for proper enzymatic reactions to take place in the human body and are classified into two different groups by chemical polarity or solubility: water-soluble and fat-soluble. **Water-soluble** vitamins have polar groups, such as OH (negative charge; hydroxyl group) and COOH ("neutral" charge, carboxylic group), that make them soluble to the aqueous environment within all body fluids, tissues, and cells. Most water-soluble vitamins and enzymes are not primarily stored in the body (limited amounts are stored in the lean tissue of the body, such as vitamin C in muscles), and any excess water-soluble vitamins are excreted through the urine. Therefore water-soluble vitamins are imperative as part of a daily regime, preferentially through mindful diet and daily supplementation. Examples of water-soluble vitamins include B-complex vitamins (e.g., B3, B6, B12) and vitamin C. These vitamins are absorbed along with water in the gastrointestinal tract.

The **fat-soluble** vitamins are nonpolar compounds that are soluble in the fat (lipid) components of the body, such as liver, fat deposits, and cell membranes. Fat-soluble vitamins (A, D, E, and K) bind to ingested lipids and are absorbed through entry to the blood through lymph channels in the intestinal wall. Many fat-soluble vitamins travel in body fluids through the body only under conjugation by proteins that act as carriers.

Minerals and **trace mineral micronutrients** are needed for functionality for all cellular and metabolic processes. Approximately 4% of the body's mass consists of minerals, which cannot be made in the body. Major minerals and electrolytes include magnesium, sodium, potassium, calcium, phosphorus, manganese, sulfur, cobalt, and chlorine. Trace minerals are iron, zinc, copper, selenium, iodine, fluorine, and chromium. They provide physiologic support, for example, for optimal processing in the brain, such as transmitting nerve impulses and maintaining a healthy heart rhythm. They are required for proper hormone regulation, modulation of cellular activity, and overall bone structure and health. For example, minerals support the development of bone strength with calcium, phosphorus, and magnesium. Vitamins, such as A, D, E and K, also work synergistically, combining naturally with minerals magnesium, calcium, selenium, and zinc. The body generally uses minerals and trace minerals as enzyme cofactors involved in a variety of biochemical reactions, including processes including metabolism, anabolism, catabolism, and oxidation reactions.

Some of the earth's naturally occurring minerals have debilitating effects on the body when present in excess. These minerals include mercury, lead, copper, flouride, and arsenic, which can lead to inflammation, pain, illness, severe dehydration, and death are not properly regulated. (UNICEF, 2010).

NATURAL SOURCES OF VITAMINS AND NUTRIENTS
Food and Water
Food enables a human to live by carrying out all life functions. The several purposes of food include providing energy for life processes, building and repairing cell

protoplasm, and regulating body processes. Organic foods are produced by living organisms that contain carbohydrates (sugars and starches), fats, and proteins needed for transportation of minerals, vitamins, and micronutrients in the body. Organic produce and other ingredients are grown on many local farms without pesticides, synthetic fertilizers, sewage sludge, genetically modified organisms, or radiation.

"Inorganic" foods can be used to refer to foods that contain pesticides and other unwanted chemicals. It may also traditionally refer to foods that come from rocks, soils, and seawater that contain minerals, such as calcium, phosphorus, iron, sulfur, iodine, magnesium, and copper. Found naturally in food as well, these minerals are needed to assist in cell building and repairing (especially bone, teeth, and muscle tissue), as well as general functionality of the body.

More discussion into food production and food-based vitamins and how they may affect inflammation and pain in the body is provided under "Food Production."

WATER AND HYDRATION
WATER AND FLUORIDATION

Although not classified as "food," water is a compound essential to all body functions and also present and abundant in foods. All organisms rely on growth, repair, maintenance, and reproduction, and water is the primary medium required for all these actions to take place. Water makes up at least 5% and up to 95% of every cell and is most commonly found in the range 65% to 75%. Outside the cells, nutrients are dissolved in water (extracellular fluids); inside the cells, water provides the medium for life-sustaining chemical reactions. This molecular compound of hydrogen and oxygen dissolves food, nutrients, oxygen, and wastes that make up a significant portion of the blood.

Chemicals, volatile organic compounds (VOCs), and toxins that are part of the final product present in our drinking water and found in most of our foods are leading to hazardous health outcomes that affect brain, body, and major disruptions at the cellular level. Later in the chapter, we will examine water's properties and the additives (chemicals that are added to the water) that affect inflammation and acute and chronic pain. First, the next section discusses the history and discovery of vitamins and how they relate to population health today.

ENTER THE NUTRITIONAL ERA

History relates the discovery of vitamins beginning with the long sea voyages that were part of Europeans' "discovery" of Africa, Asia, and the Americas. For example, what can be recognized as nutritional deficiencies were reported on the part of Ferdinand Magellan's crew in 1519 during the first circumnavigation of the globe when their explorations reached the Pacific Ocean. During most of the ensuing Mercantile and Colonial periods, sailors lived on salted meats and dried breads, when after a few weeks of sailing, they would become ill and many eventually died. It was eventually discovered that sailors who were given juice from lemons and limes did not succumb to *scurvy*, an illness resulting from serious vitamin C deficiency. Symptoms of scurvy include muscle and joint *pain*, bleeding of the gums, tiredness, and unpleasant red dots on the skin. Although British Navy officials were unaware of the nutritional reason for the sailor's illness, they observed how to treat it empirically with limes and lemons. Royal Navy officials ordered that every ship must carry lemons and limes for the crew's consumption. This provision in turn became a more widespread law and tremendously helped the prevention of scurvy (and led to the slang term for British sailors as "limeys").

Around the same time it was discovered that Japanese and Chinese sailors who were out at sea began developing a serious deficiency called "beriberi" (Japanese for "I cannot! I cannot!"). The disease results from a lack of thiamine pyrophosphate, the active form of the vitamin thiamine or vitamin B1 (also spelled thiamin). The disease affects the muscles, weakening them and eventually paralyzing them. The symptoms of beriberi include increasing overall body pain, abdominal pain, difficulty breathing, tingling or loss of feeling in the feet and hands, numbness, paralysis, mental confusion, and vomiting.

Japanese doctors observed that beriberi could be relieved and prevented by consuming vegetables, meat, and whole, unpolished rice (such as brown rice, in which only the "hull," the outermost layer of the rice kernel, is removed, leaving the vitamin-rich bran layer). White rice usually contains no healthy hulls, bran, germ, or husks after milling. This deficiency is still one example of the effects of inadequate production of mainstream foods today. Intensive agriculture and milling, as in the case of white rice, is more costly, takes longer to harvest and produce, and significantly reduces the nutritional content by removing superior nutrients, such as fiber and essential vitamins.

DISCOVERY OF VITAMINS

In the 1880s the disease beriberi reached endemic proportions in the Dutch colonies in the East Indies (currently Indonesia). Typical of rice-intensive agriculture, the indigenous people produced enough quantities of rice to provide carbohydrate and calories to support a large population but were relatively lacking in foods with protein and essential nutrients, such as B vitamins. Christiaan Eijkman, a Dutch military physician, worked in Java and was assigned many responsibilities for controlling beriberi disease. One of his responsibilities was to conduct research to help to determine what was accountable for beriberi. He tried injecting blood from native soldiers with the disease into animals (to test an infectious theory of the disease). He also worked within animal models for experiments. He observed that chickens developed some of the symptoms of beriberi, such as leg weakness, also known as *polyneuritis*. He noticed that chickens fed cooked "white" rice succumbed with these symptoms. In essence, his studies led to uncovering the significant nutritional properties of brown rice and he eventually used brown rice to restore sick chickens back to health. In Europe and Asia scientists saw these experiments as a gateway for further research and began to isolate rice "polishings" (hulls, bran, and husks) to identify their vitamin constituents and, furthermore, ultimately to synthesize them.

Casimir Funk, a biochemist from Poland, was considered the "father of vitamin therapy." He reported in 1911 that he had isolated the active factor in rice polishings and went on to recognize this active factor belonged to a group called "amines" (containing nitrogen). He went on to suggest that diseases, such as pellagra (vitamin deficiency of B3 or niacin), scurvy (vitamin C deficiency), and rickets (vitamin D deficiency), were caused by specific nutritional deficiencies not yet identified. One of the earliest patent products containing vitamins was "Oscodal," a vitamin concentration of vitamin A and D, the first vitamin preparation accepted by the American Medical Association as an ethical product. Research led to the discovery of a total of 13 vitamins, including eight forms of vitamin B and vitamins C, A, D, E, and K (Spedding, 2013).

Funk coined the term "vitamine" because these components were attentively "vital amines" and also because of their meaning. "Vita" means life in Latin, and "amine" means a nitrogenous substance essential for life. For this purpose "amine" was used because Casimir Funk thought all vitamins contained amino acids. Amine also refers to a chemical term in which there are known organic derivatives of ammonia. Vitamines later was changed to "vitamins" because the amines group became considered as its own distinct category (as in amino acids), and the term vitamin was accepted into the scientific community in 1912.

Frederick Hopkins, an early biochemist, was well known in the medical field for isolating amino acids. His work heavily contributed to experimental research on vitamins. In 1929, Christiaan Eijkman, along with Sir Frederick Hopkins, won the Noble Prize in Physiology or Medicine for the discovery of vitamins, specifically vitamin B1 and growth stimulating vitamins.

TRAVELING BACK IN TIME

Medical texts have been around since the ancient Chinese civilizations during the Han, Tang, and other dynasties more than 2000 years ago. Ancient physicians used foods and herbs (and incidentally the nutrients they contain) to relieve health problems and to alleviate pain and inflammation, treat diseases, and aid digestion.

Ancient Greece had its own set of medicinal theoretical systems and ideological beliefs on medicinal uses of natural remedies for pain and disease found in historical texts written by Hippocrates of Cos and others in 4th century BC. Hippocrates, known in the West as the "Father of Modern Medicine," was recorded to use trial and observation of these affects (after the earlier Egyptians and Sumerians). According to *Dorland's Illustrated Medical Dictionary*, nearly 90% of medical terms and botanical material medica used today have Greek or Latin roots. For example, the sea buckthorn *(Hippophae)*, also known as sea berry, is a small tree that was documented in classical medical texts to help to decrease pain and inflammation and treat chronic gastric ulcers. This herb was used for centuries in Asia (see Chapter 23 for more herbal remedies).

Greece had powerful influences on the later Romans and their medicinal texts on herbs and natural remedies. Centuries later (as we saw in the Colonial period during the British and Dutch Empires' introduction of modern nutrition and vitamines), it was an important time for the foundations of fundamental experimental research on vitamins and a healthy diet.

Sea buckthorn is becoming as popular as similar berries, such as pomegranate and acai berry, because of its nutrition contains vitamins A, B1, B2, B6, and C. Contrary to its name, it does not come from the sea but grows in mountainous and coastal areas of Asia and Europe. Currently sea buckthorn is found helpful for a variety of symptoms, including chronic pain, fibromyalgia, arthritis, heart disorders including chest pain, reducing illness due to cancer, as well as limiting the toxicity of chemicals that are present in cancer therapy. Sea buckthorn can help to deter the growth of tumors (Geetha et al., 2005; Larmo, Alin, Salminen, Kallio, & Tahvonen, 2008; Suryakumar & Gupta, 2011; Upadhyay et al., 2009).

Contemporary Research

Ongoing vitamin and mineral research has contributed greatly to the awareness of mind and body connection and the benefits of vitamin and mineral supplementation. New initiatives in the paradigm of health and healing, such as so-called alternative and complementary medicine therapies, vitamins, natural herbal remedies, and organic foods (as well as yoga, meditation, and the shift of mindfulness practices), have all contributed to potential transformation for the 21st century and the intention for a lifetime of exceptional health.

In the next section regarding water, we will see where some initiatives for public health and hygiene have failed. We will then cover some best practices for individuals to be better-educated consumers and how food production affects everyday vitamin intake, as well the role of general vitamin supplementation.

Factors Contributing to Vitamin Deficiency: "The Death" of Water

Natural Salts Found in Water

Water contains natural and organic minerals, such as calcium, potassium, magnesium, manganese, iron, and sodium. These minerals, also known as salts, or electrolytes, help the body to replenish quickly especially when minerals are lost when sweating occurs after an exercise regime.

Salt is a building block of human life. Terrestrial life emerged from the sea approximately 300 million years ago—and terrestrial life carried all that salty seawater along with it. Biologists believe the human body's natural salt levels reflect the levels found in the earth's oceans all those millions of years ago. The seawater ocean also has its natural benefits when the body is submerged. Research shows that taking a bath in Dead Sea salt has been shown to reduce inflammation in atopic dry skin and enhance skin hydration (Proksch, Nissen, Bremgartner, & Urquhart, 2005).

Blood cells and internal organs swim in a sea of salt water, so regular salt intake is critical for metabolism, physiology, and hydration. However, when people think of salt, they may think of common table salt, which is 99.9% sodium chloride. Natural sea salt is the far better choice—for cooking or adding additional minerals to water lacking these nutrients—and is just 84% sodium chloride. It contains other key electrolytes and important minerals, such as iodine and zinc. Your body needs these critical mineral nutrients for bones, as well as general health. Sodium is a major electrolyte in the body, which must continually maintain a careful balance between sodium and other minerals. **Sea salt** is a superior choice because it already contains numerous other minerals that are natural to the body from biologic history.

A too low-salt diet can actually be deadly. One study showed that older people with the lowest salt consumption had the highest risk of early death, and researchers have consistently found more dangers of low-salt diets (O'Donnell et al., 2011).

In one study, researchers looked at the connections between dietary salt and cardiovascular disease among 2937 men with high blood pressure. Those with the lowest level of salt intake had a more than 4 times greater rate of heart attacks compared with those with the highest level of salt intake. According to the authors, most important was the finding that subjects consuming the highest amount of sodium did *not* experience more heart attack events than did those consuming a low-sodium diet (Alderman, Madhavan, Cohen, Sealey, & Laragh, 2015).

Rain and Water Cycle

All plants and animals require water to carry out the activities of living. Plants secure water through their roots, and excess water vapor is given off into the atmosphere during a process called "transpiration". "Aerosol therapy," discussed in Chapters 23 and 24, reveals how plant oils are released into the air based on the impact of raindrops when they hit the ground (and in essence, soils and plants). This action enables a process called "aerosol generation" and produces a subtly "sweet" smell in the air from the plant oils (petrichor). This process usually happens when rainwater is clean and does not contain unwanted chemicals or additives because these pollutants can cover and disrupt the plant oils from being released into the atmosphere and onto the earth.

Animals that feed directly or indirectly on plants still take in a good amount of water from the high water content of vegetation. Animals take in some water vapor from the air and replace it into the atmosphere during the process of respiration. Thus water is found in the air we breathe, plants, soil, and the production of other processed foods. Water vapor in the air eventually condenses and finds its way back to the soil, where the cycle continues. When there are large amounts of chemicals and heavy metal concentrations in the soil, it can affect the rain cycle. Chemicals and molecules in every raindrop disperse and are immediately absorbed into the earth. Unwanted and excessive chemicals in rain can affect plants and the animals that eat the vegetation.

Global Drinking Water Supply

The lack of clean and healthy drinking water has become an international crisis. Developing nations have come a long way toward rehabilitating their water supplies; however, there is still much concern. Unsafe water, poor sanitation, and inadequate hygiene create a high-risk environment for infection, inflammation, illness, disease, and death. More than 884 million people do not have access to clean drinking water, and more than 2300 people per day die from severe dehydration due to diarrhea and other causes (Prüss-Ustün et al., 2014). There are many developing countries and regions, such as Bangladesh, India, Africa, and Kenya, that suffer nutritional deficiencies, malnutrition, illnesses, and death from drinking poor-quality water or having no regular access to water at all. For example, Bangladesh has very high amounts of the chemical poison arsenic released from human activities and found naturally on earth (UNICEF, 2010). Exposure to more than 50 µg arsenic can lead to death from cancers, cardiovascular disease, infectious disease, diarrheal disease, severe dehydration, and neurological impairment in children (UNICEF, 2010). Waterborne diseases are also of main concern. Pathogenic microbes can spread in already poor water supplies and cause malnutrition, inflammation, abdominal pain, severely affected organs, skin infections, and severe diarrhea that usually leads to death from dehydration (CDC, 2012; WHO, 2001).

Chemicals and Heavy Metals

What is in drinking water? Marketing and other advertisements of healthy drinking water notwithstanding, the quality of water supplies may be eroding since the 1940s. "New York has the best drinking water on the planet." This appears to be more a conditioned reinforcement than a factual statement. The mountainous regions of New York supply its immediate surrounding areas with superb, clean, mineral-enhanced drinking water. However, when carrying water through lead and copper pipes over hundreds of miles to reach city and urban areas, such as New York City (and this goes for anywhere in the world), the beginning water changes drastically to where it ends up being consumed and what is in the final "by-product."

Fluoride (as well as chlorine) increases the erosion of lead and copper in water pipes, thus increasing concentrations of lead and copper in drinking water (Cantor, Park, & Vaiyavatjamai, 2000; Schweitzer, 1994). Drinking water is typically used for showering and bathing and is another method of "ingesting" water into the bloodstream through skin pores (where typically absorption is maximized in warm or hot conditions). *The American Journal of Public Health* stated that up to two thirds of VOCs and harmful chlorine exposure may be due to skin absorption and inhalation while showering (Brown, Bishop, & Rowan, 1984). Studies show that spending only minutes in the shower can cause blood levels of trihalomethanes (THMs) (common disinfection by-product—DBP) to greatly increase (Gordon et al., 2006; Grazuleviciene et al., 2011; Nuckols et al., 2005; Rivera-Núñez et al., 2012). In addition, steam inhaled during the shower can lead to 20 times the concentration of chlorine and other chemicals. Another study showed that THM exposure in drinking water may alter fetal growth in pregnant women, depending on the internal dose (Grazuleviciene et al., 2011).

The Centers for Disease Control and Prevention (CDC) states (completely apart from the issue of fluoridation of water): "When water sits in leaded pipes for several hours, lead can leach into the water supply (CDC, 2016), and people can still be exposed to high amounts of lead through the drinking water supply" (ATSDR, 2015). Lead inhibits vitamin and mineral absorption, such as iron (Abbaspour, Hurrell, & Kelishadi, 2014; Goyer, 1993; Hegazy, Zaher, Abd El-Hafez, Morsy, & Saleh, 2010). Somewhat ironically, the CDC also holds that iron is one of the largest micronutrient deficiencies in the United States. Despite efforts to combat lead toxicity levels in the 20th century, after increasing in the 19th century, the use of lead piping to transport and supply water currently continues. In the 19th century many medical treatments of the day included lead. During the 20th century lead was used in paints, pigments, and gasoline.

Many cities that have suffered widespread lead-contaminated homes and schools include Boston, Massachusetts; Durham, South Carolina; and Camden, New Jersey (Boston Globe, 1988, 2005; Rabin, 2008). More than half the homes in Washington, DC, exceeded the Environmental Protection Agency (EPA) level of lead contamination of 15 parts per billion (ppb) (Rabin, 2008). Most homes were built with lead piping until the 1960s and 1970s (Rabin, 2008). In 2004, cities manipulated results of tests to detect lead in water, thereby putting millions at risk by contamination (Leonnig, Becker, & Nakamura, 2004). New York City, the nation's largest water provider, had for years assured its nearly 10 million customers that its water was safe because the lead content fell below federal limits and declined paperwork that provided test results for more than 2 years (Leonnig et al., 2004).

In addition to the pipes that carry most of the drinking water in the United States, there are chemical additives intentionally added to the water supply around the globe since the United States began the practice in the 1940s. However, some countries have completely outlawed chemicals that officials continue to minimally regulate and use in the United States. Some of these additives include chlorine and fluoride.

Let us take a closer look at some of these additives still found in the United States and some other countries—such as three distinct types of fluoride. Fluoride not only relates to acute and chronic inflammation and pain but also, over time, can affect vitamin levels and how vitamins are absorbed in the body. Because more than 70% of the United States contains fluoridated water, which affects upwards of 190 million people, it is important to note the long- and short-term effects of what is going into the body and blood stream and how it affects vitamin intake and overall health (see http://www.cdc.gov/fluoridation/statistics/2010stats.htm).

MANY FACETS OF FLUORIDE

A number of inorganic fluoride compounds are used in conjunction with nuclear power plants, water supplies, pesticides, pharmaceuticals, fabric conditioners, and other industrial uses. The United States produces approximately 80% hydrofluoric acid in a continued annual variation in potential uses. One of these uses is for drinking water as an additive in the United States, Canada, and other countries since the use of fluoridated water in the United States began in 1945. Fluoride has been an ongoing public health, government, and political debate since this chemical was first added to drinking water in the United States.

Many believe fluoride aids in bone strength, reducing dental cavities and strengthening tooth enamel. However, multiple studies show that fluoride can have the opposite effect. Prior to 1945 fluoride was known as a toxin and for developmental disturbances in animals and humans. The *Journal of the American Medical Association* stated "fluorides are general protoplasmic poisons that change the permeability of the cell membrane by certain enzymes" (JAMA, 1943). In 1944, the American Dental Association stated the "harm" of fluoridation outweighs the "benefits." A 1936 issue of the *Journal of the American Dental Association* stated that fluoride at the 1 parts per million (ppm) concentration is as toxic as arsenic and lead (Journal of American Dental Association, 1936).

A number of much more recent studies published during the year 2015 alone show no correlation of fluoride protecting people against adverse health effects. The Cochrane Collaborative Review, The York Report, and The National Academy of Sciences (NAS) all reported that fluoridation does not show any correlation with healthy teeth and gums and does not improve strength of teeth nor decrease dental cavities (The National Academy of Sciences, 2006; Treasure, Chestnutt, Whiting, McDonagh, Wilson, & Kleijnen, 2002).

Some countries that have banned fluoride in drinking water include Switzerland, Sweden, France, Germany, Denmark, Iceland, Israel, Norway, and Japan (Cheng, Chalmers, & Sheldon, 2007; Peckham & Awofeso, 2014). Less than 2% to 3% of Europeans drink fluoridated water, whereas approximately two thirds of the US population has fluoridated public water, according to the CDC (CDC, 2012). The recitation of fluoride's putative benefits appears to have become a conditioned reinforcement repeated by public health officials and certain health practitioners who are not nutritional scientists.

Ninety percent of the chemicals used in fluoridation in the United States do not occur naturally on earth. The natural form of mineral fluoride found both in nature and in teeth and bones is called "apatite" (calcium fluoro-chloro-hydroxyl phosphate)."Fluorides" are chemical toxins known to enhance concentrations of other heavy metals and chemicals when mixed. The word "fluoride" resembles a "semantic sanitation" due to political debacles governed by health coordinators and managers that are in large part affected by the strong conditional reinforcement of fluoride that in turn affects the larger public and demographics. However qualified, many experts appear to remain unaware of the present dangers in distributing fluoride additives in drinking-water supplies.

Inflammation

Scientific studies have clearly demonstrated that fluoride is a *proinflammatory* agent, an inhibitor of adenosine triphosphate (ATP) in cells (compromising energy production, and ironically undermining cellular hydration), and it promotes extreme oxidative stress in white blood cells (Gutowska, Baranowska-Boasiacka, Goschorskab, Kolasac, Łukomskaa, Jakubczyka, 2015; Gutowska, Baranowska-Bosiacka, Baśkiewicz, Milo, Siennicka, & Marchlewicz, 2010). Long-term exposure to fluoride can affect many enzyme activities, which may increase risks of digestive issues, irritable bowel syndrome, and prevent the absorption of nutrients (Gutowska et al., 2015; Gutowska, Baranowska-Boasiacka, Siennicka, Baśkiewicz, Machaliński, Stachowska, & Chlubek, 2011). Fluoride has been shown to enhance *inflammation* and proliferation of monocytes and macrophages that usually enable processes to help the body to heal from injury or illness (Gutowska et al., 2015). However, even when there is no frank chronic inflammatory illness, but the body is under a constant stimulus of creating high counts of monocytes and macrophages (white blood cells), fluoride can cause acute and chronic pain, as well as a number of diseases, such as stroke, heart disease, Crohn's disease, rheumatoid arthritis, and scleroderma (Edwards, 2005). In addition, this acute and chronic inflammation can cause anemia and the loss of iron absorption from cytokines attacking erythropoietin production (Gasche, Lomer, Cavill, & Weiss, 2004).

Neurotoxic Effects

A recent study conducted at Harvard University shows fluoride in drinking water is of "concern" and that "further research is warranted" (Choi, Sun, Zhang, & Grandjean, 2012). The same study also brought to light fluoride's neurotoxic effects on children and how it dramatically interferes with brain development and causes later neurological impairment. There have been studies associating iodine deficiency (and thus thyroid deficiency and associated neurological deficits; see later) with fluoride exposure (Lin Fa-Fu et al., 1991). "Average" amounts of fluoride exposure, as little as 1 to 2 ppm, can increase the neurological effects of iodine deficiency and in turn lower overall cognitive capacity (Lin, Aihaiti, Zhai, & Lin, 1991; Yang, Wang, Guo, & Hu, 1994).

Bone Cancer and Bone Diseases

In 1992 Cohn found osteosarcoma rates to be up to 6 times higher in young men living in fluoridated versus unfluoridated areas in New Jersey (Cohn, 1992). Recently Kharb et al. found that osteosarcoma was directly linked to fluoride intake in patients and that fluoride had an overall effect on bone growth (Kharb, Sandhu, & Kundu, 2012). In 2001, researcher at Harvard University published a study in *Cancer Causes and Control* that found that boys between the ages of 6 to 8 years who consumed fluoridated water had an increased risk of osteosarcoma (bone cancer) of 5.5% over boys with a lower or no consumption of fluoride. It was noted that no effect was seen in girls (Bassin, Wypij, Davis, & Mittleman, 2006; DeNoon, 2006). However, in 2009, another study found that fluoride affected cortical bone density in girls (Levy, Eichenberger-Gilmore, Warren, Letuchy, Broffitt, & Marshall, 2009). Fluoride accumulates in bones over time and has been shown to increase *joint pain* and cause *arthritis-like symptoms* (Czerwinski, Nowak, Dabrowska, Skolarczyk, Kita, & Ksiezyk, 1988). The NAS found that fluoride causes severe changes in bone density that lead to joint stiffness and bone *pain* (The National Academy of Sciences, 2006).

Thyroid Function

Decreased thyroid function is a common symptom from fluoride exposure, which can slow down metabolism, inhibit proper hormone release, and keep the metabolism out of balance. Fluoride was used in medicine during the 1930s through 1950s in Europe to treat patients with *overactive* thyroid glands or hyperthyroidism (Stecher, Finkel, & Siegmund, 1960) to decrease thyroid activity. Nowadays, millions suffer from an underactive thyroid gland or hypothyroidism. Hypothyroidism can affect mood and cause depression, exhaustion and fatigue, weight gain, muscle cramps, aches, swelling of joints and joint *pains*, increase cholesterol levels, and contribute to heart disease (National Center for Biotechnology Information, 2014). According to the US National Research Council, fluoride has an effect on thyroid function and is an endocrine disruptor (National Research Council, 2006). Synthroid, also known as levothyroxine, used to treat an underactive thyroid, continues to be the most prescribed drug in the United States and Canada (Brogan, 2013; Medscape, 2014).

People who suffer from various medical conditions are even more prone to fluoride toxicity. People increasingly vulnerable to the toxic effects are those who already suffer from micronutrient deficiencies of calcium, magnesium, vitamin C, vitamin D, and/or iodine (Institute of Medicine, 2001). People who suffer from malnutrition and protein-poor diets are also vulnerable. The Agency for Toxic Substances and Disease Registry (ATSDR) found infants, children, and the elderly to be the most affected of all groups, most likely because they are at the extremes in the life cycle (ATSDR, 1993). Adults who suffer kidney disease are vulnerable because the kidneys must act as filtration systems for the fluoridated water we drink. Children who have diabetes insipidus are found to be more easily affected by fluoride toxicity (Greenburgh, Nelson, & Kramer, 1974; Klein, 1975).

Inhibition of Enzymes

Fluoride inhibits a large number of very important enzyme reactions, such as enolase (a catalyst of glycolysis), lipase, and amylase (Gambino, 2013; Gumińska & Sterkowicz, 1976; Hara & Yu, 1995; Mikesh & Bruns, 2008; Shearer & Suttie, 1970). Fluoride strongly inhibits enolase in the presence of inorganic phosphate, which is heavily used in fluoridated water (Qin, Chai, Brewer, Lovelace, & Lebioda, 2006). Glycolysis, in turn, is responsible for producing ATP and regulating and supporting energetic processes in the cells of the brain and body. Glucose levels, responsible for the brain and body's energy, are functionally reduced by fluoride (Bueding & Goldfarb, 1941; Lee et al., 2009). Other enzymes inhibited by fluoride include lipase, which is responsible for digestion of fats in the gastrointestinal tract (Loevenhart & Peirce, 1906). Inhibition of lipase can lead to obesity and type 2 diabetes (Klannemark, Orho, Langin, Laurell, Holm, & Reynisdottir, 1998; Tucci, Boyland, & Halford, 2010). Lipase function is critical for those who suffer from celiac disease, in which gluten damages the intestinal tract and can cause abdominal pain and extreme fatigue (Ehrlich, 2015). A study published in the *New England Journal of Medicine* found that pancreatic enzymes, including lipase, increase the absorption of nutrients in patients suffering from cystic fibrosis (FitzSimmons et al., 1997). Chronic pain, chest pain, lung infections, and inflamed nasal passageways are common symptoms of people who have cystic fibrosis (Mayo Clinic, 2015; Ravilly, Robinson, Suresh, Wohl, & Berde, 1996). Inorganic phosphate has been shown to increase muscle fatigue, inhibit enolase and glycolysis, and affect glucose levels in the body (Mikesh & Bruns, 2008; Westerblad, Allen, & Lännergren, 2002).

Fluoride Accumulation

Healthy adults excrete approximately 50% of the fluoride ingested each day (Marier & Rose, 1977). Fluoride that is not excreted increases calcification in the bones and other areas, such as the brain. One area important for hormone regulation is the pineal gland. The pineal gland can become calcified from fluorides, inhibiting its function as a melatonin producer (Luke, 1997, 2001). Melatonin is needed for deep sleep, and the lack of melatonin also contributes to thyroid problems that affect the entire endocrine system. Fluoride binds to other heavy metals that can then cross the blood-brain barrier (Lubkowska et al., 2004). Ekstrand observed infant's and children's absorption rates of fluoride to be more than 80% in their bones (Ekstrand, et al., 1994). Fluoride levels in the bones, blood plasma, and body increase over time (National Research Council, 2006). Fluoride intake on an individual basis is not monitored.

Fluoride Regulation

Fluoride, although a hazardous chemical, is not regulated by the US Department of Agriculture or the US Food and Drug Administration (FDA). Fluoride levels in water depend on regulations and recommendations that are expressed in "not-to-exceed" levels in air, water, soil, or food that are usually based on dangerous levels that affect animals, and then they are subsequently adjusted under the assumption they help to protect people (ATSDR, 2003).

In 1986 the EPA started to regulate fluoride in water using ppm units to represent the highest concentration of fluoride that are allowed to be added to US drinking water. Studies have shown as little as 0.3 ppm can severely affect cognitive ability (Ding et al., 2011). Currently the maximum contaminant level is 4 mg/L (4 ppm). If one surpasses that amount, it may result in bone disease and pain and tenderness of bones; and children may develop mottled teeth (US EPA, 2016). The EPA also allows states the option to follow a secondary standard because fluoride in excess of 2 ppm causes tooth and skin discoloration, as well as aesthetic effects, such as taste or odor alterations in water (US EPA, 2016).

The EPA mandates "naturally occurring" fluoride levels in communal water supplies. At higher levels, as seen in 1978 and 2010 in southern Iceland, for example, fluoride is extremely toxic to animal and human health (The National Academy of Sciences, 2006; BBC News, 2010). However, the EPA relies on "state-by-state" fluoride monitoring and reporting for artificial fluoride materials added to the drinking water, including populations served, fluoride concentrations, and fluoride sources (CDC, 2008).

Sources of Natural and Artificial Fluoride

Fluoride is present on earth both inorganically and organically. Organically, fluoride comes from an abundance of phosphate, or phosphoritic rock. Fluoride is the negative ion of the halogen element **fluorine**. Fluorine is found naturally and is the 13th most abundant element in the earth's crust (Weinstein & Davison, 2004). Fluorine (not fluoride) is found on the periodic table of elements as a halogen written as letter F. Phosphorite is primarily used for manufacturing phosphate fertilizer (CDC, 2014). Phosphorite quickly takes on synthetic forms when mixed vigorously with such chemicals as calcium phosphate, limestone minerals, and sulfuric acid. This mixture is heated together and later becomes phosphoric acid-gypsum or calcium sulfate ($CaSo_4$). The initial heating process releases hydrogen fluoride (HF) and silicon tetrafluoride (SiF_4) gases. These gases eventually liquefy to approximately 23% fluorosilicic acid (FSA) solution. More than 95% of FSA used for water fluoridation comes from this artificial industrial chemical process (CDC, 2014). The remaining 5% of FSA is produced in manufacturing hydrogen fluoride or from the use of hydrogen fluoride to etch silicates and glasses when manufacturing solar panels and electronics. Sodium fluorosilicate and sodium fluoride are dry additives that come from FSA. FSA can be partially balanced by either table salt (sodium chloride) or caustic soda to get sodium fluorosilicate. Caustic soda can be added to balance fluorosilicate, and the product is **sodium fluoride**. Approximately 90% of the sodium fluoride used in the United States comes from FSA (CDC, 2014). Caustic soda is a dangerous, hazardous, and highly corrosive chemical that can seriously affect health (New Jersey Department of Health, 2010).

Molecular Levels in Fluoride Mixtures
An *ion* is an atom or group of atoms that have an electrical charge because of a loss or gain of electron(s).

Atoms are typically linked together into chemical structures called "molecules", and two or more atoms of the same kind form a dimer molecule of a single element. Stable gases like oxygen (O_2) and nitrogen (N_2) typically exist in the atmosphere in this form. An ozone ion is chemically represented as O_3 and is of course highly chemical reactivity (e.g., forming the ozone layer). Atoms of different kinds, of two or more different elements, also become linked together, resulting in a compound. Any compound that contains the fluoride ion whether it is organic or inorganic is also known as a fluoride. A "mixture" is the result of combinations of two or more elements or of elements and molecular compounds in such a way that each substance retains its own identity. However, a compound is a result of a combination of two or more elements that absolutely lose their identity to form a third, new substance. This chemical factor may be the reason why there is overall concern and uncertainty regarding fluoride and fluoride additives in water. When fluoride is mixed in water, the compounds separate and retain their own identities, defeating the identities of the original chemical binding.

The three most abundant chemicals used by the United States for water fluoridation are fluorosilicic acid (H_2SiF_6), sodium silicofluoride (Na_2SiF_6), and sodium fluoride (NaF) (Urbansky, 2002). Again, these chemicals are often used interchangeably when referred to generally as "fluorides." Sodium fluoride is a negative ion because, after fluorine gains an electron from sodium, it becomes a negatively charged ion. Elemental atoms generally lose, gain, or share electrons with other atoms to achieve exact structures and measurements produced in the gaseous elemental field. After fluorine gains an electron, ions containing the fluoride ion are then similarly called "fluorides" (e.g., bifluoride, or hydrofluoric acid, HF_2, which has been used to etch glass since the 1670s). Thus, fluorine is an element, and fluoride is an ion or a compound that contains the fluoride ion. When fluoride is mixed in water, it becomes hydrofluorosilic acid and is considered a "mixture" of chemicals because the chemicals separate.

FLUORIDE ADDITIVES

Fluorosilicic acid is a water-based solution used by most water systems in the United States. Fluorosilicic acid is also referred to as hydrofluorosilicate, FSA, or HFS.

Sodium fluorosilicate is a dry additive, dissolved into a solution before being added to water.

Sodium fluoride is also a dry additive, typically used in smaller water systems, dissolved into solution before being added to water. Sodium fluoride that dissolves in water forms hydrofluoric acid.

Organically Derived Fluoride—Fluorine

Large deposits and concentrations of fluoride are found near or on volcanoes and rock dust and infrequently traced in water, but there have been a lack of appropriate studies. Volcano ash has an unusually high soluble fluorine concentration and can be deposited over large geographical areas, affecting these areas with high concentrations for years (Araya, Wittwer, & Villa, 1993). Ash fall has been shown to have devastating effects on agricultural crops and animals, including the consumption of contaminated vegetables and drinking water. Volcanic ash can travel great distances in the upper atmosphere and spread over vast areas far away from the erupting volcano. Some factors that should be investigated in determining fluoride toxicity in a specific area where volcano ash is present include ash thickness, type and growing condition of a crop, presence of soluble fluoride in the ash, and intensity of rainfall carrying fluoride. Poisoning and death of animals have been known consequences of environmental fluoride toxicity (Ranjan & Ranjan, 2015). Domestic and wild animals that drink water contaminated with volcano ash may also suffer from severe fluorosis, dental lesions, and decay (Araya, Wittwer, Villa, & Ducom, 1990; Ranjan & Ranjan, 2015).

Fluoride has also been shown to affect precipitation and weather patterns. A 2-year study (2010 to 2011) of fluoride in atmospheric precipitation was conducted in Wielkopolski National Park (west-central Poland). The findings of this study, after measuring factors such as air, precipitation in specific proximities, and concentrations of fluoride, revealed that high concentrations of fluoride can be carried for long distances and that the direction of airflow revealed which countries may be polluting with fluoride sources to the greatest extent (Walna, Kurzyca, Bednorz, & Kolendowicz, 2012). Fluoride compounds are considered to be significant environmental pollutants because of dangerous effects on wildlife and major ecosystems (ATSDR, 2003; Divan et al., 2008; Liteplo & Gomes, 2002; Walna et al., 2012; Weinstein & Davison, 2004.) Anthropogenic sources include aluminum smelters, inorganic fertilizers, and industrial activities, such as manufacturing of brick, cement, and pottery.

At the local level, many communities and municipalities are beginning to question the need for adding fluoridation to drinking water supplies. It represents an additional cost and step in the supply of water. To the extent it is not necessary and even represents a health hazard besides, it is another example of government waste with counterproductive effects on the health and well-being of the citizens. Local votes being held about continuing the practice of fluoridation typically are influenced by local dentists and other public health authority figures whose grasp of the science and research may be woefully lacking, advising a public that has been the repository of received conventional wisdom without rigorous scientific examination.

Chapter 21 discusses the role of hydration and water as a basic nutrient together with other recognized nutrients in human diet and nutrition.

REFERENCES

Abbaspour, N., Hurrell, R., & Kelishadi, R. (2014). Review on iron and its importance for human health. *Journal of Research in Medical Sciences, 19,* 164–174. http://www.ncbi.nlm.nih.gov/pmc/articles/PMC3999603/#ref57.

Agency for Toxic Substances and Disease Registry (ATSDR). (1993). *Toxicological Profile for fluorides, hydrogen fluoride, and fluorine (F).* US Department of Health & Human Services, Public Health Service. ATSDR/TP-91/17.

Agency for Toxic Substances and Disease Registry (ATSDR). (2003). *Public health statement for fluorides, hydrogen fluoride, and fluorine.* http://www.atsdr.cdc.gov/phs/phs.asp?id=210&tid=38.

Agency for Toxic Substances and Disease Registry (ATSDR). (2015). *Public health statement for lead.* http://www.atsdr.cdc.gov/PHS/PHS.asp?id=92&tid=22.

Alderman, M. H., Madhavan, S., Cohen, H., Sealey, J. E., & Laragh, J. H. (2015). Low urinary sodium is associated with greater risk of myocardial infarction among treated hypertensive men. *Hypertension.* http://hyper.ahajournals.org/content/25/6/1144.short.

Araya, O., Wittwer, F., & Villa, A. (1993). Evolution of fluoride concentrations in cattle and grass following a volcanic eruption. *Veterinary and Human Toxicology, 35*, 437–440. http://www.ncbi.nlm.nih.gov/pubmed/8249268.

Araya, O., Wittwer, F., Villa, A., & Ducom, C. (1990). Bovine fluorosis following volcanic activity in the southern Andes. *The Veterinary Record, 126*(26), 641–642.

Bassin, E. B., Wypij, D., Davis, R. B., & Mittleman, M. A. (2006). Age-specific fluoride exposure in drinking water and osteosarcoma (United States). *Cancer Causes and Control, 17*(4), 421–428.

BBC News. (19 April 2010). *Toxic ash threatens Iceland animals: Farmers in southern Iceland have been racing to protect their animals from being poisoned by volcanic dust.* http://news.bbc.co.uk/2/hi/europe/8629241.stm

Boston Globe. (1988). *Lead Confirmed in School Water* (p. 1).

Boston Globe. (2005). *Concerns raised on lead levels MWRA study cites pipes in 4500 homes.* http://www.boston.com/news/local/massachusetts/articles/2005/11/17/concerns_raised_on_lead_levels/.

Brown, H. S., Bishop, D. R., & Rowan, C. A. (1984). The role of skin absorption as a route of exposure for volatile organic compounds (VOCs) in drinking water. *American Journal of Public Health, 74*, 479–484. http://ajph.aphapublications.org/doi/abs/10.2105/AJPH.74.5.479.

Bueding, E. & Goldfarb, W. (1941). *The effect of sodium fluoride and sodium iodoacetate on glycolysis in human blood.* http://www.jbc.org/content/141/2/539.full.pdf.

Cantor, F. A., Park, J. K., & Vaiyavajatai, P. (2000). *The effect of chlorine on corrosion in drinking water systems.* http://mtac.isws.illinois.edu/mtacdocs/corrosionfinrpt/corrosnfnlrpt00.pdf.

Centers for Disease Control and Prevention. (2012). *Global WASH-related diseases and contaminants.* http://www.cdc.gov/healthywater/wash_diseases.html.

Centers for Disease Control and Prevention. (2016). *Lead, Water.* https://www.cdc.gov/nceh/lead/tips/water.htm.

Centers for Disease Control and Prevention. (2008). *Populations receiving optimally fluoridated public drinking water—United States, 1992–2006.* http://www.cdc.gov/mmwr/preview/mmwrhtml/mm5727a1.htm.

Centers for Disease Control and Prevention. (2014). *Water fluoridation additives fact sheet: Types of fluoride additives/sources of fluoride additive.* http://www.cdc.gov/fluoridation/factsheets/engineering/wfadditives.htm.

Cheng, K. K., Chalmers, I., & Sheldon, T. A. (2007). Adding fluoride to water supplies. *British Medical Journal, 335*, 699–702. https://www.ncbi.nlm.nih.gov/pmc/articles/PMC2001050/.

Choi, A. L., Sun, G., Zhang, Y., & Grandjean, P. (2012). Developmental fluoride neurotoxicity: A systematic review and meta-analysis. *Environmental Health Perspectives, 120*, 1362–1368. http://www.ncbi.nlm.nih.gov/pmc/articles/PMC3491930/.

Cohn, P. D. (1992). An epidemiologic report on drinking water and fluoridation. *New Jersey Department of Health, Environmental Health Service, 8.*

Czerwinski, E., Nowak, J., Dabrowska, D., Skolarczyk, A., Kita, B., & Ksiezyk, M. (1988). Bone and joint pathology in fluoride-exposed workers. *Archives of Environmental Health, 43*, 340–343. http://www.ncbi.nlm.nih.gov/pubmed/3178291.

DeNoon, D. J. (2006). *Study examines boyhood drinking of fluoridated water and possible links to osteosarcoma.* http://www.webmd.com/cancer/news/20060406/does-fluoridation-up-bone-cancer-risk.

Ding, Y., Sun, H., YanhuiGao, Han, H., Wang, W., Ji, X., et al. (2011). The relationships between low levels of urine fluoride on children's intelligence, dental fluorosis in endemic fluorosis areas in Hulunbuir, Inner Mongolia, China. *Journal of Hazardous Materials, 186*, 1942–1946. http://www.ncbi.nlm.nih.gov/pubmed/21237562.

Divan, A. M., Jr, Oliva, M. A., Ferreira, F. A. (2008). Dispersal fluoride accumulation in eight plant species. *Ecological Indicators, 8*, 454–461. http://dx.doi.org/10.1016/j.ecolind.2007.04.008.

Edwards, T. (2005). Inflammation, pain, and chronic disease: An integrative approach to treatment and prevention. *Alternative Therapies in Health and Medicine, 11*, 20–27. http://www.ncbi.nlm.nih.gov/pubmed/16320856.

Ehrlich, S. D. (2015). *Lipase.* https://umm.edu/health/medical/altmed/supplement/lipase.

Ekstrand, J., et al. (1994). Fluoride pharmacokinetics in infancy. *Pediatric Research, 35*, 157–163.

FitzSimmons, S. C., Burkhart, G. A., Borowitz, D., Grand, R. J., Hammerstrom, T., Durie, P. R., et al. (1997). High-dose pancreatic-enzyme supplements and fibrosing colonopathy in children with cystic fibrosis. *New England Journal of Medicine.* http://www.nejm.org/doi/full/10.1056/NEJM199705013361803.

Gambino, R. (2013). Sodium fluoride: An ineffective inhibitor of glycolysis. *Annals of Clinical Biochemistry*, *50*, 3–5. http://www.ncbi.nlm.nih.gov/pubmed/23129725.

Gasche, C., Lomer, M. C., Cavill, I., & Weiss, G. (2004). Iron, anaemia, and inflammatory bowel diseases. *Gut*, *53*, 1190–1197. http://www.ncbi.nlm.nih.gov/pmc/articles/PMC1774131/.

Geetha, S., Singh, V., Ram, M., Ilavazhagan, G., Banerjee, P. K., & Sawhney, R. C. (2005). Immunomodulatory effects of seabuckthorn (Hippophae rhamnoides L.) against chromium (VI) induced immunosuppression. *Molecular and Cellular Biochemistry*, *278*, 101–109. http://www.ncbi.nlm.nih.gov/pubmed/16180095.

Gordon, S. M., Brinkman, M. C., Ashley, D. L., Blount, B. C., Lyu, C., Masters, J., et al. (2006). Changes in breath trihalomethane levels resulting from household water-use activities. *Environmental Health Perspectives*, *114*, 514–521. http://www.ncbi.nlm.nih.gov/pmc/articles/PMC1440773/.

Goyer, R. A. (1993). Lead toxicity: Current concerns. *Environmental Health Perspectives*, *100*, 177–187.

Grazuleviciene, R., Nieuwenhuijsen, M. J., Vencloviene, J., Kostopoulou-Karadanelli, M., Krasner, S. W., Danileviciute, A., et al. (2011). Individual exposures to drinking water trihalomethanes, low birth weight and small for gestational age risk: A prospective Kaunas cohort study. *Environmental Health*, *10*, 32. http://www.ncbi.nlm.nih.gov/pmc/articles/PMC3100244/.

Greenberg, L. W., Nelsen, C. E., & Kramer, N. (1974). Nephrogenic diabetes insipidus with fluorosis. *Pediatrics*, *54*, 320–322.

Gumińska, M. & Sterkowicz, J. (1976). Effect of sodium fluoride on glycolysis in human erythrocytes and Ehrlich ascites tumour cells in vitro. *Acta Biochimica Polonica*, *23*, 285–291. http://www.ncbi.nlm.nih.gov/pubmed/1035019.

Gutowska, I., Baranowska-Bosiacka, I., Baśkiewicz, M., Milo, B., Siennicka, A., Marchlewicz, M., et al. (2010). Fluoride as a pro-inflammatory factor and inhibitor of ATP bioavailability in differentiated human THP1 monocytic cells. *Toxicology Letters*, *196*, 74–79. http://www.ncbi.nlm.nih.gov/pubmed/20399260.

Gutowska, I., Baranowska-Boasiacka, I., Siennicka, A., Baśkiewicz, M., Machaliński, B., Stachowska, E., et al. (2011). Fluoride and generation of pro-inflammatory factors in human macrophages. *Fluoride*, *44*(3), 125–134.

Gutowska, I., Baranowska-Bosiacka, M., Goschorskab, A., Kolasac, A., Łukomskaa, K., Jakubczyka, K., et al. (2015). Fluoride as a factor initiating and potentiating inflammation in THP1 differentiated monocytes/macrophages. *Toxicology in Vitro*, *29*, 1661–1668. http://www.sciencedirect.com/science/article/pii/S0887233315001605.

Hara, K., & Yu, M.-H. (1995). Effect of fluoride on human salivary amylase activity. *Fluoride*, *28*(2), 71–74.

Hegazy, A. A., Zaher, M. M., Abd El-Hafez, M. A., Morsy, A. A., & Saleh, R. A. (2010). Relation between anemia and blood levels of lead, copper, zinc and iron among children. *BMC Research Notes*, *3*, 133. http://www.ncbi.nlm.nih.gov/pmc/articles/PMC2887903/.

Brogan, I. M. S. (2013). *Top 20 dipensed drugs in 2012*. http://www.imshealth.com/deployedfiles/imshealth/Global/North%20America/Canada/Home%20Page%20Content/Pharma%20Trends/Top20Dispensed_En_12.pdf.

Institute of Medicine. (2001). *Dietary reference intakes for vitamin A, vitamin K, arsenic, boron, chromium, copper, iodine, iron, manganese, molybdenum, nickel, silicon, vanadium and zinc*. Washington, DC: National Academy Press.

Journal of American Medical Association. (1943). Chronic fluorine intoxication. *Journal of American Medical Association*, *123*(3), 150–152. http://jama.jamanetwork.com/article.aspx?articleid=263874.

Journal of American Dental Association. (1936). *Fluorine in relation to bone and tooth*. 23:568.

Kharb, S., Sandhu, R., & Kundu, Z. S. (2012). Fluoride levels and osteosarcoma. *South Asian Journal Cancer*, *1*, 76–77.

Klannemark, M., Orho, M., Langin, D., Laurell, H., Holm, C., Reynisdottir, S., et al. (1998). The putative role of the hormone-sensitive lipase gene in the pathogenesis of type II diabetes mellitus and abdominal obesity. *Diabetologia*, *41*, 1516–1522. http://link.springer.com/article/10.1007/s001250051099.

Klein, H. (1975). Dental fluorosis associated with hereditary diabetes insipidus. *Oral Surgery, Oral Medicine, and Oral Pathology*, *40*(6), 736–741.

Larmo, P., Alin, J., Salminen, E., Kallio, H., & Tahvonen, R. (2008). Effects of sea buckthorn berries on infections and inflammation: a double-blind, randomized, placebo-controlled trial. *European Journal of Clinical Nutrition, 62*(9), 1123–1130.

Lee, Y. W., Cha, Y. J., Chae, S. L., Song, J., Yun, Y. M., Park, H. I., et al. (2009). Effectiveness of sodium fluoride as a glycolysis inhibitor on blood glucose measurement: Comparison of blood glucose using specimens from the Korea National Health and Nutrition Examination survey. *Korean Journal of Laboratory Medicine, 29*, 524–528. http://www.ncbi.nlm.nih.gov/pubmed/20046083.

Leonnig, C. D., Becker, J., & Nakamura, D. (2004). *Lead levels in water misrepresented across US.* http://www.washingtonpost.com/wp-dyn/articles/A7094-2004Oct4.html.

Levy, S. M., Eichenberger-Gilmore, J., Warren, J. J., Letuchy, E., Broffitt, B., Marshall, T. A., et al. (2009). Associations of fluoride intake with children's bone measures at age 11. *Community Dentistry and Oral Epidemiology, 37*(5), 416–426.

Lin Fa-Fu, Aihaiti, Hong-Xin, Zhao, Jin, Lin, Ji-Yong, Jiang, Maimaiti, Aiken, et al. (1991). The relationship of a low-iodine and high-fluoride environment to subclinical cretinism in Xinjiang. *Endemic Disease Bulletin, 6*(2), 62–67 (republished in *Iodine Deficiency Disorder Newsletter* 7(3):24–25).

Liteplo, R., Gomes, R., Howe, P., & Malcolm, H. (2002). Fluorides: environmental health criteria 227. Geneva: WHO, United Nations Environment Programme, International Labour Organization.

Loevenhart, A. S. & Peirce, G. (1906). The inhibiting effect of sodium fluoride on the action of lipase. *Journal of Biological Chemistry, 2*, 397. http://www.jbc.org/content/2/5/397.full.pdf.

Lubkowska, A., Chlubek, D., Machoy-Mokrzyńska, A., Noceń, I., Zyluk, B., & Nowacki, P. (2004). Concentrations of fluorine, aluminum and magnesium in some structures of the central nervous system of rats exposed to aluminum and fluorine in drinking water. *Annales Academiae Medicae Stetinensis, 50*, 73–76. http://www.ncbi.nlm.nih.gov/pubmed/16892590.

Luke, J. (1997). *The effect of fluoride on the physiology of the pineal gland.* University of Surrey, Guildford. Ph.D. Thesis.

Luke, J. (2001). Fluoride deposition in the aged human pineal gland. *Caries Research, 35*(2), 125–128.

Marier, J. & Rose, D. (1977). Environmental fluoride. In: *National Research Council of Canada. Associate Committe on Scientific Criteria for Environmental Quality.* NRCC No. 16081.

Mayo Clinic. (2015). *Cystic fibrosis.* http://www.mayoclinic.org/diseases-conditions/cystic-fibrosis/basics/symptoms/con-20013731.

Medscape Medical News Top 100 Most Prescribed, Top Selling Drugs. Megan Brooks. May 13, 2014. http://www.medscape.com/viewarticle/825053.

Mikesh, L. M. & Brunsa, D. E. (2008). *Clinical Chemistry, 54*(5), 930–932. http://www.clinchem.org/content/54/5/930.long.

National Center for Biotechnology Information. (2014). *Underactive thyroid: Overview.* http://www.ncbi.nlm.nih.gov/pubmedhealth/PMH0072785/.

National Research Council. (2006). *Fluoride in drinking water: A scientific review of EPA's standards.* (pp. 507). Washington, DC: National Academies Press.

New Jersey Department of Health. (2010). *Hazardous substance fact sheet: Sodium hydroxide.* http://nj.gov/health/eoh/rtkweb/documents/fs/1706.pdf.

Nuckols, J. R., Ashley, D. L., Lyu, C., Gordon, S. M., Hinckley, A. F., & Singer, P. (2005). Influence of tap water quality and household water use activities on indoor air and internal dose levels of trihalomethanes. *Environmental Health Perspectives, 113*, 863–870. http://www.ncbi.nlm.nih.gov/pmc/articles/PMC1257647/.

O'Donnell, M. J., Yusuf, S., Mente, A., Gao, P., Mann, J. F., Teo, K., et al. (2011). Urinary sodium and potassium excretion and risk of cardiovascular events. *Journal of American Medical Association, 306*, 2229–2238. http://jama.jamanetwork.com/article.aspx?articleid=1105553.

Peckham, S. & Awofeso, N. (2014). Water fluoridation: A critical review of the physiological effects of ingested fluoride as a public health intervention. *Scientific World Journal,* 293019. http://www.ncbi.nlm.nih.gov/pmc/articles/PMC3956646/.

Proksch, E., Nissen, H. P., Bremgartner, M., & Urquhart, C. (2005). Bathing in a magnesium-rich Dead Sea salt solution improves skin barrier function, enhances skin hydration, and reduces inflammation in atopic dry skin. *International Journal of Dermatology, 44*, 151–157. http://onlinelibrary.wiley.com/ doi/10.1111/j.1365-4632.2005.02079.x/abstract;jsessionid=257435324216CF57A80030AE1579D97B. f03t03?userIsAuthenticated=false&deniedAccessCustomisedMessage.

Prüss-Ustün, Bartram, J., Clasen, T., Colford, J. M., Jr., Cumming, O., Curtis, V., et al. (2014). Burden of disease from inadequate water, sanitation and hygiene in low- and middle-income settings: A retrospective analysis of data from 145 countries. *Tropical Medicine and International Health, 19*, 894–905. http://www.ncbi.nlm.nih.gov/pmc/articles/PMC4255749/pdf/tmi0019-0894.pdf.

Qin, J., Chai, G., Brewer, J. M., Lovelace, L. L., & Lebioda, L. (2006). Fluoride inhibition of enolase: Crystal structure and thermodynamics. *Biochemistry, 45*, 793–800. http://www.ncbi.nlm.nih.gov/ pmc/articles/PMC2566932/.

Rabin, R. (2008). The lead industry and lead water pipes "a modest campaign". *American Journal of Public Health, 98*, 1584–1592. http://dx.doi.org/10.2105/AJPH.2007.113555.

Ranjan, R. & Ranjan, A. (2015). *Fluoride toxicity in animals.* (pp. 11–12). New York: Springer.

Ravilly, S., Robinson, W., Suresh, S., Wohl, M. E., & Berde, C. B. (1996). Chronic pain in cystic fibrosis. *Pediatrics, 98*, 741–747. http://www.ncbi.nlm.nih.gov/pubmed/8885955.

Rivera-Núñez, Z., Wright, J. M., Blount, B. C., Silva, L. K., Jones, E., Chan, R. L., et al. (2012). Comparison of trihalomethanes in tap water and blood: A case study in the United States. *Environmental Health Perspectives, 120*, 661–667. http://www.ncbi.nlm.nih.gov/pmc/articles/PMC3346785/.

Schweitzer, P. A. (1994). *Corrosion-resistant piping systems* (p. 261). CRC Press.

Sheare, T. R. & Suttie, J. W. (1970). Effect of fluoride on glycolytic and citric acid cycle metabolites in rat liver. *The Journal of Nutrition, 100*, 749–756. http://jn.nutrition.org/content/100/7/749.full.pdf.

Spedding, S. (2013). Vitamins are more funky than Casimir thought. *Australasian Medical Journal, 6*, 104–106. http://www.ncbi.nlm.nih.gov/pmc/articles/PMC3593520/.

Stecher, P., Finkel, M., & Siegmund, O. (1960). *The Merck index of chemicals and drugs* (p. 352). Rahway, NJ: Merck & Co., Inc.

Suryakumar, G. & Gupta, A. (2011). Medicinal and therapeutic potential of Sea buckthorn (*Hippophae rhamnoides L.*). *Journal of Ethnopharmacology, 138*, 268–278. http://www.ncbi.nlm.nih.gov/pubmed/21963559.

The National Academy of Sciences. (2006). *Fluoride in drinking water: A scientific review of EPA's standards.* http://dels.nas.edu/resources/static-assets/materials-based-on-reports/reports-in-brief/fluoride_brief_final.pdf.

Treasure, E. T., Chestnutt, I. G., Whiting, P., McDonagh, M., Wilson, P., & Kleijnen, J. (2002). The York review—A systematic review of public water fluoridation: A commentary. *British Dental Journal, 192*, 495–497. http://www.nature.com/bdj/journal/v192/n9/full/4801410a.html.

Tucci, S. A., Boyland, E. J., & Halford, J. C. G. (2010). The role of lipid and carbohydrate digestive enzyme inhibitors in the management of obesity: A review of current and emerging therapeutic agents. *Diabetes Metabolic Syndrome and Obesity, 3*, 125–143. http://www.ncbi.nlm.nih.gov/pmc/articles/ PMC3047983/.

UNICEF. (2010). *Arsenic mitigation in Bangladesh.* http://www.unicef.org/bangladesh/Arsenic_ Mitigation_in_Bangladesh.pdf.

Upadhyay, N., Kumar, R., Mandotra, S. K., Meena, R. N., Siddiqui, M. S., Sawhney, R. C., et al. (2009). Safety and healing efficacy of Sea buckthorn (*Hippophae rhamnoides L.*) seed oil on burn wounds in rats. *Food and Chemical Toxicology, 47*, 1146–1153. http://www.ncbi.nlm.nih.gov/pubmed/19425187.

Urbansky, E. T. (2002). Fate of fluorosilicate drinking water additives. *Chemical Reviews, 102*, 2837–2854. http://cof-cof.ca/wp-content/uploads/2012/08/Urbansky-Fate-Of-Fluorosilicate-Drinking-Water-Additives-American-Chemical-Society-Chem.-Rev.-2002-102-2837-2854.pdf.

US Environmental Protection Agency (US EPA). (2016). *Drinking Water Contaminant Human Health Effects Information: Drinking Water Standards and Advisory Tables.* https://www.epa.gov/ dwstandardsregulations/drinking-water-contaminant-human-health-effects-information.

Walna, B., Kurzyca, I., Bednorz, E., & Kolendowicz, L. (2012). Fluoride pollution of atmospheric precipitation and its relationship with air circulation and weather patterns (Wielkopolski National Park, Poland). *Environmental Monitoring and Assessment, 185*, 5497–5514. http://www.ncbi.nlm.nih.gov/ pmc/articles/PMC3667360/.

Weinstein, L. H. & Davison, A. (2004). *Fluorides in the environment: Effects on plants and animals.* (pp. 6–7). Cambridge, MA: CABI Press.

Westerblad, H., Allen, D. G., & Lännergren, J. (2002). Muscle fatigue: Lactic acid or inorganic phosphate the major cause? *News in Physiological Sciences, 17,* 17–21. http://physiologyonline.physiology.org/content/17/1/17.

World Health Organization (WHO). (2001). *Water-related diseases* (p. 477). http://www.who.int/water_sanitation_health/diseases/hepatitis/en/.

Yang, Y., Wang, X., Guo, X., & Hu, P. (1994). The effects of high levels of fluoride and iodine on intellectual ability and the metabolism of fluoride and iodine. *Chinese Journal of Epidemiology, 15*(4), 296–298 (republished in Fluoride 2008; 41:336-339).

Suggested Readings can be found on the companion website, http://www.micozzipainconditions.com.

Chapter 21

Nutrition and Hydration
Part Two: Micronutrient Deficiencies and Dietary Supplementation

Malnutrition is a growing epidemic, and there are numerous campaigns to help with malnutrition, as there are with world hunger. Awareness of malnutrition in the developing world is high. However, specific micronutrient deficiencies are rarely discussed but are very serious, not only worldwide but currently in the United States. The groups of people most affected are usually not affluent but include people with low and middle incomes. These groups have limited access to organic foods, dietary supplements (which are not considered by the government as medical expenses or deductions), and simply cannot afford the extra cost of essential nutrition.

Four major physiologic factors that exacerbate vitamin and mineral deficiencies nowadays include (1) decreased absorption, (2) decreased intake, (3) increased loss, and (4) increased utilization. Some of these factors are related to a specific disease, such as the inability to digest nutrients adequately or "malabsorption." This condition is seen in patients with Crohn's disease, irritable bowel syndrome, obesity, disordered microbiome or gut bacteria, diabetes, and liver or kidney disease (Krajmalnik-Brown, Ilhan, Kang, & DiBaise, 2012; Mayo Clinic Staff, 2014; Mercadante, 1996; Rendell, 2004). In addition, negative habitual behaviors, such as stress reactions, heavy use of antibiotics, addictions to alcohol or drugs, anorexia, and excess smoking, can all interfere with vitamin and mineral absorption by displacing good, healthy bacteria (probiotics) in the stomach lining and the intestines. Other substances, such as refined sugars and carbohydrates, can also lead to deficiencies.

Increased vitamin loss may occur due to the effects of prescription drugs, such as metformin, which causes loss of B vitamins. Increased vitamin loss is often cited as an effect of smoking on antioxidants, such as vitamin C. Decreased intake is a common problem due to poor food choices and declining nutrient content even of foods considered healthy. All of these factors point to the need for sensible dietary supplementation.

FOOD PRODUCTION

Not having a proper diet or access to nutrient-dense foods can lead to severe vitamin deficiencies that drastically affect health. What is happening to the majority of food in the world?

Much of the food grown is shared among industrialized countries, shipped frozen, and transported globally for weeks or months at a time. By the time many foods reach the grocery store, whether meat, dairy, or vegetables and fruits, they have already been sitting for weeks or months. This stagnation and aging results in the loss of vital nutrients. What kind of food a person eats depends to a large extent on what kind of food they are buying. Millions of people currently rely on the food they buy in grocery stores. Heavily processed foods, which are widely available in the easy-to-access center sections in retail stores, are typically high in calories and contain insignificant amounts of micronutrients. These foods contribute to the widespread micronutrient deficiencies, as well as caloric excess, that exist in many Americans.

Most of the vegetables and fruits are grown in such large quantities at the national scale, and mass agricultural practices result in the depletion of nutrients. Lack of nutrients in the soils in which foods are grown inhibits people from truly receiving all the nutrients that should be naturally "packaged" in their foods.

The plant usually receives nutrients through the soil from an abundance of solids and gases that eventually dissolve in soil-water solution and are then taken up in aqueous solution as water moves into the plant through the roots and stems. When there are little to no nutrients in the soil and water, they are the same low quantities that will be found in the plants grown. The declining content and composition of nutrients in fruits and vegetables from industrial-driven farms have resulted in less nutrient-dense plants than are found among organic food because of fertilization, irrigation, and other environmental means (Crinnion, 2010). For these reasons the agricultural practices that result in reducing nutrients in soil and water also accompany the decrease of natural vitamins and minerals present in the crops grown.

In 1981 Jarrell and Beverly cleverly discovered the decrease of nutrient concentrations in foods and reviewed the evidence for this research. They referred to the decreased concentrations of mineral and vitamin content in these foods as the "dilution effect" (Jarrell & Beverly, 1981). Similar studies thereafter show that foods grown over the past 160 centuries show a progressive, drastic decline in overall nutrient content (Fana et al., 2008; Farnham, Grusak, & Wang, 2000).

A study conducted by Donald Davis and researchers at the University of Texas in 2004 analyzed nutrition data from the US Department of Agriculture (USDA). This research updated analyses conducted by the author (Micozzi) with National Institutes of Health (NIH) and USDA colleagues in the mid-1980s. Between the years 1950 and 1999, researchers studied 43 different vegetables and fruits, finding increasingly rapid declines in vitamins and protein, year after year, decade after decade. They searched for declines in protein, calcium, phosphorus, iron, riboflavin (vitamin B2), and vitamin C over the past half century. They found significant alterations in the nutrient content and composition. Overall they concluded the nutritional value of vegetables and fruits continued to decline based on lack of nutrients in soils due to agricultural practices and intensive farming (Davis, Epp, & Riordan, 2004). Other vitamins and minerals, such as magnesium, zinc, and vitamins B6 and E, which were not initially studied in 1950, also appear to have decreased in nutrient value based on the accuracy of evidence from this study.

A similar study of British nutrient data from 1930 to 1980 published in the *British Food Journal* found among 20 vegetables that the average calcium content had declined 19%, iron 22%, and potassium 14% (Mayer, 1997). According to the World Watch Institute, less nutrition per calorie in more crops means that food now contains 10% to 25% less iron, zinc, protein, calcium, vitamin C, and other nutrients (Herro, 2013). In essence, we would have to eat eight oranges today to derive the same amount of vitamin C as our grandparents would have obtained from eating only one.

Researchers from Washington State University analyzed 63 spring wheat cultivars grown between 1842 and 2000 over 160 years. Mineral nutrients tested include calcium (Ca), copper (Cu), iron (Fe), magnesium (Mg), manganese (Mn), phosphorus (P), selenium (Se), and zinc (Zn). They found significant reductions in all eight minerals over time. Researchers found an 11% decline in iron content, a 16% decline in copper, a 25% decline in zinc, and a 50% decline in selenium (Murphy & Jones, 2007).

Furthermore, obtaining vitamins or minerals from these food sources is based on consuming plants and herbs that already contain lower concentrations. How vitamins and minerals are measured and food quality and sources will be addressed in the next section.

PAIN, CHRONIC INFLAMMATORY DISEASES, AND MICRONUTRIENT DEFICIENCIES

As the numbers of acute and chronic pain sufferers increase, dietary supplement sales increase in parallel. Sales of vitamins, minerals, and supplements totaled nearly $23 billion in the United States in 2012, according to Euromonitor International. Per capita consumption of vitamin supplementation is significantly rising, contributing to the 5% to 7% annual growth rate. In annual studies since 2004, more than 3 billion of the world's population are malnourished in terms of vitamins and other micronutrients (Welch & Graham, 2004). In 2004 there were 6.4 billion people living on the planet and malnourished individuals accounted for approximately half of the population. And according to the World Health Organization nowadays, not much has changed since 2004 (Black, Allen, Bhutta, 2008; Pimentel & Wilson, 2004; WHO, 2015). The United States also currently has a fairly large population of *malnourished* and *micronutrient-deficient* individuals, which was estimated to cost the United States $157 billion annually (Abbott, 2014). There are more than 90% of Americans who lack essential vitamins, including children. According to the *Journal of Nutrition*, more than half of American children do not get enough of vitamins D and E, and more than a quarter do not get enough vitamin A, calcium, or magnesium (FOA, 2011). These deficiencies can result in children with compromised immune systems, stunted physical growth, reduced mental ability, chronic diseases, and even death.

Populations in Chronic Pain

As the Earth's population grows, so does the populations of acute and chronic pain sufferers. The US Census Bureau's annual projections for the United States in 2015 well exceeded 320 million people, and the rest of the planet more than 7.2 billion (United States Census Bureau, 2014). In 2011 the Institute of Medicine (IOM) reported more than 100 million Americans suffering from chronic pain and that pain costs the United States approximately 700 million per year (Institute of Medicine, 2011). These numbers have continued to drastically rise annually because the treatment of pain in America is clearly a major public health challenge that accounts for more than 70% of the states.

Newborns, Toddlers, and Children

More than just adults feel chronic pain on a daily basis. It affects people of all ages and is often challenging to diagnose. More than 3 million children suffer from chronic pain. Until the 1980s doctors did not know that babies felt pain. A recent study found that untreated pain in infancy could have a lifelong effect on how a person feels and reacts to pain (Fitzgerald & Walker, 2009). Treatment for children suffering from chronic pain in the United States costs approximately 19.5 billion health care dollars per year. The parents report these children receiving more medication, missing more school, and having a lower quality of life (Huguet & Miró, 2008). There is also reporting of increased anxiety and family dysfunction (Logan & Scharff, 2005). In the United States a baby is born every 8 seconds. According to scientists, babies are highly vulnerable to micronutrient deficiency up to 2 to 3 years of age, which can cause a number of developmental problems, such as increased pain perception, impaired cognition, and mental and physical developmental delays, thus pointing out the importance of breast-feeding infants by mothers, assuming they are well nourished themselves. Dietary vitamin and mineral supplements given to children 5 years of age or younger show positive correlations in overall health and reduced perceptions of pain and general pain syndromes (Rivera, Hotz, González-Cossío, Neufeld, & García-Guerra, 2003; Morandi et al., 2015).

Growing Problem

Malnourished and micronutrient-deficient individuals are found to suffer general increases in pain, as well as increases in the perception of pain, acute and chronic pain symptoms, abdominal pain, muscle pain, bone and joint pain, depression, chronic obstructive pulmonary disease (COPD), coronary heart disease, restless leg syndrome, and dementia (Ahmed & Haboubi, 2010; Chiplonkar & Agte, 2007; Dowling, Klinker, Amaya, Paulus, & Liebetanz, 2009; Ferdous et al., 2013; Wells & Dumbrell, 2006).

QUALITY OF VITAMIN SUPPLEMENTS

The quality of vitamin supplements depends on many factors, including where and how they are derived. Some are obtained from foods, such as vitamin K from kale or fat-soluble vitamins A and D from fish oil. In essence, these are "good" quality vitamins from good manufacturing companies that extract the vitamins in plants, vegetables, fruits, and other organic and natural sources. Fat-soluble vitamins (A, D, and E) should always come from natural sources, but the majority of these vitamins in the market are not supplied in natural forms. Some vitamins are combined with foods and **herbs** to provide the consumer with "food vitamins." These supplements are all considered vitamins that are naturally sourced.

The buffering process of a vitamin has a huge effect on the absorbency rate in the gut that leads into the blood stream. For example, most forms of vitamin C supplements are present as ascorbic acid. People have a more difficult time digesting this acidic form, so manufacturers may "buffer" the vitamin by adding additional micronutrients, such as magnesium and potassium. When there is buffering of any vitamin, this means it has been chemically altered. When there is no "buffered" version of vitamin C on the front of the label, check the label on the back to see if it contains any magnesium or potassium because this finding may signal it has indeed been buffered.

Magnesium in the form of magnesium *chelate* helps the survival of this important nutrient intact through the passage from the stomach to the small intestines. Because of this process, more magnesium from the chelated variety will be absorbed in the intestinal tract compared with magnesium that is nonchelated.

Other standard ingredients found on many vitamin labels are sodium citrate, dicalcium phosphate, cellulose, and silica. These are considered harmless "fillers" that help to keep the vitamin supplement together and intact.

SYNTHETIC VITAMINS

Other vitamins are sourced in laboratories and are synthetic. They are not processed or broken down in the body the same way as are natural vitamins. These vitamins may be "labeled" natural, but they are only made from "natural" precursors of the original, healthy vitamin. For example, a label that has "d, l-alpha" shows a synthetic form of vitamin E. This mixture of "d" and "l" forms is biochemically different from natural vitamin E, which is labeled "d-alpha." This kind of labeling relates to the presence of different chemical stereoisomers that are either dextrorotatory (d) versus levorotatory (l) in nature—meaning that the same chemical composition of the molecule may bend light to the right (d) or to the left (l), which has implications for its metabolic activities although chemically "identical." When one takes a synthetic vitamin, for example vitamin E, one risks having it interrupt the metabolism of natural vitamin E that is present in some foods and can be stored in the liver.

Big pharmaceutical and mainstream food companies are buying some smaller nutritional supplement companies to participate in the billions of US sales. For example, Wyeth, a huge billion-dollar pharmaceutical company, makes the multivitamin

Centrum and other supplements. Daily multivitamins typically contain "everything but the kitchen sink" mixtures based more on marketing studies than scientific research. They consistently rank low in industry evaluations of quality. In the lifelong experience and scientific review by the authors, it is impossible to obtain optimal doses of all essential daily vitamins and minerals in any single little daily pill. There simply is not enough room—even if they were of high quality, which they typically are not.

Vitamin and Herbal Industrial Formulations

Larger companies tend to seek bulk ingredient suppliers from less developed countries, and quality is thus severely compromised. Earlier in 2015 GNC and other popular drug and retail stores were accused of selling adulterated herbal supplements. An investigation earlier that year conducted by the New York State Attorney General's office found store-operated supplement brands to be illegitimate and hazardous to public health. These alleged to be dangerous supplements were found at four large national retailers: GNC, Target, Walgreens, and Wal-Mart. All four were sent cease-and-desist letters demanding they stop selling a number of their dietary supplements, few of which were found to contain the actual ingredients listed on the labels, but many of which included potential allergens not listed that may have been affecting millions of people unknowingly. These vitamin tests were conducted using DNA barcoding, which identifies individual ingredients. The US Food and Drug Administration (FDA) is tasked to ensure that supplement products are safe and accurately labeled; however, they are not entirely governed, managed, or regulated appropriately or safely. In October 2012 the Department of Health and Human Services advised that awareness and oversight needs to be heavily emphasized and improved because of the significant evidence of potential public-health problems in regard to the regulation of dietary and herbal supplements (US Department of Health and Human Services, 2012). In 1994 Congress passed the Dietary Supplement Health and Education Act (DSHEA), which was heavily supported by the dietary supplements industry, as well as by consumers. However, they defined herbal supplements and botanicals as **dietary supplements**, and DSHEA removed them from the more intense, rigorous standards used by the FDA in regulating food, medicine, drugs, and medical devices (Braman, 1999). To some extent the entire supplement industry has been regulating itself. Some perceive that loopholes have been left in this growing and important health industry and have created lack of sufficient oversight in an ever-expanding and profitable market. In terms of what is not supposed to be present, among lower-quality supplements, are potential allergens that may be dangerous in vitamins, which may have affected millions of people. These allergens can cause serious inflammation and destabilize insulin, influencing blood sugar levels. Severe inflammation can also lead to pain conditions, including joint pain, overheating, redness, and swelling (Jenkins et al., 2015).

Vitamin Units of Measurement

Vitamins are measured according to the metric system, which is internationally standardized. Every vitamin is usually expressed in micrograms (mcg, ug, or µg), milligrams, or International Units (IUs). The IU is used by many supplement manufacturers (instead of measures of mass) to indicate the presence of the functional activity of a vitamin on an organism or its potency. IU is also a standard measurement for certain daily vitamin recommendations; however, the measurements can be confusing to consumers. There is an international "agreement" specifying the biologic effect of a substance when the dose administered is equal to 1 IU. Therefore the IU as a measure of functional activity or potency has no direct conversion to simple measurements of mass in grams and milligrams. For example, 1 IU for vitamin A is equal to 0.3 µg, but for vitamin D, 1 IU is equal to 25 nanograms (ng). One nanogram is equal to 0.001 µg, and 1 mg is equal to 1,000,000 ng. One microgram is one millionth of a gram, and one thousandth of a milligram. The IU is an international unit, usually used to measure fat-soluble vitamins, including vitamins A, D, and E. Vitamin C is expressed in milligrams. Some B vitamins are expressed in milligrams, such as B6, whereas others are expressed in micrograms, such as B12. Vitamin K and some forms of folate are indicated in micrograms.

Folate is a water-soluble B vitamin naturally present in some foods and can also be taken as a dietary supplement; 10 to 30 mg is stored in the body, and approximately half of this amount is present in the liver (Bailey & Gregory, 2006; Carmel, 2005). Folate is an essential nutrient, key for preventing heart disease, anemia, brain diseases, and birth defects. It comes in two forms: dietary folate, which is from such foods as beans, leafy greens, citrus fruits, and cruciferous vegetables like broccoli, and folic acid, which is the form often used in dietary supplements. In recent years the FDA has progressively changed how to measure folate in dietary supplements. It appears to be based largely on just a single study of nonpregnant women and not representative of the entire population. The FDA is also proposing that supplements contain only folic acid and not folate. This unaccountable step essentially allows government regulatory bureaucrats to restrict folate in its natural form solely to drug company use. The new FDA supplement labeling rule will change the unit of measurement for folic acid from simple metric micrograms to "micrograms dietary folate equivalent" (or µg DFE). *One microgram DFE is equivalent to only 0.6 µg of folic acid* (Box 21.1).

BOX 21.1 *Simple Equation for Converting Micrograms Into Milligrams*

Folate, which is usually measured in micrograms (µg), can be converted into milligrams by dividing the microgram amount by 1000 to determine the required amount in milligrams. In this example, 320 µg of folate is equivalent to 0.32 mg of folate. This calculation would serve as a general equation for converting any vitamin expressed in µg into mg.

However, with the new FDA labeling rule for *folate*, one would take 320 µg and multiply it by 0.6, leaving 192 and then subtract 192 from the original 320.

$$320\,\mu g\,DFE \times 0.6 = 192$$

$$320 - 192 = 128\mu g \times 1000 = 0.128 mg$$

Recommended Daily Allowances Standards Determination

The Recommended Daily Allowances (RDAs) are set to prevent frank nutritional deficiency diseases and to prevent or treat disease. These values are prepared by the Food and Nutrition Board of the US National Academy of Sciences and branch of the IOM. RDAs are "designed" to represent the average daily dietary intake level that is sufficient to meet the nutrient requirements in nearly the entire population and to enhance the social and psychologic needs of healthy individuals. These factors were initially established during World War II to determine what nutrients would be needed in case of possible wartime shortages of food and food rationing and to ensure that adequate nutrition of the public would be protected. The first known RDA was published in 1943 and was intended as a guide to plan and procure food supplies for national defense. The Food and Nutrition Board of the National Research Council initially established the RDAs in the 1940s. The members of this board come from the National Academy of Sciences, National Academy of Engineering, and IOM.

There are other measurements that work together with setting the RDA, such as adequate intake (AI), tolerable upper intake level (UL), and estimated average requirement (EAR). All of these measurements use sets of data to determine nutrient intakes for different groups of healthy people, research on adverse health effects of the general population, and the highest level of nutrient intake of at least half of a healthy study group. For example, UL is based on speculation that as the nutrient intake of a vitamin increases above the RDA, there is an increase in adverse health effects, as if nutrients were drugs. This approach is based on faulty theories and studies because most vitamins (such as water-soluble vitamins) when present in excess, and not being used in the body, are simply excreted through the urine. Fat-soluble vitamins are intentionally stored and kept in the muscles, tissues, and fat cells. Although not readily excreted, they are very difficult to build up to toxic levels in the body.

Iron is a common mineral micronutrient that commonly shows adverse health effects when excess iron stores are present in the body, as demonstrated and published by the author (Micozzi) working with Nobel laureate Baruch Blumberg and colleagues, (published in the *New England Journal of Medicine* and the *International Journal of Epidemiology*). Ironically, iron is the one micronutrient that has been consistently pushed for years by both public health authorities and mainstream medical practitioners.

Another real problem with RDA measurements is that the standard RDAs for all vitamins are geared toward a healthy population (not a widely deficient population) in a particular life stage group, along with other specific demographics, such as age, gender, and pregnancy. For example, the EAR works closely with setting the RDA for any one vitamin. The EAR is the daily intake value of a nutrient that is estimated to meet the nutrient requirement of half the healthy individuals in a life stage and gender group. If an EAR cannot be determined, there is no sufficient RDA. These estimates are usually delivered after a short study with limited research in one specific group of healthy individuals.

As we can see from this chapter, the majority of the population is deficient in one or more vitamins. Even the FDA's recommended daily intakes of the most important vitamins and minerals necessary for proper physical and mental development are in reality *not* actually consumed by nearly 90% of Americans. This lapse means there is little evidence or statistics on the amount of vitamins people are taking or the specific brands (which is a determining factor of quality). Available information suggests that people are following the "lowball" RDAs but are still deficient in one or more vitamins. Again, the RDA is not specific to each individual but set as a nutrient value based only on studies for groups of healthy individuals. These factitious standards pose a serious threat to the health of the population because of insufficient data on *unhealthy* individuals and *malnourished* individuals, which appears to potentially include almost everyone from an optimal nutrition standpoint.

Vitamin D

Another example of the misguided RDAs comes from two independent researchers from Edmonton University who published a paper in the *Journal of Nutrients* showing that IOM made a huge calculation error in the RDA for vitamin D (Veugelers & Ekwaru, 2014). Instead of the 600 to 700 IU per day they currently recommend, the daily requirement published in many articles should be 10 times higher—6000 to 7000 IU. Medical doctors who have hands-on experience in this field have observed for the past 30 years that 5000 to 10,000 IU vitamin D per day is necessary for superior benefits in health. Allowing for 1000 to 2000 IU per day from diet and sun exposure, for those who actually still get healthy sun exposure, that leaves room for the same 5000 IU per day dietary supplement recommendation that many other astute medical professionals have already been making for years.

Early in November 2014 the US Preventive Services Task Force (USPSTF), another quasi-government group that weighed in on the question, released a report claiming lack of evidence supporting the benefits of taking supplemental vitamin D. Part of the problem is that government committees have focused only on vitamin D's effects on bone health, based on discoveries starting during the 1920s. The USPSTF now joins other quasi-government committees that developed the RDAs. These RDAs are still focused on preventing 19th-century nutritional-deficiency diseases when the problem then was not the poor nutrient quality of food, as we have today, but the lack of food availability and distribution.

Scientists have more recently gone on to show that vitamin D is critical for every cell, tissue, and organ in the body—not just the bones. Studies have shown higher levels of vitamin D can prevent many common cancers and increase survival time and quality of life, such as *reduced pain*, in cancer patients. An adequate supply of vitamin D can help to *reduce bone pain*, prevent heart disease, multiple sclerosis, depression, and other common problems. Thousands of medical research studies have discovered convincing scientific evidence of the perils of vitamin D deficiency. And many more doctors are seeing vitamin D deficiency in real patients every day.

Based on all this information, there is a good chance that there are more examples of vitamins for which the RDA should be dramatically increased, perhaps where there is no error in calculation but in the fundamentally flawed ways in which the data are assessed and healthy populations are used to set standards.

ENERGETIC PROPERTIES OF MICRONUTRIENTS

Every cell in the human body requires enough energy to power thousands of processes just to make it through every second of every minute of every single day. This energy must be available to the cells immediately and must be present in all the trillions of cells that make up the human body. It is in the mitochondria that nutrient energy is released and where "energy" is contained in all cells.

Vitamins help to support the cellular mitochondria, the basic energy factories of the body. Mitochondria are present in all cells, where they produce adenosine triphosphate (ATP) for metabolic energy and enzymatic reactions. They also support all organ functions and the immune system. In the brain they help neurons to perform and to help cope with stress and remain calm. Vitamins support mitochondria, so the body will have the needed physical and emotional energy to endure hardship and stress, as well as the daily requirements of metabolism and homeostasis.

ATP is produced in the mitochondria using energy stored in food macronutrients. Each kind of food contains a specific amount of calories that provide a measurement for the amount of energy present in the food. ATP carefully stores and transfers this energy in appropriate amounts to the specific needs of each individual cell. Energy release of ATP when uncoupled to other cellular processes results in the output of heat or thermogenesis. This output of heat results in the dissipation of calories to the environment.

When food contains synthetic ingredients, the body must break them down. Sometimes the chemical bonding needed to produce ATP and provide energy to the cells is not available with synthetic chemicals. This requirement results in a waste of energy trying to break down a chemical that the body cannot use metabolically, and therefore it can remain and accumulate in the body tissues over an extended period of time. The body may eventually identify these molecules as foreign particles or free radicals, contributing to chronic inflammation. Some of these free radicals are eventually excreted from the body. However, many foreign particles and free radicals stay in the body and cause damage to the cells by attacking their macromolecules. Over time, free radicals cause severe cellular damage by destroying healthy cells. Free radicals can also lead to cellular mutation and DNA damage, contributing to cancers.

Vitamin Micronutrient Deficiency Tests

Testing for the presence of minerals in foods is a theoretically simple exercise: burn the food and a gray-white ash appears that does not burn any further. This residue indicates the presence of carbon and minerals. Testing for the presence of *vitamins* in food is not a simple matter and usually needs to be completed in a specialized laboratory. Health professionals typically do not have a laboratory in the office or clinic to test for the presence of vitamins in foods or in body fluids of patients. There are other ways to measure vitamins in diet and in the body.

Intracellular Nutrient Analysis

Commercial laboratories offer panel tests evaluating intracellular levels of micronutrients through microscopic blood analysis. Testing for the presence of a few, selected vitamins in the body can also be completed at certain clinical labs, or samples can be sent to appropriate laboratory(ies) through blood-testing services. It will usually be necessary to ask for the test(s) and the results because they are not supplied as part of a routine medical check-up. Advocacy groups, such as the Alliance to Advance Patient Nutrition, are encouraging more health care institutions to provide nutrition screenings to assess patient risk in the hospital and impact all 50 states in the United States. "Nutrient panel testing," or nutrient analysis, simply educates the consumer on whether they are receiving enough nutrients. The test measures current levels of vitamins, minerals, antioxidants, and organic, fatty, and amino acids. Other possible uses for the test include screening for major nutritional deficiencies of individuals suffering from a chronic diseases of pain and inflammation.

REFERENCES

Abbott. (2014). *Impact of malnutrition in U.S. at $157 billion annually*. http://abbott.mediaroom. com/2014-12-04-Impact-of-Malnutrition-in-U-S-at-157-Billion-Annually.

Ahmed, T. & Haboubi, N. (2010). Assessment and management of nutrition in older people and its importance to health. *Clinical Interventions in Aging, 5*, 207–216. http://www.ncbi.nlm.nih.gov/pmc/articles/PMC2920201/.

Bailey, L. B. & Gregory, J. (2006). *Present knowledge in nutrition*. http://www.ilsi.org/PKN10/Pages/Home.aspx.

Black, R. E., Allen, L. H., Bhutta, Z. A., et al. (2008). Maternal and child undernutrition: Global and regional exposures and health consequences. *The Lancet, 371*(9608), 243–260.

Braman, J. K. (1999). Food for port or Faustian bargain: Regulating performance enhancing dietary supplements. *Cleveland State Law Review*. Engaged Scholarship@CSU, http://engagedscholarship. csuohio.edu/cgi/viewcontent.cgi?article=1491&context=clevstlrev.

Carmel, R. (2005). Folic acid. In M. Shils, M. Shike, A. Ross, B. Caballero, & R. Cousins (Eds.), *Modern nutrition in health and disease* (pp. 470–481). Baltimore, MD: Lippincott Williams & Wilkins.

Chiplonkar, S. A. & Agte V. V. (2007). Association of micronutrient status with subclinical health complaints in lactovegetarian adults. *Scandinavian Journal of Food and Nutrition, 51*(4), 159–166. http://www.ncbi.nlm.nih.gov/pmc/articles/PMC2606995/.

Crinnion, W. J. (2010). Organic foods contain higher levels of certain nutrients, lower levels of pesticides, and may provide health benefits for the consumer. *Alternative Medicine Review, 15*(1), 4–12. http://www.ncbi.nlm.nih.gov/pubmed/20359265.

Davis, D. R., Epp, M. D., & Riordan, H. D. (2004). Changes in USDA food composition data for 43 garden crops, 1950 to 1999. *Journal of the American College of Nutrition, 23*(6), 669–682. http://www.ncbi.nlm.nih.gov/pubmed/15637215.

Dowling, P., Klinker, F., Amaya, F., Paulus, W., & Liebetanz, D. (2009). Iron-deficiency sensitizes mice to acute pain stimuli and formalin-induced nociception. *Journal of Nutrition, 139*(11), 2087–2092. http://jn.nutrition.org/content/139/11/2087.full.

Fana, M. S., Zhaoa, F. J., Fairweather-Taitc, S. J., Poultona, P. R., Dunhama, S. J., & McGratha, S. P. (2008). Evidence of decreasing mineral density in wheat grain over the last 160 years. *Journal of Trace Elements in Medicine and Biology, 22*(4), 315–324. http://www.sciencedirect.com/science/article/pii/S0946672X08000679.

Farnham, M. W., Grusak, M. A., & Wang, M. (2000). Calcium and magnesium concentration of inbred and hybrid broccoli heads. *Journal of the American Society for Horticultural Science, 125*(3), 344–349. http://journal.ashspublications.org/content/125/3/344.short.

Ferdous, F., Das, S. K., Ahmed, S., Farzana, F. D., Latham, J. R., Chisti, M. J., et al. (2013). Severity of diarrhea and malnutrition among under five-year-old children in rural Bangladesh. *The American Journal of Tropical Medicine and Hygiene, 89*(2), 223–228. http://www.ncbi.nlm.nih.gov/pmc/articles/PMC3741240/.

Fitzgerald, M. & Walker, S. M. (2009). Infant pain management: A developmental neurobiological approach. *Nature Clinical Practice Neurology, 5*(1), 35–50. http://www.ncbi.nlm.nih.gov/pubmed/19129789.

Food and Agriculture Organization of the United Nations (FAO). (2001). *The state of food insecurity in the world.* Rome, Italy: FAO.

Herro, A. (2013). *Crop yields expand, but nutrition is left behind.* Worldwatch Institute. http://www.worldwatch.org/node/5339.

Huguet, A. & Miró, J. (2008). The severity of chronic pediatric pain: An epidemiological study. *Journal of Pain, 9*(3), 226–236. http://www.jpain.org/article/S1526-5900%2807%2900903-0/abstract.

Institute of Medicine. (2011). *Report brief: Relieving pain in America: A blueprint for transforming prevention, care, education, and research.* http://iom.nationalacademies.org/Reports/2011/Relieving-Pain-in-America-A-Blueprint-for-Transforming-Prevention-Care-Education-Research/Report-Brief.aspx&gt.

Jarrell, W. M. & Beverly, R. B. (1981). The dilution effect in plant nutrition studies. (pp. 197–224). In N. C. Brady (Ed.), *Advances in agronomy. Vol. 34.* New York, NY: Academic Press.

Jenkins, D. J. A., Kendall, C. W. C., Augustin, L. S. A., Franceschi, S., Hamidi, M., Marchie, A., et al. (2015). Glycemic index: Overview of implications in health and disease. *The American Journal of Clinical Nutrition, 76*(1), 266S–273S. http://ajcn.nutrition.org/content/76/1/266S.full.pdf+html?cnn=yes.

Krajmalnik-Brown, R., Ilhan, Z. E., Kang, D. W., & DiBaise, J. K. (2012). Effects of gut microbes on nutrient absorption and energy regulation. *Nutrition in Clinical Practice, 27*(2), 201–214. http://www.ncbi.nlm.nih.gov/pmc/articles/PMC3601187/.

Logan, D. E. & Scharff, L. (2005). Relationships between family and parent characteristics and functional abilities in children with recurrent pain syndromes: An investigation of moderating effects on the pathway from pain to disability. *Journal of Pediatric Psychology, 30*(8), 698–707. http://www.ncbi.nlm.nih.gov/pubmed/16093517.

Mayer, A. M. B. (1997). Historical changes in the mineral content of fruits and vegetables. *British Food Journal, 99*(6), 207–211. http://www.researchgate.net/publication/235318646_Historical_changes_in_the_mineral_content_of_fruits_and_vegetables.

Mayo Clinic Staff. (2014). *Crohn's disease.* http://www.mayoclinic.org/diseases-conditions/crohns-disease/basics/definition/con-20032061.

Mercadante, S. (1996). Nutrition in cancer patients. *Supportive Care in Cancer, 4*(1), 10–20. http://www.ncbi.nlm.nih.gov/pubmed/8771288.

Morandi, G., Maines, E., Piona, C., Monti, E., Sandri, M., Gaudino, R., et al. (2015). Significant association among growing pains, vitamin D supplementation, and bone mineral status: Results from a pilot cohort study. *Journal of Mineral and Bone Metabolism, 33*(2), 201–206. http://www.ncbi.nlm.nih.gov/pubmed/24633492.

Murphy, K. & Jones, S. (2007). *Sustaining the Pacific Northwest nutritional value of winter and spring wheat: A comparison of historic and modern varieties.* http://csanr.wsu.edu/publications/SPNW/SPNW-v5-n2.pdf.

Pimentel, D. & Wilson, A. (2004). World population, agriculture, and malnutrition. *World Watch Magazine, 17*(5). http://www.worldwatch.org/node/554.

Rendell, M. (2004). Advances in diabetes for the millennium: Drug therapy of type 2 diabetes. *Medscape General Medicine, 6*(3 Suppl.), 9.

Rivera, J. A., Hotz, C., González-Cossío, T., Neufeld, L., & García-Guerra, A. (2003). The effect of micronutrient deficiencies on child growth: A review of results from community-based supplementation trials. *Journal of Nutrition, 133*(11), 4010S–4020S. http://jn.nutrition.org/content/133/11/4010S.full.

United States Census Bureau. (2014). *Census Bureau Projects U.S. and world populations on New Year's Day.* http://www.census.gov/newsroom/press-releases/2014/cb14-tps90.html.

US Department of Health and Human Services. (2012). *CMS fiscal year 2012 performance budget.* Baltimore, MD: Centers for Medicare and Medicaid Services. https://www.cms.gov/About-CMS/Agency-Information/PerformanceBudget/downloads/CMSFY12CJ.pdf.

Veugelers, P. J. & Ekwaru, J. P. (2014). A statistical error in the estimation of the recommended dietary allowance for vitamin D. *Nutrients, 6*(10), 4472–4475. http://www.mdpi.com/2072-6643/6/10/4472&gt.

Welch, R. & Graham, R. D. (2004). Breeding for micronutrients in staple food crops from a human nutrition perspective. *Journal of Experimental Botany, 55*(396), 353–364. http://jxb.oxfordjournals.org/content/55/396/353.abstract?ijkey=f7ea2f6bb17a88f9760830f9caedb2df8d610618&keytype2=tf_ipsecsha.

Wells, J. & Dumbrell, A. C. (2006). Nutrition and aging: Assessment and treatment of compromised nutritional status in frail elderly patients. *Clinical Interventions in Aging.* http://www.ncbi.nlm.nih.gov/pmc/articles/PMC2682454/.

World Health Organization. (2015). *Micronutrient deficiencies.* http://www.who.int/nutrition/topics/ida/en/.

Suggested Readings can be found on the companion website, http://www.micozzipainconditions.com.

Chapter 22

Nutrition and Hydration
Part Three: Management of Pain and Inflammation with Micronutrients and Foods

This chapter provides information on topical and internal use of superior natural vitamins and minerals, classified as dietary supplements, for everyday health and prevention of pain. This chapter also provides information about the most common vitamin and mineral deficiency conditions and their symptoms including chronic pain and chronic inflammation.

An early simple telephone survey of more than 2000 English-speaking adults in the late 20th century found that more than 40% had used at least one alternative therapy, of which dietary supplements use was the most common form. In the same survey, nearly 20% of adults who regularly took prescription medications also reported the concurrent use of at least one herbal product or high-dose vitamin. Fewer than 40% of those surveyed who saw an alternative health practitioner discussed their experience with their regular physician. These findings are significant because interaction problems may arise when dietary supplements are combined with prescription or over-the-counter drugs, usually due to the more powerful effects of the drugs and the known and otherwise accepted side effects of prescription drugs.

The pharmacologic effect of dietary supplements is not surprising because many of the drugs in clinical practice are also derived from plants but are designed for greater potency. Lidocaine and novocaine are derived from the coca plant *(Erythroxylum coca)*, opioid pain relievers (e.g., morphine and codeine) from the poppy *(Papaver somniferum)*, and aspirin from the white willow *(Salix alba)* and meadowsweet *(Spiraea ulmaria)*, whence the "spir" part of aspirin's name derives. Digoxin comes from foxglove *(Digitalis lanata)*, and warfarin is a derivative of dicoumarin found in sweet clover *(Melilotus officinalis)*.

A large proportion of herbal remedy and dietary supplement use currently in the United States involves products that include therapeutic actions or effects on the brain and central nervous system (CNS), including treatment of mood and pain.

Vitamins, amino acids, and other dietary supplements are also popular. Studies indicate that dietary supplements are safe and effective for the management of pain and several neurologic problems.

IRON

According to the World Health Organization (WHO), iron deficiency is the most common nutritional disorder in the world. Iron deficiency symptoms correlate with the severity of the nutrient. Chronic pain, chest pain, headache, backache, abdominal pain, weakness, fatigue, shortness of breath, soreness of the tongue, and frequent infections are common symptoms of iron deficiency and should be taken seriously (Mulari, Mustonen, & Sotaniemi, 1996; National Heart, Lung and Blood Institute, 2014). In early 2012, excess iron was linked to an increased glaucoma risk, which can lead to total blindness. However, studies show that greater intake of whole foods that are higher in iron (e.g., greens, eggs, and lean red meat) did not show an effect on the development of glaucoma. Indeed, men and women who ate high-nutrient foods had a lower risk of developing glaucoma. Foods with high iron content also have high content of other nutrients, and the body is best equipped to metabolize nutrients (including iron) that are taken into the body in whole foods. The American Academy of Ophthalmology (AAO) meeting report concludes that dietary intake of foods must indeed be different biologically from supplement intake. Chances are very good that most people do not need iron supplements or multivitamins with iron. It is necessary only when people are specifically diagnosed by their doctor as having iron-deficiency anemia. Otherwise, it can potentially accumulate in heart muscle and other tissues, eventually leading to organ failure in some people. On a population basis, excess body iron stores have long been associated with increased risks of cancers, infections, and heart disease (Sempos, Looker, Gillum, & Makuc, 1994; Stevens, Jones, Micozzi, & Taylor, 1988).

VITAMINS B1, B2, B3, B5, B6, AND B12

When the body is stressed, water-soluble B vitamins are usually the first things that are "used" up by the brain and nervous system. Stress exhausts a huge amount of energy in the body and the brain, and B vitamins are important for maintaining daily energy levels. B vitamins are water-soluble nutrients found in many foods, primarily animal-based products, such as red meat, poultry, eggs, fish, and dairy. They cannot be produced or stored by the body and therefore must be consumed through the daily diet. They include B1 (thiamine), B2 (riboflavin), B3 (nicotinic acid), B6 (pyridoxine), B12 (cobalamin), and folate (folic acid). These nutrients contribute to a wide array of physiological functions, such as red blood cell production, nerve cell function, metabolism of carbohydrates and fats, energy production, and immune system function. Deficiency can occur from a poor diet or due to medical conditions that interfere with absorption of B vitamins from the gastrointestinal tract or from drugs such as Metformin used to treat chronic medical conditions like diabetes mellitus type 2. Abnormalities in the stomach or small intestine can interfere with the biochemical "intrinsic factor" (IF), which must bind with B12 to be absorbed in the small intestine along with other nutrients.

B vitamin deficiency, particularly B12, can contribute to several ailments, such as sore tongue or mouth, weight loss, pale skin, weak immunity, rapid heart rate, diarrhea, menstrual dysfunction, burning foot pain, pernicious anemia, and even tumor development. There are also specific diseases that cause B vitamin deficiency, such as autoimmune diseases, inflammatory bowel disease, and multiple sclerosis. In the aging, deficiency is usually caused from malabsorption. Significant early data have shown that B vitamins also play a role in cancer prevention. A study published in *Cancer Epidemiology Biomarkers & Prevention* in 1999 reported an association of low levels of B12 with breast cancer in postmenopausal women (Lajous, Romieu, Sabia, Boutron-Ruault, & Clavel-Chapelon, 2006). Another study published in the *Annals of Internal Medicine* in 1998 has shown a protective effect of dietary folate against the development of colon cancer (Giovannucci et al., 1988).

In terms of pain and pain processing, B vitamins also play a significant role in protecting the nervous system and spinal cord. Vitamin B12 is critical for the fatty myelin tissues that protect nerve and brain cells. B vitamins along with natural nutrients, such as berberine, lutein, and choline (l-α-glycerylphosphorylcholine [GPC] or alpha-GPC), help to maintain healthy brain function and normal central pain processing as well as other critical CNS functions (see Chapter 23).

VITAMIN C

Research indicates that vitamin C may contribute significantly to lowering blood pressure, maintaining muscle mass, and preventing cancer and associated pain. Researchers at Johns Hopkins found sufficient evidence from research studies that a 500-mg daily dose of vitamin C can lower blood pressure by 5 mm Hg. Although it cannot take the place of medications, it may be a very useful supplement in the process of cutting back on the amount of medication one has to take, something each individual should consult a physician to do safely.

With regard to muscle mass, the entire musculoskeletal system accounts for approximately 85% of the body's weight, mass, and size. Vitamin C is a collagen builder and extremely important for the regeneration of every cell in the body, not just for bones and joints. It may be used to support bone and joints and reduce common joint pain. This nutrient is so important in so many ways that most animals make their own as part of normal metabolism. Indeed, all animals make their own vitamin C except for two: humans and guinea pigs. (This is one reason why guinea pigs originally became such an important laboratory model in early scientific experiments.)

There has been more evidence on the potential health benefits of vitamin C than almost any other nutrient. And yet, the National Cancer Institute not only failed to conduct large-scale clinical trials on its cancer-preventing abilities, but they went further to claim it had actually been "given a bad name" by two-time Nobel prize winner Linus Pauling's efforts to promote vitamin C's benefits for preventing everything from cancer to the common cold.

VITAMIN D

The term vitamin D actually refers to a pair of biologically inactive precursors of a critical micronutrient. They are vitamin D3, also known as cholecalciferol, and vitamin D2, also known as ergocalciferol. Cholecalciferol is produced in the skin by a photoreaction on exposure to ultraviolet B light from the sun (wavelength 290 to 320 nm). Ergocalciferol is produced in plants and enters the human diet through consumption of plant sources. Once present in the circulation, both D2 and D3 enter the liver and kidneys, where they are hydroxylated to form both 25-hydroxyvitamin D (25-OH-D) and 1,25-dihydroxyvitamin D. The former, 25-OH-D, is relatively inactive and represents the storage form of vitamin D. By contrast, 1,25-dihydroxyvitamin D is highly active metabolically, and its levels are tightly controlled. Vitamin D has many critical metabolic functions. There has been confusion in the literature regarding differences in relative abundance, availability, and effects of vitamins D2 and D3, which have been reconciled by thoughtful investigation.

The major circulating form of vitamin D3 in human blood is 25-hydroxyvitamin D3, and therefore it is the form measured by physicians to evaluate vitamin D status in people worldwide. However, it takes a long time for this form to work on calcium absorption and mobilization, and it must be converted or metabolized to the more active 1,25-dihydroxyvitamin D for effectiveness in the body.

Knowledge of the role of vitamin D metabolic activity, its role in human health, and identification of the forms and metabolic pathways for vitamin D had been building for many decades but only became fully elucidated during the 1970s. Although nutrition is fundamental in human health, understanding of nutritional metabolism has generally lagged behind the pace of medical investigation and practice focusing on factors external to the host, such as infectious microorganisms.

VERSATILITY

The first major functions of vitamin D to be recognized were (1) enhancement of calcium absorption from the diet through the intestine and (2) mobilization and reabsorption of calcium from bone, which represents the major store of calcium (or "calcium bank") in the body (Fig. 22.1). Calcium (a divalent cation, with chemical symbol Ca^{++}), in turn, is critical for cellular metabolism and membrane actions, enzymatic reactions, muscle function, skeletal structure, and a host of activities needed to sustain life and maintain homeostasis. Because vitamin D has long been recognized for its role in calcium metabolism, it has long been used to treat patients with renal failure and bone diseases. It also has an important role in the treatment of postmenopausal osteoporosis and the current epidemic of bone fractures in the elderly.

However, in 1979, DeLuca found that vitamin D is actually recognized by every tissue in the body. Every cell has receptors for vitamin D. Since then vitamin D has been used to treat hyperproliferative skin diseases, such as psoriasis.

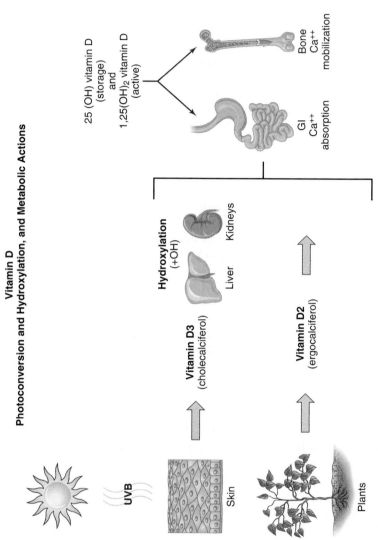

FIG 22.1 | Sources and photoconversion of vitamin D.

Regarding *inflammation,* in the immune system the large white blood cell macrophages activate vitamin D. The activated vitamin D in turn causes macrophages to make a peptide that specifically kills infective agents, such as tuberculosis mycobacteria. Vitamin D also has a role in helping to prevent autoimmune diseases, such as multiple sclerosis, rheumatoid arthritis, and diabetes.

Vitamin D's activity in the kidney has long been recognized, and it has been found to affect the production of renin and angiotensin, the major regulators of blood pressure, in the kidney. There is a direct correlation between higher (further from the equator) latitudes (where both sunlight and vitamin D levels are lower) and higher blood pressure in both the northern and southern hemispheres of the earth. People at high latitudes with high blood pressure experience a return to normal blood pressure levels after exposure to ultraviolet B light in a tanning bed three times a week for 3 months and restoration of active vitamin D levels.

Vitamin D is also thought to have an important role in cancer. As early as the 1940s it was noted that living at higher latitudes is associated with a higher incidence of several cancers (whereas only skin cancer specifically has a lower incidence at higher latitudes). Recent epidemiological observations have continued to bear out this association. A high frequency of sunbathing before age 20 was found to reduce the risk of non-Hodgkin's lymphoma.

Although sun exposure is related to an increased incidence of malignant melanoma skin cancer, it was also found to be associated with increased survival from melanoma in a recent study. It appears that basic nutrients like vitamin D can regulate cell growth and gene expression and have a role where conventional therapies have failed for generations.

Research has studied the effect of vitamin D3 (and an analogue of vitamin D) on preventing progression of ductal carcinoma in situ (DCIS) to invasive ductal carcinoma (IDC). DCIS may never progress to cause symptoms of actual breast cancer—but is nonetheless used by the mainstream cancer industry as justifications for breast surgery, including mastectomy, as well as chemotherapy and radiation. Cells in culture can form "mammosphere" groups of breast cells. The mammosphere cell culture system included breast cancer stem cells along with normal breast cells. When given vitamin D, the mammosphere culture transformed from disorganization and irregular patterns to more organized and symmetrical shapes as formed by normal breast cells. We will see these kinds of "cellular" results in the next study as well.

New Kinds of Cancer

A 2015 in vitro study published in the *Journal of Steroid Biochemistry and Molecular Biology* identified a new type of cancer cell called "cancer stem cells". Researchers believe these stem cells play a pivotal role in the formation of breast cancer, its progression toward malignant cancer, and its resistance to conventional treatments.

According to this research, there appear to be "mother" stem cells capable of infinitely renewing themselves and producing many "daughter" cells. Theoretically the presence of even a small number of mother breast cancer stem cells can cause recurrence of breast cancer. These mothers are resistant to conventional cancer treatments. Conventional treatments, such as surgery, radiation, and chemotherapy, can actually increase their numbers because they do not address the root cause of the cancer.

Researchers found that more aggressive treatment measures, such as double mastectomies, do not improve mortality rates in women with breast cancer. Women who underwent aggressive treatments of early cancer ended up having the exact same mortality rate as women who received no treatment. Perhaps those aggressive measures do not change the outcomes because they do not address the root cause of the cancer.

Research studied the effect of vitamin D3 (and an analogue of vitamin D) on preventing the progression of an early form of "abnormal cells" called DCIS into IDC. For this study, they applied a vitamin D3 compound to DCIS cells to see what would happen and noted three important outcomes.

First, the mother breast cancer stem cells decreased in number. (Remember— conventional cancer therapies can actually increase their populations.) Second, the daughter cells started to behave in a more "normal" way. Cells in culture (in a petri dish) can form "mammosphere" groups of breast cells. In this case, the mammosphere cell culture included breast cancer stem cells along with normal breast cells. After the researchers applied the vitamin D3, the mammosphere culture transformed from disorganization and irregular patterns into more organized and symmetrical shapes formed by normal breast cells. Third, the vitamin D3 reduced the cells' chemical markers associated with cancer (Wahler et al., 2015).

These three discoveries all point to one big benefit for cancer patients: vitamin D may be a more effective (and safer) treatment than any of the conventional therapies. It is much more selective and safe than surgery, radiation, and chemotherapy because it targets cancer at the cellular level, the ultimate source of breast cancer. Also, vitamin D does not cause damaging side effects, unlike conventional cancer therapies. The "side effects" of vitamin D include a long list of other health benefits.

Vitamin D is naturally made by converting a key cholesterol metabolite using ultraviolet B light (from the sun) in the skin. Cholesterol and sunlight are the natural keys and are the two natural elements against which mainstream medicine has been researching for decades. There is an epidemic of vitamin D deficiency—and epidemics of cancer, dementia, and neurological and other diseases associated with inadequate vitamin D levels.

FOODS THAT REDUCE CHRONIC INFLAMMATION AND CANCER

Research shows women have a much lower risk of developing breast cancer (as well as most other cancers) if they eat more of five key foods.

Broccoli

We have known about the ability of broccoli and other cruciferous vegetables to reduce cancer risk, especially breast cancer risk, for nearly 100 years. This knowledge first became available during the British Empire Cancer Campaign studies in the 1920s.

Nowadays most experts (including at the National Cancer Institute) understand broccoli is a potent anticancer agent. But it is not enough to know broccoli protects you against cancer. They want to know how and why it works. Most current research focuses on two classes of broccoli's biologically active components—indoles and sulforaphanes—that promote healthy cell growth and have "anticancer" activities.

Olive Oil

Olive oil also gets a lot of attention for its anti-inflammatory and anticancer properties. Scientists speculate that olive oil's "antioxidant" properties also contribute to its other benefits, such as reducing cardiovascular diseases (CVDs) and preventing heart attacks and strokes. Of course, it also helps to balance blood lipids (blood fats), which could possibly help to account for heart and other benefits. Chronic inflammation is a critical factor in the pathogenesis of many inflammatory disease states including CVD, cancer, diabetes, degenerative joint diseases, and neurodegenerative diseases, and olive oil has been shown to reduce inflammation and have many therapeutic actions (Lucas, Russell, & Keast, 2011). Olive oil resembles ibuprofen in its healing abilities (Lucas et al., 2011).

Salmon

Salmon contains anti-inflammatory properties, promotes healthy cell growth, and helps to prevent breast cancer. In a study published in 2015 a team of researchers investigated salmon as a potential inflammatory agent. They found that a protein in salmon inhibited acute inflammation in mice (Saigusa, Nishizawa, Shimizu, & Saeki, 2015).

Salmon also has many other health benefits, such as omega-3 fatty acids, which play a critical role in supporting the brain, heart, and immune system. In addition, like other healthy fish and meat, it has high levels of bioavailable B vitamins and vitamin D, which are very difficult to get from even the most healthful vegetables.

Always make sure to buy wild-caught salmon. Farm-raised salmon can have as little as one tenth of the key nutrients. In addition, they often contain high levels of heavy metals, such as mercury and other toxins.

Unfortunately, virtually all Atlantic salmon is currently farm-raised, whether from Scotland or Nova Scotia, so make sure your salmon comes from the Pacific.

COPING WITH PAIN AND STRESS: VITAMINS B AND D

Stress and anxiety, as discussed throughout this book, are major components of pain. Processing of pain is perceived as a stress, which induces anxiety, and anxiety influences the perception of pain. In 2010 a magnitude 7.1 earthquake struck Christchurch, New Zealand. Through the rubble, observers noticed the survivors who used micronutrient supplements reduced and prevented the mental health problems typically associated with the stress of living through such a disaster. It also

NEUROLOGICAL DISORDERS OF TASTE AND SMELL

Acute, severe zinc deficiency can cause decreased sensitivity of taste. Two studies found that taking 50 mg of elemental zinc a day significantly improved sense of taste. A study of more than 100 patients with loss of taste found that 100 mg zinc taken daily resulted in improvements. Zinc may be effective only in those individuals with low serum zinc levels. Nearly 100 patients in one study were divided into four groups, depending on the cause (zinc deficient, idiopathic, drug induced, and other). All received zinc gluconate (22.6 mg twice per day) for 4 months. Zinc benefited the zinc-deficient and idiopathic groups but not the groups of patients whose conditions were drug induced or fell into other categories.

In another study, patients with sensory-neural olfactory disorder were treated with usual drug therapy, zinc sulfate, or both. Of patients with posttraumatic olfactory disorder, those in the zinc sulfate groups had significantly greater improvements. For patients with disorders of postviral or unknown etiology, there were no significant differences in improvement among the three groups.

Surgical and medical treatments for head and neck cancer often cause taste alterations. In a randomized, placebo-controlled study, patients receiving external radiation to the head and neck were randomly chosen to receive zinc sulfate (45 mg twice per day) or placebo at the onset of taste alterations. The treatment was continued for 1 month after the radiation therapy had ended. Patients treated with placebo experienced a greater loss in taste acuity during radiation treatment compared with those treated with zinc. In addition, those treated with zinc had a faster recovery of taste acuity than those receiving placebo.

gave researchers an idea: give disaster victims much-needed nutritional support, and they will better cope with stress.

In June 2013 a devastating spring flood hit Alberta, Canada, and caused more than 100,000 residents to evacuate. In the midst of the flooding and evacuation, researchers contacted residents through social media to participate in a trial on the potential benefits of nutritional supplements to reduce anxiety and stress. Fifty-six men and women—whose homes were damaged by the flood—agreed to participate. They ranged in age from 22 to 66 years old. They received 1000 IU of vitamin D daily, a vitamin B-complex daily, or a daily broad-spectrum multivitamin-mineral four times daily. The study continued for 6 weeks, with a 93% compliance rate.

All participants selected scored at least one point higher than the standard limits on the Depression, Anxiety, and Stress Scale. In other words, they all had to show marked symptoms of depression, anxiety, and stress. None of the participants had been on psychiatric medications for at least 4 weeks prior to the start of the study.

During the 6 weeks, participants in all groups showed improvements in anxiety and stress levels. Those who took the daily B-complex or the broad-spectrum multivitamin-mineral experienced significantly greater improvements compared with those who took only 1000 IU of vitamin D.

A national spokesperson for the American Society of Nutrition commented on these findings. She noted that government and health officials typically think of supplying water and basic food items after a natural disaster, but they should also think about actual nutrition, especially when you consider most people will have a poorer diet and further reduced nutrient intake following natural disasters. In addition, most people do not have good nutritional status to begin with, according to many other studies.

According to a new study's author, Bonnie J. Kaplan, PhD, "It is so cheap to give people extra supplements after a hurricane or whatever, to strengthen their ability to cope with the stressors—and so expensive to treat them all as psychiatric patients" (Kaplan, Rucklidge, Romijn, & Dolph, 2015).

Vitamin E

Research shows this nutrient is crucial for every stage of life—from helping normal fetal development to staving off Alzheimer's disease. It is important for heart, eyes, and immune system and vital for brain health.

It is critical for pregnant women to consume adequate vitamin E because it is essential for normal fetal development. Lack of vitamin E during pregnancy is associated with anemia, infections, stunting, and overall poor outcomes for both infant and mother. During childhood, not getting enough vitamin E can cause neurological disorders, along with abnormalities of skeletal and heart muscles (Linus Pauling Institute, 2014).

Later in life, vitamin E appears to have an important role in preventing or managing Alzheimer's disease and dementia. A recent study revealed that taking 2000 IU of vitamin E per day reduced symptoms of dementia and improved cognitive function in a group of older Americans. The Alzheimer's drug memantine showed no effect in this study. The drug even appeared to negate the benefits of vitamin E in the people who received both the drug and the nutrient (Dysken et al., 2014). This dose may seem "high" when compared to the RDA but in this case it was used for reversing a devastating "incurable" chronic disease, compared to an ineffective drug.

Throughout life, there is evidence that vitamin E is important for supporting the brain and improving cognition. An interesting study reported that people who have higher levels of vitamin E (together with B, C, and D) throughout their lives not only have better cognitive function—they actually have bigger brains when they are older (Bowman et al., 2012).

Studies suggest that vitamin E appears to protect the functions of essential omega-3 fatty acids, which are important for brain and eye health, heart health, and supporting a balanced immune system. One study cited in the *Advances in Nutrition Review* showed that people who had the highest levels of docosahexaenoic acid (DHA)—a component of omega-3—cut their risk of dementia nearly in half (Traber, 2014).

TREATMENT OF PAIN AND PAIN-RELATED CONDITIONS

This section addresses specific pain and pain-related conditions, as well as inflammation, and provides evidence for the role vitamins, minerals, foods, and their dosages that can be used for treatment.

INFLAMMATION AND INFLAMMATORY CONDITIONS

Vitamins A, B, C, D, and E have been shown to have anti-inflammatory properties, and these vitamins have also shown effectiveness in the treatment of inflammatory dermatoses, acne, and pigmentation disorders as well as wound healing (Burgess, 2008). Additional benefits have been recorded when vitamins are taken together rather than individually. Vitamin A has been shown to decrease inflammation and be closely involved in the prevention of disease (Reifen, 2002). Vitamins B3, B6, B9, and B12 have been shown to have anti-inflammatory effects in the body.

Vitamin C can help to repair damaged tissue and cushion the body's joints and protect them from damage. Vitamin C essentially helps to rebuild collagen.

Increased levels of vitamin D (6000 to 8000 IU/day) were shown to improve inflammation and muscular function, control blood pressure, and improve levels of glucose in the body.

Vitamin E (50 mg/day), as far back as 1967, has shown its powerful anti-inflammatory properties. More recently, in studies published in 2005, 2011, and 2015, the researchers found that a combination of vitamin E lowers inflammation (Rossato, Hoffmeister, Tonello, de Oliveira Ferreira, & Ferreira, 2015; Singh, Devaraj, & Jialal, 2005; Tahan et al., 2011). Vitamin E also prevents oxidative stress and improves the body's ability to use insulin with an increase in glucose metabolism (Barbagallo, Dominguez, Tagliamonte, Resnick, & Paolisso, 1999).

Vitamin E has been shown to significantly decrease inflammation in bowel disease. In a study in 2011, researchers found vitamin E was a powerful antioxidant, decreasing free radicals, and it may be a promising therapeutic action for ulcerative colitis (Tahan et al., 2011).

MIGRAINE HEADACHE, PREMENSTRUAL SYNDROME, AND MENSTRUAL CRAMPS

Vitamins and minerals have been shown to be helpful for the related conditions in women of migraine headache, premenstrual syndrome, and menstrual cramps. **Magnesium** is beneficial to both treat and prevent migraine headache attacks. Magnesium is essential for more than 300 biochemical reactions in the brain and body using adenosine triphosphate (ATP). It is the fourth most prevalent cation (or positive ion: Na^+, K^+, Ca^{++}, Mg^{++}) in the body, after Ca^{++}, and the second most common divalent cation (carrying two positive charges, chemical symbol Mg^{++}). However, dietary magnesium deficiency is quite common. According to estimates of magnesium intake based on the Third US National Health and Nutrition

Examination Survey (1988 to 1994), magnesium intake was lower than the recommended daily allowance (RDA) in both males and females between 12 and 60 years of age in all racial and ethnic groups, except non-Hispanic white males. The incidence of deficiency is even higher among hospitalized patients; 65% of those in intensive care, up to 12% in general wards, and 30% of hospitalized alcoholics have low magnesium.

Several studies indicate that magnesium supplementation may be helpful for treatment of *migraine*, as well as *tension-type headaches* (Bigal, Bordini, Tepper & Speciali, 2002; Blumenthal, Weisz, Kelly, & Mayer 2003; Pittler & Ernst 2004). Although the exact mechanism of action of magnesium's effects is unclear, it may interrupt the process at the vasoconstriction stage by interacting with serotonin and *N*-methyl-D-aspartate receptors, nitrous oxide synthesis and release, other migraine-related receptors, and neurotransmitters.

Increased magnesium causes diarrhea, a side effect seen in every trial in which these data were collected. Inorganic forms of magnesium (magnesium oxide, magnesium chloride) may be more likely to cause diarrhea than organic forms (magnesium citrate, magnesium aspartate), but diarrhea can result from administration of any preparation.

In another study, adult migraine patients, with an average attack frequency rate of four headaches per month, received oral magnesium for 12 weeks to *prevent migraine* attacks. In the last 4 weeks, migraine attacks were reduced by nearly 50%. The number of days with migraine was also significantly decreased. Diarrhea was reported in 18% and gastric irritation in 4% of patients receiving magnesium.

Researchers have also long noted lower levels of magnesium in the red blood cells of women with *premenstrual syndrome* (Rosenstein, Elin, Hosseini, Grover, & Rubinow, 1994; Sherwood, Rocks, Stewart, & Saxton, 1986). Studies have demonstrated the effectiveness of magnesium for relief of *menstrual pain*. Magnesium also reduced the need for pain medication (Wilson & Murphy, 2002).

In a study of *menstrual migraines*, women received 360 mg/day of magnesium pyrrolidine carboxylic acid or placebo from the 15th day of their cycles until menses. Women receiving magnesium had significantly less pain than the placebo group, and the number of days with headache decreased only in the magnesium group. The effects were so dramatic that for ethical reasons, after 2 months, the study was changed to an "open-label trial" in which magnesium was given to all patients for an additional 2 months. Significant decreases in pain were seen in both groups between the second and fourth months.

Riboflavin is a B vitamin, or "neurovitamin," needed in the production of ATP as energy source for all the cells in the body. Outright riboflavin deficiency is relatively rare in Western countries, but marginal deficiency (insufficiency) is relatively common, especially among older adults and adolescents. A study of *migraine headaches* found that 400 mg of riboflavin taken daily was superior to placebo in reducing attack frequency and headache days. The dose of riboflavin used in this trial was quite high—about 300 times higher than the RDA. However, riboflavin is quite safe and any excess is excreted in the urine.

CARPAL TUNNEL SYNDROME

Studies on **vitamin B6** and carpal tunnel syndrome show that it is useful as adjunctive treatment to conservative, nonsurgical therapy. In one study, patients took large doses of **omega-3 fatty acids** daily from 2400 to 7200 mg/day of EPA-DHA. The patients suffered from nerve pain due to carpal tunnel syndrome and experienced "clinically significant pain reduction" for up to 19 months following the initial treatment.

DIABETIC NEUROPATHY AND PAIN

In a study of type 2 diabetes and **vitamin E,** given for 6 months, nerve conduction in the median motor nerve fibers improved significantly in the treatment group.

In Tanzania, diabetic peripheral neuropathy is associated with **thiamine** deficiency. In a study comparing thiamine (25 mg/day) and pyridoxine (50 mg/day) therapy with placebo (containing 1 mg each thiamine and pyridoxine), significant improvements in pain, numbness, tingling, and impairment of sensation in the legs were noted in the treatment group. The severity of signs of peripheral neuropathy decreased 50% in the treatment group compared with 11% in the placebo group.

In a study on **alpha-lipoic acid** for diabetic neuropathy, patients with type 2 diabetes and symptomatic peripheral neuropathy were randomly selected to receive placebo or three different doses of intravenous alpha-lipoic acid (1200, 600, or 100 mg) over 3 weeks. Total symptoms were significantly reduced in groups receiving 600 or 1200 mg alpha-lipoic acid.

NERVE AND NEUROPATHIC PAIN

Omega-3 fatty acids are key nutrients found in fatty fish varieties, such as herring, salmon, bluefish, lake trout, and mackerel, and are available as supplements. Omega-3 fatty acids have heart-health benefits, and they also have an anti-inflammatory effect, making them helpful in treating irritable bowel syndrome (IBS). Omega-3 fatty acids appear to work especially well for *nerve pain*. If supplementing with fish oil, 1 to 2 g is recommended.

Biochemical studies have shown that high doses of omega-3 fatty acids lead to the incorporation of these compounds into the neuronal membrane phospholipids, which are crucial for cell signaling.

Dietary supplementation with large amounts of omega-3 fatty acids is related to a general dampening of signal transduction pathways. An association between *depression* and *multiple sclerosis* is consistent with essential fatty acid depletion in both brain and nerve white matter and in blood plasma. DHA is apparently absent in the adipose tissue of patients with multiple sclerosis. Relations between abnormal concentrations of omega-3 and omega-6 fatty acids and the occurrence of other neurologic disorders also have been noted.

In a research study, patients with neuropathic pain took large doses of omega-3 fatty acids daily. This dose varied from 2400 to 7200 mg/day of EPA-DHA. The patients suffered from nerve pain due to carpal tunnel syndrome, fibromyalgia, and other conditions. According to the results of the study, the patients experienced "clinically significant pain reduction" for up to 19 months following the initial treatment.

Although individual vitamins and minerals can be obtained in dietary supplements, they are all available in healthy foods together with many other biologically active constituents that are not necessarily classified as "vitamins" or micronutrients.

Restless Legs Syndrome

Iron deficiency, whether or not it results in anemia, appears to be an important factor in the development of *restless legs syndrome* (RLS) in older adults. In one study, patients with severe RLS had iron (as ferritin) levels less than 50 µg/mL. Lower ferritin levels correlated with greater severity of RLS symptoms and decreased *sleep* efficiency. In another study, serum ferritin levels were lower in RLS patients. Lower serum ferritin levels correlated significantly with greater RLS severity, and improvement was noted after iron repletion.

It must be kept in mind that excess body iron stores, or iron overload, is associated with increased risk of cancer and other chronic diseases, most likely related to the free radical generating properties of unbound, free iron in the body.

Cerebral Stroke

Recent findings about vitamin D relate to CVD, the most common health problem currently. Previous studies had established a connection between low vitamin D and CVD. However, in these earlier studies, researchers typically took just one blood sample to test for vitamin D, and they did not look at the differences between fatal and nonfatal CVD events. In other words, they looked only at the number of cardiovascular events overall. They did not look at who died and, just as important, who did not die.

The most recent German study is much stronger because researchers measured vitamin D levels at three different times and looked at the differences between who died and who did not die after suffering a heart attack or stroke.

For the study, researchers followed a cohort of nearly 10,000 adults ages 50 to 74 years for more than 10 years. They measured the amount of vitamin D (25-OH-D) in the participants' blood at the outset of the study. Then, they measured it again after 5 years and one last time after 8 years. They found that 59% of women and men in the study had inadequate vitamin D levels (Perna, Schöttker, Holleczek, & Brenner, 2013). The researchers defined "inadequate" as anything lower than 50 nanomoles per liter. Over the next 10 years, 854 participants had a nonfatal CVD event; 460 of them suffered nonfatal heart attacks and 313 had nonfatal strokes. However, 176 participants had a fatal CVD event. (There were 79 fatal heart attacks and 41 fatal strokes.) Overall, men and women with low vitamin D levels had a 27% greater risk of suffering a heart attack or stroke.

A NEW STROKE FOR STROKE

In an innovative, new study, Japanese researchers found an effective and noninvasive way to help cerebral stroke victims to cope with poststroke pain. For the past century, fundamental sciences—such as physics and quantum mechanics, biology, and ecology—have begun to look at energetic interactions. These energetic interactions form a common basis for health and healing. Thus, in this view, all the other therapies just access the body's energy in ways that influence health and healing. With this new understanding about energy, the medicine of the future may learn to bypass invasive drugs and surgeries, as well as ingested foods, micronutrients and dietary supplements. They will go straight to the source of energetic healing. Transcranial magnetic stimulation (TMS) is already available (see Chapter 10). TMS is a noninvasive procedure that uses magnetic fields to stimulate nerve cells in the brain. Doctors use TMS to help to treat *depression, anxiety, migraines*, and now—*pain*. For the procedure itself, doctors place an electromagnetic coil against the scalp near the forehead. The electromagnet used in TMS creates electric currents that stimulate nerve cells in the region of the brain involved in pain. A study involved 18 patients who had experienced a blood clot or bleeding in one side of the brain, called "unilateral ischemic" or "hemorrhagic strokes". Several weeks into recovery, patients began to experience *severe hand or leg pain* because of brain damage from the stroke. Indeed, stroke can cause severe pain sensations, such as uncomfortable numbness, prickling or tingling, as well as other pain.

All the patients in the study received repetitive TMS treatments—called rTMS—to the primary motor cortex for at least 12 weeks. After 12 weeks of rTMS, 11 patients achieved satisfactory-to-excellent pain relief. Researchers defined "satisfactory" relief when a patient achieved a 40% to 69% reduction in pain scores (Kobayashi, Fujimaki, Mihara, & Ohira, 2015). They defined "excellent" relief when a patient achieved a 70% or greater pain reduction. The six study patients who continued treatment for 1 year achieved permanent pain relief. The researchers for this study urge neurologists and pain management specialists to take an interest in this effective method, which has minimal side effects. Indeed, none of the 18 patients reported any serious side effects from the weekly sessions.

NEUROLOGICAL DISORDERS, DEPRESSION, DEMENTIA, AND DEMYELINATING MYELOPATHY

Folate and **vitamin B12** are required for the methylation of homocysteine to methionine and for the synthesis of S-adenosylmethionine. S-adenosylmethionine plays a role in numerous methylation reactions involving proteins, phospholipids, deoxyribonucleic acid, and neurotransmitter metabolism. Folate and vitamin B12 deficiency may cause similar neurologic and psychiatric disturbances, including *depression, dementia, and a demyelinating myelopathy*. B vitamin supplementation may be beneficial.

A study that evaluated nutritional status and cognitive function in men and women older than 60 years who had no known physical illnesses and were taking no medications showed that subjects with low blood levels of **vitamins C** or **B12** had generally lower functions. Subjects with low levels of **riboflavin** or **folic acid** also had lower readings for some cognitive functions. These differences were significant. Studies compared high-dose **vitamin E** (2000 IU) to a drug and to placebo for treatment of dementia. Vitamin E showed remarkable benefits, whereas the drug showed no effect. However, when the drug was given with vitamin E, it negated the benefits of vitamin E alone. Another study showed benefits of **vitamin D** for dementia. The daily dose of vitamin D required for good health is 10 times the RDA of 600 to 700 IU. Two studies exposed that the calculations of the RDA for vitamin D are off by a factor of 10. Therefore daily vitamin D intake should be 5000 IU, accounting for the 1000 to 2000 IU that is obtained from the diet.

Omega-3 polyunsaturated fatty acids are long-chain, polyunsaturated fatty acids (PUFAs) found in plant and marine sources. These essential fatty acids, particularly DHA, are necessary for cell membrane function and may be factors in *depression, bipolar disorder, schizophrenia,* and other mood and neurologic disorders. The Western diet contains considerably high amounts of omega-6 fatty acids but lesser amounts of omega-3 fatty acids. Fish oil is high in PUFAs, DHA, and eicosapentaenoic acid. Nerve membranes contain high concentrations of DHA, as well as arachidonic acid (AA). Neurotransmitter receptors lie embedded in the nerve membrane, and their three-dimensional conformation is dependent on the fatty acids that give structure to the membrane.

FOODS AND PHYTOCHEMICALS

Scientists have long been aware that many organic fruits, vegetables, and legumes appear to reduce the risk of heart disease and cancer and help to manage pain and other conditions. It has been hypothesized that these activities are present because they contain antioxidants (vitamins, minerals, and other constituents that protect cells from being damaged by oxidation). In addition, organic fruits and vegetables are not contaminated with pesticides that may contain fluoride and other harmful toxins and chemicals that may inhibit vitamin absorption of food that is already poor in nutrients. For example, fluoride is reduced with **vitamin D** or **vitamin E** supplementation and decreases reproductive toxicity from fluoride (Kumar et al., 2012). Fluoride decreases the absorption of vital vitamins and nutrients. Precautions for fluoride include appropriate water filtration systems and adding a pinch (1/3 tsp) of organic Himalayan or sea salt to increase mineral content in water.

Another group of disease-fighting nutrients has been identified: phytochemicals, some of which are known commercially as "nutraceuticals."

Phytochemicals are thought to fight chronic inflammation, cancer, and other conditions by keeping disease-causing substances from latching onto healthy cells and by removing toxins before they can cause harm. There are many thousands of phytochemicals—tomatoes alone contain 10,000 different kinds—each with slightly different functions. **Genistein**, for example, which is found in soybeans, prevents the formation of the capillaries needed to nourish tumors. **Indoles**, which increase immune function, are found in members of the *Brassica* family, such as broccoli and cauliflower. **Bioflavonoids** found in lemons, limes, and other citrus fruits prevent certain cancer-causing hormones from attaching to the body's cells. Much as an earlier generation of scientists sought to identify and synthesize vitamins, researchers nowadays are working to isolate and manufacture phytochemicals. However, it is unlikely that they will be able to reproduce the rich mix of beneficial substances found in a single tomato or a handful of vegetables.

Two examples are popularized and commonly used as foods, spices, and remedies.

Garlic *(Allium sativum)* has been widely promoted as a remedy for anti-inflammatory and antifungal purposes, in addition to warding off colds, coughs, flu, chronic bronchitis, whooping cough, ringworm, asthma, intestinal worms, fever, and digestive, gallbladder, and liver disorders. Investigators have explored its use as a treatment for mild hypertension and hyperlipidemia.

Unlike many other herbal remedies, garlic is also a biologically active food with medicinal properties, including possible anticancer effects. Clinical studies of garlic in humans address three areas: (1) effect on cardiovascular system-related disease and risk factors, such as lipid levels, blood pressure, glucose level, atherosclerosis, and thrombosis; (2) protective associations with cancer; and (3) clinical adverse effects.

Scant data, primarily from case-control studies, suggest that dietary garlic consumption is associated with decreased risk of laryngeal, gastric, colorectal, and endometrial cancer and adenomatous colorectal polyps.

Cholesterol levels have also been related to the use of garlic. There is high consumer use of garlic as a health supplement. Garlic preparations studied have included standardized dehydrated tablets, "aged garlic extract," oil macerates, distillates, raw garlic, and combination tablets.

Side effects of oral ingestion of garlic are "smelly" breath and body odor. Other possible effects include flatulence, esophageal and abdominal pain, small intestinal obstruction, contact dermatitis, rhinitis, asthma, and bleeding. How frequently adverse effects occur with oral ingestion of garlic as a food and whether they vary for particular garlic preparations have not been established. Adverse effects of inhaled garlic dust include allergic reactions, such as asthma, rhinitis, urticaria, angioedema, and anaphylaxis. Adverse effects of topical exposure to raw garlic include contact dermatitis, skin blisters, and ulcerative lesions. Whether adverse effects are specific to particular preparations, constituents, or dosages should be elucidated. In particular, adverse effects related to bleeding and interactions with other drugs, such as aspirin and anticoagulants, warrant further study.

Ginger, like garlic, can be considered as both a popular ingredient in prepared foods and beverages and as an effective medicinal plant remedy. Ginger has long been known and used for its *anti-inflammatory*, antinausea effects, and calming properties on the stomach—thus the traditional popular beverages ginger ale and ginger beer. It is particularly useful for nausea associated with pregnancy and with chemotherapy, for which acupuncture is also a useful alternative therapy.

PROBIOTICS

Probiotics have *anti-inflammatory* activity. There are specifically types of normal bacteria found naturally inside the intestines that aid in digestion. Probiotics have been found to specifically help to reduce inflammation in the intestine (Mengheri, 2008).

According to Frye, "There is plausible rationale for why these would be helpful. If altered bacteria in the gut aren't the cause of the IBS, it certainly is an effect." Probiotics can be found in some yogurts with active cultures and other cultured foods, or they may be taken in capsule form, but make sure they are truly active and effective probiotic supplement. Eating certain foods also has probiotic effects in the gastrointestinal tract.

Digestive Enzymes

Bromelain, an enzyme derived from pineapple, is a potent source of digestive enzymes. A recent study found evidence that bromelain may have beneficial effects in the gastrointestinal tract for people with IBS. A good serving of fresh pineapple or pineapple juice provides bromelain in a food matrix together with other nutrients.

Coffee, Type 2 Diabetes, and Inflammation

A new study shows men and women who drink moderate amounts of coffee run a significantly lower risk of developing type 2 diabetes. First, drinking coffee also benefits the brain, over both short and long terms. Second, coffee helps to detoxify the body and acts as an old-fashioned "tonic." Third, it helps to support the cardiovascular system. Coffee is full of antioxidants that have the same anticancer and anti-inflammatory properties as green tea, the darling of the natural health world, but apparently at much higher levels.

In this study, researchers followed 1300 men and women in Athens, Greece, for 10 years. The participants in the study provided the researchers with dietary information, including information about their coffee-drinking habits. The researchers classified anyone who drank fewer than 1.5 cups of coffee a day a "casual" coffee drinker. "Habitual" drinkers drank more than 1.5 cups per day. In the study, there were 816 casual drinkers, 385 habitual drinkers, and 239 nondrinkers.

After 10 years, 191 people had developed type 2 diabetes (13% of men and 12% of women in the original groups). Overall, habitual coffee drinkers were 54% less likely to develop type 2 diabetes compared with nondrinkers. That strong association held up even after the researchers accounted for smoking, high blood pressure, family history, and total caffeine intake. Researchers also found coffee drinkers had lower levels of inflammation. Many researchers believe the active ingredient in caffeine from coffee may increase a hormone called "adiponectin". This hormone affects insulin and blood sugar levels. Natural compounds like coffee have many different physiologic activities.

These effects of natural compounds on pain, pain-related conditions, and chronic inflammation illustrate the roles of foods and vitamin and mineral micronutrients. Chapter 23 addresses the potent pain-relieving properties and anti-inflammatory activities of other natural constituents considered as herbal remedies and also classified as dietary supplements.

REFERENCES

Barbagallo, M., Dominguez, L. J., Tagliamonte, M. R., Resnick, L. M., & Paolisso, G. (1999). Effects of vitamin E and glutathione on glucose metabolism. *Hypertension, 34*, 1002–1006. http://hyper.aha-journals.org/content/34/4/1002.full.

Bigal, M. E., Bordini, C., Tepper, S. J., & Speciali, J. G. (2002). Intravenous magnesium sulphate in the acute treatment of migraine without aura and migraine with aura. A randomized, double-blind, placebocontrolled study. *Cephalalgia, 22*, 345–353.

Blumenthal, H. J., Weisz, M. A., Kelly, K. M., Mayer, R. L., & Blonsky, J. (2003). Treatment of primary headache in the emergency department. *Headache, 43*(10), 1026–1031.

Bowman, G. L., Silbert, L. C., Howieson, D., Dodge, H. H., Traber, M. G., Frei, B., et al. (2012). Nutrient biomarker patterns, cognitive function, and MRI measures of brain aging. *Neurology, 78*(4), 241–249.

Burgess, C. (2008). Topical vitamins. *Journal of Drugs in Dermatology, 7*(Suppl 7), S2–S6. http://www.ncbi.nlm.nih.gov/pubmed/18681152.

Dysken, M. W., Sano, M., Asthana, S., Vertrees, J. E., Pallaki, M., Liorente, M., et al. (2014). Effect of vitamin E and memantine on functional decline in Alzheimer disease: The TEAM-AD VA cooperative randomized trial. *Journal of the American Medical Association, 311*(1), 33–34.

Giovannucci, E., Stampfer, M. J., Colditz, G. A., Hunter, D. J., Fuchs, C., Rosner, B. A., et al. (1988). Multivitamin use, folate, and colon cancer in women in the Nurses' Health Study. *Annals of Interal Medicine, 129*(7), 517–524.

Kaplan, B. J., Rucklidge, J. J., Romijn, A. R., & Dolph, M. (2015). A randomised trial of nutrient supplements to minimise psychological stress after a natural disaster. *Psychiatry Research, 228*(3), 373–379. http://www.psy-journal.com/article/S0165-1781%2815%2900393-5/abstract.

Kobayashi, M., Fujimaki, T., Mihara, B., & Ohira, T. (2015). Repetitive transcranial magnetic stimulation once a week induces sustainable long-term relief of central poststroke pain. *Neuromodulation, 18*(4), 249–254. http://onlinelibrary.wiley.com/doi/10.1111/ner.12301/abstract.

Kumar, N., Sood, S., Arora, B., Singh, M., Beena & Roy, P. S. (2012). To study the effect of vitamin D and E on sodium-fluoride-induced toxicity in reproductive functions of male rabbits. *Toxicology International, 19*(2), 182–187. http://www.ncbi.nlm.nih.gov/pmc/articles/PMC3388764/.

Lajous, M., Romieu, I., Sabia, S., Boutron-Ruault, M. C., & Clavel-Chapelon, F. (2006). Folate, vitamin B12 and postmenopausal breast cancer in a prospective study of French women. *Cancer Causes & Control, 17*(9), 1209–1213.

Linus Pauling Institute. (2014). *Vitamin E intake critical during "the first 1000 days".* http://lpi.oregonstate.edu/news/vitaminE1000days.html.

Lucas, L., Russell, A., & Keast, R. (2011). Chronic inflammation is a critical factor in the pathogenesis of many inflammatory disease states including cardiovascular disease, cancer, diabetes, degenerative joint diseases and neurodegenerative diseases. *Current Pharmaceutical Design, 17*(8), 754–768. http://www.ncbi.nlm.nih.gov/pubmed/21443487.

Mengheri, E. (2008). Health, probiotics, and inflammation. *Journal of Clinical Gastroenterology, 42*(Suppl 3), S177–S178.

Mulari, S., Mustonen, M., & Sotaniemi, E. A. (1996). Iron deficiency anemia, backache, and abdominal pain attacks during sexual intercourse in a 42-year-old woman. *Scandinavian Journal of Gastroenterology, 31*(6), 622–623. http://www.ncbi.nlm.nih.gov/pubmed/8789904.

National Heart, Lung and Blood Institute. (2014). *What are the signs and symptoms of iron-deficiency anemia?* http://www.nhlbi.nih.gov/health/health-topics/topics/ida/signs.

Perna, L., Schöttker, B., Holleczek, B., & Brenner, H. (2013). Serum 25-hydroxyvitamin D and incidence of fatal and nonfatal cardiovascular events: A prospective study with repeated measurements. *The Journal of Clinical Endocrinology and Metabolism, 98*(12), 4908–4915. http://press.endocrine.org/doi/full/10.1210/jc.2013-2424.

Pittler, M. H. & Ernst, E. (2004). Dietary supplements for body-weight reduction: a systematic review. *American Journal of Clinical Nutrition, 79*(4), 529–536.

Reifen, R. (2002). Vitamin A as an anti-inflammatory agent. *Proceedings of the Nutrition Society, 61*(3), 397–400. http://www.ncbi.nlm.nih.gov/pubmed/12230799.

Rosenstein, D. L., Elin, R. J., Hosseini, J. M., Grover, G., & Rubinow, D. R. (1994). Magnesium measures across the menstrual cycle in premenstrual syndrome. *Biol Psychiatry*, *35*(8), 557–561.

Rossato, M. F., Hoffmeister, C., Tonello, R., de Oliveira Ferreira, A. P. & Ferreira, J. (2015). Anti-inflammatory effects of vitamin E on adjuvant-induced arthritis in rats. *Inflammation*, *38*(2), 606–615. http://www.ncbi.nlm.nih.gov/pubmed/25120238.

Saigusa, M., Nishizawa, M., Shimizu, Y., & Saeki, H. (2015). In vitro and in vivo anti-inflammatory activity of digested peptides derived from salmon myofibrillar protein conjugated with a small quantity of alginate oligosaccharide. *Bioscience, Biotechnology, and Biochemistry*, *79*(9), 1518–1527. http://www.ncbi.nlm.nih.gov/pubmed/25884412.

Sempos, C. T., Looker, A. C., Gillum, R. F., & Makuc, D. M. (1994). Body iron stores and the risk of coronary heart disease. *N Engl J Med*, *330*, 1119–1124.

Sherwood, R. A., Rocks, B. F., Stewart, A., & Saxton, R. S. (1986). Magnesium and the premenstrual syndrome. *Ann Clin Biochem*, *23*, 667–670.

Singh, U., Devaraj, S. & Jialal, I. (2005). Vitamin E, oxidative stress, and inflammation. *Annual Review of Nutrition*, *25*, 151–174. http://www.ncbi.nlm.nih.gov/pubmed/16011463.

Stevens, R. G., Jones, D. Y., Micozzi, M. S., & Taylor, P. R. (1988). Body iron stores and the risk of cancer. *New England Journal of Medicine*, *319*(16), 1047–1052.

Tahan, G., Aytac, E., Aytekin, H., Gunduz, F., Dogusoy, G., Aydin, S., et al. (2011). Vitamin E has a dual effect of anti-inflammatory and antioxidant activities in acetic acid-induced ulcerative colitis in rats. *Canadian Journal of Surgery*, *54*(5), 333–338. http://www.ncbi.nlm.nih.gov/pubmed/21933527.

Traber, M. G. (2014). Vitamin E inadequacy in humans: Causes and consequences. *Advances in Nutrition*, *5*, 503–514.

Wahler, J., So, J. Y., Cheng, L. C., Maehr, H., Uskokovic, M., & Suh, N. (2015). Vitamin D compounds reduce mammosphere formation and decrease expression of putative stem cell markers in breast cancer. *Journal of Steroid Biochemistry and Molecular Biology*, *148*, 148–155. http://www.ncbi.nlm.nih.gov/pubmed/25445919.

Wilson, M. L. & Murphy, P. A. (2002). Dietary magnesium intake for primary and secondary dysmenorrhea. *Cochrane Database Syst Rev*, *1*, CD000121.

Suggested Readings can be found on the companion website, http://www.micozzipainconditions.com.

Chapter 23

Plant-Based Treatments
Part One: Herbal Remedies for Pain, Inflammation, and Diseases of Chronic Inflammation

INTRODUCTION: HERBAL REMEDIES

Herb as a word has an ancient pedigree, originating with the Latin word *herba*, which refers to green crops and grasses and could also mean the same as meant by **herb** today *(Oxford English Dictionary)*. Herbs and plants comprise an integral and higher-order part of life on Earth. Herbs are any plants composed of little or no woody tissue and usually perish at the end of the growing season where and when cold temperatures interrupt plant growth. As their history as food and medicine demonstrates, herbs are potent and can be used for aromatic, culinary, and/or medicinal purposes. The natural affinities of herbs are primarily geographical and are based on plants grown in similar climates. As such, they form an important part of the natural herbal remedies available to different and distinctive ethnomedical traditions globally (see Section IV on Asian Medical Systems). Collections of indigenous herbal remedies in traditional ethnomedical use can be referred to as "pharmacopeia."

Pharmacopeial standards for verifying the composition, identity, purity, quality, and strength (potency) of a botanical substance are developed based on an intended analysis. In principle, the protocol of assigning quality and grade of herbs should be representative of the traditionally specified standards for the intended uses of medicinal herbs.

New and modernized pharmacopeial standards for medicinal plants originate from specific systems of traditional medicine (e.g., Traditional Chinese Medicine, Ayurvedic medicine [North India], Jamu medicine, Kampo medicine [Japan], Siddha medicine [South India], and Unani medicine [Middle East]). Standards developed outside of the botanical species' geographical and cultural contexts may or may not correspond to certain qualities defined in traditional medicine formularies and pharmacopoeias. For example, one of these qualities is associated with superior clinical efficacy in studies.

There are consequences of introducing botanical species to cultivation in eco-systems that are significantly different from their indigenous origins. These trans-planted plants (or literally, "trans-plants") may manifest measurable differences in chemical composition and strength and may even change how the plant physically appears and tastes. For example, the latitude (and altitude) of an herb's location de-termines the number of daylight hours and amount of sunshine to which the herb is exposed during the year. The number of daylight hours is one of the key compo-nents influencing the concentration and composition of bioactive substances and therefore the overall features of the herb. Furthermore, agricultural cultivation and collection practices and postharvest processes (even in the same climates) that dif-fer significantly from the traditional practices in geographical origin often result in measurable or observable differences when compared against geo-authentic spec-imens. This circumstance is especially true in the case of botanicals traditionally subjected to special processes or treatments specified in the formularies and phar-macopoeias used in systems of traditional medicine (Brinckman, 2013).

HERBAL AUTHENTICITY

Herbs qualified as **daodi** herbs have an important role in Traditional Chinese Medicine, for example, unique as one of the Chinese medicinal materials (CMM). In CMM, daodi means good quality, high yield, special processing techniques, and, most importantly, usually produced only in a specific geographic region. The sci-entific principles implied by the Chinese word daodi, or "geo-authenticity," should be taken into consideration because in Chinese medicine theory and practice, geo-authentic medicinal herbs are regarded as superior in quality and effects by com-parison to the same species introduced to cultivation in other regions (Zhao et al, 2012). Daodi herbs are grown in specific environments and have received notable attention in recent years due to the high correlation with the practice of Chinese medicine and its superior economic value throughout China and other countries. In contrast, with more than 500 most commonly used Chinese crude herbs, approx-imately 200 are recognized as daodi, or less than half. Yet these herbs account for more than 80% of total usage in Traditional Chinese Medicine. Nonetheless, plants are now being cultivated throughout North America, parts of Europe, and Africa as well (Huang, Guo, Ma, Gao, & Yuan, 2011).

The current national and international protocol for the specifying of geograph-ical indication is called "botanicals." A geographically indicated botanical is named after a geographical area, indicating that it is produced within a particular area, and its quality and characteristics depend on natural, historical, and cultural factors. Cultural factors may include how the plant is cultivated and harvested. Historical factors may include how the herb was harvested and prepared for specific medicinal purposes. There are also locally grown herbs (i.e., medicinal plants cultivated away from their native origins and closer to where they will be processed and used) in clinical practice and in formulation of herbal medicinal products, such as dietary supplements.

BOX 23.1 *Current United States Legislative and Regulatory Environment*

Under the US DSHEA of 1994 the US FDA presently has power to regulate herbal remedies and dietary supplements in the following ways:

1. Institute "GMPs," including practices addressing identity, potency, cleanliness, and stability (although the FDA did not finally promulgate GMPs until 13 years after passage of DSHEA; long after the science-based sector of industry had implemented and/or exceeded anticipated GMPs)
2. Refer for criminal action for the sale of toxic or unsanitary products
3. Obtain injunction against the sale of products making false claims
4. Seize products that pose an unreasonable risk of illness and injury
5. Sue any company making a claim that a product "cures" or "treats" disease (regardless of scientific investigations, evidence and peer-reviewed publications)
6. Stop sale of an entire class of products if they pose an imminent health hazard
7. Stop products from being marketed if the FDA does not receive sufficient safety data in advance (under "GRAS" provisions)

DSHEA, Dietary Supplement Health and Education Act; *FDA*, Food and Drug Administration; *GMPs*, good manufacturing practices; *GRAS*, generally recognized as safe.

The daodi verification process is often impossible to replicate in the United States. However, using United States Pharmacopeial (USP) Convention, verified dietary supplements could help to eliminate concerns about herbal supplements where integrity and quality have been growing in awareness for the consumer. These herbal supplements have been submitted to the USP Dietary Supplement Verification Program and have successfully met the program's stringent testing and extensive quality criteria. The more potent an herb, the higher the nutritional value, and less amount is needed to be consumed for effective and potent dosages.

CONTEMPORARY HERBALISM

Herbalism is the contemporary study and practice of using plant material for food, medicine, and health promotion. This field includes not only treatment of disease but also enhancement of quality of life, both physically and spiritually. A fundamental principle of herbalism is to promote preventive care and guided, simple treatment for the general population. An "herbalist" or "herbal practitioner", is someone who has undertaken specific study and supervised practical training to achieve competence in treating patients. Herbal medicines are recommended by physicians in the practice of integrative medicine and by other practitioners within the pharmacopeia of their traditions.

There is an eclectic practice of herbal medicine in Europe and North America that draws on herbs from many different ethnomedical healing traditions and has been called "Western herbalism". These practices have resulted in further modification and mandatory regulations during the past 3 decades (Box 23.1).

Herbs for Pain Relief

Herbs have been used for thousands of years and are documented as early as 3000 BC. Since ancient times, spices have been used to season food and yield medicinal compounds for response to sickness or disease. In the medieval era, pain relief came from a variety of different herbs, and it was an era focused on what nowadays would be called "polypharmacy," or the use of more than one type of herbal medication for an adult (usually more than four). This polypharmacy approach is still common in the contemporary practice of Chinese and Ayurvedic medicine, for example (see Section IV). Herbs for pain relief and inflammation most used during this time were rosemary, balm, basil, horehound, bay leaves, sage, and thyme. Yarrow and chamomile were used to treat headaches. There are currently numerous studies on the effects of herbs on pain and inflammation. Specifically in the United States, Americans spend billions annually on herb and vitamin supplements to treat inflammation, pain, and other symptoms and conditions.

Inflammation: A Root Cause of Physical Pain

Inflammation is a normal part of the response to injury and the healing process. Physicians know the visible effects of inflammation and often refer to them as the four cardinal signs of pain, redness, heat, and swelling (Latin: *dolor, rubor, calor,* and *tumor*). People experience these symptoms usually after an injury, such as twisting an ankle or pulling a muscle. In these cases, the inflammatory process is the first step toward self-healing. Inflammation is a complex process involving various types of immune cell responses, clotting proteins, and signaling molecules, in a sequence over time to help to stabilize the immediate situation. However, prolonged, chronic inflammation becomes a crucial factor behind chronic diseases. *Chronic inflammation* is suspected as a leading cause of a wide array of health problems, including but not limited to chronic pain, obesity, peripheral neuropathy, diabetes, depression, heart disease, stroke, migraine headaches, thyroid conditions, dental problems, anxiety, chronic fatigue, fibromyalgia, irritable bowel, phantom pain, posttraumatic stress, ulcers, and even cancer.

Immune System in Action: Acute Inflammation After Injury

The white blood cells, known as leukocytes and macrophages, are versatile cells of the immune system that help to fight infection by over-riding invader cells toxic to the body or by engulfing or literally "swallowing" infected or dead cells. Most blood cells in the adult are produced in the bone marrow. Exercise has been shown to promote white cell survival and cell proliferation in bone marrow (De Lisio, Baker, & Parise, 2013). Lymphocytes, antibodies, neutrophils, monocytes and adult monocytes, called "macrophages", are all immune system cells recognized at sites following injury. High white blood cell counts in the circulating blood indicate the presence of infection, stress, inflammation, trauma, allergy, or specific chronic diseases.

TESTING FOR PRESENCE OF CHRONIC INFLAMMATION

The liver produces C-reactive protein (CRP) and the level of CRP helps to determine how much inflammation is present in the body. It is very important for doctors to check for the CRP test. The test is completed through a venipuncture procedure, and the levels of CRP are measured in the blood. If CRP numbers are too high, it indicates excessive, harmful inflammation somewhere in the body. Measurement of CRP in the blood does not determine the exact location of the inflammation.

DISEASES OF CHRONIC INFLAMMATION

Chronic inflammation contributes to the many leading causes of death in the United States. Causes of chronic inflammation include mitochondrial dysfunction, increased blood sugar levels, and other variables, such as significant oxidation that leads to cellular damage. As we have read so far, many of the herbs discussed have anti-inflammatory properties and can enhance the cellular energy factories—the mitochondria—and reduce oxidative stress in cells. Many common diseases nowadays are caused by, or thought related to, chronic inflammation. Some include heart disease, cancer, diabetes, stroke, Alzheimer's disease, kidney disease, and chronic lower respiratory disease. Herbal remedies active against inflammation also have activities that appear to directly benefit diseases associated with chronic inflammation.

More broadly, people feel *chronic pain* as a result of many chronic diseases, such as Parkinson's disease, Crohn's disease, multiple sclerosis, rheumatoid arthritis (RA), migraines, dental issues, and cancer. Much of the material covered under the individual specific herbs, and in the herbal activity tabular content presented, illustrate the common connections among disorders and plant-based remedies that can help to treat them.

TREATING PAIN, INFLAMMATION, AND DISEASES OF CHRONIC INFLAMMATION

Many safe, effective natural compounds help to reduce inflammation in the body and therefore help to alleviate pain. Indeed, many natural compounds appear to work like natural COX-2 inhibitors but without the dangers that drugs engender.

Human physiology is a product of nature, and plants are the predominant feature of the environment in which humans developed. Therefore to be effective, a drug would be expected to have properties that are naturally found in plants. However, the isolated, synthetic chemical nature of drugs typically makes them less safe (and sometimes even less effective) than natural plant ingredients.

For example, COX-2 inhibitor drugs hit the market during the late 1990s. They work by preventing the formation of certain prostaglandin hormones that cause pain. There was a rush to market these new drugs, but their side effects were so

> Some herbs work like natural COX-2 inhibitors but without the dangerous side effects. The following herbal remedies are listed with research regarding their effects on inflammation, pain, and related neurologic conditions, as well as diseases of chronic inflammation.

intense that one of them, Vioxx, was soon taken off the market in 2004 because of its toxic effects on the heart.

Aloe Vera

Research suggests that aloe vera may be helpful in treating *inflammation, pain,* diabetes, hyperlipidemia, topical burns, frostbite, pressure ulcers, herpes simplex lesions, and ulcerative colitis. It is also useful for upper gastrointestinal (GI) complaints, such as gastroesophageal reflux disease (GERD) and gastritis. Aloe latex (from the inside lining of the leaf) belongs to the anthraquinone family of laxatives, which cause increased mucus secretion and peristalsis in the mucus membranes, increased motility of the colon, increased propulsion, and reduced transit time through the colon. Aloe also seems to have antibacterial, antifungal, and antioxidant properties, along with inhibiting synthesis of thromboxane A2, decreasing levels of prostaglandin E2, and interleukin (IL)-8.

Black Cohosh: *Cimicifuga racemosa*

Black cohosh is a tall, flowering plant found in rich, shady woods in eastern areas of North America. It is part of the buttercup family and is also known as black snakeroot, bugbane, bugwort, and squawroot. Its rhizomes and roots (both underground parts of the plant) are used for medicinal purposes. Black cohosh contains glycosides (sugar compounds), isoferulic acids (substances with *anti-inflammatory* effects), and possibly phytoestrogens (plant-based estrogens), among several other active substances.

Black cohosh has been used safely and effectively in the treatment of *painful menopausal* symptoms, irritability, and mood swings (Geller & Studee, 2005; Ross, 2012). It has been commercially available in Germany since the mid-1950s, where it has been used to manage painful menopause symptoms. The principal active ingredient is the triterpene glycosides, and the postulated presence of isoflavones has not been proven. The mechanism for its estrogen-like effects is unknown because black cohosh does not bind to estrogen receptors, upregulate estrogen-dependent genes, or stimulate the growth of estrogen-dependent tumors in vitro. Black cohosh does not affect endometrial tissue or hormone levels, such as estradiol, luteinizing hormone (LH), follicle-stimulating hormone (FSH), or prolactin. It has been shown to decrease symptoms of menopause, such as hot flashes, night sweats, insomnia, nervousness, and irritability, versus an antidepressant drug, such as Prozac. Although symptoms of menopause improve, there are no estrogenic effects in women; thus, black cohosh should be used only for symptom control and not for hormone replacement. Black cohosh combined with St. John's wort has been shown to significantly reduce menopausal symptoms. Preliminary studies suggest that black cohosh may help to reduce inflammation associated *osteoarthritis* and *RA*.

Boswellia: *Boswellia sacra*

Boswellia, also known as *Boswellia sacra*, or frankincense, is a traditional Ayurvedic remedy with potent *anti-inflammatory* and *pain-relieving* effects. Boswellia trees grow in African and Arabian regions, including Yemen, Oman, Somalia, and

Ethiopia. A variety also comes from a gum tree that grows in South Asia. In Christian belief, it was one of the traditional gifts brought from the East by the Three Magi at Epiphany. These three wise men brought it for the birth of the Messiah 2000 years ago. And these wise men traveling for thousands of miles could be expected to know a little something about joint pain. Boswellic acids are reported to have significant *analgesic, anti-inflammatory*, and *complement-inhibitory* properties.

It is used for pain-erasing ailments, especially for *osteoarthritis*. Researchers recruited 30 patients with osteoarthritis of the knee (Kimmatkar, Thawani, Hingorani, & Khiyani, 2003). They randomly divided the subjects into two groups. One group took boswellia extract for 8 weeks. The other group took a placebo. Then there was a washout period in which both groups took nothing. After that, the groups crossed over and received the opposite treatment for the next 8 weeks. One hundred percent of the patients reported decreases in knee pain when taking the boswellia extract. They also increased their knee flexibility and walking distance when taking the extract. The frequency of swelling in the knee joint also decreased. Any natural remedy for joints should include an effective dose of boswellia, 400 to 500 mg/day.

In another study conducted in 2013 researchers compared a combination of the herbs turmeric and boswellia to the nonsteroidal, anti-inflammatory, COX-2 inhibitor drug Celebrex (celecoxib). For the study, researchers divided 30 patients with knee osteoarthritis into two groups. One group received 500 mg daily of a combined turmeric and boswellia supplement. The other group received 100 mg of Celebrex twice daily. After 12 weeks the researchers found that the turmeric and boswellia combination reduced pain significantly better than Celebrex. The men and women who took the herbs experienced dramatic improvements in pain and joint tenderness. Both groups increased their range of motion and increased the distance they could walk. Overall, the researchers concluded that the herbal combination is as effective as the drug in treating osteoarthritis with fewer adverse effects (Kizhakkedath, 2013).

In 2003 a double-blind, placebo-controlled study of men and women with *knee pain* demonstrated that 333 mg of boswellia taken 3 times per day promoted a healthy inflammatory response. After only 8 weeks every study subject reported they could climb up and down stairs with ease, walk further, and walk at a steady gait—which in turn have been strongly associated with longevity in other studies.

Capsaicin: *Capsicum annum*

Capsaicin (or *Capsicum annum*, also known by many as cayenne pepper) originally comes from the chili pepper of South America. Capsaicin has the ability to reduce the brain's perception of pain. Capsaicin is an effective, natural pain reliever most often applied topically over painful joints or by taking it internally. Topical creams are usually in 0.025% and 0.075% strengths.

As a topical treatment, capsaicin depletes or interferes with a chemical called "substance P". This chemical transmits pain impulses to the brain. This property makes capsaicin an ideal treatment option for *neuralgia* (i.e., *shingles*), *osteoarthritis, RA,* and *diabetic neuropathy* (Sayanlar, Guleyupoglu, Portenoy, & Ashina, 2012).

Eating chili pepper seeds may make patients want to stop eating them because of the immediate local reaction of heat and pain experienced. This property also protects the plants' innate ability to spread seeds and survive in regions such as North and South America by discouraging predators from consuming and destroying the seeds, allowing them to spread naturally instead by dispersal in wind, rain and soil. The word chili in the United States has been used to refer to culinary items prepared with them, such as the dish *chili con carne* (Spanish: chili peppers with meat). Chilies are native to South America (including, in fact, parts of Chile), where people have been cultivating and trading them for at least 6000 years. Chilies belong to the genus *Capsicum*, a member of the Solanaceae, or nightshade, family that also includes important foods: tomatoes, peppers, potatoes, and eggplant.

Perception of Pain

Applied externally, chili causes a sensation of burning on the skin. This process occurs when capsaicin activates in nerves in the skin. When the exposure to capsaicin is "marinated" for an extended period of time, the "pain" that is usually felt through nerve cells become exhausted. Naturally exposed to capsaicin for long enough, these pain nerve cells become refractory to further stimulation (exhausted), having depleted their internal chemical neurotransmitter stores. After this segment, the nerve cells are no longer able to respond to capsaicin in the same way, so pain is no longer felt, and these cells are no longer able to perceive pain. Therefore ongoing exposure to capsaicin acts as an *analgesic.*

In one study in 2014, a man who was injured in a bomb explosion experienced an 80% reduction in pain symptoms after using a capsaicin (8%, known as high concentration) patch (Zis, Apsokardos, Isaia, Sykioti, & Vadalouca, 2014). Topical treatment with 0.025% (low-concentration) capsaicin cream has long been found to relieve pain associated with *osteoarthritis*, with 80% of patients experiencing a reduction in pain after 2 weeks of 4-times-daily treatment (Deal et al., 1991).

Capsaicin also has antioxidant and *anti-inflammatory* properties, which are important in chronic diseases. It has been shown to activate cell receptors in the intestinal lining and initiate a reaction that lowers the risk of tumors. Research has shown that capsaicin suppresses the growth of human prostate cancer cells by inducing an antiproliferation effect while leaving normal cells intact (Díaz-Laviada, 2010).

Capsaicin was also shown to help to reduce or eliminate burning, stinging, itching, and redness of skin associated with moderate-to-severe *psoriasis* (Bernstein, Parish, Rapaport, Rosenbaum, & Roenigk, 1986). In a 2011 study capsaicin nasal spray significantly reduced *nasal allergy* symptoms from nonallergic rhinitis (Bernstein et al., 2011). The term nonallergic implies there is no apparent cause from the allergy symptoms; however, sinus pain, sinus pressure, hay fever, headache, and extreme nasal congestion result (Bernstein et al., 2011). Chronic rhinitis can result from inflammatory or noninflammatory symptoms of rhinitis. Inflammatory rhinitis includes seasonal or perennial allergic rhinitis (AR), entopic (localized intranasal specific immunoglobulin E) rhinitis, and nonallergic rhinitis eosinophilic syndrome.

In a 1991 study patients with RA and osteoarthritis rubbed capsaicin cream or a placebo cream on their knees 4 times a day for 4 weeks. After only 2 weeks, 80% of patients who used the capsaicin cream reported significant pain relief. The cream appeared to work slightly better for patients with RA compared with those with osteoarthritis.

One does not need a prescription for capsaicin, and there are affordable products containing capsaicin in local drugstores. For pain relief, usually apply capsaicin 3 or 4 times a day. Rub the cream or gel into the painful area until it is no longer visible on the skin. Patients given capsaicin may experience a mild burning sensation, so washing hands thoroughly after applications is beneficial, and it is important to avoid touching the eyes.

Cloves: *Syzygium aromaticum*

Cloves consist of the kernels of a dried flower taken from a highly aromatic evergreen tree that can grow up to 30 feet in height found in such areas as India, Indonesia, and Sri Lanka. Cloves are used in the forms of an herb or as an *essential oil* that is mostly made up of eugenol and beta-caryophyllene, which constitute approximately 78% and 13% of the oil, respectively. Cloves are observed to show *anti-inflammatory* effects, and its potency has been ranked among the most potent 24 common herbs (Dearlove, Greenspan, Hartle, Swanson, & Hargrove, 2008). Researchers at the University of Delhi, India, found that cloves reduce and relieve general pain and *neuropathic pain* and also increase memory retention (Cortés-Rojas, Fernandes de Souza, & Oliveira, 2014; Guénette, Ross, Marier, Beaudry, & Vachon, 2007; Halder, Mehta, Mediratta, & Sharma, 2012; Prashar, Locke, & Evans, 2006). Nowadays clove oils are used in *dental care* as an antiseptic and *analgesic*. Since the 13th century cloves have been repeatedly noted to be useful for *toothaches* and *joint pain*.

Cranberry: *Vaccinium macrocarpon*

Cranberry juice can be used for prevention of urinary tract infection (UTI) and inflammation and as a urinary deodorizer for people with incontinence. Studies have shown that cranberry juice appears to reduce urinary odors when given orally on a regular basis to patients with urinary incontinence. Daily consumption of 10 oz (300 mL) of cranberry juice seems to prevent recurrent UTIs in both young and elderly women; however, it is generally considered that there is not enough evidence to show that cranberry juice alone can treat UTIs. Cranberry juice does not seem to prevent UTIs related to neurogenic bladder in adults or children. Preliminary trials suggest cranberry may help people following urostomy and enterocystoplasty to keep their urine clear of mucus buildup and reduce the risk of UTIs.

Cranberries contain proanthocyanidins (also formerly known as condensed tannins), which appear to interfere with bacterial adherence to the urinary tract epithelial cells. Cranberry juice has shown antibacterial activity in culture medium against bacteria *Escherichia coli, Staphylococcus aureus, Klebsiella pneumoniae, Pseudomonas aeruginosa,* and *Proteus mirabilis.* Cranberry, as well as many other fruits and vegetables, contains significant amounts of salicylic acid, the active metabolite of aspirin, which has *anti-inflammatory,* antiplatelet, and antitumor effects. One liter of cranberry juice contains approximately 7 mg of salicylic acid. The average cardiovascular prophylactic dose of aspirin for heart disease is 81 mg or 325 mg for pain and inflammation.

Curcumin: *Curcuma longa*

Curcumin *(Curcuma longa)* is a bioactive ingredient in turmeric. Turmeric may very well be the embodiment of the ancient Greek medicinal concept of "panacea," or "all-heal." Turmeric has been found particularly effective in cancer, cardiovascular disease, diabetes, dementia, depression, and osteoarthritis, as well as *pain* and *inflammation*. It also promotes healthy brain and GI functions. The common dose is approximately 500 mg/day.

> Turmeric gets many of its health properties from curcumin, its antioxidant ingredient that is also responsible for the spice's yellow color. It is one of the three or four common components of traditional curry spice (together with coriander and cumin, and sometimes red chili pepper).

It is an ancient Ayurvedic remedy for pain and is a prime example of a natural and effective COX-2 inhibitor. Curcumin reduces pain and joint inflammation. Curcumin appears to work especially well for RA patients. In a recent study, patients who took curcumin significantly improved their pain. It reduces inflammation as effectively as the potent prescription drug phenylbutazone (Butazolidine). According to some natural medicine experts, using the right dose of curcumin provides the most effective pain relief treatment. More than 6000 studies have shown that turmeric and its active ingredient curcumin have the potential to help treat virtually any condition. Researchers have uncovered 175 different ways this spice affects the body, as well as more than 600 potential therapeutic applications. Some of these studies suggest it reduces pain even when drugs are ineffective. In one study, curcumin was found to be as potent an anti-inflammatory as aspirin, ibuprofen (Motrin), naproxen (Aleve), steroids, COX-2 inhibitors such as Celebrex, and the breast cancer drug tamoxifen (Takada, Bhardwaj, Potdar, & Aggarwal, 2004).

Researchers discovered that curcumin also improves the health of the cells that line blood vessels, reducing atherosclerosis, inflammation, and oxidative stress. The researchers concluded that curcumin does the same thing as claimed for the popular statin drug Lipitor but without all of the crippling drug side effects (Usharani, Mateen, Naidu, Raju, & Chandra, 2008). Like aspirin, curcumin also works as a blood thinner, which can help to prevent blood clots that could lead to heart attacks or stroke.

Among dozens of natural substances that can treat multidrug-resistant cancers (considered by many to be related to chronic inflammation), curcumin tops the list. It is as effective as the breast cancer drug tamoxifen. Other research shows it compares favorably with the chemotherapy drug oxaliplatin as well (Kim, Davis, Zhang, He, & Mathews, 2009). Studies also report that curcumin causes cancer cell death or sensitizes drug-resistant cancer cells to chemotherapy and radiation—theoretically reducing the doses of these toxic cancer treatments that would be required (Somasundaram et al., 2002).

With each passing year, we learn more and more about the role that this ancient spice turmeric (curcumin) can play in preventing and treating breast cancer. One study from southeast Asia shows that women who eat more turmeric have a lower risk of metastatic breast cancer.

According to a comprehensive report from 2013 in the *Journal of Breast Cancer,* we now know turmeric incites cancer cell death and inhibits tumor cell growth. It also inhibits the movement of breast cancer cells along known pathways in the body, perhaps related to its known potent anti-inflammatory activity (Liu & Chen, 2013).

In the study comparing curcumin to the cancer chemotherapy drug oxaliplatin, researchers also observed that the spice was at least 500 times as potent as the diabetes drug metformin in lowering blood sugar in the treatment of type 2 diabetes, of which a major complication is *peripheral neuropathy* and *diabetic nerve pain* (and for which there has been a proliferation of new drugs). Curcumin is thought to activate an enzyme that increases muscles' and other tissues' ability to extract glucose from the blood, and suppress glucose production in the liver. Both of these actions can reduce the risk of developing diabetes in the first place (Ng et al., 2006).

Curcumin is capable of crossing the blood-brain barrier and therefore may also have neuroprotective capabilities. Research shows that curcumin helps to protect brain and nervous tissues. It has also been shown to prevent the clumping of a specific protein in the brain—a process that has been considered to be one of the causes of Alzheimer's disease and age-related dementia (Ng et al., 2006). Animal research suggests another bioactive compound in turmeric called "aromatic-turmerone" can increase neural stem cell growth in the brain by as much as 80% at certain concentrations. It has the ability to inhibit microglia activation, a feature that may be useful in treating neurodegenerative disease. The findings suggest aromatic-turmerone may help in the recovery of brain function in neurodegenerative diseases such as Alzheimer's disease (Hucklenbroich et al., 2014). In addition, a recent study shows that curcumin can improve memory, boost attention span, and reduce mental fatigue in people older than age 60 (Cox, Pipingas, & Scholey, 2014). Animal research shows that curcumin has neurochemical effects on the brain that are similar to antidepressant drugs—but without all of the dangerous side effects (Sanmukhani, Anovadiya, & Tripathi, 2011). Chronic inflammation has also been implicated in some models of neurodegeneration and dementia.

Curcumin has also been found to show neuroprotective properties in animal models of Parkinson's disease and alleviated the effects of glutathione depletion that in turn causes oxidative stress (Jagatha, Mythri, Vali, & Bharath, 2008; Zbarsky et al., 2005). Curcumin crosses the blood-brain barrier and is able to penetrate the brain and provide significant antioxidant activities.

Osteoarthritis Remedy

Considering turmeric's potent anti-inflammatory effects, this herb has been shown to be highly effective for joint pain, as well as the chronic diseases in which chronic inflammation is considered to play a role. Research shows that a combination of turmeric and boswellia (frankincense) reduced knee osteoarthritis symptoms more effectively than the popular—and dangerous—drug celecoxib (Kizhakkedath, 2013).

Any nonsteroidal anti-inflammatory drug (NSAID), including osteoarthritis drugs, is associated with significantly increased risks of GI bleeding, kidney damage, and heart problems. No adverse effects were reported with a turmeric and boswellia combination.

Elderberry: *Sambucus nigra*

Elderberries have been used for years as a food to make wine, pastries, and lemonade. European herbalists have used this herb as a poultice to promote healing of soft-tissue injuries. Modern research has shown that elderberry juice has been effective in reducing the symptoms of influenza. Elderberry contains flavonoids, including quercetin, which have antioxidant, anti-inflammatory, and immunomodulating effects.

The typical adult dose for treating influenza is to take 15 mL (1 tablespoon) 4 times daily elderberry juice-containing syrup daily for 3 to 5 days. In children, a dose of 15 mL (1 tablespoon) twice daily for 3 days has been used. This treatment works best if taken within 48 hours of symptom onset. Elderberry juice is well tolerated when taken for 5 days.

Evening Primrose Oil: *Oenothera biennis*

Evening primrose oil (EPO) is produced from the seeds of the evening primrose plant. The oil contains gamma-linoleic acid (GLA), linoleic acid, and vitamin E. The GLA is thought to have many anti-inflammatory properties, such as reducing production of IL-1β and possible antiestrogenic effects. Theoretically EPO's anti-inflammatory properties are thought to be helpful in diseases such as RA, Sjodren, and other autoimmune disorders. It has also been used for premenstrual syndromem, atopic eczema, ADHD, and multiple sclerosis (MS), but current research supports only its use in the treatment of mastalgia and osteoporosis.

The standard dose is 3 to 4 g daily and is generally well tolerated. Theoretically it can increase risk of bleeding when taken along with other anticoagulant and antiplatelet drugs and also lower seizure threshold in patients taking phenothiazines. Care should be used when using with other medications that affect platelet aggregation, such as garlic, ginger, and turmeric.

Garlic: *Allium sativum*

Garlic's use has been described in the Bible and Talmud. In ancient China, garlic has been used in remedies since 2700 BC. It is currently used in many cultures in cuisine and as a medicine. Garlic has been claimed to have many health benefits, including anti-inflammatory properties, antioxidative and antiatherosclerotic effects, prevention of colon and stomach cancer, treatment of hypertension, and as a topical treatment for dermal fungal infections (Schäfer & Kaschula, 2014). It is also prescribed as an antibiotic, antimicrobial, and antiviral and is used for ear infections, *muscle pain, nerve pain, arthritis, and sciatica* (Dartmouth University, 2010). Garlic appears to influence and affect important cellular functions, creating a balanced immune system. Some of these cell types that are enhanced by garlic are macrophages, lymphocytes, natural killer (NK) cells, dendritic cells, and eosinophils (Arreola et al., 2015).

Garlic is a key nutrient that perpetuates the prevention of inflammation in the body (Lee et al., 2012). This effect may also occur due to garlic's ability to increase the effects NSAIDs that a patient may take to manage pain. As much as garlic may increase the effects of drugs such as aspirin—it may also decrease certain drugs effects—such as protease inhibitors, which are a set class of medications for HIV infection and hepatitis (Piscitelli, Burstein, Welden, Gallicano, & Falloon, 2002). In contrast, garlic oil may decrease how quickly garlic breaks down certain medications, thereby perhaps increasing their effects and side effects. The anticancer effects of garlic have been shown through prevention of colon, stomach, and prostate cancers and now in the brain. The presence of allyl sulfur in garlic can slow down the progress of cancerous cell growth. Organo-sulfur compound properties decrease brain cancer cells in glioblastoma, a deadly brain tumor (Das, Banik, & Ray, 2007).

The pharmacological effects of garlic are attributed to the sulfur compound allicin, ajoene, and other organosulfur constituents, such as *S*-allyl-L-cysteine. Fresh garlic typically contains 1% alliin, but aged garlic typically contains only 0.03% alliin. Garlic has been found to inhibit platelet aggregation, increase fibrinolysis, and reduce atherosclerosis. Garlic also has a mild antihypertensive and antioxidant effect. Although earlier studies prompted enthusiasm for treatment of hyperlipidemia, recent clinical trials have shown that garlic does not have a significant effect on lowering cholesterol and triglycerides. Garlic has antibacterial, antiviral, and antifungal activity in vivo, but currently it is not suggested to be substitute for antibiotics. The topical version of garlic has been proven to treat tinea cruris, tinea corporis, and tinea pedis as effectively as 1% terbinafine. Human population studies suggest a benefit in preventing esophageal, stomach, and colon cancer. Usual doses that have been studied are fresh garlic (1 to 2 cloves) per day and garlic extract (200 to 400 mg) 2 to 3 times per day. The topical garlic constituent ajoene can be found in concentrations of 0.4% cream, 0.6% gel, and 1.0% gel for the treatment of tinea. The most common adverse effects of taking garlic orally include breath and body odor, mouth and GI burning or irritation, heartburn, flatulence, nausea, vomiting, and diarrhea. Some of these effects can be mitigated by taking encapsulated forms of garlic.

Ginkgo: *Ginkgo biloba*

The ginkgo (GBE) tree is one of the oldest living plant species and is indigenous to Japan, Korea, and China but can now be found all over the world. The use of ginkgo has greatly increased since 1994, when Germany approved a standardized form of leaf extract (EGb 761) for the treatment of dementia. The standardized extract contains 22% to 27% flavonoid glycosides (including quercetin and kaempferol and their glycosides) and 5% to 7% terpene lactones (consisting of 2.8% to 3.4% ginkgolides A, B, and C and 2.6% to 3.3% bilobalide). GBE is used in cognitive therapy and enhances the effects of gamma aminobutyric acid (GABA) release in the brain (Johnston, 2003).

Research published over the past 30 years consistently shows that GBE enhances memory and cognitive function. Initially, researchers thought GBE worked because it increases blood flow to the brain. Newer studies suggest that it protects nerve cells from damage that may also be useful in certain kinds of pain, such as neuropathic pain.

A study of more than 300 patients with Alzheimer's disease or multi-infarct dementia found that patients who received EGb 761 (120 mg/day) from ginkgo scored higher on the Alzheimer's Disease Assessment Scale-Cognition subscale (ADAS-Cog). After 1 year of treatment, nearly one third of patients receiving ginkgo showed an improvement on the test compared with half that proportion of those receiving placebo. A 6-month study of 216 patients with Alzheimer's disease or multi-infarct dementia found that patients who were given 240 mg/day of a standardized ginkgo extract had significant improvements in memory, attention, psychopathology, and behavior.

In another study of 40 Alzheimer's disease patients, those given 240 mg/day of standardized ginkgo extract for 3 months showed significant improvements in memory, attention, and psychopathology after 1 month. Ginkgo may also have beneficial effects on memory impairment that is not related to Alzheimer's disease. In one double-blind study, 31 outpatients who were older than 50 years and had mild-to-moderate memory impairment were given 120 mg of ginkgo a day. Researchers noted a beneficial effect of the therapy after 12 and 14 weeks. A recent analysis attempted a summary of all published studies in which ginkgo was given for dementia. The patients were sufficiently characterized with a diagnosis of Alzheimer's disease by either the *Diagnostic and Statistical Manual of Mental Disorders* or DSM-III or National Institute of Neurological Disorders and Stroke-Alzheimer's Disease and Related Disorders Association criteria, or the article contained enough clinical detail for the reviewer to assign diagnosis. The trials excluded patients with depression or other neurologic disease and excluded use of other central nervous system (CNS)-active medications. They included studies that used standardized ginkgo extract at any dose, had at least one outcome measure that was an objective assessment of cognitive function, and contained sufficient statistical information for analysis. Although more than 50 articles were identified, the majority did not meet inclusion criteria because of a lack of clear diagnoses of dementia and Alzheimer's disease. Of the four studies that met all inclusion criteria, there were 212 subjects in each of the placebo and ginkgo treatment groups. The authors concluded that 3 to 6 months of treatment with 120 to 240 mg ginkgo has a small but significant effect on objective measures of cognition in patients with Alzheimer's disease.

In another study, German researchers followed more than 13,000 patients prescribed with ginkgo biloba extract. Approximately 7000 of them were taking a capsule that contained 120 mg of GBE. A little more than 6000 of them were taking a capsule that contained less than 120 mg of GBE. And just 430 of them were taking the "ideal" dose of 240 mg per capsule. Interestingly, 240-mg capsules of GBE only became available in 2008 in Germany, so most doctors are still not familiar with prescribing the larger, optimal dose. After 6 months, researchers found that just 23% of the 240-mg capsule groups were still taking their daily dose and 6% in the 120-mg group maintained their regimen. Practically no one in the group that took less than 120 mg maintained it. So, after the optimal 6 months, very few dementia patients remained under treatment. This study helps to explain why we rarely see success with GBE in the pharmaceutical world. Most patients simply do not take a strong enough dose for a long enough period of time, and when no results are achieved in a timely manner, people stop taking it.

Pain is frequently a component of chronic diseases like cancer. Researchers at Georgetown University Medical Center found anticancer properties after careful extraction from the leaves of the *Ginkgo biloba* tree. The researchers found that an extract from the leaves reduce the risk of aggressive cancer in animal experiments. Mice that were treated with ginkgo biloba extract had decreased expression of a cell receptor associated with invasive cancer.

Ginkgo extract slowed the growth of breast tumors by 80% for as long as the extract was used and also reduced the size of brain tumors. However, the brain tumors were inhibited for only 50 days, despite continuous treatment.

It has been well known for some time that ginkgo interacts with a peripheral-type benzodiazepine receptor (PBR) that carries cholesterol into the mitochondria, helping to regulate growth in some cells. Some highly invasive cancer cells overexpress PBR, which may help to explain why ginkgo is effective against some forms of cancer.

MITOCHONDRAIL EFFECTS

Mitochondria are responsible for most of the energy needed by the body and brain to sustain life and support growth. When there is improper regulation of sodium, potassium, and molecules like cholesterol, there is less energy generated within the cell. Cell injury and cell death may follow and when repeated throughout the body, immunity is compromised. Diseases of the mitochondria appear to cause the most damage to cells of the brain, heart, liver, skeletal muscles, kidney, and the endocrine and respiratory systems. According to the United Mitochondrial Disease Foundation, depending on which cells are affected, symptoms may include loss of motor control, muscle weakness and pain, GI disorders and difficulty swallowing, poor growth, cardiac disease, liver disease, diabetes, respiratory complications, seizures, visual and hearing problems, lactic acidosis, developmental delays, and susceptibility to infection. Many active herbs for pain and inflammation appear to influence the mitochondria as well.

Hearing and Tinnitus

Ten ear, nose, and throat specialists conducted a study involving more than 100 patients with tinnitus over a 3-month treatment period. Patients were comparable in regard to duration and intensity of symptoms and degree of impairment. A significantly greater percentage of the ginkgo-treated group experienced either resolution of symptoms or distinct improvement, regardless of the duration of symptoms, whether the tinnitus was bilateral or unilateral, and whether symptoms were constant or intermittent.

There are overall mixed results on the efficacy of ginkgo in patients with tinnitus. There is a possibility that ginkgo may have significant potential only in patients with recent-onset tinnitus.

In a therapeutic trial of acute deafness, EGb 761 (320 mg/day) and a standard drug (alpha-blocker, nicergoline) were each given for 1 month. The rationale for the study was that lack of blood flow might underlie acute deafness, regardless of the triggering event. From the 10th day until the end of the trial, improvement appeared to be greater in the ginkgo group, although both groups improved. The gain in the ginkgo group ranged between 6 and 15 dB greater than in the nicergoline drug group.

In another study, 80 patients with sudden hearing loss were used for a study (of no more than a 10-day duration). EGb 761 (175 mg intravenous infusion plus 160 mg oral per day) was compared with the standard drug used for this condition (a vasodilating, antiserotonergic drug, naftidrofuryl). After 1 week of observation, 40% of the patients in each group showed a complete remission of hearing loss, consistent with expected rates of spontaneous recovery. After 2 and 3 weeks of observation, there was no difference between groups in relative hearing gain, yet there was a borderline benefit of ginkgo ($p = 0.06$) over the drug naftidrofuryl. Although no side effects were attributed to ginkgo, some patients in the naftidrofuryl drug group developed blood pressure changes, headache, or sleep disturbances (Table 23.1).

Kava: *Piper methysticum*

Kava *(Piper methysticum)* is a psychoactive member of the pepper family; the root of the kava plant is used widely in Polynesia, Micronesia, and Melanesia as a ceremonial, tranquilizing beverage. Kava has long been traditionally used in Tonga, Hawaii, Fiji, Samoa, Vanuatu, and other exotic locations and parts of Polynesia as an effective antianxiety agent. It is commonly used medicinally for anxiety and insomnia in Europe and the United States and is approved and registered in Germany for the treatment of "states of nervous anxiety, tension, and agitation" in doses of 60 to 120 mg of kavalactones for up to a 3-month duration. Currently, new research shows kava's amazing abilities to help to prevent cancer. Kava appears to be a safe herbal remedy for short-term relief of stress and anxiety.

In one study patients with various anxiety and neurotic disorders as diagnosed per the International Classification of Diseases received 70 mg of kavalactones 3 times daily for 4 weeks. The kava group demonstrated a significant reduction in

TABLE 23.1 *Common Herbs for Pain and Inflammation*

Genus, Species Common English Name	Conditions and Results
Allium sativum Garlic	Hyperlipidemia. Results in improved levels of lipids (lipid lowering, antithrombotic, antihypertensive, immunomodulatory)
Boswellia serrata Frankincense	Arthritis. Some reports of beneficial effects (anti-inflammatory)
Capsicum annuum Chili pepper, paprika	Cluster headaches, neuropathy, and arthritis. Improvement reported in some studies External: Rubefacient, blocks pain neurotransmitter—substance P, depletes substances P, desensitizes the sensory neurons Internal: Reduces platelet aggregation and triglycerides, and improves blood flow
Curcuma longa Turmeric	Functional gall bladder problems (increase in secretin and bicarbonate output); hyperlipidemia. Some studies report improvement in cholesterol levels. (Fatty acid metabolism alteration and decrease in serum lipid peroxide levels) Osteoarthritis. Some studies report positive results. (anti-inflammatory)
Commiphora guggulu Guggulipid	Hyperlipidemia. Improved lipid levels noted (antagonist of farnesoid X receptors)
Withania somnifera Winter cherry	Arthritis. Some studies report improvement (anti-inflammatory)
Zingeber officinale Ginger	Antiemetic (carminative, local effect on stomach). Reduces nausea Osteoarthritis. Some studies report benefit. (Anti-inflammatory; inhibits cyclo-oxygenase pathways, prostaglandin PGE2) and leukotriene (LTB4) synthesis

anxiety. In a second study, 101 outpatients with anxiety disorders (agoraphobia, specific phobia, generalized anxiety disorder, or adjustment disorder with anxiety) as diagnosed per the third, revised *Diagnostic and Statistical Manual of Mental Disorders* (DSM-IIIR) were treated with a kava extract for 24 weeks. The results showed significant reductions in anxiety. Several other studies on kava extracts or the isolated compound DL-kawain have been published in the Germany. In one placebo-controlled trial, 58 patients with anxiety received 210 mg kava or placebo daily for 1 month (Kinzler, Kromer, & Lehmann, 1991). Compared with those receiving placebo, those receiving kava had significantly greater reductions in Hamilton Anxiety Scale (HAMA) scores, with improvements beginning within 1 week.

Approximately 10 years ago there was a false "scare" about possible liver toxicity of kava. Jorg Gruenwald et al. in Germany showed there was no specific evidence pointing to kava for liver toxicity. Gruenwald found that it was prescription drugs that were likely responsible for the cases of liver toxicity that were observed.

The new study showed the ability of an extract of kava to prevent cancer in 99% of lung tumors in laboratory animals studied. A cancer prevention rate of 99% is unprecedented among cancer prevention studies using "chemopreventive agents."

To qualify for interest and research funding in more costly human studies, National Cancer Institute experts get excited about a putative ability to reduce cancer by 4 times, 3 times, or even 2 times (like the typical range of many vitamins and minerals). However, here is a finding that reduces cancer by 100 times.

Lab animals were given a kava-derived dietary supplement on a daily basis. This supplement prevented formation of tumors in 99% of lab animals in lung tumorigenesis model. In these lab models multiple lung tumors are chemically induced, and they are, routinely used for predicting the ability to cause lung cancer in humans. Some mice given kava developed no tumors at all. The types of DNA changes and effects that are typically associated with heavy tobacco use were also significantly reduced.

This lab evidence of kava shows that people living in the South Pacific have dramatically lower rates of lung cancer. Rates of cancer in the South Pacific Islands of Fiji, Vanuatu, and Western Samao are dramatically lower than in countries with no kava consumption, despite comparable rates of tobacco use. In Fiji, the rate of lung cancer is only 5% to 10% of the US lung cancer rate. That is a reduction in lung cancer of 10 to 20 times, potentially just from using kava. That means that kava can reduce the risk of lung cancer as much or more than cigarette smoking is said to increase it.

The new study also showed no effects on liver toxicity. The University of Minnesota research team is pursuing development of kava-derived drugs that may aid in both the prevention and treatment of lung and other types of cancer. A new patent-pending kava supplement enriched with cancer-preventive extracts is also planned to be used in human clinical trials. New research from the University of Minnesota revealed kava's anticancerous preventative effects on cigarette smoke-induced lung cancer and was published in *Cancer Prevention Research* (University of Minnesota, 2014).

Red Wine: Resveratrol

Resveratrol is a prominent constituent of red wine and a potent antioxidant found in certain fruits, such as red grape skins, berries (e.g., raspberries), pomegranate, mulberries, vegetables, peanuts, and raw cacao. It also appears to block pain receptors. A study shows one way in which resveratrol acts by inhibiting sphingosine kinase and phospholipase D, two molecules known to trigger inflammation (Issuree, Pushparaj, Pervaiz, & Melendez, 2009).

Resveratrol is notable among antioxidants because it can cross the blood-brain barrier to help to protect the brain and nervous system. Resveratrol may also help cells from free radical damage, inhibiting the growth of cells that lead to cancer (especially prostate), lower blood pressure, and help to prevent Alzheimer's disease perhaps by helping to normalize inflammatory response. Resveratrol is a natural chemosensitizer—a substance that can help overcome resistance to chemotherapy drugs—and a radiation sensitizer, increasing the effectiveness of radiation therapy (Gupta, Kannappan, Reuter, Kim, & Aggarwal, 2011).

Researchers from the University of Arizona School of Medicine published a study on resveratrol in the medical journal *Molecular Pain* (Tillu et al., 2012). Resveratrol profoundly inhibits two important pathways involved in the sensitization of *peripheral pain* receptors.

In addition, resveratrol may one day help faster *recovery from surgery*. Patients used to be sent home after surgery with a prescription for a week's worth of opioid painkillers, but in light of the US government's "war" against prescription painkillers, some patients have become more reluctant to take an effective prescription painkiller following surgery, and doctors more afraid to prescribe them. This circumstance points up the increasing need for safe and effective natural alternatives to pain relief.

Researchers at the University of Arizona found that resveratrol injections effectively prevented *acute postsurgical pain*. In addition, it prevented the development of *chronic pain at the incision site*. In the United States, doctors perform more than 45 million surgeries annually, and up to 75% of patients experience some form of acute pain after surgery. Pain at the incision site usually causes the most trouble. Appropriate use of herbal remedies may help to solve the problems of postsurgical pain and the use and abuse of narcotic pain-relieving drugs.

Rooibos (Aspal): *Aspalathus linearis*

Rooibos, an indigenous plant that grows in South Africa, is used as an herb, tea, and powder. It has gained attention as an herb that reduces or relieves nervous tension, allergies, digestive problems, and enhances hydration (Bramati et al., 2002). It has trace minerals such as magnesium (essential for the nervous system), calcium and manganese (essential for strong teeth and bones), zinc (important for metabolism), and iron (which helps the blood and muscles to distribute oxygen). Rooibos also contains powerful anti-inflammatory agents, such as the flavonoid quercetin, and antioxidative abilities, as well as antioxidants and polyphenols (Baba et al., 2009; Fukasawa, Kanda, & Hara, 2009). Anti-inflammatory mechanisms, along with its antidiabetic and antiallergy activities, may help to reduce the effects of drinking fluoridated water and other chemicals in drinking water.

Rooibos is naturally free of caffeine, oxalic acid, and tannins. Water fortified with powdered rooibos helps cells to make their own water. This activity mediates hydration inside cells at the micro level and maintains hydration for the rest of the body because most of the water inside cells must be made solely by each cell. When cells are not hydrated, it can help stimulate inflammation signaling and promote diseases, such as atherosclerosis and cardiovascular disease (Dmitrieva & Burg, 2015).

In a cell, glucose (carbohydrate) combines with oxygen to create energy. The by-product of this process, called "cellular respiration", is carbon dioxide and water. The water formed by cellular respiration is the primary source of water inside the cells—also known as "cellular hydration". Cells cannot become hydrated just by drinking fluids and electrolytes. The cells must also produce their own water. However, drinking a beverage that contains powdered extract of South African red bush, or rooibos, is like throwing more wood into these cellular "hearths." Rooibos helps more sugar get into the cells, which creates more energy and consequently more water for cellular hydration. That observation also explains research showing rooibos lowers blood sugar and helps to reduce the risk of type 2 diabetes (Kawano et al., 2009). In addition, the cells' increased energy and hydration improves muscle performance (as it improves performance of all other cells and tissues). When a cell is burning more sugar and getting more energy, it sends signals not to store energy in the form of fat. In turn, it helps muscles to better use carbohydrates and lowers blood sugar. This effect influences the process of inhibiting cells from storing extra fat, which helps to keep weight down.

It is important to note the quality of teas are significantly reduced when fluoride is present in the stems and leafs and reduces nutrients, polyphenols, and amino acids (Lu, Guo, & Yang, 2004). As fluoride levels increase the quality of tea (green tea, oolong tea, black tea, and jasmine tea collected from six provinces), nutrients decrease, thereby indicating the role of research on fluoride as a quality indicator of herbal teas (see Chapter 20).

Thunder God Vine: *Tripterygium wilfordii*

Thunder god vine is a perennial vine native to China, Japan, and Korea and is incorporated as part of Chinese Medicine. It has been used in China for health purposes and to treat a spectrum of inflammatory diseases for centuries. It is used for conditions involving inflammation or overactivity of the immune system. It is used to relieve *menstrual pain* and *autoimmune diseases*, such as RA, multiple sclerosis, and lupus. Extracts are prepared from the skinned root of thunder god vine.

In 2009 researchers at the National Institutes of Health, the University of Texas, and nine rheumatology clinics around the country randomly assigned RA patients to take either 60 mg of thunder god vine root extract 3 times per day for 6 months or 1 g of a prescription RA medication 2 times a day for 6 months (Goldbach-Mansky et al., 2009). The patients each had six or more painful and swollen joints. All study participants were also allowed to take prednisone and NSAIDs. Patients in both groups experienced side effects, with stomach complaints and digestive symptoms being the most common. Approximately half of the participants dropped out of the study before it was completed. However, more dropped out of the prescription drug group than from the thunder god vine group. Of the patients who continued treatment for the full 6 months, 65% of the thunder god vine group saw improvements in *joint pain, joint function, and inflammation*. Only 36% of those who took the prescription drug experienced improvements.

Valerian: *Valeriana officinalis*

Valerian *(Valeriana officinalis)* is a popular European medicine used for its mild sedative and tranquilizing properties and help with insomnia. The ancient Greeks, Romans, and Chinese recorded valerian for healing purposes. Early herbalists and physicians, such as Hippocrates, noted the sedative and digestive properties of valerian, advocating its use as a muscle relaxant, diuretic, expectorant, and wound healer (Plushner, 2000). The drug's CNS activity is largely ascribed to the constituents of the volatile oils. The German Commission E recommends 2 to 3 g of the dried root one or more times a day for "restlessness and nervous disturbance of sleep." Valerian is a popular sleep remedy in patients with or without pain.

Valerian has stimulating effects in the brain that effect GABA, a relaxing neurotransmitter in the brain and a major neurotransmitter for fast inhibitory synaptic transmission (Olsen, 2002; Yuan et al., 2004). GABA exhibits anti-inflammatory functions related to antiapoptotic cellular effects and further influences beta cells, which are found in the pancreas and are responsible for maintaining blood sugar levels in the blood (Li et al., 2015). In as many as three preclinical studies the administration of GABA prevented type 1 diabetes and exhibited strong anti-inflammatory and immunosuppressive activities (Prud'homme, 2014). Because there is such a large amount and use of GABA throughout the body, it is considered to be involved in functions of the CNS, as well as in chronic diseases. In essence, valerian has the ability to enhance, prevent, or reduce the breakdown of GABA in the brain and highly influences proper release (Johnston, 2003). Normalization of GABA produces better brain waves associated with longer and deeper sleep (Johnston, 2003). In addition, when GABA levels are balanced, less anxiety, stress, and nervousness are a result. Research conducted in India shows that valerian is a cognitive enhancer and is an agent used for depressive symptoms and mood stabilization (Tabassum, Rasool, Malik, & Ahmad, 2011). Studies on rats show that valerian acts as a neuromodulator and balances metabolic adaptations to long-term pain stimulations (Ignatov & Andreev, 1992). Neuromodulators have a controlling influence on the excitability of a population of neurons.

One study of 128 subjects compared the effects of an herbal preparation containing *Valeriana officinalis* as one of a mixture of herbs, a valerian-only extract (400 mg), and placebo in subjects with varying sleep difficulties. Both valerian preparations produced a significant decrease in subjectively evaluated sleep latency scores and improved sleep quality. In another study, patients with sleep difficulties received two pills that they took on consecutive nights. Both pills contained hops and lemon balm, but one pill contained only 4 mg of valerian and the other contained a full 400-mg dose. Seventy-eight percent of the subjects preferred full-dose valerian, 15% preferred the low-dose valerian, and 7% had no preference.

A study published in 2001 found that people who suffer from stress and insomnia can find relief in the herbs valerian and kava. In that study, adults who had suffered from stress-induced insomnia for more than 15 years first received 120 mg daily of kava for 6 weeks. Then, after 2 weeks off treatment, they received 600 mg of valerian daily for another 6 weeks. Overall, the participants reported that both herbs significantly relieved their overall symptoms of stress and insomnia (Wheatley, 2001).

Winter Cherry: *Withania somnifera*

Winter cherry *(Withania somnifera)* is also known as "ashwagandha root" the name in Sanskrit for "mare sweat," which may relate to the aroma of the root of this plant. It is a small evergreen perennial herb that grows approximately 5 feet tall. Another common name for *Withania somnifera* (Latin botanical name) is "Indian ginseng". This plant is another Ayurvedic remedy with potent anti-inflammatory and pain-relieving effects. Ashwagandha is also a potent adaptogen, meaning it adapts in the body to support good health and helps the body to react to physical and mental stress.

Winter cherry is commonly used to treat *back pain* because it also helps to nourish muscle and bone tissues. It also has a relaxing effect on the CNS. The dose is 500 mg/day to relieve pain.

Kulkarni originally found ashwagandha helpful with both control of *pain* and *inflammation* in *osteoarthritis* study participants. Pain scores and disability scores in this study dropped significantly (Kulkarni, Patki, Jog, Gandage, & Patwardhan, 1991). In 2004 Indian researchers conducted a 32-week randomized, placebo-controlled clinical trial using a standardized form of winter cherry (Chopra, Lavin, Patwardhan, & Chitre, 2004). For the study, the researchers recruited patients with *chronic arthritic knee pain.* They gave half the patients a standardized form of winter cherry for 32 weeks. The other half received a placebo. None of the patients in either group were allowed to take NSAIDs or steroids for pain relief. After 32 weeks, the winter cherry group experienced "significantly superior" pain scores. They reported very mild side effects.

In 2012 Chopra demonstrated ashwagandha in an herbal combination with other Ayurvedic herbs called "Shunthi-Guduchi" for relief of pain using an activity questionnaire pain score. A reduction in urinary cartilage collagen breakdown products was also a consequence. Remarkably a drop in serum hyaluronic acid levels, IL-1β, IL-6, and tumor necrosis factor-alpha (TNF-α) (inflammatory markers) was noted as a result (Chopra et al., 2012).

Wolfberry: *Lycium barbarum*

Wolfberry (goji, goji berry, *Lycium barbarum*) is a sweet red berry that has been often used traditionally as an herb and food supplement in Chinese medicine. Wolfberry has definite anti-inflammatory, antioxidative, antiviral and antiaging properties (Cheng et al., 2014). Goji berries contain vitamin C, vitamin B2, vitamin A, iron, zinc, copper, selenium, and other antioxidants (notably polysaccharides), which are used in many neurological (brain) and immunity studies (Bucheli et al., 2011; Chang & So, 2008; Chiu et al., 2010). Goji berries are high in phytochemicals, which offer protection against cancer, dementia, and heart disease.

In a 2012 study, researchers found that inflammation was reduced in mice and expression of a gene encoding for glutathione peroxidase, which protects cells from oxidative damage (caused by free radicals), was greatly increased (Philippe et al., 2012). Wolfberry is shown to protect the liver from injuries due to exposure to toxic chemicals and other harmful substances and significantly reduce of toxicities in organs exposed to chemotherapy (Cheng et al., 2014). In addition, wolfberry expresses antitumor activities against various types of cancer cells and inhibits tumor growth (Cheng et al., 2014).

Wolfberry protects against neuronal injury and aids in memory and learning, specifically affecting the neurogenesis of the hippocampus and subventricular zones (Cheng et al., 2014). Wolfberry has neuroprotective elements specific to ganglion cells (send visual stimulation signals to the brain) in the brain, and further studies show its effects for enhancing synaptic plasticity in the brain (Chiu, Macmillan, & Chen, 2009; Nelson, Ramberg, Best, & Sinnott, 2012).

DISEASES OF CHRONIC INFLAMMATION

Chronic inflammation contributes to the many leading causes of death in the United States. Causes of chronic inflammation include mitochondrial dysfunction, increased blood sugar levels, and other variables, such as significant oxidation that leads to cellular damage. As we have read so far, many of the herbs discussed have anti-inflammatory processes and even enhance the cellular energy factories—the mitochondria—and reduce oxidative stress in cells. Many common diseases nowadays are caused by, or thought related to, chronic inflammation. Some of them include heart disease, cancer, diabetes, stroke, and Alzheimer's disease, kidney disease, and chronic lower respiratory disease. Herbal remedies active against inflammation also have activities that appear to directly benefit diseases associated with chronic inflammation.

More broadly, people feel chronic pain as a result of the many chronic diseases, such as Parkinson's disease, Crohn's disease, multiple sclerosis, RA, migraines, dental issues, and cancer. Much of the material covered under the individual specific herbs is presented as herbal activity tabular content and should illustrate the common connections among disorders and plant-based remedies that can help to treat them.

LATEST RESEARCH ON PRACTICAL PAIN SUPPLEMENTS AND SYNERGIES

Of course relative to other natural approaches discussed in this text, for busy people it can be highly efficient and effective to take a daily treatment orally, but one does not have to rely on drugs. Powerful and proven ancient remedies are available for pain and inflammation referred to as "the ABCs" for pain, especially for joint pains: ashwagandha, boswellia, and curcumin. Ashwagandha is found as winter cherry, as discussed previously. These three pain powerhouses continue to come under increasing scientific scrutiny not only for their benefits for pain and inflammation, but for a host of other health benefits for brain and body. One new study looked at use of a boswellia extract compared with standard medical treatment for management of knee osteoarthritis symptoms. Compared with standard medical treatment, the patients given boswellia had as good a reduction of pain, restoration of function, better overall emotional and social functions, and overall physical performance (Belcaro et al., 2015).

The effectiveness of curcumin has been established in a wide range of inflammatory conditions. A new laboratory study used a novel approach loading lipid (fat) nanoparticles into a curcumin supplement, which markedly improved pain and molecular measures of inflammation (Arora, Kuhad, Kaur, & Chopra, 2015). Another study on a curcumin extract in a large general population of patients with osteoarthritis showed improvements in pain, mobility, and quality of life within the first 6 weeks. More than half of the patients were able to discontinue drugs for pain and inflammation (Appelboom, Maes, & Albert, 2014).

Of course, many herbal remedies, including these "ABCs," are even more potent when all three ingredients are taken together in the same supplement. A new clinical trial study gave boswellia and curcumin together to patients following highly painful tendon repair, compared with standard drug treatment. Boswellia and curcumin alleviated short-term and mid-term pain better than drugs alone but not long-term pain—for which researchers advised increasing dosage over the first 4 weeks and extending treatment by 1 to 2 months (Merolla, Dellabiancia, Ingardia, Paladini, & Porcellini, 2015).

In addition to the use of specific broad-based herbal remedies, following a healthy diet will help the physical and spiritual body, mind, behavior, mood, and nervous system—all of which are critical for prevention, perception, and management of pain. In addition, there are many vitamins and minerals micronutrients, available as dietary supplements (see Chapters 20 and 21) as well as common foods (see Chapter 22) that help to manage pain and pain-related conditions. Plants hold natural answers to pain, inflammation, and diseases of chronic inflammation. They are effective against pain and inflammation as foods, and as sources of vitamins, minerals, phytonutrients, and herbal constituents, as well as essential oils, the latter of which is discussed in Chapter 24 (Table 23.2).

TABLE 23.2 *Herbal Activities for Pain, Inflammation, and Diseases of Chronic Inflammation*

Herb	Common Uses	Activity	Adverse Effects and Contraindications	Doses	Drug Interactions
Aloe vera—*Aloe vera*	Orally—constipation, ulcerative colitis, gastroesophageal reflux, gastritis, peptic ulcer disease. Topically—psoriasis, minor cuts and burns	Orally the anthraquinone has a powerful cathartic properties. Also has antibacterial, antifungal, and antioxidant properties	General pain, abdominal pain and cramps, reduces inflammation. Long-term use or abuse can cause diarrhea, weight loss, albuminuria, hematuria, and potassium depletion	Orally 100–200 mg aloe or 50 mg aloe extract daily. Topically 0.5% aloe extract cream applied to area TID	Caution in patients on digoxins prolonged use can lead to hypokalemia
Bilberry—*Vaccinium myrtillus*	Diabetic and hypertensive retinopathy	Flavonoid complex (anthocyanoside)		160 mg BID for retinopathy	—
Black cohosh—*Cimicifuga racemosa*	Menopausal symptoms (hot flashes) and mood disturbances	Estrogen-like effects without estrogenic activity	GI upset, rash, headache, dizziness. Avoid in patients with hepatitis, breast cancer	Remifemin 20 mg tablet BID	No well-known drug interactions
Cranberry—*Vaccinium macrocarpon*	UTI prevention, urinary deodorizer	Proanthocyanidins seem to interfere with bacterial adherence to urinary tract epithelial cells. Mild anti-inflammatory, antiplatelet, and antitumor effects	Excessive use (>1 L/d) over a prolonged period of time could lead to uric acid kidney stone formation	1 8-oz glass/d	Daily ingestion of 250 mL cranberry juice can increase serum and urine salicylate level
Echinacea—*Echinacea angustifolia*	Decrease symptoms of common cold, diminishes recurrence of vaginal yeast infections	Immune stimulant	Nausea, abdominal pain, diarrhea, and vomiting. Caution in patients with autoimmune disorders	A tablet of 300 mg of Echinacea dosed as 1-2 tablets TID	Theoretically can interfere with immunosuppressant meds

Herb	Indications	Properties/Effects	Adverse Effects	Dosage	Drug Interactions
Elderberry—*Sambucus nigra*	Influenza	Antioxidant, anti-inflammatory, and immunomodulating effects	—	Adult 15 mL QID for 3-5 days, child's dose is 15 mL (1 tbsp) TID	Can potentiate effects of antiplatelet/anticoagulant drugs
Evening primrose oil—*Oenothera biennis*	Mastalgia, osteoporosis, atopic dermatitis, neuropathy	GLA—anti-inflammatory properties, possible anti-estrogenic effects	Avoid in patients taking phenothiazines	3-4 g daily	—
Garlic—*Allium sativum*	Hypertension, atherosclerosis, prevention of stomach and colon cancer. Topical treatment of dermal fungal infections (tinea corporis, tinea cruris, and tinea pedis)	Pharmacological effects attributed to allicin, ajoene, and other organosulfur constituents such as S-allyl-L-cysteine	Orally: breathe and body odor, mouth and gastrointestinal burning or irritation, heartburn, nausea, flatulence, vomiting, and diarrhea. Topically: dermatitis, eczema, blisters, and scarring.	Fresh garlic (1-2 cloves/day), garlic extract (200-400 mg) 2-3 times/d, topical garlic constituent ajoene at 0.4% cream, 0.6% gel, and 1.0% gel for the treatment of tinea	May potentiate effects of antiplatelet/anticoagulant drugs. May decrease concentrations of INH and HIV meds
Ginger—*Zingiber officinale*	Morning sickness, motion sickness, nausea/vomiting, arthritis	Antiemetic, anti-inflammatory, anti-hypertensive, antiplatelet, antipyretic, and antitussive properties	Rare—abdominal discomfort, heartburn, diarrhea, and a pepper-like irritant effect in the mouth and throat	250 mg QID prn for morning sickness, 500-1000 mg 30 min before travel for motion sickness, 500-1000 mg 2-3 times a day for arthritis	Theoretically ginger can potentiate the effects of antiplatelet and anticoagulant drugs

(Continued)

TABLE 23.2 *Herbal Activities for Pain, Inflammation, and Diseases of Chronic Inflammation—cont'd*

Herb	Common Uses	Activity	Adverse Effects and Contraindications	Doses	Drug Interactions
Ginkgo— *Ginkgo biloba*	Age-related memory impairment, improving cognitive function, dementia, diabetic retinopathy, glaucoma, intermittent claudication, PMS, Raynaud's syndrome, vertigo, tinnitus, sexual dysfunction related to SSRIs	Anti-inflammatory, reduces pain, antioxidant, free radical scavenger, inhibits platelet aggregation, protects cell membranes, erythrocytes, neurons, and retinal tissue	Mild gastrointestinal upset, headache, dizziness, palpitations, constipation, and allergic skin reactions. Rare cases of spontaneous bleeding and seizures	120-240 mg divided TID	Can potentiate effects of antiplatelet/anticoagulant drugs
Ginseng— *Panax ginseng*	Adaptogen, improving cognition, nourishing stimulant, aphrodisiac, treatment of diabetes, treatment of erectile dysfunction and premature ejaculation	Ginsenosides or panaxosides	Generally well tolerated, most common side adverse effect is insomnia	200-500 mg daily. For erectile dysfunction, 900 mg TID	None known to exist, but there are several potential theoretical drug interactions
Grape seed— *Vitis vinifera*	Venous insufficiency, ocular stress, atherosclerosis, hypertension	Antioxidant, vasodilating, anti-lipoperoxidant, and antiplatelet effects	—	360-720 mg/d	Induces cytochrome P450 and may decrease plasma levels of common prescription drugs such as warfarin, clopidogrel, and propranolol

Herb	Indications	Properties/Mechanism	Side Effects	Dosage	Cautions/Interactions
Kava Kava—*Piper methysticum*	Anxiety, social anxiety disorder, cancer	Attributed to the kavalactones, which have anxiolytic, sedative, anticonvulsant, spasmolytic, anti-inflammatory, and analgesic properties	Concern about potential hepatotoxicity has caused it to be banned from several countries including Germany	100 mg TID (100 mg—standardized to contain 70% kavalactones)	Caution should to taken to avoid use with CNS depressants, such as benzodiazepines, alcohol, and barbiturates
Milk thistle—*Silybum marianum*	Type 2 diabetes, alcohol-induced liver damage and hepatitis B or C infection	Silymarin — antioxidant, free-radical scavenger, inhibitor of lipid peroxidation, TNF inhibitor, decreases insulin resistance	—	Silymarin 200 mg TID	Might inhibit cytochrome P450
Olive leaf—*Olea europaea*	Hyperlipidemia, hypertension, prevention of CAD, osteoarthritis, rheumatoid arthritis	Anti-inflammatory, antiplatelet, antioxidant effects	—	2-3 tbsp/d added to diet	—
Red clover—*Trifolium pretense*	Hot flashes, menopausal symptoms, hyperlipidemia	Contains isoflavones, acts as a alterative	Myalgia, headache, nausea, vaginal spotting	40-160 mg/d of standardized extract, 1-2 tsp dried flowers to make a cup of tea, or 2-4 mL of tincture TID	Theoretical interactions with birth control pills, estrogen replacement hormonal products, tamoxifen, blood thinners, and diabetes meds

(Continued)

TABLE 23.2 *Herbal Activities for Pain, Inflammation, and Diseases of Chronic Inflammation—cont'd*

Herb	Common Uses	Activity	Adverse Effects and Contraindications	Doses	Drug Interactions
Saw palmetto— *Serenoa repens*	BPH, alopecia	Antiandrogenic, antiproliferative, and anti-inflammatory	Dizziness, headache, nausea, vomiting, constipation. One case report of excessive bleeding during surgery - ? anti-platelet effect	160 mg BID or 320 mg once daily for BPH	Theoretically can potentiate effects of antiplatelet/anticoagulant drugs
Soy— *Glycine max*	Hyperlipidemia, menopausal symptoms, osteoporosis, cardiovascular disease	Contains phytoestrogens, known as isoflavones and lignans. Rich in calcium, iron, potassium, amino acids, vitamins, and fiber	May cause endometrial hyperplasia.	20-100 g/day of soy protein. 50-120 mg/day of concentrated soy isoflavones	Tofu and soy sauce contain tyramine—avoid with MAOIs. Can interfere with absorption of oral thyroid hormone replacement.
St. John's Wort— *Hypericum perforatum*	Depression, somatization disorder, menstrual symptoms	Inhibits reuptake of serotonin, dopamine, and norepinephrine	Insomnia, vivid dreams, restlessness, anxiety, agitation, irritability, and mild GI complaints	300 mg TID	Multiple drug interactions, probably due to it being a potent inducer of cytochrome P450. Can decrease levels of common important drugs (digoxin, OCPs, phenobarbital, phenytoin, and cyclosporine, etc). Can also potentiate serotonin effects when taken with other SSRIs, demerol, tramadol)

Valerian— *Valeriana officinalis*	Insomnia, anxiety	GABA agonist	—	400-900 mg taken up to 2 h before bedtime	Can theoretically potentiate effects of other CNS depressants such as benzodiazepines, alcohol, and opiates
Yohimbe— *Pausinystalia yohimbe*	Erectile dysfunction, sexual dysfunction	MAOI, calcium channel blocking, and peripheral serotonin receptor blocking effects	Excitation, tremor, insomnia, anxiety, hypertension, tachycardia, dizziness, gastric intolerance, salivation, sinusitis, irritability, headache, urinary frequency, fluid retention, rash, nausea, and vomiting. Avoid in patients with CAD, HTN, BPH, anxiety	15-30 mg daily	Can potentiate MAOIs, TCAs, phenothiazenes, and stimulant drugs. Also antagonizing effects with antihypertensive drugs

BID, Twice a day; *BPH*, benign prostatic hyperplasia; *CAD*, coronary artery disease; *CNS*, central nervous system; *GABA*, gamma aminobutyric acid; *GI*, gastrointestinal; *GLA*, gamma-linoleic acid; *HTN*, hypertension; *INH*, isonicotinic acid hydrazde; *MAOI*, monoamine oxidase inhibitor; *OCPs*, oral contraceptive pills; *PMS*, premenstrual syndrome; *prn*, as needed; *QID*, four times a day; *SSRIs*, selective serotonin reuptake inhibitor; *TCA*, tricyclic antidepressants; *TID*, three times a day; *TNF*, tumor necrosis factor; *UTI*, urinary tract infection; ?, unknown.

REFERENCES

Appelboom, T., Maes, N., & Albert, A. (2014). A new curcuma extract (flexofytol) in osteoarthritis: Results from a Belgian real-life experience. *The Open Rheumatology Journal, 8,* 77–81.

Arora, R., Kuhad, A., Kaur, I. P., & Chopra, K. (2015). Curcumin loaded solid lipid nanoparticles ameliorate adjuvant-induced arthritis in rats. *European Journal of Pain, 19*(7), 940–952.

Arreola, R., Quintero-Fabián, S., López-Roa, R. I., Flores-Gutiérrez, E. O., et al. (2015). Immunomodulation and anti-inflammatory effects of garlic compounds. *Journal of Immunology Research, 401630,* 1–13. http://doi.org/10.1155/2015/401630.

Baba, H., Ohtsuka, Y., Haruna, H., Lee, T., Nagata, S., Maeda, M., et al. (2009). Studies of anti-inflammatory effects of Rooibos tea in rats. *Pediatrics International, 51*(5), 700–704. http://www.ncbi.nlm.nih.gov/pubmed/19419525.

Belcaro, G., Dugall, M., Luzzi, R., Ledda, A., Pellegrini, L., Hu, S., et al. (2015). Management of osteoarthritis (OA) with the pharma-standard supplement FlexiQule (Boswellia): A 12 week registry. *Minerva Gastroenterologica e Dietologica.* [epub ahead of print].

Bernstein, J. A., Davis, B. P., Picard, J. K., Cooper, J. P., Zheng, S., & Levin, L. S. (2011). A randomized, double-blind, parallel trial comparing capsaicin nasal spray with placebo in subjects with a significant component of nonallergic rhinitis. *Annals of Allergy, Asthma, and Immunology, 107*(2), 171–178. http://www.annallergy.org/article/S1081-1206%2811%2900383-8/fulltext.

Bernstein, J. E., Parish, L. C., Rapaport, M., Rosenbaum, M. M., Roenigk, H. H., Jr. (1986). Effects of topically applied capsaicin on moderate and severe psoriasis vulgaris. *Journal of the American Academy of Dermatology, 15*(3), 504–507. http://www.ncbi.nlm.nih.gov/pubmed/3760276.

Bramati, L., Minoggio, M., Gardana, C., Simonetti, P., Mauri, P., & Pietta, P. (2002). Quantitative characterization of flavonoid compounds in Rooibos tea (Aspalathus linearis) by LC-UV/DAD. *Journal of Agricultural and Food Chemistry, 50*(20), 5513–5519. http://www.ncbi.nlm.nih.gov/pubmed/12236672/.

Brinckman, J. A. (2013). Emerging importance of geographical indications and designations of origin— Authenticating geo-authentic botanicals and implications for phytotherapy. *Phytotherapy Research, 27*(11), 1581–1587.

Bucheli, P., Gao, Q., Redgwell, R., Vidal, K., Wang, J., & Zhang, W. (2011). Biomolecular and clinical aspects of Chinese wolfberry. In I. F. F. Benzie & S. Wachtel-Galor (Eds.), *Herbal medicine: Biomolecular and clinical aspects* (2nd ed.). Boca Raton, FL: CRC Press/Taylor & Francis. http://www.ncbi.nlm.nih.gov/books/NBK92756/.

Chang, R. C. & So, K. F. (2008). Use of anti-aging herbal medicine, *Lycium barbarum*, against aging-associated diseases. What do we know so far? *Cellular and Molecular Neurobiology, 28*(5), 643–652. http://www.ncbi.nlm.nih.gov/pubmed/17710531.

Cheng, J., Zhou, Z. W., Sheng, H. P., He, L. J., Fan, X. W., He, Z. X., et al. (2014). An evidence-based update on the pharmacological activities and possible molecular targets of *Lycium barbarum* polysaccharides. *Drug Design, Development and Therapy, 9,* 33–78. http://www.ncbi.nlm.nih.gov/pmc/articles/PMC4277126/.

Chiu, Y. H., Macmillan, J. B., & Chen, Z. J. (2009). RNA polymerase III detects cytosolic DNA and induces type I interferons through the RIG-I pathway. *Cell, 138*(3), 576–591.

Chiu, K., Zhou, Y., Yeung, S. C., Lok, C. K., Chan, O. O., Chang, R. C., et al. (2010). Up-regulation of crystallins is involved in the neuroprotective effect of wolfberry on survival of retinal ganglion cells in rat ocular hypertension model. *Journal of Cellular Biochemistry, 110*(2), 311–320. http://www.ncbi.nlm.nih.gov/pubmed/20336662.

Chopra, A., Lavin, P., Patwardhan, B., & Chitre, D. (2004). A 32-week randomized, placebo-controlled clinical evaluation of RA-11, an Ayurvedic drug, on osteoarthritis of the knees. *Journal of Clinical Rheumatology, 10*(5), 236–245. http://www.ncbi.nlm.nih.gov/pubmed/17043520.

Chopra, A., Saluja, M., Tillu, G., Venugopalan, A., Narsimulu, G., Sarmukaddam, S., et al. (2012). Evaluating higher doses of Shunthi–Guduchi formulations for safety in treatment of osteoarthritis knees: A Government of India NMITLI arthritis project. *Journal of Ayurveda and Integrative Medicine, 3*(1), 38–44. http://www.ncbi.nlm.nih.gov/pmc/articles/PMC3326794/.

Cortés-Rojas, D. F., Fernandes de Souza, C. R., & Oliveira, W. P. (2014). Clove (*Syzygium aromaticum*): A precious spice. *Asian Pacific Journal of Tropical Biomedicine, 4*(2), 90–96. http://www.ncbi.nlm.nih.gov/pmc/articles/PMC3819475/#b42.

Cox, K. H., Pipingas, A., & Scholey, A. B. (2014). Investigation of the effects of solid lipid curcumin on cognition and mood in a healthy older population. *Journal of Psychopharmacology, 29*(5), 642–651. http://dx.doi.org/10.1177/0269881114552744.

Dartmouth University. (2010). *Garlic.* http://cancer.dartmouth.edu/pf/health_encyclopedia/d04411a1.

Das, A., Banik, N. L., & Ray, S. K. (2007). Garlic compounds generate reactive oxygen species leading to activation of stress kinases and cysteine proteases for apoptosis in human glioblastoma T98G and U87MG cells. *Cancer, 110,* 1083–1095. http://dx.doi.org/10.1002/cncr.22888.

De Lisio, M., Baker, J. M., & Parise, G. (2013). Exercise promotes bone marrow cell survival and recipient reconstitution post-bone marrow transplantation, which is associated with increased survival. *Experimental Hematology, 41*(2), 143–154. http://www.ncbi.nlm.nih.gov/pubmed/23063724.

Deal, C. L., Schnitzer, T. J., Lipstein, E., et al. (1991). Treatment of arthritis with topical capsaicin: A double-blind trial. *Clinical Therapeutics, 13*(3), 383–395. http://www.ncbi.nlm.nih.gov/pubmed/1954640.

Dearlove, R. P., Greenspan, P., Hartle, D. K., Swanson, R. B., & Hargrove, J. L. (2008). Inhibition of protein glycation by extracts of culinary herbs and spices. *Journal of Medicinal Food, 11*(2), 275–281. http://www.ncbi.nlm.nih.gov/pubmed/18598169?ordinalpos=2&itool=EntrezSystem2.PEntrez.Pubmed.Pubmed_ResultsPanel.Pubmed_RVDocSum.

Díaz-Laviada, I. (2010). Effect of capsaicin on prostate cancer cells. *Future Oncology, 6*(10), 1545–1550. http://www.ncbi.nlm.nih.gov/pubmed/21062154.

Dmitrieva, N. I. & Burg, M. B. (2015). Elevated sodium and dehydration stimulate inflammatory signaling in endothelial cells and promote atherosclerosis. *PLoS One, 10*(6), e0128870. http://www.ncbi.nlm.nih.gov/pubmed/26042828.

Fukasawa, R., Kanda, A., & Hara, S. (2009). Anti-oxidative effects of rooibos tea extract on autoxidation and thermal oxidation of lipids. *Journal of Oleo Science, 58*(6), 275–283. http://www.ncbi.nlm.nih.gov/pubmed/19430189.

Geller, S. E. & Studee, L. (2005). Botanical and dietary supplements for menopausal symptoms: What works, what doesn't. *Journal of Womens Health (Larchmt), 14*(7), 634–649. http://www.ncbi.nlm.nih.gov/pmc/articles/PMC1764641/.

Goldbach-Mansky, R., Wilson, M., Fleischmann, R., Olsen, N., Silverfield, J., Kempf, P., et al. (2009). Comparison of *Tripterygium wilfordii* Hook F versus sulfasalazine in the treatment of rheumatoid arthritis: A randomized trial. *Annals of Internal Medicine, 151*(4), 229–240. http://www.ncbi.nlm.nih.gov/pubmed/19687490.

Guénette, S. A., Ross, A., Marier, J. F., Beaudry, F., & Vachon, P. (2007). Pharmacokinetics of eugenol and its effects on thermal hypersensitivity in rats. *European Journal of Pharmacology, 562*(1–2), 60–67.

Gupta, S. C., Kannappan, R., Reuter, S., Kim, J. H., & Aggarwal, B. B. (2011). Chemosensitization of tumors by resveratrol. *Annals of the New York Academy of Sciences, 1215,* 150–160. http://onlinelibrary.wiley.com/doi/10.1111/j.1749-6632.2010.05852.x/full.

Halder, S., Mehta, A. K., Mediratta, P. K., & Sharma, K. K. (2012). Acute effect of essential oil of Eugenia caryophyllata on cognition and pain in mice. *Naunyn-Schmiedeberg's Archives of Pharmacology, 385*(6), 587–593. http://www.ncbi.nlm.nih.gov/pubmed/22453493.

Huang, L., Guo, L., Ma, C., Gao, W., & Yuan, Q. (2011). Top-geoherbs of traditional Chinese medicine: Common traits, quality characteristics and formation. *Frontiers of Medicine, 5*(2), 185–194. http://www.ncbi.nlm.nih.gov/pubmed/21695624.

Hucklenbroich, J., Klein, R., Neumaier, B., et al. (2014). Aromatic-turmerone induces neural stem cell proliferation in vitro and in vivo. *Stem Cell Research Therapy, 5*(4), 100.

Ignatov, IuD. & Andreev, B. V. (1992). Role of the GABA system in adaptation to long-term pain stimulation. *Patologicheskaia Fiziologiia i Eksperimental'naia Terapiia,* (4), 66–70. http://www.ncbi.nlm.nih.gov/pubmed/1303507.

Issuree, P. D. A., Pushparaj, P. N., Pervaiz, S., & Melendez, A. J. (2009). Resveratrol attenuates C5a-induced inflammatory responses in vitro and in vivo by inhibiting phospholipase D and sphingosine kinase activities. *The FASEB Journal, 23*(8), 2412–2424. http://www.fasebj.org/content/23/8/2412.abstract.

Jagatha, B., Mythri, R. B., Vali, S., & Bharath, M. M. (2008). Curcumin treatment alleviates the effects of glutathione depletion in vitro and in vivo: Therapeutic implications for Parkinson's disease explained via in silico studies. *Free Radical Biology and Medicine, 44*(5), 907–917. http://www.ncbi.nlm.nih.gov/pubmed/18166164.

Johnston, G. A. R. (2003). Dietary chemicals and brain function. *Journal and Proceedings of the Royal Society of New South Wales, 35,* 57–71. http://sydney.edu.au/medicine/pharmacology/adrien-albert/images/pdfs/RefsPDFs/355.pdf.

Kawano, A., Nakamura, H., Hata, S., Minakawa, M., Miura, Y., & Yagasaki, K. (2009). Hypoglycemic effect of aspalathin, a rooibos tea component from Aspalathus linearis, in type 2 diabetic model db/db mice. *Phytomedicine, 16*(5), 437–443. http://www.ncbi.nlm.nih.gov/pubmed/19188054.

Kim, T., Davis, J., Zhang, A. J., He, X., & Mathews, S. T. (2009). Curcumin activates AMPK and suppresses gluconeogenic gene expression in hepatoma cells. *Biochemical and Biophysical Research Communications, 388*(2), 377–382.

Kimmatkar, N., Thawani, V., Hingorani, L., & Khiyani, R. (2003). Efficacy and tolerability of Boswellia serrata extract in treatment of osteoarthritis of knee–a randomized double blind placebo controlled trial. *Phytomedicine, 10*(1), 3–7. http://www.ncbi.nlm.nih.gov/pubmed/12622457.

Kinzler, E., Kromer, J., & Lehmann, E. (1991). Wirksamkeit eines Kava- Spezial-Extraktes bei Patienten mit Angst-, Spannungs-und Er- regungszustanden nicht-psychotischer Genese. *Arzneimittel-Forschung/Drug Research, 41,* 584–588.

Kizhakkedath, R. (2013). Clinical evaluation of a formulation containing *Curcuma longa* and *Boswellia serrata* extracts in the management of knee osteoarthritis. *Molecular Medicine Reports, 8*(5), 1542–1548. http://dx.doi.org/10.3892/mmr.2013.1661.

Kulkarni, R. R., Patki, P. S., Jog, V. P., Gandage, S. G., & Patwardhan, B. (1991). Treatment of osteoarthritis with a herbomineral formulation: A double-blind, placebo-controlled, cross-over study. *Journal of Ethnopharmacology, 33*(1–2), 91–95. http://www.ncbi.nlm.nih.gov/pubmed/1943180.

Lee, D. Y., Li, H., Lim, H. J., Lee, H. J., Jeon, R., & Ryu, J. H. (2012). Anti-inflammatory activity of sulfur-containing compounds from garlic. *Journal of Medicinal Food, 15*(11), 992–999. http://www.ncbi.nlm.nih.gov/pubmed/23057778.

Li, J., Zhang, Z., Liu, X., Wang, Y., et al. (2015). Study of GABA in healthy volunteers: Pharmacokinetics and pharmacodynamics. *Frontiers in Pharmacology, 6,* 260.

Liu, D., & Chen, Z. (2013). The effect of curcumin on breast cancer cells. *Journal Breast Cancer, 16*(2), 133–137.

Lu, Y., Guo, W. F., & Yang, X. Q. (2004). Fluoride content in tea and its relationship with tea quality. *Journal of Agricultural and Food Chemistry, 52*(14), 4472–4476. http://www.ncbi.nlm.nih.gov/pubmed/15237954.

Merolla, G., Dellabiancia, F., Ingardia, A., Paladini, P., & Porcellini, G. (2015). Co-analgesic therapy for arthroscopic supraspinatus tendon repair pain using a dietary supplement containing Boswellia serrate and Curcuma longa: A prospective randomized placebo-controlled study. *Musculoskeletal Surgery, 99*(Suppl. 1), S43–S52.

Nelson, E. D., Ramberg, J. E., Best, T., & Sinnott, R. A. (2012). Neurologic effects of exogenous saccharides: A review of controlled human, animal, and in vitro studies. *Nutritional Neuroscience, 15*(4), 149–162. http://www.ncbi.nlm.nih.gov/pmc/articles/PMC3389826/.

Ng, T. P., Chiam, P. C., Lee, T., Chua, H. C., Lim, L., & Kua, E. H. (2006). Curry consumption and cognitive function in the elderly. *American Journal of Epidemiology, 164*(9), 898–906. http://www.ncbi.nlm.nih.gov/pubmed/16870699.

Olsen, R. W. (2002). GABA. In K. L. Davis, D. Charney, & J. T. Coyle (Eds.), *Neuropsychopharmacology: The fifth generation of progress* (pp. 159–168). Philadelphia: Lippincott Williams & Wilkins.

Philippe, D., Brahmbhatt, V., Foata, F., Saudan, Y., Serrant, P., Blum, S., et al. (2012). Anti-inflammatory effects of Lacto-Wolfberry in a mouse model of experimental colitis. *World Journal of Gastroenterology, 18*(38), 5351–5359. http://www.ncbi.nlm.nih.gov/pmc/articles/PMC3471103/.

Piscitelli, S. C., Burstein, A. H., Welden, N., Gallicano, K. D., & Falloon, J. (2002). The effect of garlic supplements on the pharmacokinetics of saquinavir. *Clinical Infectious Diseases, 34*(2), 234–238.

Plushner, S. L. (2000). Valerian: Valeriana officinalis. *American Journal of Health-System Pharmacy, 57*(4), 328.

Prashar, A., Locke, I. C., & Evans, C. S. (2006). Cytotoxicity of clove *(Syzygium aromaticum)* oil and its major components to human skin cells. *Cell Proliferation, 39*(4), 241–248. http://www.ncbi.nlm.nih.gov/pubmed/16872360.

Prud'homme, G. J. (2014). 5th World Congress on diabetes and metabolism. *Journal of Diabetes and Metabolism, 5*(10), 122. http://www.omicsonline.org/2155-6156/2155-6156.S1.026-072.pdf.

Ross, S. M. (2012). Menopause: A standardized isopropanolic black cohosh extract (remifemin) is found to be safe and effective for menopausal symptoms. *Holistic Nursing Practice, 26*(1), 58–61. http://www.ncbi.nlm.nih.gov/pubmed/22157510.

Sanmukhani, J., Anovadiya, A., & Tripathi, C. B. (2011). Evaluation of antidepressant like activity of curcumin and its combination with fluoxetine and imipramine: An acute and chronic study. *Acta Poloniae Pharmaceutica, 68*(5), 769–775.

Sayanlar, J., Guleyupoglu, N., Portenoy, R., & Ashina, S. (2012). Trigeminal postherpetic neuralgia responsive to treatment with capsaicin 8% topical patch: A case report. *Journal of Headache and Pain, 13*(7), 587–589. http://www.ncbi.nlm.nih.gov/pubmed/22717586.

Schäfer, G. & Kaschula, C. H. (2014). The immunomodulation and anti-inflammatory effects of garlic organosulfur compounds in cancer chemoprevention. *Anti-Cancer Agents in Medicinal Chemistry, 14*(2), 233–240. http://www.ncbi.nlm.nih.gov/pubmed/24237225.

Somasundaram, S., Edmund, N. A., Moore, D. T., et al. (2002). Dietary curcumin inhibits chemotherapy-induced apoptosis in models of human breast cancer. *Cancer Research, 62*(13), 3868–3875.

Tabassum, N., Rasool, S., Malik, Z. A., & Ahmad, F. (2011). Natural cognitive enhancers. *Journal of Pharmacy Research, 5*(1), 153–160. http://www.researchgate.net/publication/221676516_Natural_Cognitive_Enhancers.

Takada, Y., Bhardwaj, A., Potdar, P., & Aggarwal, B. B. (2004). Nonsteroidal anti-inflammatory agents differ in their ability to suppress NF-kappaB activation, inhibition of expression of cyclooxygenase-2 and cyclin D1, and abrogation of tumor cell proliferation. *Oncogene, 23*(57), 9247–9258.

Tillu, D. V., Melemedjian, O. K., Asiedu, M. N., Qu, N., De Felice, M., Dussor, G., et al. (2012). Resveratrol engages AMPK to attenuate ERK and mTOR signaling in sensory neurons and inhibits incision-induced acute and chronic pain. *Molecular Pain, 8*, 5. http://www.ncbi.nlm.nih.gov/pubmed/22269797.

University of Minnesota. (2014). *University of Minnesota research finds kava plant may prevent cigarette smoke-induced lung cancer.* http://www.health.umn.edu/news-releases/university-minnesota-research-finds-kava-plant-may-prevent-cigarette-smoke-induced.

Usharani, P., Mateen, A. A., Naidu, M. U., Raju, Y. S., & Chandra, N. (2008). Effect of NCB-02, atorvastatin and placebo on endothelial function, oxidative stress and inflammatory markers in patients with type 2 diabetes mellitus: A randomized, parallel-group, placebo-controlled, 8-week study. *Drugs in R&D, 9*(4), 243–250.

Wheatley, D. (2001). Kava and valerian in the treatment of stress-induced insomnia. *Phytotherapy Research, 15*(6), 549–551.

Yuan, C. S., Mehendale, S., Xiao, Y., Aung, H. H., Xie, J. T., & Ang-Lee, M. K. (2004). The gamma-aminobutyric acidergic effects of valerian and valerenic acid on rat brainstem neuronal activity. *Anesthesia & Analgesia, 98*(2), 353–358. http://www.ncbi.nlm.nih.gov/pubmed/14742369.

Zbarsky, V., Datla, K. P., Parkar, S., Rai, D. K., Aruoma, O. I., & Dexter, D. T. (2005). Neuroprotective properties of the natural phenolic antioxidants curcumin and naringenin but not quercetin and fisetin in a 6-OHDA model of Parkinson's disease. *Free Radical Research, 39*(10), 1119–1125. http://www.ncbi.nlm.nih.gov/pubmed/16298737.

Zhao, Z., Guo, P., & Brand, E. (2012). The formation of daodi medicinal materials. *Journal of Ethnopharmacology, 140*, 476–481.

Zis, P., Apsokardos, A., Isaia, C., Sykioti, P., & Vadalouca, A. (2014). Posttraumatic and postsurgical neuropathic pain responsive to treatment with capsaicin 8% topical patch. *Pain Physician, 17*(2), E213–E218. http://www.ncbi.nlm.nih.gov/pubmed/24658488.

Suggested Readings can be found on the companion website, http://www.micozzipainconditions.com.

Chapter 24

Plant-Based Treatments
Part Two: Aromatherapy and Plant Essential Oils

Essential plant oils are involved in the living interactions among earth, soil, light, and air. Aromatherapy may be defined as the selected use of essential oils and related products of plant origin with the general goal of improving health and wellness and relieving stress, infections, inflammation, and pain. Aromatherapy has a twofold method of delivery, systemically through the blood (physiological) and olfactory through the nervous system route (psychological). It has built into its application an ideal multifaceted approach. The word *aromathérapie* was first used in a 1937 publication by the French perfumer and chemist René-Maurice Gattefossé (1881–1950), who with Jean Valnet (1920–95) and Marguerite Maury (1895–1968) are largely responsible for revival of interest in the use of essential oils for therapeutic purposes. Their efforts founded the modern science of aromatherapy.

René-Maurice Gattefossé was a French chemist and scholar who began describing aromatherapy as a particular branch of science and therapeutics in 1928. The term aromathérapie was coined by Gattefossé in 1928 (his book of the same name was published in 1937). This term became used to describe the use of aromatic oils for treating physical or emotional problems.

He first became interested in the study of essential oils after an accident in his laboratory when Gattefossé burnt his hand badly in a chemical explosion. He applied lavender essential oil that was close at hand. The burn healed with remarkable speed and without infection or scarring. Amazed at this result, Gattefossé began to investigate the properties of essential oils. He was first to analyze and record the individual chemical components in each oil, classifying the oils according to their therapeutic properties (e.g., analgesic, antitoxic, antiseptic, tonifying, stimulating, calming) (Franchomme & Pénoël, 1990).

Gattefossé carried out experiments in military hospitals during World War I (1914–18). WWI provided an opportunity for great advances in aromatherapies

Acknowledgments to Caroline Hoffman and Rhiannon Harris Lewis for prior contributions in Micozzi, M.S. (Ed.), (2016). *Fundamentals of commentary and alternative medicine* (5th ed.). St Louis: Elsevier Health Sciences/Saunders.

since it was used as a part of routine practice by medical professionals, including doctors, nurses, massage therapists, physiotherapists, and other health care providers. He achieved results using essential oils to prevent gangrene, cure burns, and obtain cicatrization far more quickly than usual. After the war his methods came under professional scrutiny and were largely left behind (Maury, 1964). Gattefossé has been considered by many to be the founder of the modern scientific use of essential oils.

During the mid-20th century, aromatherapy was brought to the United Kingdom from France by Madame Marguerite Maury, who was born in Austria. She was the first layperson to study and use the effects of essential oils absorbed through the skin. Her research was based on that of Gattefossé and her own work with her husband, a French homoeopathic doctor. She promoted the 20th-century use of massage with essential oils, aromatherapy massage, and began teaching aromatherapy to beauticians. This training has gradually filtered from the cosmetic into the therapeutic domain. It is increasingly being used by nurses, physiotherapists, and other health care professionals. The food and perfume industries currently remain the largest users of essential oils. Some reservations about the therapeutic potential of aromatherapy may be due to the connection with the cosmetic industry; however, by definition, aromatherapy links essential oils to treatment of specific ailments. Aromatherapy became widely utilized in the United States during the 1980s (Figures 24.1 and 24.2).

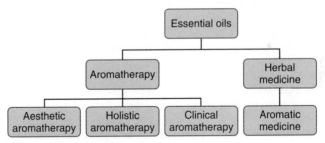

FIG 24.1 | Different styles of aromatherapy.

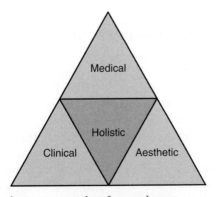

FIG 24.2 | Interdependence among styles of aromatherapy.

ETHNOMEDICAL AND HISTORICAL USES

Essential oils have been used for therapeutic purposes for nearly 6000 years. The ancient Chinese, Indians, Egyptians, Greeks, and Romans used them in rituals and as perfumes and drugs. They were used in spiritual, therapeutic, and hygienic practices to deliver relaxing, sedating, refreshing, and stimulating effects.

The ancient Greeks used aromatic essences both for potent medicines and for perfumes. Hippocrates wrote that having a daily bath filled with plant oils and a scented massage is the key to maintaining health and well-being. Aristotle argued that pleasant smells also contribute to well-being. The Romans are famous for the magnificent baths they built, inspired by the more simple baths constructed by the ancient Greeks. Touch and smell typically engender heart-brain emotional reactions. The Roman poet Lucretius described the "particles" of pleasant smells as being "smooth and round," whereas particles of unpleasant smells were "barbed and prickly."

Native American shamans were familiar with the use of herbs and aromatics. The Latin American *perfumeros,* or healers, bathed their patients in scents. By the skillful use of perfumes, they transformed what is today called the "auric field"—the energetic or emotional envelope that surrounds a person. The blowing of tobacco smoke over a person, combined with a perfume, also was seen as having curative powers. The use of fragrances facilitated transformations in religious, magical, and healing rituals. An ancient connection exists between fumigating and perfuming (Steele, 1992). Native American tribes, such as the Cheyenne in the midwest or central west of the United States, used a medicine wheel, sometimes called the "sacred hoop" with different uses of indigenous plants. The Navajo tribes in the Rocky Mountain regions of the Southwest used osha root, also known as "bear root." The legend states that they learned of the osha root from brown bears because bears consume it as a repellant against harmful parasites and infections, and also digest the root after hibernation periods. Isolation of bear root phthalides reveals a lactone, together with complex compounds of natural oils, proven to be anti-inflammatory. It also has antinociceptive or pain-reducing effects (Deciga-Campos, González-Trujano, Navarrete, & Mata, 2005; Del-Ángel, Nieto, Ramírez-Apan, & Delgado, 2015).

AROMATHERAPY AND BREATHING IN THE 21ST CENTURY

In modern-day aromatherapy the therapist uses these fragrant and active substances to affect the body-mind via a number of administration methods, such as external, inhalational, and internal. Every aromatic oil has its own individual constituents, and they in turn interact with the body's chemistry to have specific therapeutic effects. Always take caution before administration of essential oils by mouth or, in certain cases, externally without specific instruction from a trained and qualified specialist, such as massage therapists, clinicians, and certified aromatherapists. When essential oils are integrated into medical environments to address particular patient challenges alongside mainstream care, the practice is often termed clinical aromatherapy (Table 24.1).

TABLE 24.1 *Health Care Settings Where Aromatherapy Is Being Integrated*

Cancer Care	Critical Care	Drug Rehabilitation
Mindfulness	Meditation	Yoga
Elderly care	HIV/AIDS care	Midwifery
Neurology	Pediatrics	Palliative care
Postoperative care	Preprocedural care	Prison/young offenders units
Psychiatry	Pain clinics	Pneumology/ ENT
Rheumatology	Special needs	Sports rehabilitation
Wound care	Therapy for staff and carergivers	

ENT, Ear, nose and throat specialist.

People in pain often hold their breath for short periods of time without even realizing it. Breathing through the nose (to actually use the sensory receptors that pick up scent) is also the most important way for breathing optimally. Breathing patterns directly influence the heart-rhythm's patterns and virtually every part of the body. An irregular heartbeat can cause neck and shoulder pain, discomfort, numbness, and other symptoms. Nasal breathing gives the highest potential of aromatherapy's benefits in general. Breathing through the nose also helps to prevent sleep apnea and related disorders, such as snoring and sinus congestion. It also delivers a full amount of oxygen into the lungs for proper blood regulation. During respiration, the nose and other passages of the nasopharynx perform humidification, heat transfer, and filtration.

Nose breathing stimulates the nose's bitter receptors that react to chemicals that bacteria use to communicate. These receptors stimulate nitric oxide production that kills bacteria and triggers innate immunity responses (Lee et al., 2014). Genetic variability in receptors from person to person may help to explain why certain individuals are more susceptible to developing gram-negative bacterial infections and inflammation.

EXTRACTION OF OILS FROM PLANTS

Essential oils are concentrated extracts taken from the stems, roots, leaves, seeds, or blossoms of plants. These highly concentrated and fragrant substances of plant origin have complex chemical composition, the totality of which determines the essential oil's aroma and therapeutic potential. Essential oils carry biologically active volatile compounds in a highly concentrated form that can provide therapeutic benefits in minute amounts (Box 24.1).

In addition to the biologically active chemicals in plants (phytochemicals) that are important for health, the essential oils or volatile oils in plants also have important ecological effects. These volatile oils are normally released from the plant into the air and are responsible for the fragrance of the plant (see Chapter 23).

BOX 24.1 *Commonly Used Essential Oils in Clinical Environments (Latin Name and Common Name)*

Boswellia carterii, frankincense
Cananga odorata, ylang ylang
Chamaemelum nobile, Roman chamomile
Citrus aurantium var. *amara flos.,* neroli
Citrus aurantium var. *amara fol.,* petitgrain
Citrus bergamia, bergamot
Citrus paradisii, grapefruit
Citrus sinensis, sweet orange
Cupressus sempervirens, cypress
Cymbopogon martinii, palmarosa
Cymbopogon citratus, lemongrass
Eucalyptus radiata, eucalyptus
Lavandula angustifolia, lavender
Lavandula latifolia, spike lavender
Matricaria recutita, German chamomile
Melaleuca alternifolia, tea tree
Mentha citrata, bergamot mint
Mentha × piperita, peppermint
Origanum majorana, sweet marjoram
Pelargonium × asperum, geranium
Piper nigrum, black pepper
Rosa damascena, rose
Rosmarinus officinalis, rosemary
Sabinyl acetate, juniper
Santalum album, sandalwood
Zingiber officinale, ginger
Vetiveria zizanioides, vetiver

The concept of the "whole oil," as opposed to one that has been rectified, chemically concentrated by deterpenation, or otherwise chemically altered, is fundamental to most aromatherapists. They believe that there is inherent synergy among the chemical components that needs to be preserved as much as possible. This concept of synergy has some evidence in terms of antimicrobial and *anti-inflammatory* effects, as also seen with anti-microbial herbal remedies. A number of studies have demonstrated synergy among major active components and minor, less active components in an individual essential oil (Harris, 2002).

Aroma impacts the body-mind via the olfactory sense, with direct connections to parts of the brain, including the limbic system and higher brain connections. These connections influence emotions, memory, mood, desire, basic drive, libido, and hormonal responses. The olfactory neurons travel directly to the frontal portions of the brain. For these reasons, inhalation of essential oil fragrance is considered a key aspect of an aromatherapy treatment. A systematic review addressing the psychophysiological effects on mood, cognition, behavior, performance, physiology of fragrant substances (Herz, 2009) confirmed that they can significantly impact the body-mind via inhalation. Ongoing research at Brain Performance and Nutrition Research Centre at Northumbria University, United Kingdom, found that aromas influence mood, cognition, and behavior (Moss, Hewitt, Moss, & Wesnes, 2008; Moss, Rouse, Wesnes, & Moss, 2010).

Oils may be extracted from leaves (eucalyptus, peppermint), flowers (lavender, rose), blossoms (orange blossom or neroli), fruits (lemon, mandarin), grasses (lemongrass), wood (camphor, sandalwood), barks (cinnamon), gum (frankincense), bulbs (garlic, onion), roots (calamus), or dried flower buds (clove). Varying amounts of essential oil can be extracted from a particular plant; 220 pounds of rose petals will yield less than 2 ounces of the essential oil, whereas other plants, such as lavender, lemon, or eucalyptus, give much greater proportions. This variation helps to account for the differences in price among essential oils.

The process of distillation uses steam, which is considered the best way to obtain essential oils for use in aromatherapy. However, the steam distillation method produces varying oil qualities dependent upon the temperature, pressure, and time used for distillation. The lower temperature carbon dioxide (CO_2) extraction process was not available when aromatherapy was first becoming popular and documented. The CO_2 extraction process may produce superior oil that has not been altered by the high heat associated with steam distillation. Higher temperature and thermal energy involved in the steam extraction process changes the molecular composition of the plant matter and prevents further denaturing and decomposition. The use of heat in the distillation process changes the molecular composition of the essential oil. Application of heat is also important for uses in lung care, colds, congestion, or tension, in which steam inhalation of essential oils warms and moistens the membranes and opens and relaxes the airways.

VIBRATIONAL FREQUENCY INFLUENCES FROM PLANTS

Plants have crystalline structures that flow with natural bioenergy and have some of the highest vibrational frequencies of any measured natural substance. Essential oils and plant extracts are also thought to be able to impact the individual at a very subtle or vibrational level. Many therapists refer to essential oils as the "life force" of the plant and believe that their vibrational energetic qualities are able to influence the individual on a subtle level. Practices that include different forms of energy medicine, such as Traditional Chinese Medicine and Ayurvedic medicine, may also use essential oils (Holmes 2007, 2008; Miller & Miller, 1995; Mojay, 1996). During the Ayurvedic detoxification or purification process of pañchakarma, application of essential oils is central (see Chapter 18).

Everything around us vibrates—including all matter—as well as every atom in the universe. The vibrational frequency of the human mind-body is governed by states of vibrations whereby all atomic particles in the universe are in constant flux and therefore emit a frequency. This frequency is much like a resonating sound somewhat similar to what researchers have found with the sun, earth, and planets in our solar system (see Gehl & Micozzi, 2017).

Einstein wrote, "Everything in the universe vibrates," and nowadays researchers are demonstrating these subtle vibrational states in atoms. Atoms, which make up all matter, are connected and bonded to neighboring atoms through interatomic attractive forces, which can be visualized as springs. A defined finite temperature influences the fixed kinetic energy in atoms stored as vibrations. The vibrational frequencies are set by the mass of the atoms, the "stiffness" of the bonds, or "springs," that connect the atoms, and the temperature. In solids these atoms are relatively fixed and do not move freely, which differs from atoms in a physical state of liquid or gas, which move or vibrate more frequently than solids. Solids, liquids, and gases are physical states present in the human body—and the atoms vibrate under different conditions. From these and other observations it is reasonable to conclude that the human body has its own specific frequencies (Trigo et al., 2013). Frequencies can change based on emotional states, such as mood, as well as which foods (which have aroma) are consumed and how certain smells are sensed and perceived.

Every periodic motion has a frequency determined by the number of oscillations per second (motion that repeats itself regularly and can be measured in Hertz—see Chapter 3). Every element, including different vibrational states of water (which constitutes over 70% of the human body), has specific vibratory frequencies that can be measured. Food and nutrient elements are broken down by digestive and metabolic enzymes. Likewise, when essential oils are internally consumed or inhaled, there are enzymes that break them down. These enzyme molecules also have their own unique crystalline forms with specific vibratory frequencies. The overall energetic imprint is based on the frequency of an essential oil (as well as plants and vegetation, including foods consumed). It is said to reflect the energetic "life force," as well as the integrity of the producer's original intent.

The exact mechanisms by which humans detect smells or aromas may be based on something similar to the vibrational frequency of a plant oil. Most smell researchers think the way aromas are detected has to do only with the stochastic shapes of odiferous molecules matching those of receptors in the nose. This 20th, century concept is quite similar to notions of the "shapes" of medicinal drugs or hormones that stochastically fit into cell receptors and/or interact with neurotransmitters, and then react chemically, whether the substance is organic or synthetic. Dr. Luca Turin, a biophysicist from France, believes that the way smell molecules vibrate is responsible for aroma, involving a quantum effect called "tunneling". His study suggests that the olfactory apparatus recognizes molecules' vibrations, or energetic imprints, not only their molecular shapes (Gane et al., 2013). The five atomic elements responsible for different smells are carbon, nitrogen, hydrogen, oxygen, and sulfur. Scientists have been able to "copycat" smells, such as perfumes, based on their molecular and vibrational structures.

Providing aesthetic pleasure, from aromas such as perfume fragrance, is not the only role of plants. By taking carbon dioxide from the atmosphere and water from soil, along with light energy from the sun, plants then convert this "food" to carbohydrates through photosynthesis. Plants are the ultimate production machine, purifying the air and providing food and medicine for humans and animals. Plants provide a conduit for the earth's vast chemical potential, converting carbon dioxide to oxygen, acting essentially as the "lungs" of the earth, and maintaining breathing. According to recent research, plants are not the only places where photosynthesis occurs. Research at the University of California shows that oxygen molecules can form without the botanical process of plant photosynthesis with the shortest wavelength

THE CYCLE OF RAIN, WATER, AND NATURAL AROMATHERAPY

There is a distinct odor in the air before and after it rains, although water itself is colorless and odorless. The characteristic "smell of rain" actually occurs when the rainwater "activates" plant oils, phytochemicals, and nutrients in the plants and soil. (Similarly, water can "activate" compounds in water-soluble herb-vitamin mixes—see Chapter 23.) In the natural world, a chemical process actually begins in the atmosphere before the rainfall.

In the atmosphere, both oxygen and nitrogen atoms are usually bound to each other in two-atom molecules for chemical stability. In stormy weather, electricity in the air can split apart molecules into single "free radical" atoms of oxygen. Then, the free oxygen atoms combine with other diatomic oxygen molecules to form ozone. (These are the same kind of free radicals responsible for "oxidation," when we discuss "antioxidants," such as vitamins and other plant constituents, because they are chemically reactive.) The reactive ozone layer in the upper atmosphere filters out some dangerous solar radiation. During a rainstorm, winds also drive ozone down toward the surface of the Earth. This chemical part of the process gives the air that characteristic smell when it is about to rain.

Then when the rain actually begins to fall on plants, the aroma in the air changes again. The rainwater releases oils that plants have produced during dry, dormant periods. Plants actually produce some of these chemicals during dry spells to inhibit growth. These chemicals reduce the plant's need to compete for limited moisture and prevent the plant from using up all available water in the soil.

Scientists call this mix of plant oils released by new rain "petrichor." The word "petrichor," coined in 1967 by two Australian researchers, occurs from tiny bubbles that drift into the air after it escapes the rain particles that hit porous surfaces.

Plants and other organisms found in the ground soil often secrete oils. During dry spells, these organisms and plants secrete more oils. With a longer period of drought comes more oil buildup in the ground soil. When water comes in contact with this oil buildup during rain, it gets released in the air. Then when the rain seeps into the soil, it affects bacteria in the soil and produces another well-recognized smell. When soil gets wet, it releases small amounts of a chemical called "geosmin" into the air. Humans are extremely sensitive to the aroma of this chemical and can detect its presence at levels of only five parts per million. (That is approximately 1 teaspoon in 200 Olympic-sized swimming pools.) It is the chemical that gives the "earthy" smell to beets, for example.

of ultraviolet light or "vacuum ultraviolet light" (University of California, Davis, 2014). This form of light energy in essence breaks apart the carbon dioxide molecules. There is synergy among plants, earth, and air. Their long-lasting effects on the atmosphere and the air animals breathe provide oxygen, the essential element needed for cellular mitochondrial respiration (which produces energy and water, for animal life on earth). We next discuss how water interacts with the earth, soil, and plants to produce aromas with relaxing effects naturally whenever it rains.

AEROSOL THERAPIES

The lung serves a portal to the body for oxygen, as well as inhaled aerosol agents, which may be given as intended for systemic effects, such as pain control. Aerosol therapies have two distinct and very different applications. Ultrasonic aerosols can produce a significant alteration in airway mechanics and are used to help the lungs to heal from certain ailments, such as asthma. Aerosols have also been used for treating common symptoms and relieving pain and since the 19th century to treat lung afflictions. The application of aerosols, formulating drugs, and administering medications effectively to the desired site(s) of action constitute the science of respiratory drug delivery.

Aerosols are also found in nature. Aerosols are defined as the mixture of liquid or solid particles/droplets that are stably suspended in air. When carrying a certain amount of negative electrical charge, they are defined as negatively charged aerosols. Such droplets also fall as they descend from clouds in the atmosphere. Therapeutically, negatively charged aerosol therapy can accelerate wound healing and improve the healing of injuries, alleviating pain symptoms (Xie, Chen, Zhang, Shi, & Xie, 2013).

Inhaled aerosol therapy has been tested in human and veterinary clinical trials and used, for example, in equine medicine. Horses have shown benefits from aerosol therapy for illnesses of the lungs, such as pleural pneumonia, which usually engenders suffering from a substantial amount of pain and severe inflammation.

Aromas in the Brain and Central Nervous System

Aromas, fragrances, and smells have powerful effects on the brain and are hardwired into memory. Sense of smell is the strongest memory-holder. The sense of smell is most powerful in terms of memory—approximately 10,000 times stronger than other senses. The olfactory nerves are also responsible for most taste sensation, due to aromas that travel into the nasopharynx during chewing and the early stages of digestion. Aromatic sensations are detected by the olfactory nerves, which travel from the nose up directly into the brain through a finely porous entry in the skull (cribriform plate of the frontal bone). In the brain the olfactory nerves gather together in the olfactory bulb located right in the middle of the brain tissue.

In research studies the olfactory senses have been tied to the dorsal posterior insula, the pain center of the brain, during odor identification and olfactory stimulation (Kareken et al., 2004; Kareken, Mosnik, Doty, Dzemidzic, & Hutchins, 2003).

These studies show the powerful direct connection between scent stimuli and the pain center of the brain.

Certain aromas and smells have powerful effects, conjuring up strong memories and feelings. The presence of a mere four scent-bearing molecules is enough for the brain recognize a familiar smell. This ability is no doubt part of the biological equipment that protects humans and animals in learning and reacting to the environment.

When people and animals recognize odors, they react. The nose's smell receptors are directly connected to the deepest and most primal regions of the brain, including the hippocampus and amygdala, which store memory and link it to emotional expression. In prehistoric times this property allowed human ancestors to instantly identify and respond to such significant scents associated with predators and prey. Nowadays the sense of smell protects people from eating spoiled food or leaving the gas on in the oven (natural gas, or methane, and propane are odorless but manufacturers add a little potent methyl mercaptan, or other sulfur-containing gas, to allow people to detect the smell).

Smell is also considered a large part of physical attraction, one of the reasons that perfume-making currently remains nearly a $5 billion industry. There is considerable debate among scientists about the vomeronasal organ, also called Jacobson organ. This structure in the nose is used to sniff out pheromones emitted by a potential mate. It is found in amphibians, reptiles, and mammals, but scientists are pretty sure that the structure is nonfunctioning in humans, so beware of products with "human pheromones" that supposedly increase one's attraction to the opposite (or same) sex. Human pheromones do not appear to be the reason for the various varieties of sexual attraction among people.

The powerful connections among sense of smell and emotional responses is one important way that aromatherapy can improve physical, emotional, and mental health. Inhaling, absorbing, and ingesting plant-based essential oils have been effective in treating infections, inflammation, pain, stress, and other conditions. Lack of more clinical trials hampers acceptance in the conventional medical community. However, aromatherapy's widespread use by consumers and health care practitioners, for everything from the pain of burns to boosting the immune system, provides a place among natural plant-based remedies in the United States and Europe.

TREATMENT OF PAIN, INFLAMMATION, AND RELATED CONDITIONS

Essential oils are pharmacologically active and can be administered via different routes, according to the specific needs of the individual.

Herbs in modern aromatherapy provide a new method for modulating immune system reactions, as well as neural processes. Aromatherapy using **turmeric** has the ability to inhibit microglia activation, a property that has been shown to treat neurodegenerative diseases and to support nerve regeneration (Hucklenbroich et al., 2014). Neural stem cells have been shown to proliferate in the subventricular zone and hippocampus region.

Science says that what makes us "happy" and alleviates pain symptoms is by means of neural and hormonal reactions that involve four categories of

BOX 24.2 *Reasons to Administer Aromatherapy*

Alleviating pain and discomfort
Eliminating insomnia and restlessness
Enhancing self-image
Healing infections and wounds
Insomnia and restlessness
Relaxation; relieving stress and anxiety
Treating burns
Treatment for constipation
Stimulating immune function

neurochemicals: dopamine, serotonin, oxytocin, and endorphins. They are the quartet of "happy" markers that interact with the brain's opiate and other receptors to help to reduce or eliminate pain and stress, as well as the central processing and perception of both (Sprouse-Blum, Smith, Sugai, & Parsa, 2010). These neuropeptides and hormones also influence the release of chemicals associated inflammation, such as cortisol and norepinephrine. For example, the smell of lavender and vanilla has been shown to promote the release of endorphins (Butje, Repede, & Shattell, 2008). Modern medicine treats patients to influence the release or retention of these active chemicals using drugs and over-the-counter medicines. However, just the power of scent can promote basic and complex components of relaxation, stress, and pain reduction via direct neurological and neurochemical pathways (Box 24.2).

Various essential oils that are used in aromatherapy practice are listed here.

Anti-inflammatory Effects:

Lavender

Chamomile

Eucalyptus

Ginger

Clove

Anxiety, Depression, and Overall Mood Enhancers:

Bergamot

Lavender

Neroli

Rosemary

Peppermint

Jasmine

Clary Sage

Geranium

Sandalwood

Chronic Tension:

Orange

Neroli

Lemon
Grapefruit
General Pain Relief (arthritis, back pain, etc.):
Lavender
Chamomile
Frankincense
Eucalyptus
Thyme
Wintergreen
Spruce
Ginger
Headaches, Tension, Migraines, Insomnia:
Marjoram
Wintergreen
Eucalyptus
Rosemary
Pine
Peppermint
Grapefruit
Benzoin
Labor Pains:
Salvia
Frankincense
Rose
Menstrual Pain Relief:
Rose
Geranium
Clary Sage
Neurological Diseases and Memory:
Lavender
Turmeric
Perception of Pain:
Vanilla
Lavender
Premenstrual Cramps:
Rose
Jasmine
Clary Sage
Sleep Enhancers:
Rose
Sandalwood
Lavender
Ylang Ylang
Chamomile

Plants are a prominent part of the terrestrial environment. Plants are responsible for converting solar energy to food sources that support all life on earth. Botanical processes in plants provide a blueprint by which biological processes in animals have developed and adapted their physiology and metabolism, In addition, plants provide foods, energy, vitamin and mineral micronutrients, as well as active herbal remedies and essential oils that have therapeutic properties when ingested, inhaled or applied topically. Their systematic application to human health is at once age old, as well as providing innovative new approaches for the 21st century.

REFERENCES

Butje, A., Repede, E., & Shattell, M. M. (2008). Healing scents: An overview of clinical aromatherapy for emotional distress. *Journal of Psychosocial Nursing and Mental Health Services, 46*, 46–52. http://libres. uncg.edu/ir/uncg/f/M_Shattell_HealingScents_2008.pdf.

Del-Ángel, M., Nieto, A., Ramírez-Apan, T., & Delgado, G. (2015). Anti-inflammatory effect of natural and semi-synthetic phthalides. *European Journal of Pharmacology, 752*, 40–48. http://www.ncbi.nlm. nih.gov/pubmed/25622553.

Deciga-Campos, M., González-Trujano, E., Navarrete, A., & Mata, R. (2005). Antinociceptive effect of selected Mexican traditional medicinal species. *Proceedings of the Western Pharmacological Society, 48*, 70–72. http://www.ncbi.nlm.nih.gov/pubmed/16416665.

Franchomme, P. & Penoel, D. (1990). *Aromatherapie exactement*. Paris: Roger Jollois.

Gane, S., Georganakis, D., Maniati, K., Vamvakias, M., Ragoussis, N., Skoulakis, E. M., et al. (2013). Molecular vibration-sensing component in human olfaction. *PLoS ONE, 8*, e55780. http://journals. plos.org/plosone/article?id=10.1371/journal.pone.0055780.

Gehl, J. & Micozzi, M. S. (2017). *Science of planetary signatures in medicine*. Rochester, VT: Healing Arts Press/Inner Traditions.

Harris, R. (2002). Synergism in the essential oil world. *International Journal of Aromatherapy, 12*(4), 179.

Hertz, R. (2009). Aromatherapy facts and fictions: a scientific analysis of olfactory effects on mood, physiology and behaviour. *International Journal of Neuroscience, 119*, 263–290.

Holmes, P. (2007). *The energetics of Western herbs* (Vols. 1-2; 4th ed.). Boulder, CO: Snow Lotus Press.

Holmes, P. (2008). *Clinical aromatherapy*. Cotati, CA: Tigerlily Press.

Hucklenbroich, J., Klein, R., Neumaier, B., Graf, R., Fink, G. R., Schroeter, M., et al. (2014). Aromatic-turmerone induces neural stem cell proliferation in vitro and in vivo. *Stem Cell Research and Therapy, 5*, 100. http://www.ncbi.nlm.nih.gov/pmc/articles/PMC4180255/.

Kareken, D. A., Mosnik, D. M., Doty, R. L., Dzemidzic, M., & Hutchins, G. D. (2003). Functional anatomy of human odor sensation, discrimination, and identification in health and aging. *Neuropsychology, 17*, 482–495. http://www.ncbi.nlm.nih.gov/pubmed/12959514.

Kareken, D. A., Sabri, M., Radnovich, A. J., Claus, E., Foresman, B., Hector, D., et al. (2004). Olfactory system activation from sniffing: Effects in piriform and orbitofrontal cortex. *NeuroImage, 22*, 456–465. http://citeseerx.ist.psu.edu/viewdoc/download?doi=10.1.1.420.8842&rep=rep1&type=pdf.

Lee, R. J., Kofonow, J. M., Rosen, P. L., Siebert, A. P., Chen, B., Doghramji, L., et al. (2014). Bitter and sweet taste receptors regulate human upper respiratory innate immunity. *Journal of Clinical Investigation, 124*, 1393–1405. http://www.ncbi.nlm.nih.gov/pmc/articles/PMC3934184/.

Maury, M. (1964). *Marguerite Maury's guide to aromatherapy: The secret of life and youth*. England: C.W. Daniel Company.

Miller, L. & Miller, B. (1995). *Ayurveda and aromatherapy: the earth essential guide to ancient wisdom and modern healing*. Twin Lakes, WI: Lotus Press.

Mojay, G. (1996). *Aromatherapy for healing the spirit*. New York: Henry Holt.

Moss, M., Hewitt, S., Moss, L., & Wesnes, K. (2008). Modulation of cognitive performance and mood by aromas of peppermint and ylang-ylang. *International Journal of Neuroscience, 118*, 59–77.

Moss, L., Rouse, M., Wesnes, K. A., & Moss, M. (2010). Differential effects of the aromas of Salvia species on memory and mood. *Human Psychopharmacology: Clinical and Experimental, 25*, 388–396.

Sprouse-Blum, A. S., Smith, G., Sugai, D., & Parsa, F. D. (2010). Understanding endorphins and their importance in pain management. *Hawaii Medical Journal, 69*, 70–71. http://www.ncbi.nlm.nih.gov/pmc/articles/PMC3104618/.

Steele, J. J. (1992). The anthropology of smell and scent in ancient Egypt and South American Shamanism. In S. Van Toller & G. H. Dodd (Eds.), *Fragrance: The psychology and biology of perfume*. Barking, UK: Elsevier Science Publishers Ltd.

Trigo, M., Fuchs, M., Chen, J., Jiang, M. P., Cammarata, M., Fahy, S., et al. (2013). Fourier-transform inelastic X-ray scattering from time- and momentum-dependent phonon–phonon correlations. *Nature Physics, 9*, 790–794. http://www.nature.com/nphys/journal/v9/n12/full/nphys2788.html.

University of California, Davis. (2014). *Making oxygen before life*. http://phys.org/wire-news/173783397/making-oxygen-before-life.html.

Xie, X., Chen, L., Zhang, Z. Q., Shi, Y., & Xie, J. (2013). Clinical study on the treatment of chronic wound with negatively-charged aerosol. *International Journal of Clinical and Experimental Medicine, 6*, 649–654. http://www.ncbi.nlm.nih.gov/pmc/articles/PMC3762619/.

Suggested Readings can be found on the companion website, http://www.micozzipainconditions.com.

Psychometrics of Pain

INTERACTIVE TOOLS FOR INDIVIDUALIZED PATIENT PAIN MANAGEMENT

This Appendix provides the interactive tools for conducting individual assessments of each patient's "boundary" or "emotional" psychometric type.

In discussing pain with patients, four important points are useful to keep in mind.

1. Most chronic pain results from the *reception* of pain signals by pain sensors in the **body** and the *perception* and processing of pain sensation in the **mind** through nerve circuits in the brain and through various levels of *consciousness*.

2. Furthermore, the **reception** and the **perception** of pain occur in a feedback loop, each continually influencing, and potentially aggravating, the other until chronic pain may be *permanently* cemented in place.

3. The many mind-body therapies presented in this book can each work for most chronic pain conditions because they address these vital linkages, and feedback loops, between the mind and the body.

4. However, not every mind-body therapy works equally well for everyone with chronic pain.

That last point brings us to a clinical *breakthrough* in managing pain by being able to choose, from among all these safe and effective therapies, the ones more likely to work best for each unique individual patient, and for their specific pain condition(s).

We can now apply an important way of understanding how the mind-body perceives and processes pain, as well as emotions, moods, and other feelings that affect and reflect our health. Researcher Ernst Hartmann at Tufts University in Boston worked over his long career on identifying and understanding the psychological and personality **boundaries** that effect how people process feelings and sensations.

Hartmann found that peoples' boundaries exist along a continuum of thin boundary to thick boundary on a spectrum of feelings and experiences—how feelings are experienced and how experiences are felt.

Since the 1990s with Michael Jawer (now with the American Academy of Naturopathic Physicians), one of us (Micozzi) has researched how people with different boundary types are more susceptible to different diseases and chronic pain conditions. Micozzi has reviewed of thousands of research studies on natural therapies for his textbook, *Fundamentals of Complementary & Alternative Medicine* (now going into a 6th edition) over the past 25 years. Together with understanding of the Hartmann-Jawer boundary types, this work has enabled us to help determine and predict which therapies will work for each individual patient based upon where they lie on this mind-body boundary type spectrum. This approach is the same in concept to the widespread use of the Spiegel Hypnotic Susceptibility Scales. The Hartman-Jawer boundary types consistently include evaluation of hypnosis but go well beyond it to several other major common natural therapies.

A simple survey questionnaire allows each individual to quickly answer and score his or her boundary type. The following questionnaire can be used to administer to pain patients.

THE BOUNDARY QUESTIONNAIRE

Before taking the Boundary Questionnaire (BQ), here is a brief explanation of the personality boundary concept. The original BQ was developed by Ernest Hartmann, MD, a researcher at Tufts University, based on research he conducted starting in the 1980s. The full version consists of 146 questions grouped into a dozen categories, reflecting themes such as "Interpersonal," "Thoughts/Feelings/Moods," "Childhood/Adolescence/Adult," and "Sleep/Dream/Waking." Thus an individual patient can be scored as a thin or thick boundary person overall and score different places along the boundary spectrum within each of these categories. No one is reducible to a single "spot" on the boundary spectrum. Each individual is likely to be thin in some respects, thick in others (Hartmann, 1998).

Where an individual places on the boundary spectrum is not strictly permanent over a lifetime. People tend to develop thicker boundaries as they age, but everyone is different. A person may instead develop thinner boundaries as she or he gets older, based on her or his unique experiences. Someone's boundaries can even thicken or become thinned based on the medications she or he takes or depending on how tired the person happens to be (Hartmann, 1998). However, as a general personality trait, boundary type would not vary too much from day to day, or year to year.

A short form of the BQ is provided. It consists of 18 questions and usually takes less than 10 minutes to complete and score. For a quick way to assess her/his boundary type, the short-form BQ is the most direct route (Jawer & Micozzi, 2012).

We find that this subset of 18 questions through factor analysis captures most of the spectrum variability that is obtained with the complete, much lengthier survey. That is, each of these particular questions in the short survey is highly correlated to the overall results of the sum of answers to all questions on the other 128 possible questions on the long survey. Furthermore, the precision of this short survey is comparable to the precision of the research studies that assessed the effectiveness of different mind-body therapies for different pain conditions and that were used in evaluating their association with a specific boundary type.

Please note instructions to patients: There are no "right" or "wrong" responses. Consider these statements merely as prompts intended to understand where you are at this time in your life. Please rate each of the statements from 0 to 4 (0 indicates "not at all true of me"; 4 indicates "very true of me"). Try to respond to all of the statements as quickly as you can.

OBTAINING YOUR SCORE

To obtain your score, simply add up the scores (0–4) for all questions.

CAUTION: the scores for questions 5, 6, 7, and 16 are scored backwards (i.e., for these questions an answer of "0" is scored as 4, "1" is scored as 3, "2" is scored as 2, "3" is scored as 1, and "4" is scored as 0).

1. My feelings blend into one another. 0 1 2 3 4

2. I am very close to my childhood feelings. 0 1 2 3 4

3. I am easily hurt. 0 1 2 3 4

4. I spend a lot of time daydreaming, fantasizing, or in reverie. 0 1 2 3 4

5. I like stories that have a definite beginning, middle, and end. 0 1 2 3 4

6. A good organization is one in which all the lines of responsibility are precise and clearly established. 0 1 2 3 4

7. There is a place for everything, and everything should be in its place. 0 1 2 3 4

8. Sometimes it is scary when one gets too involved with another person. 0 1 2 3 4

9. A good parent has to be a bit of a child too. 0 1 2 3 4

10. I can easily imagine myself as an animal or what it might be like to be an animal. 0 1 2 3 4

11. When something happens to a friend of mine or to a lover, it is almost as if it happened to me. 0 1 2 3 4

12. When I work on a project, I do not like to tie myself down to a definite outline. I rather like to let my mind wander. 0 1 2 3 4

13. In my dreams, people sometimes merge into each other or become other people. 0 1 2 3 4

14. I believe I am influenced by forces that no one can understand. 0 1 2 3 4

15. There are no sharp dividing lines between normal people, people with problems, and people who are considered psychotic or crazy. 0 1 2 3 4

16. I am a down-to-earth, no-nonsense kind of person. 0 1 2 3 4

17. I think I would enjoy being some kind of creative artist. 0 1 2 3 4

18. I have had the experience of someone calling me or speaking my name and not being sure whether it was really happening or whether I was imagining it. 0 1 2 3 4

SCORE

For additional copies, and to take this survey on-line, please go to http://www.drmicozzi.com and take the "Emotional Type" quiz on landing page and automatically get your score.

Scores less than 30 are considered definitely "thick," and scores greater than 42 are considered definitely "thin." Find out where you are on the spectrum:

THICK BOUNDARY............................MIDDLE............................THIN BOUNDARY								
0	9	18	27	36	45	54	63	72

FINDING THE RIGHT TREATMENTS FOR EACH PATIENT

Boundary type is related to the effectiveness of each of several common mind-body treatments for pain disorders, based upon review of available research and scientific evidence. As learned from reading this book, there are many "alternative" mind-body medical treatments and natural approaches being studied and applied for pain. Each of the common treatments presented here are well-established, safe, and effective treatments that are, or rapidly becoming, widely available. The effectiveness of each of these treatments for pain is evaluated on the basis of what has been shown by scientific evidence. This information is provided as a useful clinical guide. We do not get into any experimental or controversial treatments but address only evidence-based treatments that are widely available and have been used for decades, if not longer. The benefit is that now you can help determine which treatments are best for an individual patient based upon psychometric boundary type. If a treatment appears on this list, it is a reasonable and safe choice for patients to try.

APPROPRIATE TREATMENTS FOR EACH PSYCHOMETRIC TYPE

Listed here is each of seven major treatments for common and significant pain disorders by their **effectiveness** as indicated by published clinical studies. Then we scored the degree of **specificity** for each treatment for each boundary type. Armed with this guide and knowledge of boundary type, you have an additional tool to begin selecting the most promising and appropriate treatments suited to each patient's pain condition.

The following chart shows the thick and thin boundary disorders and the anxiety and depression that typically accompany these disorders, as well as the relative evidence-based effectiveness of each therapeutic modality for each of these conditions. Based on the available science and research, the effectiveness and potencies of these treatments are ranked on a scale of 1 to 5, relative to each other, and relative to the most potent treatments regular medicine has to offer in terms of drugs, procedures, and surgery. (Even when drugs and surgery are successful—which often they are not—they are far more dangerous than any of these seven treatments in terms of known complications and side effects.)

Disorder	Hyp	Acu	BioF	Med-Yoga	Relax.	Imag
Thick						
Arthritis	—	3	3	4	3	—
CFS	—	4	3	3	—	3
Phantom pain	1	3	2	2	—	—
Thin						
Fibro	—	—	—	3	3	—
Migraine	3	—	5	3	2	3
PTSD	2	—	2	3	3	—
Common						
Depression/Anxiety	4	3	5	3	3	—
Chronic pain	4	5	5	3	3	—

Acu, Acupuncture; *biof,* biofeedback; *CFS,* chronic fatigue syndrome; *Fibro,* fibromyalgia; *hyp,* hypnosis; *imag,* guided imagery; *Med-Yoga,* meditation-yoga; *PTSD,* post-traumatic stress disorder; *relax,* relaxation-stress reduction therapies.
Where no number appears it generally means there was insufficient data to evaluate it.

Pain Relief

The symptom of chronic pain, shown at the bottom, typically accompanies these specific disorders, and virtually all of these therapies can be highly potent and effective for pain when matched to the right type. These treatments can be equal (and acupuncture, for one, may actually exceed) to treatments typically available in mainstream medical treatment for pain. They are highly effective and extremely safe and interfere minimally with life compared with many other pain management treatments. Furthermore, unlike effective narcotic drug medications, they are not regulated to the same extent and degree by government agencies, such as the US Food and Drug Administration (FDA) and US Drug Enforcement Administration (DEA), which may place regulatory law enforcement concerns in substitution or preemption of medical judgment and ethics regarding effective pain management for suffering patients.

Some of these conditions remain difficult to manage by any means, such as chronic fatigue syndrome (CFS) and fibromyalgia (FM), and the effectiveness and potencies of these active treatments do not reach the highest levels of 4 or 5, although they are usually still quite helpful. Regular medicine neither has had much to offer for decades for CFS or FM, most doctors long telling these millions of sufferers that it was "all in their heads." Now that drug companies have developed drugs purportedly for these disorders, suddenly they actually do exist to the world of modern mainstream medicine. We made another observation in working on these data. FM-CFS also exists along a spectrum, and a thin boundary type person is more likely to fall on the FM side of this syndrome, whereas a thick boundary type is more likely to fall on the CFS side of the manifestation of symptoms.

For many conditions, there is a choice of effective treatments. It is interesting that several of the therapies are useful for treating both thick and thin, as well as the common conditions of anxiety and depression. However, hypnosis generally does better treating thin boundary conditions, whereas guided imagery, meditation-yoga, and relaxation-stress management generally do better with thick boundary conditions. Biofeedback appears equally effective with both, and acupuncture appears to be a potent across the board for these conditions, although even more effective for thin boundary type.

A "POINT" ABOUT ACUPUNTURE

Just when one might have thought that it was not possible to say anything new about acupuncture, a medical tradition that is 2000 years old, this approach to boundary type also shed some new light on this ancient and effective treatment.

One important reason acupuncture does not always work for everyone is because modern "cookbook" recipes and texts for the way acupuncture is frequently practiced by Westerners do not capture the full scope of available approaches and potencies available in the full spectrum of Classical Chinese Medicine. It is not only that individuals vary in their sensitivities to acupuncture by thick or thin boundary type or some other characteristic.

When in research or practice we have observed that "acupuncture just does not work" or it "does not work for this person," we simply have taken it at face value in light of general acceptance that complementary and alternative medicine (CAM) and natural approaches are just not as "potent" as Western biomedicine. However, it is also the case that many writers and practitioners of acupuncture have taken an incomplete approach to using all the complete knowledge that is indeed available to us from the ancient Chinese sources.

Much of acupuncture practice in the West is incomplete or incorrect because it has been based upon particularistic, or idiosyncratic, interpretations typically taking into account only part of the rich body of knowledge available from all the ancient Chinese medical classics. The result can be a somewhat "watered down," Western version that is less potent, or less broad, in its applications to different individual people and their pain conditions, particular patients with difficult conditions to treat (for which there is an entire relatively neglected classical Canon of Chinese Medicine).

When therapeutic problems are encountered with a particular condition, or in a particular individual, too often there is an inability to pursue the next steps by consulting the solutions that are available, but have remained hidden, in the original Chinese medical writings. When your regular doctor tries a treatment that does not work, does she or he then send you away? No. She or he keeps trying. The same is true for what might occur as a lack of initial response in Chinese medicine, if we truly know what else to try, rather than relying only on standard recipes with incomplete, idiosyncratic knowledge or understanding.

It is also remarkable to note, in addition to the improved therapeutic options provided by a full and complete reading of the authentic Chinese sources, the remarkable depth of diagnostic information available. Although the Chinese diagnostics are literally "foreign" to us, they provide a rich, internally consistent, and complete description of the clients' complaints and experiences not reduced to a series of numbers from standardized biomedical tests performed on only a subset of relevant information. Likewise, understanding of these mind-body boundary types helps to complete the picture for our understanding of pain and the modern pain disorders addressed in this book.

Spectrum of Treatments Along Boundary Lines

THIN ------------------------------ MIDPOINT ------------------------------ THICK

| HYPNOSIS | ACUPUNCTURE | BIOFEEDBACK | GUIDED IMAGERY | STRESS REDUCTION | MEDITATION & YOGA |

This picture shows the treatments that are most specific to thin boundary conditions on the left, with those most specific to thick boundary conditions on the right, and arranged in between as to their degree of specificity for one or the other. In terms of general treatments for your boundary type, the most strongly specific treatments for thick personality boundaries (in this order) are: guided imagery, relaxation-stress management, meditation-yoga. For thin boundary, hypnosis is the therapy of choice when effective for your condition, followed by acupuncture. Biofeedback is exceptional for thick or thin boundaries.

Pain Treatment Profile

It is notable that the origins of many chronic pain disorders have remained a mystery to mainstream medical science, and effective treatments have remained elusive. It is well established in medicine that sometimes it is ultimately the "treatment profile" of a disease that ultimately provides clues to help backtrack to its "etiology," or origins ("reverse analysis"). That is, after effective *treatments* are found clinically, it often leads to a better understanding of the *causes* of the disease. After we figure out how to cure or effectively treat a disease, it gives clues as to what is really causing it in the first place.

Now that we can apply the thin and thick boundary concepts to disorders and their treatments, we have another window into what causes these disorders in the first place.

Hypnosis: A 250-Year-Old Mystery Investigated

Hypnosis provides a good example of what is conveyed in this book. Like the other "mind-body" therapies, the "mechanism of action" has never been known or understood. Again, there is a good reason why this important and effective therapy has remained of unknown mechanism of action: the view of neuroscience regarding the brain, mind, and body remains incomplete. It has been disregarding critical scientific observations, clinical experiences, and everyday awareness, all of which are central to how the mind-body truly functions.

First developed in the late 18th century by Franz Anton Mesmer in Vienna and brought to Paris in the court of Louis XVI, the use of "animal magnetism" to help people with mind-body disorders proved compelling. However, "mesmerism," "animal magnetism," and "magnetic healing" of the 19th century were all once consigned to the dustbin of history by the self-proclaimed "scientific medicine" of the 20th century. The potency of hypnotism for problems for which drugs or psychosurgery (such as the notorious frontal lobotomies of the 20th century) had no answers nonetheless led serious contemporary psychiatrists and psychologists to again develop and use hypnotism to help their patients.

In the absence of a complete understanding of how hypnotism and mind-body medicine really work, Drs. Spiegel, father and son, at Stanford University in Palo Alto, California, developed "hypnotic susceptibility scales" to be able to predict who would benefit with what types of disorders. This breakthrough provided the comfort of proving statistical associations where a more fundamental "mechanistic" science was lacking.

We have now observed that the susceptibility of individuals to hypnosis also relates to psychometric boundary type, again based upon statistical associations. Furthermore, new understandings of boundary type can be applied to six other common and effective natural, mind-body treatments considered in this book. These observations provide another tool for seeking better, more effective treatments that are suited to each individual patient—providing some real, simple tools for an era of true "individualized medicine."

INDIVIDUALIZED MEDICINE: GUIDE TO MANAGING PAIN

This appendix provides a clear guide as to which type of treatment(s) you would probably want to recommend depending upon the patient's boundary type and medical condition(s).

A thin boundary personality would probably want to try hypnosis or acupuncture first for FM or migraine headache, knowing there are also other treatments to try for almost all of these conditions if need be. We also found that, like the personality and emotional type boundaries themselves, FM-CFS exists along a spectrum. We observed that a thick boundary type is more likely to experience symptoms more toward the CFS end of the spectrum. A thin boundary type is more likely to experience the syndrome more on the FM end of the spectrum.

Seen also as spiritual problems in the context discussed in this book, it is clear that accompanying anxiety and depression are amenable to every modality of treatment as well that may be used to directly address the primary pain condition.

ALL things being equal, one might begin with the highest number ratings (for effectiveness) to see which treatments appear to work best for a given medical condition; then proceed with the effective treatment that best matches boundary type; and then go from there as needed.

As with other things in life, really knowing your boundaries is an important key to health, healing, and happiness, as well as treating common pain conditions.

REFERENCES

Hartmann, E. (1998). *Dreams and nightmares* (p. 228). New York and London: Plenum Press.

Jawer, M. & Micozzi, M. S. (2012). *Your emotional type*. Rochester, VT: Park Street Press/Inner Traditions.

Appendix *II*

Patient Monitoring Pain and Related Symptoms

Participants can self-monitor pain by noting and recording symptoms of pain and related anxiety or stress. They can record symptoms at the time they occur and rate their severity on a scale of 1 to 10, using a pain symptom monitoring form (see sample form). For many patients it may be a useful tool to become more familiar with their own symptoms and experiences of pain.

A pain symptom monitoring form may show each day of the week divided into four periods: morning, afternoon, evening, and night. Participants record their activities and circumstances and then rate the severity of symptoms on a scale of 0 to 10 (0 for no pain to 10 for worst pain).

Practitioners may believe that they can elicit all relevant information from the patient about pain, symptoms, or the factors that aggravate it. However, patients are able to later recall, during a clinical visit, only when pain symptoms or related limitations became distracting or intolerable. The form provides an overview of pain symptoms and circumstances.

At the outset, both patient and practitioner can simply note the facts, without trying to interpret the symptoms. The patient registers only when and under what circumstances pain occurs and its severity. Registering the symptoms may be a painful or frustrating experience because it draws attention to the pain. Realizing and recording the very existence of the pain and related symptoms may make the patient unhappy or upset, and patients may try to avoid thinking about them.

However, to best find ways to control pain symptoms, it is useful to discover and consider when and in what circumstances they arise. Therefore patients can be encouraged to monitor symptoms using a simple portable form, as in the example. It is also important in the process of remembering and recalling pain to also note those times when and circumstances under which the pain is gone and when patients are feeling better.

Weekly Pain Monitoring Form

Day	Date	Morning	Afternoon	Evening	Night
1.					
2.					
3.					
4.					
5.					
6.					
7.					

Note the severity of pain symptoms using the following scale:

0 = No pain symptoms; 1, 2, 3, 4, 5, 6, 7, 8, 9; 10 = worst imaginable pains symptoms.

For each entry, record a word or phrase describing your circumstances or situation at the time. For example: Wednesday morning: busy at work, with a headache (2–3). Afternoon: went home, took nap, headache persists (1–2). Evening: quiet, headache (1). Night: sleep, fitful, headache gone on waking (0).

Illustration Credits

Fig. 4.1

From Williams, P. L. (1995). *Gray's anatomy*, Edinburgh: Churchill Livingstone.

Figs. 7.1, 12.4, 24.1, and 24.2

From Micozzi, M. S. (2015). *Fundamentals of complementary & alternative medicine* (5th ed.). St Louis: Elsevier.

Fig. 9.1

Table constructed by Sebhia M. Dibra, July 2016.

Fig. 10.2

From Collection BIU Santé Médecine; Courtesy Bibliothèque Interuniversitaire de Médecine, Paris. http://www.biusante.parisdescartes.fr/histmed/image?01883.

Figs. 12.1, 12.2, and 12.3

Courtesy Palmer College of Chiropractic.

Fig. 13.1

Courtesy The Wellcome Trustees, London.

Figs. 13.2, 13.4, and 13-6

Modified from Salvo, S. (2016) *Massage therapy: principles and practice* (5th ed.). St Louis: Elsevier.

Figs. 13.3, 13. 5, and 13.9

Modified from Salvo, S. (2007). *Massage therapy: principles and practice* (3rd ed.). St Louis: Saunders.

Figs. 13.7, 13.8, and 13.10

Borrowed with permission from Chaitow, L. & DeLany, J. (2008). *Clinical application of neuromuscular techniques* (Vol. 1; 2nd ed.). Edinburgh: Churchill Livingstone.

Fig. 16.1

From Micozzi, M. S. (2011). *Fundamentals of complementary & alternative medicine* (4th ed.). St Louis: Elsevier.

Fig. 22.1

Sources and photo conversion of vitamin D; original artwork by Marc S. Micozzi, redrawn by Elsevier.

Index

Note: Page numbers followed by *f* indicate figures, *t* indicate tables, and *b* indicate boxes.